PDR®-for all of your drug information needs.

2005 Physicians' Desk Reference®
Physicians have turned to the PDR for the latest word on prescription drugs for 59 years. Today, PDR is still considered the standard prescription drug reference and can be found in virtually every physician's office, hospital and pharmacy in the United States. You can search the more than 4,000 drugs by using one of many indices and look at more than 2,100 full-color photos of drugs cross-referenced to the label information.

2005 PDR® Companion Guide
This unique 1,900-page all-in-one clinical companion to the PDR ensures safe, appropriate drug selection with eight critical checkpoint indices including *Indications, Side Effects, Interactions,* and much more.

PDR® Pharmacopoeia Pocket Dosing Guide – Fifth Edition 2005
This pocket dosing guide brings important dispensing information to the practitioner's fingertips. Organized in tabular format, this small, 300-page quick reference is easy to navigate and gives important FDA-approved dosing information, black box warning summaries and much more, whenever it is needed. At the point of care, rely on PDR Pharmacopoeia for quick dosing information.

PDR® for Nutritional Supplements – 1st Edition
The definitive information source for more than 300 nutritional supplements. This unique, comprehensive, unbiased source of solid, evidence-based information about nutritional supplements provides practitioners with more than 700 pages of the most current and reliable information available.

2005 PDR® for Nonprescription Drugs and Dietary Supplements
This acknowledged authority offers full FDA-approved descriptions of the most commonly used OTC medicines in four separate indices within more than 400 pages. Plus, it includes a section on supplements, vitamins and herbal remedies.

PDR® for Herbal Medicines – 3rd Edition
The third edition of PDR for Herbal Medicines, adding a new section on Nutritional Supplements and new information aimed at greatly enhancing patient management by medical practitioners. All monographs have been updated to include recent scientific findings on efficacy, safety and potential interactions; clinical trials (including abstracts); case reports; and meta-analysis results. This new information has resulted in greatly expanded Effects, Contraindications, Precautions and Adverse Reactions, and Dosage sections of each monograph.

2005 PDR® for Ophthalmic Medicines
The definitive reference for the eye-care professional offers 230 pages of detailed information on drugs and equipment used in the fields of ophthalmology and optometry. With five full indices and information on specialized instruments, lenses and much more, this guide is the most comprehensive of its kind.

PDR® Medical Dictionary – 2nd Edition
The second edition reflects the thorough revision performed by 44 medical consultants as well as a team of skilled editors and lexicographers. This fully updated edition, with more than 2,100 pages, includes 1,000 images, numerous tables, an innovative Genus Finder to help you find the genus of organisms, and much more!

PDR® Drug Guide for Mental Health Professionals – 2nd Edition
The *PDR® Drug Guide for Mental Health Professionals* was created to help you understand the beneficial effects—and the dangerous side effects—of today's potent psychotherapeutic medications. Over 75 common psychotropic drugs are profiled by brand name. All this vital information is presented in an easy-to-read format, written in nontechnical language, and drawn from the FDA-approved PDR database.

PDR® Monthly Prescribing Guide™
This portable monthly digest provides healthcare professionals with the most up-to-date prescribing information for over 2,000 commonly prescribed medications. Each monograph includes clear and concise prescribing details, cross-referenced to the annual PDR.

Complete Your 2005 PDR® Library NOW! Enclose payment and save shipping costs.

Code	Item	Price	$
260000	_____ copies **2005 Physicians' Desk Reference®**	$92.95 ea.	$ _____
260018	_____ copies **2005 PDR® Companion Guide**	$71.95 ea.	$ _____
260059	_____ copies **PDR® Pharmacopoeia Pocket Dosing Guide***	$8.95 ea.	$ _____
260133	_____ copies **PDR® for Nutritional Supplements, 1st EDITION!**	$59.95 ea.	$ _____
260026	_____ copies **2005 PDR® for Nonprescription Drugs and Dietary Supplements**	$59.95 ea.	$ _____
260125	_____ copies **PDR® for Herbal Medicines, 3rd EDITION!**	$59.95 ea.	$ _____
260034	_____ copies **2005 PDR® for Ophthalmic Medicines**	$67.95 ea.	$ _____
260158	_____ copies **PDR® Medical Dictionary, 2nd EDITION!**	$49.95 ea.	$ _____
260117	_____ copies **PDR® Drug Guide for Mental Health Professionals 2nd EDITION!**	$39.95 ea.	$ _____
	_____ copies **PDR® Monthly Prescribing Guide™ (yearly subscription)**	$49.00 ea.	$ _____
	Shipping & Handling (Add $9.95 S&H per book if paying later*)		$ _____
	Sales Tax (FL, IA, & NJ)		$ _____
	Total Amount of Order		$ _____

(*Shipping and handling is $1.95 for PDR Pharmacopoeia)

Mail this order form to: **PDR**, P.O. Box 10689, Des Moines, IA 50336-0689
e-mail: PDR.customerservice@ thomson.com

**For Faster Service—FAX YOUR ORDER (515) 284-6714
or CALL TOLL-FREE (888) 859-8053**
Do not mail a confirmation order in addition to this fax.
Valid for 2005 editions only, prices and shipping & handling higher outside U.S.

PLEASE INDICATE METHOD OF PAYMENT:
Payment Enclosed (shipping & handling FREE)
☐ Check payable to PDR
☐ VISA   ☐ MasterCard
☐ Discover   ☐ American Express

_____
Account No.

_____
Exp. Date

_____
Telephone No.

_____
Signature

_____
Name

_____
Address

_____
City

_____
State/Zip

☐ **Bill me later** (Add $9.95 per book for shipping and handling*)

SAVE TIME AND MONEY EVERY YEAR AS A STANDING ORDER SUBSCRIBER
☐ Check here to enter your standing order for future editions of publications ordered. They will be shipped to you automatically, after advance notice. As a standing order subscriber, you are **guaranteed** our lowest price offer, earliest delivery and FREE shipping and handling.

KEY 773580

Announcing the new PDR® for Herbal Medicines *3rd Edition.*

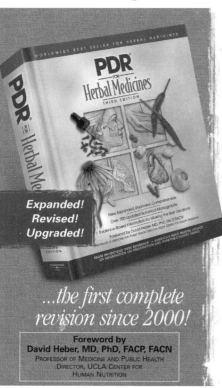

**Expanded!
Revised!
Upgraded!**

...the first complete revision since 2000!

**Foreword by
David Heber, MD, PhD, FACP, FACN**
PROFESSOR OF MEDICINE AND PUBLIC HEALTH
DIRECTOR, UCLA CENTER FOR
HUMAN NUTRITION

Patients who use herbals — prescribed or otherwise — are a daily reality for virtually every physician. But the herbal's contribution to a patient's health can be unclear and hard to assess. To make the best call for your patient, you need an authoritative, trustworthy reference that answers all your questions. It's here — the new updated PDR for Herbal Medicines *3rd Edition*.

Respected, comprehensive and current!
This new *3rd Edition* is the definitive guide to current herbal practices. With more than 700 monographs, a new section on the most popular nutritional supplements, and new information on clinical management of interactions, this edition is the ultimate source for accurate, evidence-based, trustworthy herbal information.

New interactions added
When herbal mixes with prescription, concerns over interactions are paramount. This new edition offers the most current, exhaustive interaction data available for the most extensive list of herbals assembled in one reference.

The most popular nutritional supplements added
Consumption of nutritional supplements has increased in the last decade as well. Therefore monographs of some of the most popular supplements make a logical addition to this guide.

New clinical management of interactions
At last, there's evidence-based guidance for managing herbal medicines with the most frequently prescribed drugs. This important section helps you make thoroughly informed decisions.

An herbal guide you can trust
In a field where scientific standards are not always applicable, a guide's source information is even more important. Here are three reasons why the PDR for Herbal Medicines *3rd Edition* is the world's most authoritative herbal reference:

1 The foundation for this edition continues to be the extensive herbal database of the **PhytoPharm U.S. Institute of Phytopharmaceuticals.** This resource provides extensive pharmacological and indication details that are generally not available from other sources.

2 The findings of the **German Regulatory Authority (Commission E)** are recognized for their expert consensus in the herbal field. Their widely accepted conclusions add an additional valuable dimension for physicians looking for the best counsel.

3 Finally, this edition is assembled by the same **PDR Editorial Team** that produces all the PDR reference guides. Only after their standards had been met was the PDR for Herbal Medicines *3rd Edition* ready for publication.

A typical monograph covers these critical aspects:
- herbs are listed by common name followed by its scientific name
- a thorough description of the herb is provided, including its medicinal parts (e.g., flower and fruit, etc.); unique characteristics, and additional common names and synonyms
- a detailed summary of the active compounds and the herb's clinical effects
- indications and usage — where applicable — under five categories: Commission E Approved; Chinese Medicine; Indian Medicine; Homeopathic; Unproven
- clinical studies are cited for many monographs
- drug/herb interactions and clinical management of those interactions
- precautions, adverse reactions, and dosage information provide a comprehensive overview
- a unique bibliography of the literature

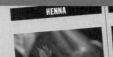

G-14/PDR FOR HERBAL MEDICINES
HENBANE | HIBISCUS | HOLLY

HENNA

HERBAL MONOGRAPHS

Arnica
Arnica montana

DESCRIPTION
Medicinal Parts: The medicinal parts of Arnica are the ethereal oil of the flowers, the dried flowers, the leaves collected before flowering and dried, the roots, and the dried rhizome and roots.

Flower and Fruit: The terminal composite flower is found in the leaf axils of the upper pair of leaves. They have a diameter of 6 to 8 cm, are usually egg yolk-yellow to orange-yellow, but occasionally light yellow. The receptacle and epicalyx are hairy. The 10 to 20 female ray flowers are lingui-form. In addition, there are about 100 disc flowers, which are tubular. The 5-ribbed fruit is black-brown and has a bristly tuft of hair.

Leaves, Stem and Root: Arnica is a herbaceous plant growing 20 to 50 cm high. The brownish rhizome is 0.5 cm thick by 10 cm long, usually unbranched, 3-sectioned and sympodial. The rhizome may also be 3-headed with many yellow-brown secondary roots. Leaves are in basal rosettes. They are in 2 to 3 crossed opposite pairs and are obovate and entire-margined with 5 protruding vertical ribs. The glandular-haired stem has 2 to 6 smaller leaves, which are ovate to lanceolate, entire-margined or somewhat dentate.

Characteristics: The flower heads are aromatic; the taste is bitter and irritating.

Habitat: Arnica is found in Europe from Scandinavia to southern Europe. It is also found in southern Russia and central Asia.

Production: Arnica flower consists of the fresh or dried inflorescence of Arnica montana or Arnica chamissonis. The flower should be dried quickly at 45° to 50°C.

Not to be Confused With: Other yellow-flowering Asteracea.

Other Names: Arnica Flowers, Arnica Root, Leopard's

Caffeic acid derivatives: including chlorogenic acid, 1,5-dicaffeoyl quinic acid

Flavonoids: numerous flavone and flavonol glycosides and their aglycones

EFFECTS
Arnica preparations have an antiphlogistic, analgesic and antiseptic effect when applied topically, due to the sesquiterpene lactone componant. The flavonoid bonds, essential oils and polyynes may also be involved. In cases of inflammation, Arnica preparations also show analgesic and antiseptic activity. The sesquiterpenes (helenalin) in the drug have an antimicrobial effect in vitro and an antiphlogistic effect in animal tests. A respiratory-analeptic, uterine tonic and cardiovascular effect (increase of contraction amplitude with simultaneous increase in frequency, i.e. positive inotropic effect) was demonstrated.

INDICATIONS AND USAGE
Approved by Commission E:
- Fever and colds
- Inflammation of the skin
- Cough/bronchitis
- Inflammation of the mouth and pharynx
- Rheumatism
- Common cold
- Blunt injuries
- Tendency to infection

Unproven Uses: External folk medicine uses include consequences of injury such as traumatic edema, hematoma, contusions, as well as rheumatic muscle and joint problems. Other applications are inflammation of the oral and throat region, furunculosis, inflammation caused by insect bites, phlebitis. In Russian folk medicine, the drug is used to treat uterine hemorrhaging. Furthermore, the drug is used in myocarditis, arteriosclerosis, angina pectoris, exhaust cardiac insufficiency, sprains, contusions and for hair due to psychological causes. While some uses are plausible, most are unproven.

Sesquiterpene lactones: particularly esters of the helenalin- and 11,13-dihydrohelenalin with short-chained fatty acids such as acetic acid, isobutyric acid, 2-methyl-butyric acid, methylacrylic acid, isovaleric acid or tiglic acid

Volatile oil: with thymol, thymol esters, free fatty acids

luted tincture, as well as nevertheless lead to sensitization.

Allergy-related skin rashes with itching, blister formation, ulcers and superficial necroses can result from repeated contact with, among other things, cosmetics containing Arnica flowers or other composites (for example, sunflowers). External application

See other side for ordering information

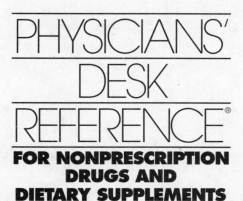

FOR NONPRESCRIPTION DRUGS AND DIETARY SUPPLEMENTS

Executive Vice President, PDR: David Duplay

Senior Vice President, PDR Sales and Marketing:
Dikran N. Barsamian
Vice President, Regulatory Affairs: Mukesh Mehta, RPh
Vice President, PDR Services: Brian Holland
Senior Directors, Pharmaceutical Solutions Sales:
Chantal Corcos, Anthony Sorce
National Solutions Managers: Frank Karkowsky,
Marion Reid, RPh
Senior Solutions Managers: Debra Goldman,
Elaine Musco, Suzanne E. Yarrow, RN
Solutions Manager: Steve Farrell
Sales Coordinators: Arlene Phayre, Janet Wallendal

Senior Director, Brand and Product Management:
Valerie E. Berger
Director, Brand and Product Management:
Carmen Mazzatta
Associate Product Managers: Michael Casale,
Andrea Colavecchio
Senior Director, Publishing Sales and Marketing:
Michael Bennett
Director, Trade Sales: Bill Gaffney
Associate Director, Marketing: Jennifer M. Fronzaglia
Senior Marketing Manager: Kim Marich
Direct Mail Manager: Lorraine M. Loening
Manager, Marketing Analysis: Dina A. Maeder
Promotion Manager: Linda Levine

Director, Operations: Robert Klein
Director, PDR Operations: Jeffrey D. Schaefer
Director, Finance: Mark S. Ritchin
Director, Client Services: Stephanie Struble
Director, Clinical Content: Thomas Fleming, PharmD
Drug Information Specialists: Michael DeLuca, PharmD;
Kajal Solanki, PharmD; Greg Tallis, RPh
Manager, Editorial Services: Bette LaGow
Senior Editor: Lori Murray

Manager, Production Purchasing: Thomas Westburgh
PDR Production Manager: Steven Maher
Production Specialist: Christina Klinger
Senior Production Coordinators: Gianna Caradonna,
Yasmin Hernández
Senior Index Editors: Noel Deloughery, Shannon Reilly
Format Editor: Michelle S. Guzman
Traffic Assistant: Kim Condon
PDR Sales Coordinators: Nick W. Clark, Gary Lew

Production Design Supervisor: Adeline Rich
Senior Electronic Publishing Designer: Livio Udina
Electronic Publishing Designers: John Castro, Bryan C. Dix,
Monika Popowitz
Production Associate: Joan K. Akerlind
Digital Imaging Manager: Christopher Husted
Digital Imaging Coordinator: Michael Labruyere

Officers of Thomson Healthcare, Inc.: *President and Chief Executive Officer:* Kevin King; *Chief Financial Officer:* Paul Hilger; *Chief Technology Officer:* Frank Licata; *Executive Vice President, Medical Education:* Jeff MacDonald; *Executive Vice President, Medstat:* Carol Diephuis; *Executive Vice President, Micromedex:* Jeff Reihl; *Executive Vice President, PDR:* David Duplay; *Senior Vice President, Business Development:* Robert Christopher; *Senior Vice President, Marketing:* Timothy Murray; *Vice President, Finance:* Joseph Scarfone; *Vice President, Human Resources:* Pamela M. Bilash

ISBN: 1-56363-501-1

FOREWORD

Physicians' Desk Reference® has been providing unparalleled drug information to doctors and other healthcare professionals for 59 years. A wider variety of *PDR®* reference options than ever before is now available and in more formats—in print, on CD, on the Internet, and for PDA.

About This Book

Physicians' Desk Reference® for Nonprescription Drugs and Dietary Supplements comprises five color-coded indices and a full-color Product Identification Guide followed by two distinct sections of product information. The first of these, entitled *Nonprescription Drug Information*, presents descriptions of conventional remedies marketed in compliance with the Code of Federal Regulations labeling requirements for over-the-counter drugs. The second section, entitled *Dietary Supplement Information*, contains information on herbal remedies and nutritional supplements marketed under the Dietary Supplement Health and Education Act of 1994. For your convenience, products in both sections are listed in the consolidated indices at the front of the book.

Physicians' Desk Reference for Nonprescription Drugs and Dietary Supplements is published annually by Thomson PDR in cooperation with participating manufacturers. The function of the publisher is the compilation, organization, and distribution of product information obtained from manufacturers. Each product description has been prepared by the manufacturer, and edited and approved by the manufacturer's medical department, medical director, and/or medical consultant. During compilation of this information, the publisher has emphasized the necessity of describing products comprehensively in order to provide all the facts necessary for sound and intelligent decision-making. Descriptions seen here include all information made available by the manufacturer. Please note that descriptions of OTC products marketed under the Dietary Supplement Health and Education Act of 1994 have not been evaluated by the Food and Drug Administration, and that such products are not intended to diagnose, treat, cure, or prevent any disease.

In organizing and presenting the material in *Physicians' Desk Reference for Nonprescription Drugs and Dietary Supplements*, the publisher does not warrant or guarantee any of the products described, or perform any independent analysis in connection with any of the product information contained herein. *Physicians' Desk Reference* does not assume, and expressly disclaims, any obligation to obtain and include any information other than that provided to it by the manufacturer. It should be understood that by making this material available, the publisher is not advocating the use of any product described herein, nor is the publisher responsible for misuse of a product due to typographical error. Additional information on any product may be obtained from the manufacturer.

Other Clinical Information Products from PDR®

For complicated cases and special patient problems, there is no substitute for the in-depth data contained in *Physicians' Desk Reference*. But for those times when you need quick access to critical prescribing information, you'll want to consult the ***PDR® Monthly Prescribing Guide™***, the essential drug reference designed specifically for use at the point of care. Distilled from the pages of *PDR*, this digest-sized reference presents key facts on more than 2,000 drug formulations, including therapeutic class, indications and contraindications, warnings and precautions, pregnancy rating, drug interactions and side effects, and, most importantly, adult and pediatric dosages. Each entry also gives the *PDR* page number to turn to for further information. In addition, a full-color insert of pill and product images allows you to correctly identify common products. Issued monthly, the guide is regularly updated with detailed descriptions of recent drugs to receive FDA approval, as well as FDA-approved revisions to existing product information. You'll also find bulletins about major new developments in the pharmaceutical industry, an overview of important new agents nearing approval, and recent clinical findings on common nutritional supplements. To learn more about this useful publication and to inquire about subscription rates, call 800-232-7379.

If you prefer to carry drug information with you on a handheld device like a Palm® or Pocket PC, you will want to know about **mobile*PDR*®**. This easy-to-use software allows you to retrieve in an instant concise summaries of the FDA-approved and other manufacturer-supplied labeling for 2,000 of the most frequently prescribed drugs, lets you run automatic interaction checks on multidrug regimens, and even alerts you to significant changes in drug labeling, usually within 24 to 48 hours of announcements. You can look up drugs by brand or generic name, by indication, and by therapeutic class. The drug interaction checker allows you to screen for interactions between as many as 32 drugs. The *What's New* feature provides daily alerts about drug recalls, labeling changes, new drug introductions, and so on. This portable electronic reference is updated daily with the latest available FDA-approved revisions to existing product information, plus the essential facts you need to make prescribing decisions for newly approved agents. Sync anytime, day or night, at your convenience, to be sure you have the most recent information available. Our auto-update feature updates the content and the software, so upgrades are easy to manage. mobilePDR works with both the Palm and Windows CE operating systems, and it's free to U.S.-based MDs, DOs, NPs, and PAs in full-time patient practice and to medical students and residents. Check it out today at www.PDR.net.

For those who prefer to view drug information on the Internet, *PDR.net* is the best online source for comprehensive FDA-approved and other manufacturer-supplied labeling information, as found in *PDR*. Updated monthly, this incredible resource allows you to look up drugs by brand or generic name, by key word, or by indication, side effect, contraindication, or manufacturer. The drug interaction checker allows you to screen for interactions between as many as 32 different drugs. The site provides an index that can be searched to find comparable drugs, and images of all products are included for easy identification. As an added benefit, *PDR.net* also gives users the option to order drug samples online. Finally, *PDR.net* hosts the download for *mobilePDR*. At this one website, you get two great *PDR* products in one. In addition to all this, *PDR.net* provides links to such useful information as *Stedman's Medical Dictionary*, MEDLINE, online CME programs, clinical trials registries, evidence-based treatment decision tools, medical newsletters, Internet directories, online formularies, and the FDA's Medwatch. A wealth of information all in one place! Registration for *PDR.net* is free for U.S.–based MDs, DOs, NPs, and PAs in full-time patient practice as well as for medical students and residents. Visit www.PDR.net today to register.

For those times when all you need is quick confirmation of a particular dosage, you will want to have a copy of the *2005 PDR® Pharmacopoeia Pocket Dosing Guide*. This handy little book can accompany you wherever you need to go, around the office or on hospital rounds. Only slightly larger than an index card and a half inch thick, it fits easily into any pocket, while providing you with FDA-approved dosing recommendations for more than 1,500 drugs. Unlike other condensed drug references, the information is drawn almost exclusively from the FDA-approved drug labeling published in *Physicians' Desk Reference*. And its tabular presentation makes lookups a breeze. The *2005 PDR Pharmacopoeia Pocket Dosing Guide* is a tool you really can't afford to be without.

To help you counsel patients who use over-the-counter supplements, the *PDR® for Nutritional Supplements* offers the latest available scientific consensus on hundreds of popular supplement products, including an array of amino acids, co-factors, fatty acids, probiotics, phytoestrogens, phytosterols, over-the-counter hormones, hormonal precursors, and much more. Focused on the scientific evidence for each supplement's claims, this unique reference offers you today's most detailed, informed, and objective overview of a burgeoning new area in the field of self-treatment. To protect your patients and ensure that they use only truly beneficial products, this book is a must.

For counseling patients who favor herbal remedies, another PDR reference may prove equally valuable. The newly updated *PDR® for Herbal Medicines Third Edition* provides you with the latest available science-based assessment of more than 700 botanicals. Indexed by scientific and common names (as well as Western, Asian, and homeopathic indications), this volume also includes a Side Effects Index, a Drug/Herb Interactions Guide, an Herb Identification Guide with nearly 400 color photos, and a Safety Guide that lists herbs to be avoided during pregnancy and herbs to be used only under professional supervision. Although botanical products are not officially regulated or monitored in the United States, *PDR for Herbal Medicines* provides you with authoritative information—the findings of the German Medicines Agency's expert committee on herbal medicines, Commission E.

To maximize the value of *PDR* itself, you'll also need a copy of the 2005 edition of the *PDR® Companion Guide*, a 1,800-page reference that augments *PDR* with eight unique decision-making tools: Interactions Index; Food Interactions Cross-Reference; Side Effects Index; Indications Index; Contraindications Index; International Drug Name Index; Generic Availability Guide; and Imprint Identification Guide. The *2005 PDR Companion Guide* includes all drugs described in *PDR*, *PDR for Nonprescription Drugs and Dietary Supplements*, and *PDR® for Ophthalmic Medicines*. It will assist you in making safe, appropriate selection of drugs faster and more easily than ever before.

PDR and its major companion volumes are also found in the *PDR® Electronic Library* on CD-ROM. This Windows-compatible disc provides users with a complete database of *PDR* prescribing information, electronically searchable for instant retrieval. A standard subscription includes *PDR's* sophisticated search software and an extensive file of chemical structures, illustrations, and full-color product photographs. For anyone who wants to run a fast double check on a proposed prescription, there's also the *PDR® Drug Interactions and Side Effects System* — sophisticated software capable of automatically screening a 32-drug regimen for conflicts, then proposing alternatives for any problematic medication. This unique decision-making tool comes free with the *PDR Electronic Library*. Optional enhancements include the complete contents of *The Merck Manual Seventeenth Edition*, *Stedman's Medical Dictionary*, and *Stedman's Spellchecker*. For more information on these or any other members of the growing family of *PDR* products, please call, toll-free, 1-800-232-7379 or fax 201-722-2680.

CONTENTS

SECTION 1

MANUFACTURERS' INDEX

This index lists manufacturers that have supplied information for this edition. Each company's entry includes the address, phone, and fax number of its headquarters and regional offices, as well as company contacts for inquiries, orders, and emergency information.

Products with entries in the Nonprescription Drug Information section are listed with their page numbers under the heading "OTC Products Described." Products with entries in the Dietary Supplement Information section are listed with their page numbers under the heading "Dietary Supplements Described." Other OTC products and dietary supplements available from the manufacturer follow these two sections.

If an entry in the index lists multiple page numbers, the first one shown refers to the photograph of the product, the last one to its prescribing information.

• The ◆ symbol marks drugs shown in the Product Identification Guide.

• *Italic page numbers* signify partial information.

A & Z PHARMACEUTICAL INC.   **758**
180 Oser Avenue, Suite 300
Hauppauge, NY 11788
Direct Inquiries to:
(631) 952-3800

Dietary Supplements Described:
D-Cal Chewable Caplets *758*

A. C. GRACE COMPANY   **602**
1100 Quitman Rd.
P.O. Box 570
Big Sandy, TX 75755
Direct Inquiries to:
(903) 636-4368
Orders Only:
(800) 833-4368

OTC Products Described:
Unique E Vitamin E Concentrate
    Capsules.......................**602**

ADAMS RESPIRATORY   **503, 602**
  THERAPEUTICS
425 Main Street
Colonial Court
Chester, NJ 07930
Direct Inquiries to:
(877) Mucinex

OTC Products Described:
◆ Mucinex 600mg
    Extended-Release Tablets ...**503, 602**
◆ Mucinex DM Tablets **503, 602**

AK PHARMA INC.   **503, 758**
P.O. Box 111
Pleasantville, NJ 08232-0111
Direct Inquiries to:
Elizabeth Klein
(609) 645-5100
FAX: (609) 645-0767
For Medical Emergencies Contact:
Alan E. Kligerman
(609) 645-5100

Dietary Supplements Described:
◆ Prelief Tablets and Powder **503, 758**

ALPHARMA   **603**
U.S. Pharmaceuticals Division
7205 Windsor Boulevard
Baltimore, MD 21244
Direct Inquiries to:
Customer Service
(800) 432-8534

OTC Products Described:
Permethrin Lotion......................**603**

ALPINE   **503, 758**
PHARMACEUTICALS
1940 Fourth Street
San Rafael, California 94901
Direct Inquiries to:
Michael J. Quinn
(888) 746-3224
FAX: (415) 451-6981
E-mail: info@alpinepharm.com
www.alpinepharm.com

For Medical Emergencies Contact:
Alpine Pharmaceuticals
(888) 746-3224
FAX: (415) 451-6981

OTC Products Described:
◆ SinEcch Capsules...............**503, 758**

ALTO PHARMACEUTICALS,   **603**
INC.
P.O. Box 271150
Tampa, FL 33688-1150
12506 Clendenning Drive
Tampa, FL 33618
Direct Inquiries to:
John J. Cullaro
Customer Service
www.altopharm.com
(800) 330-2891
(813) 968-0527

Dietary Supplements Described:
Zinc-220 Capsules **603**

AMERICAN LONGEVITY   **759**
2400 Boswell Road
Chula Vista, CA 91914
Direct Inquiries to:
Customer Service
(800) 982-3189
FAX: (619) 934-3205
www.americanlongevity.net

Dietary Supplements Described:
Noni Plus Plus Liquid **759**
Plant Derived Minerals Liquid *759*

AWARENESS CORPORATION/ dba AWARENESSLIFE   759

25 South Arizona Place, Suite 500
Chandler, AZ 85225
Direct Inquiries to:
1-800-69AWARE
www.awarecorp.com
www.awarenesslife.com

Dietary Supplements Described:

BAUSCH & LOMB   503, 604

1400 North Goodman Street
Rochester, NY 14609
Direct Inquiries to:
Main Office
(585) 338-6000
Consumer Affairs
(800) 553-5340

OTC Products Described:

BAYER HEALTHCARE LLC   605 CONSUMER CARE DIVISION

36 Columbia Road
P.O. Box 1910
Morristown, NJ 07962-1910
Direct Inquiries to:
Consumer Relations
(800) 331-4536
www.bayercare.com
For Medical Emergencies Contact:
Bayer Healthcare LLC Consumer Care
Division
(800) 331-4536

OTC Products Described:

Other Products Available:
Alka-Mints
Bactine Cleansing Spray
Bactine Cleansing Wipes
Bactine Protective Antibiotic
Bronkaid Caplets
Campho-Phenique Antiseptic Gel
Campho-Phenique Cold Sore Gel
Campho-Phenique Maximum Strength First
    Aid Antibiotic Plus Pain Reliever
    Ointment
Campho-Phenique Liquid
Concentrated Phillips' Milk of Magnesia
    (Strawberry)

BEACH PHARMACEUTICALS   761

Division of Beach Products, Inc.
EXECUTIVE OFFICE:
5220 South Manhattan Avenue
Tampa, FL 33611
(813) 839-6565
Direct Inquiries to:
Richard Stephen Jenkins, Exec. V.P.:
(813) 839-6565
Clete Harmon, Vice President Q.A.:
(864) 277-7282
Manufacturing and Distribution:
201 Delaware Street
Greenville, SC 29605
(800) 845-8210

Dietary Supplements Described:

BEUTLICH LP   607 PHARMACEUTICALS

1541 Shields Drive
Waukegan, IL 60085-8304
Direct Inquiries to:
(847) 473-1100
(800) 238-8542 in the U.S. and Canada
FAX: (847) 473-1122
www.beutlich.com
E-mail: beutlich@beutlich.com

OTC Products Described:

Dietary Supplements Described:

BOEHRINGER   503, 607 INGELHEIM CONSUMER HEALTHCARE PRODUCTS

Division of Boehringer Ingelheim
Pharmaceuticals, Inc.
900 Ridgebury Road
P.O. Box 368
Ridgefield, CT 06877
Direct Inquiries to:
(888) 285-9159

OTC Products Described:

CADBURY ADAMS USA LLC   609

182 Tabor Road
Morris Plains, NJ 07950
Direct Inquiries to:
(800) 524-2854
For Consumer Product Information Call:
(800) 524-2854

OTC Products Described:

Dietary Supplements Described:

CELLTECH   611 PHARMACEUTICALS, INC.

P.O. Box 31766
Rochester, NY 14603
Direct Inquiries to:
Customer Service Department
P.O. Box 31766
Rochester, NY 14603
(585) 274-5300
(888) 963-3382

OTC Products Described:

DANNMARIE, LLC.   762

2005 Palmer Avenue, #200
Larchmont, New York 10538
Direct Inquiries to:
(877) 425-8767
www.premcal.com
E-mail: info@premcal.com

Dietary Supplements Described:

EMINENCE LABS   762

Los Angeles, CA 90010
Direct Inquiries to:
Richard Shen
(626) 930-0254

OTC Products Described:

ENIVA CORPORATION   503, 762

Minneapolis, MN 55449
Direct Inquiries to:
www.eniva.com

Dietary Supplements Described:

4LIFE RESEARCH 763

9850 South 300 West
Sandy, UT 84070
Direct Inquiries to:
(801) 562-3600
FAX: (801) 562-3699
E-mail: productsupport@4life.com
www.4life.com

Dietary Supplements Described:

Other Products Available:
Transfer Factor

GLAXOSMITHKLINE 503, 612
CONSUMER
HEALTHCARE, L.P.

Post Office Box 1467
Pittsburgh, PA 15230
Direct Inquiries to:
Consumer Affairs
(800) 245-1040
For Medical Emergencies Contact:
Consumer Affairs
(800) 245-1040

OTC Products Described:

Dietary Supplements Described:

GREEK ISLAND LABS 767

7620 E. McKellips Road
Suite 4 PMB 86
Scottsdale, AZ 85257
Direct Inquiries to:
www.greekislandlabs.com
(888) 841-7363

Dietary Supplements Described:

HYLAND'S, INC.

(See STANDARD HOMEOPATHIC
COMPANY)

JOHNSON & JOHNSON – 506, 640
MERCK CONSUMER
PHARMACEUTICALS
CO.

7050 Camp Hill Road
Fort Washington, PA 19034
Direct Inquiries to:
Consumer Relationship Center
Fort Washington, PA 19034
(800) 775-4008

OTC Products Described:

LEGACY FOR LIFE, LLC 768

P.O. Box 410376
Melbourne, FL 32941-0376
Direct Inquiries to:
(800) 557-8477
(321) 951-8815
www.legacyforlife.net

Dietary Supplements Described:

Other Products Available:
CLA Ultra 1000 Capsules
EICO-BALANCE Omega-3 Capsules
FLEX Capsules
Legacy ESSENTIALS *for Life* Capsules
Meal Neutralizer Capsules

MANNATECH, INC. 506, 768

600 S. Royal Lane
Suite 200
Coppell, TX 75019
Direct Inquiries to:
Customer Service
(972) 471-8111
For Medical Information Contact:
Stephen Boyd, MD, PhD
(972) 471-7400
E-mail: Sboyd@mannatech.com
www.mannatech.com
(for product information)
www.glycoscience.com
(for ingredient information)

Dietary Supplements Described:

Other Products Available:
AmbroDerm Lotion
AmbroStart Beverage Mix
CardioBALANCE Heart Support Formula
    Capsules
EM•PACT Sports Drink
Emprizone Advanced Skin Care Gel
FIRM with Ambrotose Lotion
Glycentials Vitamin, Ambroglycin Mineral
    and Antioxidant Formula Tablets
Glyco•Bears Children's Chewable
    Vitamins and Minerals
GlycoLEAN Accelerator 2 Capsules
GlycoLEAN Catalyst with Ambroglycin
    Tablets
GlycoLEAN Fiber Full Capsules

MANNATECH, INC.—cont.
GlycoLEAN Glycoslim Drinks
ImmunoSTART Chewable Tablets
Manna•Bears Supplements
Manna-C Capsules
MannaCLEANSE Caplets
Mannatonin Tablets
Phyt•Aloe Capsules
Phyt•Aloe Powder
SPORT Capsules

MATRIXX INITIATIVES, INC.   **506, 642**
4742 North 24th Street
Suite 455
Phoenix, AZ 85016
Direct Inquiries to:
(602) 385-8888
FAX: (602) 385-8850
www.zicam.com

OTC Products Described:

McNEIL CONSUMER & SPECIALTY PHARMACEUTICALS   **507, 644**
Division of McNeil-PPC, Inc.
Camp Hill Road
Fort Washington, PA 19034
Direct Inquiries to:
Consumer Relationship Center
Fort Washington, PA 19034
(800) 962-5357

OTC Products Described:

Dietary Supplements Described:

MEMORY SECRET   **512, 770**
1221 Brickell Avenue
Suite 1000
Miami, FL 33131
Direct Inquiries to:
(866) 673-2738
FAX: (305) 675-2279
E-mail: intelectol@memorysecret.net

Dietary Supplements Described:

MISSION PHARMACAL COMPANY   **673**
10999 IH 10 West, Suite 1000
San Antonio, TX 78230-1355
Direct Inquiries to:
P.O. Box 786099
San Antonio, TX 78278-6099
(800) 292-7364
(210) 696-8400
FAX: (210) 696-6010
For Medical Emergencies Contact:
Mary Ann Walter

OTC Products Described:

Dietary Supplements Described:

Other Products Available:
Calcet Triple Calcium Supplement Tablets
Calcet Plus Multivitamin/Mineral Tablets
Citracal Prenatal Rx
Compete Multivitamin/Mineral Tablets
Fosfree Multivitamin/Mineral Tablets
Iromin-G Multivitamin/Mineral Tablets
Maxilube Personal Lubricant
Mission Prenatal Tablets
Mission Prenatal F.A. Tablets
Mission Prenatal H.P. Tablets
Oncovite

NOVARTIS CONSUMER HEALTH, INC.   **512, 674**
200 Kimball Drive
Parsippany, NJ 07054-0622
Direct Inquiries to:
Consumer & Professional Affairs
(800) 452-0051
FAX: (800) 635-2801
Or write to the above address

(◆) Shown in Product Identification Guide   *Italic Page Number* Indicates Brief Listing

SUNNY HEALTH CO., LTD.   775

Yaesu Center Bldg.
1-6-6 Yaesu, Chuo-Ku
Tokyo 103-0028, Japan
Direct Inquiries to:
Consumer Service
Tel. 81-33-276-5589
FAX: 81-33-276-5333
www.sunnyhealth.com

Dietary Supplements Described:

SUNPOWER   516, 776
NUTRACEUTICAL INC.

8850 Research Drive
Irvine, CA 92618
Direct Inquiries to:
Richard Lynn
(949) 553-8899
FAX: (949) 553-9084

Dietary Supplements Described:

TAHITIAN NONI   516, 777
INTERNATIONAL

333 West River Park Drive
Provo, UT 84604
Direct Inquiries to:
(801) 234-1000
www.tahitiannoni.com

Dietary Supplements Described:

UAS LABORATORIES   736

9953 Valley View Road
Eden Prairie, MN 55344
Direct Inquiries to:
Dr. S.K. Dash
(952) 935-1707
FAX: (952) 935-1650
For Medical Emergencies Contact:
Dr. S.K. Dash
(952) 935-1707
FAX: (952) 935-1650

OTC Products Described:

UPSHER-SMITH   736
LABORATORIES, INC.

6701 Evenstad Drive
Maple Grove, MN 55369
Direct Inquiries to:
Professional Services
(800) 654-2299
FAX: (763) 315-2001
For Medical Emergencies Contact:
Professional Services
(800) 654-2299
FAX: (763) 315-2001
Branch Offices:
14905 23rd Avenue N.
Plymouth, MN 55447
(763) 473-4412
FAX: (800) 328-3344
301 South Cherokee Street
Denver, CO 80223
(800) 445-8091
(303) 607-4500
FAX (303) 607-4503

OTC Products Described:

VEMMA NUTRITION   516, 778
COMPANY

8322 E. Hartford Drive
Scottsdale, AZ 85255
Direct Inquiries to:
Product Knowledge Department
(800) 577-0777
E-mail: productknowledge@govemma.com
www.govemma.com

Dietary Supplements Described:

WYETH CONSUMER   737
HEALTHCARE

Wyeth
Five Giralda Farms
Madison, NJ 07940-0871
Direct Inquiries to:
Wyeth Consumer Healthcare
(800) 322-3129 (9-5 E.S.T.)

OTC Products Described:

Dietary Supplements Described:

Other Products Available:
Junior Strength Advil Chewable Tablets
Regular Strength Anbesol Gel
Regular Strength Anbesol Liquid
Axid AR
Caltrate 600 Plus Soy Tablets
Caltrate 600 Tablets
Caltrate Colon Health Tablets
Centrum Liquid
Centrum Chewable Tablets
Centrum Kids Extra C Children's
    Chewables
Centrum Kids Rugrats Extra C Children's
    Chewables
Centrum Kids Rugrats Extra Calcium
    Children's Chewables
ChapStick All Natural

WYETH CONSUMER HEALTHCARE—
cont.
ChapStick Cold Sore Therapy
ChapStick Flava-Craze
ChapStick Lip Balm
ChapStick Lip Moisturizer
ChapStick LipSations
ChapStick Medicated
ChapStick OverNight Lip Treatment
ChapStick Ultra SPF 30
Dimetapp Cold & Allergy Tablets
Dimetapp Cold & Congestion Caplets

Dimetapp Infant Drops Decongestant
Dimetapp Maximum Strength 12 Hour
Non-Drowsy Extentabs
Children's Dimetapp Nighttime Flu Syrup
Children's Dimetapp Non-Drowsy Flu
Syrup
Dristan 12 Hour Nasal Spray
Dristan Cold Multi-Symptom Tablets
Dristan Maximum Strength Cold
Non-Drowsy Caplets
Dristan Sinus Caplets
Freelax Caplets

Orudis KT Tablets
Riopan Plus Suspension
Riopan Plus Double Strength Suspension
Robitussin Cough & Congestion Liquid
Robitussin CoughGels
Robitussin Honey Calmers Throat Drops
Robitussin Honey Cough Liquid
Robitussin Night Relief Liquid
Robitussin Pediatric Night Relief Liquid
Robitussin Sunny Orange and Raspberry
Vitamin C Supplement Drops

SECTION 2

PRODUCT NAME INDEX

This index includes all entries in the Product Information sections. Products are listed alphabetically by brand name.

If an entry in the index lists multiple page numbers, the first one shown refers to the photograph of the product, the last one to its prescribing information.

- **Bold page numbers** indicate that the entry contains full product information.

- *Italic page numbers* signify partial information.

Italic Page Number **Indicates Brief Listing**

Italic Page Number **Indicates Brief Listing**

SECTION 3

PRODUCT CATEGORY INDEX

This index cross-references each brand by pharmaceutical category. All fully described products in the Product Information sections are included.

If an entry in the index lists multiple page numbers, the first one shown refers to the photograph of the product,

the last one to its prescribing information.

The classification of each product is determined by the publisher in cooperation with the product's manufacturer or, when necessary, by the publisher alone.

ANTI-INFECTIVE AGENTS
(*see under:*
ANTI-INFECTIVE AGENTS, SYSTEMIC
SKIN & MUCOUS MEMBRANE AGENTS
ANTI-INFECTIVES)

ANTI-INFECTIVE AGENTS, SYSTEMIC
ANTHELMINTICS
Reese's Pinworm Treatments
(Reese) **516, 730**

ANTI-INFECTIVES, NON-SYSTEMIC
SCABICIDES & PEDICULICIDES
(*see under:*
SKIN & MUCOUS MEMBRANE AGENTS
ANTI-INFECTIVES
SCABICIDES & PEDICULICIDES)

ANTI-INFLAMMATORY AGENTS
(*see under:*
ANALGESICS
NONSTEROIDAL ANTI-INFLAMMATORY DRUGS (NSAIDS)
SALICYLATES
SKIN & MUCOUS MEMBRANE AGENTS
STEROIDS & COMBINATIONS)

ANTIMYCOTICS
(*see under:*
SKIN & MUCOUS MEMBRANE AGENTS
ANTI-INFECTIVES
ANTIFUNGALS & COMBINATIONS)

ANTIPRURITICS
(*see under:*
ANTIHISTAMINES & COMBINATIONS
SKIN & MUCOUS MEMBRANE AGENTS
ANTIPRURITICS)

ANTIPYRETICS
(*see under:*
ANALGESICS
ACETAMINOPHEN & COMBINATIONS
NONSTEROIDAL ANTI-INFLAMMATORY DRUGS (NSAIDS)
SALICYLATES

ANTISEPTICS
(*see under:*
SKIN & MUCOUS MEMBRANE AGENTS
ANTI-INFECTIVES
MISCELLANEOUS ANTI-INFECTIVES &
COMBINATIONS)

ANTITUSSIVES
(*see under:*
RESPIRATORY AGENTS
ANTITUSSIVES)

ARTHRITIS MEDICATIONS
(*see under:*
ANALGESICS
NONSTEROIDAL ANTI-INFLAMMATORY DRUGS (NSAIDS)
SALICYLATES
SKIN & MUCOUS MEMBRANE AGENTS
ANALGESICS & COMBINATIONS)

THROAT LOZENGES
(*see under:*
SKIN & MUCOUS MEMBRANE AGENTS
MOUTH & THROAT PRODUCTS
LOZENGES & SPRAYS)

TOPICAL PREPARATIONS
(*see under:*
NASAL PREPARATIONS
OPHTHALMIC PREPARATIONS
OTIC PREPARATIONS
SKIN & MUCOUS MEMBRANE AGENTS
VAGINAL PREPARATIONS)

V

VAGINAL PREPARATIONS
CLEANSERS AND DOUCHES
VITAMIN D ANALOGUES
(*see under:*
DIETARY SUPPLEMENTS
VITAMINS & COMBINATIONS
VITAMIN D ANALOGUES & COMBINATIONS)

VITAMINS
(*see under:*
DIETARY SUPPLEMENTS
VITAMINS & COMBINATIONS
OPHTHALMIC PREPARATIONS
VITAMINS & COMBINATIONS)

W

WOUND CARE
(*see under:*
SKIN & MUCOUS MEMBRANE AGENTS
WOUND CARE PRODUCTS)

SECTION 4

ACTIVE INGREDIENTS INDEX

This index cross-references each brand by its generic ingredients. All entries in the Product Information sections are included. Under each generic heading, all fully described products are listed first, followed by those with only partial descriptions.

If an entry in the index lists multiple page numbers, the first one shown refers to the photograph of the

product, the last one to its prescribing information.

- **Bold page numbers** indicate full product information.
- *Italic page numbers* signify partial information.

Classification of products under these headings has been determined in cooperation with the products' manufacturers or, if necessary, by the publisher alone.

Italic Page Number **Indicates Brief Listing**

SECTION 5

COMPANION DRUG INDEX

This index is a quick-reference guide to OTC products that may be used in conjunction with prescription drug therapy to reverse drug-induced side effects, relieve symptoms of the illness itself, or treat sequelae of the initial disease. All entries are derived from the FDA-approved prescribing information published by *PDR*.

The products listed are generally considered effective for temporary symptomatic relief. They may not, however, be appropriate for sustained therapy, and each case must be approached on an individual basis. Certain common side effects may be harbingers of more serious reactions. When making a recommendation, be sure to adjust for the patient's age, concurrent medical conditions, and complete drug regimen.

Consider timing as well, since simultaneous ingestion may not be recommended in all instances.

Please note that only products fully described in *Physicians' Desk Reference* and its companion volumes are included in this index. The publisher therefore cannot guarantee that all entries are totally accurate or complete. Keep in mind, too, that although a given OTC product is usually an appropriate companion for an entire class of prescription medications, certain drugs within the class may be exceptions. If you have any doubt about the suitability of a particular OTC product in a given situation, be sure to check the underlying *PDR* prescribing information and the relevant medical literature.

ARTHRITIS

May be treated with corticosteroids or nonsteroidal anti-inflammatory drugs. The following products may be recommended for relief of symptoms:

BRONCHITIS, CHRONIC, ACUTE EXACERBATION OF

May be treated with quinolones, sulfamethoxazole-trimethoprim, cefixime, cefpodoxime proxetil, cefprozil, ceftibuten dihydrate, cefuroxime axetil, cilastatin, clarithromycin, imipenem or loracarbef. The following products may be recommended for relief of symptoms:

BURN INFECTIONS, SEVERE, NUTRIENTS DEFICIENCY SECONDARY TO

Severe burn infections may be treated with anti-infectives. The following products may be recommended for relief of nutrients deficiency:

CANCER, NUTRIENTS DEFICIENCY SECONDARY TO

Cancer may be treated with chemotherapeutic agents. The following products may be recommended for relief of nutrients deficiency:

CANDIDIASIS, VAGINAL

May be treated with antifungal agents. The following products may be recommended for relief of symptoms:

CONGESTIVE HEART FAILURE, NUTRIENTS DEFICIENCY SECONDARY TO

Congestive heart failure may be treated with ace inhibitors, cardiac glycosides or diuretics. The following products may be recommended for relief of nutrients deficiency:

CONSTIPATION

May result from the use of ace inhibitors, hmg-coa reductase inhibitors, anticholinergics, anticonvulsants, antidepressants, beta blockers, bile acid sequestrants, butyrophenones, calcium and aluminum-containing antacids, calcium channel blockers, ganglionic blockers, hematinics, monoamine oxidase inhibitors, narcotic analgesics, nonsteroidal anti-inflammatory drugs or phenothiazines. The following products may be recommended:

CYSTIC FIBROSIS, NUTRIENTS DEFICIENCY SECONDARY TO

Cystic fibrosis may be treated with dornase alfa. The following products may be recommended for relief of nutrients deficiency:

DENTAL CARIES

May be treated with fluoride preparations or vitamin and fluoride supplements. The following products may be recommended for relief of symptoms:

Benadryl Allergy & Cold Tablets ...692
Ecotrin Enteric Coated Aspirin Low Strength Tablets ...616
Ecotrin Enteric Coated Aspirin Maximum Strength Tablets ...616
Ecotrin Enteric Coated Aspirin Regular Strength Tablets ...616
Goody's Extra Strength Headache Powder ...621
Goody's Extra Strength Pain Relief Tablets ...621
Hyland's Complete Flu Care Tablets ...734
Motrin IB Tablets, Caplets, and Gelcaps ...645
Children's Motrin Oral Suspension and Chewable Tablets ...647
Infants' Motrin Concentrated Drops ...647
Junior Strength Motrin Caplets and Chewable Tablets ...647
TheraFlu Cold & Cough Hot Liquid ...680
TheraFlu Cold & Sore Throat Hot Liquid ...680
TheraFlu Flu & Chest Congestion Non-Drowsy Hot Liquid ...681
TheraFlu Flu & Sore Throat Hot Liquid ...681
TheraFlu Severe Cold Non-Drowsy Hot Liquid ...683
TheraFlu Severe Cold & Cough Hot Liquid ...683
TheraFlu Severe Cold Caplets ...679
TheraFlu Severe Cold Hot Liquid ...682
TheraFlu Severe Cold Non-Drowsy Caplets ...679
Triaminic Cough & Sore Throat Softchews ...689
Regular Strength Tylenol Tablets ...655
Extra Strength Tylenol Gelcaps, Geltabs, Caplets, Cool Caplets, and Tablets ...655
Extra Strength Tylenol Adult Liquid Pain Reliever ...655
Tylenol 8-Hour Extended Release Geltabs/Caplets ...655
Tylenol Arthritis Pain Extended Relief Caplets and Geltabs ...655
Extra Strength Tylenol PM Caplets, Geltabs, and Gelcaps ...662
Maximum Strength Tylenol Sore Throat Adult Liquid ...664
Children's Tylenol Suspension Liquid and Meltaways ...666
Concentrated Tylenol Infants' Drops ...666
Junior Tylenol Meltaways ...666

FLATULENCE

May result from the use of nonsteroidal anti-inflammatory drugs, potassium supplements, acarbose, cisapride, guanadrel sulfate, mesalamine, metformin hydrochloride, methyldopa, octreotide acetate or ursodiol. The following products may be recommended:

Beano Liquid ...764
Beano Tablets ...764
Gas-X Regular Strength Chewable Tablets ...675
Gas-X Extra Strength Chewable Tablets ...675
Gas-X Extra Strength Softgels ...675
Gas-X Maximum Strength Softgels ...675
Phazyme-125 mg Quick Dissolve Chewable Tablets ...635
Phazyme-180 mg Ultra Strength Softgels ...635
Rolaids Multi-Symptom Antacid & Antigas Tablets ...708

FLU-LIKE SYNDROME

May result from the use of gemcitabine hydrochloride, interferon alfa-2b, recombinant, interferon alfa-n3 (human leukocyte derived), interferon beta-1b, interferon gamma-1b or succimer. The following products may be recommended:

Caplets ...740
Advil Caplets ...737
Advil Gel Caplets ...737
Advil Liqui-Gels ...737
Advil Tablets ...737
Children's Advil Suspension ...742
Children's Advil Chewable Tablets ...741
Advil Cold & Sinus Caplets ...739
Advil Cold & Sinus Liqui-Gels ...739
Advil Cold & Sinus Tablets ...739
Advil Flu & Body Ache Caplets ...739
Children's Advil Cold Suspension ...741
Infants' Advil Concentrated Drops ...743
Junior Strength Advil Swallow Tablets ...740
Advil Multi-Symptom Cold Caplets ...738
Aleve Tablets, Caplets and Gelcaps ...605
Aspirin Regimen Bayer Adult Low Strength 81 mg Tablets ...606
Aspirin Regimen Bayer Regular Strength 325 mg Caplets ...606
BC Powder ...612
BC Allergy Sinus Cold Powder ...612
Arthritis Strength BC Powder ...612
BC Sinus Cold Powder ...612
Benadryl Allergy & Cold Tablets ...692
Benadryl Maximum Strength Severe Allergy & Sinus Headache Caplets ...694
Benadryl D Liquid Medication ...693
Claritin-D Non-Drowsy 12 Hour Tablets ...731
Claritin-D Non-Drowsy 24 Hour Tablets ...731
Children's Dimetapp Long Acting Cough Plus Cold Syrup ...749
Children's Dimetapp ND Non-Drowsy Allergy Syrup ...749
Dimetapp Infant Drops Decongestant Plus Cough ...746
Ecotrin Enteric Coated Aspirin Low Strength Tablets ...616
Ecotrin Enteric Coated Aspirin Maximum Strength Tablets ...616
Ecotrin Enteric Coated Aspirin Regular Strength Tablets ...616
Goody's Body Pain Formula Powder ...621
Goody's Extra Strength Headache Powder ...621
Goody's Extra Strength Pain Relief Tablets ...621
Goody's PM Powder ...622
Hyland's Complete Flu Care Tablets ...734
Motrin IB Tablets, Caplets, and Gelcaps ...645
Children's Motrin Oral Suspension and Chewable Tablets ...647
Infants' Motrin Concentrated Drops ...647
Junior Strength Motrin Caplets and Chewable Tablets ...647
PediaCare Freezer Pops Long-Acting Cough-Glacier Grape and Polar Berry Blue ...706
PediaCare Long-Acting Cough Plus Cold Liquid ...704
PediaCare Long-Acting Cough Infant Drops ...705
PediaCare Multi-Symptom Cold Liquid ...704
PediaCare NightRest Cough & Cold Liquid ...704
Robitussin PM Cough & Cold Liquid ...752
Sudafed Non-Drowsy Severe Cold Tablets ...710
TheraFlu Cold & Cough Hot Liquid ...680
TheraFlu Cold & Sore Throat Hot Liquid ...680
TheraFlu Flu & Chest Congestion Non-Drowsy Hot Liquid ...681
TheraFlu Flu & Sore Throat Hot Liquid ...681
TheraFlu Severe Cold Non-Drowsy Hot Liquid ...683
TheraFlu Severe Cold & Cough Hot Liquid ...683
TheraFlu Severe Cold Caplets ...679
TheraFlu Severe Cold Hot Liquid ...682
TheraFlu Severe Cold Non-Drowsy Caplets ...679
TheraFlu Thin Strips Long Acting Cough ...684
TheraFlu Thin Strips Multi Symptom ...684
Triaminic Cough & Sore Throat Softchews ...689
Triaminic Thin Strips Cough & Runny Nose ...690
Regular Strength Tylenol Tablets ...655
Extra Strength Tylenol Gelcaps, Geltabs, Caplets, Cool Caplets, and Tablets ...655
Extra Strength Tylenol Adult Liquid Pain Reliever ...655
Tylenol 8-Hour Extended Release Geltabs/Caplets ...655
Tylenol Arthritis Pain Extended Relief Caplets and Geltabs ...655
Tylenol Cough & Sore Throat Daytime Liquid with Cool Burst ...664
Tylenol Cough & Sore Throat Nighttime Liquid with Cool Burst ...664
Extra Strength Tylenol PM Caplets, Geltabs, and Gelcaps ...662
Maximum Strength Tylenol Sore Throat Adult Liquid ...664
Children's Tylenol Suspension Liquid and Meltaways ...666
Concentrated Tylenol Infants' Drops ...666
Junior Tylenol Meltaways ...666
Pediatric Vicks 44e Cough & Chest Congestion Relief Liquid ...726
Vicks 44M Cough, Cold & Flu Relief Liquid ...722
Pediatric Vicks 44m Cough & Cold Relief Liquid ...726
Vicks DayQuil LiquiCaps/ Liquid Multi-Symptom Cold/ Flu Relief ...723
Children's Vicks NyQuil Cold/ Cough Relief ...722
Vicks NyQuil LiquiCaps/ Liquid Multi-Symptom Cold/ Flu Relief ...725

FLUSHING EPISODES

May result from the use of lipid lowering doses of niacin. The following products may be recommended:

Advil Liqui-Gels ...737
Ecotrin Enteric Coated Aspirin Low Strength Tablets ...616
Ecotrin Enteric Coated Aspirin Maximum Strength Tablets ...616
Ecotrin Enteric Coated Aspirin Regular Strength Tablets ...616
Motrin IB Tablets, Caplets, and Gelcaps ...645

GASTRITIS, IRON-DEFICIENCY SECONDARY TO

Gastritis may be treated with histamine h2 receptor antagonists, proton pump inhibitors or

INFECTIONS, SKIN AND SKIN STRUCTURE

May be treated with aminoglycosides, amoxicillin, amoxicillin-clavulanate, cephalosporins, doxycycline, erythromycin, macrolide antibiotics, penicillins or quinolones. The following products may be recommended for relief of symptoms:

IRRITABLE BOWEL SYNDROME

May be treated with anticholinergic combinations, dicyclomine hydrochloride or hyoscyamine sulfate. The following products may be recommended for relief of symptoms:

ISCHEMIC HEART DISEASE

May be treated with beta blockers, calcium channel blockers, isosorbide dinitrate, isosorbide mononitrate or nitroglycerin. The following products may be recommended for relief of symptoms:

KERATOCONJUNCTIVITIS, VERNAL

May be treated with ophthalmic mast cell stabilizers. The following products may be recommended for relief of symptoms:

MYOCARDIAL INFARCTION, ACUTE

May be treated with ace inhibitors, anticoagulants, beta blockers, thrombolytic agents or nitroglycerin. The following products may be recommended for relief of symptoms:

NASAL POLYPS, RHINORRHEA SECONDARY TO

Nasal polyps may be treated with nasal steroidal anti-inflammatory agents. The following products may be recommended for relief of rhinorrhea:

NECATORIASIS, IRON-DEFICIENCY ANEMIA SECONDARY TO

Necatoriasis may be treated with mebendazole or thiabendazole. The following products may be recommended for relief of iron-deficiency anemia:

**PEPTIC ULCER DISEASE, IRON DEFICIENCY
SECONDARY TO**

Peptic ulcer disease may be treated with histamine h2 receptor antagonists, proton pump
inhibitors or sucralfate. The following products
may be recommended for relief of iron
deficiency:

PHARYNGITIS

May be treated with cephalosporins, macrolide
antibiotics or penicillins. The following products
may be recommended for relief of symptoms:

SINUSITIS

May be treated with amoxicillin, amoxicillin-clavulanate, cefprozil, cefuroxime axetil, clarithromycin or loracarbef. The following products may be recommended for relief of symptoms:

SKIN IRRITATION

May result from the use of transdermal drug delivery systems. The following products may be recommended:

STOMATITIS, APHTHOUS

May result from the use of selective serotonin reuptake inhibitors, aldesleukin, clomipramine hydrochloride, didanosine, foscarnet sodium, indinavir sulfate, indomethacin, interferon alfa-2b, recombinant, methotrexate sodium, naproxen, naproxen sodium, nicotine polacrilex or stavudine. The following products may be recommended:

TUBERCULOSIS, NUTRIENTS DEFICIENCY SECONDARY TO

Tuberculosis may be treated with capreomycin sulfate, ethambutol hydrochloride, ethionamide, isoniazid, pyrazinamide, rifampin or streptomycin sulfate. The following products may be recommended for relief of nutrients deficiency:

Centrum Silver Tablets......................... **781**
Daily Complete Liquid.......................... **760**
Microdiet Dietary Supplement.............. **775**
Noni Plus Plus Liquid........................... **759**
Vemma Nutrition Program - Mangosteen Plus............................ **778**
Vemma Nutrition Program - Essential Minerals.......................... **778**

VAGINOSIS, BACTERIAL

May be treated with sulfabenzamide/sulfacetamide/sulfathiozole or metronidazole. The following products may be recommended for relief of symptoms:

Massengill Feminine Cleansing Wash.... **622**
Massengill Baby Powder Scent Soft Cloth Towelette......................... **622**

XERODERMA

May result from the use of aldesleukin, protease inhibitors, retinoids, topical acne preparations, topical corticosteroids, topical retinoids, benzoyl peroxide, clofazimine, interferon alfa-2a, recombinant, interferon alfa-2b, recombinant or pentostatin. The following products may be recommended:

Lubriderm Advanced Therapy Moisturizing Lotion.. **702**

XEROMYCTERIA

May result from the use of anticholinergics, antihistamines, retinoids, apraclonidine hydrochloride, clonidine, etretinate, ipratropium bromide, isotretinoin or lodoxamide tromethamine. The following products may be recommended:

Zicam No-Drip Liquid Nasal Moisturizer.................................... **643**

DRUG COMPARISON TABLES

This section provides a quick comparison of the ingredients and dosages of common brand-name drugs in seven therapeutic classes: antidiarrheals; laxatives; antacids and heartburn agents; dermatitis agents; allergy medicines; analgesics; and cough, cold, and flu preparations.

Table 1. ANTACIDS AND HEARTBURN AGENTS

BRAND NAME	INGREDIENT/STRENGTH	DOSE
ANTACID		
Gaviscon Extra Strength liquid (GSK Consumer Healthcare)	Aluminum Hydroxide/Magnesium Carbonate 254mg-237.5mg/5mL	**Adults:** 2-4 tsp (10-20mL) qid.
Gaviscon Extra Strength tablets (GSK Consumer Healthcare)	Aluminum Hydroxide/Magnesium Carbonate 160mg-105mg	**Adults:** 2-4 tabs qid.
Gaviscon Original chewable tablets (GSK Consumer Healthcare)	Aluminum Hydroxide/Magnesium Trisilicate 80mg-20mg	**Adults:** 2-4 tabs qid.
Alka-Mints chewable tablets (Bayer Healthcare)	Calcium Carbonate 850mg	**Adults & Peds:** ≥**12 yo:** 1-2 tabs q2h. **Max:** 9 tabs q24h.
Maalox Quick Dissolve Regular Strength chewable tablets (Novartis Consumer Health)	Calcium Carbonate 600mg	**Adults:** 1-2 tabs prn. **Max:** 12 tabs q24h.
Rolaids Extra Strength Softchews (Pfizer Consumer Healthcare)	Calcium Carbonate 1177mg	**Adults:** 2-3 chews q1h prn. **Max:** 6 chews q24h.
Titralac chewable tablets (3M Consumer Healthcare)	Calcium Carbonate 420mg	**Adults:** 2 tabs q2-3h prn. **Max:** 19 tabs q24h.
Titralac Extra Strength chewable tablets (3M Consumer Healthcare)	Calcium Carbonate 750mg	**Adults:** 1-2 tabs q2-3h prn. **Max:** 10 tabs q24h.
Tums chewable tablets (GSK Consumer Healthcare)	Calcium Carbonate 500mg	**Adults:** 2-4 tabs q1h prn. **Max:** 15 tabs q24h.
Tums E-X chewable tablets (GSK Consumer Healthcare)	Calcium Carbonate 750mg	**Adults:** 2-4 tabs prn. **Max:** 10 tabs q24h.
Tums Lasting Effects chewable tablets (GSK Consumer Healthcare)	Calcium Carbonate 500mg	**Adults:** 2 tabs prn. **Max:** 15 tabs q24h.
Tums Smooth Dissolve tablets (GSK Consumer Healthcare)	Calcium Carbonate 750mg	**Adults:** 2-4 tabs prn. **Max:** 10 tabs q24h.
Tums Ultra Maximum Strength chewable tablets (GSK Consumer Healthcare)	Calcium Carbonate 1000mg	**Adults:** 2-3 tabs prn. **Max:** 7 tabs q24h.
Mylanta gelcaps (Johnson & Johnson/Merck Consumer)	Calcium Carbonate/Magnesium Hydroxide 550mg-125mg	**Adults:** 2-4 caps prn. **Max:** 12 caps q24h.
Mylanta Supreme Antacid liquid (Johnson & Johnson/ Merck Consumer)	Calcium Carbonate/Magnesium Hydroxide 400mg-135mg/5mL	**Adults:** 2-4 tsp (10-20mL) qid. **Max:** 18 tsp (90mL) q24h.
Mylanta Ultra chewable tablets (Johnson & Johnson/ Merck Consumer)	Calcium Carbonate/Magnesium Hydroxide 700mg-300mg	**Adults:** 2-4 tabs qid. **Max:** 10 tabs q24h.
Rolaids Extra Strength tablets (Pfizer Consumer Healthcare)	Calcium Carbonate/Magnesium Hydroxide 675mg-135mg	**Adults:** 2-4 tabs q1h prn. **Max:** 10 tabs q24h.
Rolaids tablets (Pfizer Consumer Healthcare)	Calcium Carbonate/Magnesium Hydroxide 550mg-110mg	**Adults:** 2-4 tabs q1h prn. **Max:** 12 tabs q24h.
Alka-Seltzer Gold tablets (Bayer Healthcare)	Citric Acid/Potassium Bicarbonate/ Sodium Bicarbonate 1000mg-344mg-1050mg	**Adults:** ≥**60 yo:** 2 tabs q4h prn. **Max:** 7 tabs q24h. **Adults & Peds: >12 yo:** 2 tabs q4h prn. **Max:** 8 tabs q24h. **Peds: <12 yo:** 1 tab q4h prn. **Max:** 4 tabs q24h.
Alka-Seltzer Heartburn Relief tablets (Bayer Healthcare)	Citric Acid/Sodium Bicarbonate 1000mg-1940mg	**Adults:** ≥**60 yo:** 2 tabs q4h prn. **Max:** 4 tabs q24h. **Adults & Peds:>12 yo:** 2 tabs q4h prn. **Max:** 8 tabs q24h.
Riopan suspension (Wyeth Consumer Healthcare)	Magaldrate 540mg/5mL	**Adults:** 1-4 tsp (5-20mL) qid.
Dulcolax Milk of Magnesia liquid (Boehringer Ingelheim Consumer Healthcare)	Magnesium Hydroxide 400mg/5mL	**Adults & Peds:** ≥**12 yo:** 1-3 tsp (5-15mL) qd-qid.
Brioschi powder (Brioschi, Inc.)	Sodium Bicarbonate/Tartaric Acid 2.69g-2.43g/dose	**Adults & Peds:** ≥**12 yo:** 1 capful (6g) dissolved in 4-6 oz water q1h. **Max:** 6 doses q24h.

Brand Name	Ingredient/Strength	Dose
ANTACID/ANTIFLATULENT		
Gelusil chewable tablets *(Pfizer Consumer Healthcare)*	Aluminum Hydroxide/Magnesium Hydroxide/Simethicone 200mg-200mg-25mg	**Adults:** 2-4 tabs qid.
Maalox Max liquid *(Novartis Consumer Health)*	Aluminum Hydroxide/Magnesium Hydroxide/Simethicone 400mg-400mg-40mg/5mL	**Adults & Peds:** ≥12 yo: 2-4 tsp (10-20mL) qid. **Max:** 12 tsp (60mL) q24h.
Maalox Regular Strength liquid *(Novartis Consumer Health)*	Aluminum Hydroxide/ Magnesium Hydroxide/ Simethicone 200mg-200mg-20mg/5mL	**Adults & Peds:** ≥12 yo: 2-4 tsp (10-20mL) qid. **Max:** 16 tsp (80mL) q24h.
Mylanta Maximum Strength liquid *(Johnson & Johnson/ Merck Consumer)*	Aluminum Hydroxide/ Magnesium Hydroxide/ Simethicone 400mg-400mg-40mg/5mL	**Adults & Peds:** ≥12 yo: 2-4 tsp (10-20mL) qid. **Max:** 12 tsp (60mL) q24h.
Mylanta Regular Strength liquid *(Johnson & Johnson/ Merck Consumer)*	Aluminum Hydroxide/ Magnesium Hydroxide/ Simethicone 200mg-200mg-20mg/5mL	**Adults & Peds:** ≥12 yo: 2-4 tsp (10-20mL) qid. **Max:** 24 tsp (120mL) q24h.
Rolaids Multi-Symptom chewable tablets *(Pfizer Consumer Healthcare)*	Calcium Carbonate/Magnesium Hydroxide/Simethicone 675mg-135mg-60mg	**Adults:** 2 tabs qid prn. **Max:** 8 tabs q24h.
Gas-X with Maalox capsules *(Novartis Consumer Health)*	Calcium Carbonate/Simethicone 250mg-62.5mg	**Adults:** 2-4 caps prn. **Max:** 8 caps q24h.
Maalox Max Quick Dissolve tablets *(Novartis Consumer Health)*	Calcium Carbonate/Simethicone 1000mg-60mg	**Adults:** 1-2 tabs prn. **Max:** 8 tabs q24h.
Titralac Plus chewable tablets *(3M Consumer Healthcare)*	Calcium Carbonate/Simethicone 420mg-21mg	**Adults:** 2 tabs q2-3h prn. **Max:** 19 tabs q24h.
Riopan Plus Double Strength suspension *(Wyeth Consumer Healthcare)*	Magaldrate/Simethicone 1080mg-40mg/5mL	**Adults:** 2-4 tsp (5-20mL) qid.
Riopan Plus suspension *(Wyeth Consumer Healthcare)*	Magaldrate/Simethicone 540mg-20mg/5mL	**Adults:** 2-4 tsp (5-20mL) qid.
Riopan Plus tablets *(Wyeth Consumer Healthcare)*	Magaldrate/Simethicone 540mg-20mg	**Adults:** 2-4 tabs qid.
BISMUTH SUBSALICYLATE		
Maalox Total Stomach Relief Maximum Strength liquid *(Novartis Consumer Health)*	Bismuth Subsalicylate 525mg/15mL	**Adults & Peds:** ≥12 yo: 2 tbl (30mL) q1/2-1h. **Max:** 8 tbl (120mL) q24h.
Pepto-Bismol chewable tablets *(Procter & Gamble)*	Bismuth Subsalicylate 262mg	**Adults & Peds:** ≥12 yo: 2 tabs q1/2-1h. **Max:** 8 doses q24h.
Pepto-Bismol caplets *(Procter & Gamble)*	Bismuth Subsalicylate 262mg	**Adults & Peds:** ≥12 yo: 2 tabs q1/2-1h. **Max:** 8 doses q24h.
Pepto-Bismol liquid *(Procter & Gamble)*	Bismuth Subsalicylate 262mg/15mL	**Adults & Peds:** ≥12 yo: 2 tbl (30mL) q1/2-1h. **Max:** 8 doses (240mL) q24h.
Pepto-Bismol Maximum Strength liquid *(Procter & Gamble)*	Bismuth Subsalicylate 525mg/15mL	**Adults:** ≥12 yo: 2 tbl (30mL) q1h. **Peds: 9-12 yo:** 1 tbl (15mL) q1h. **6-9 yo:** 2 tsp (10mL) q1h. **3-6 yo:** 1 tsp (5mL) **Max:** of 8 doses (240mL) q24h.
H2-ANTAGONIST		
Tagamet HB tablets *(GSK Consumer Healthcare)*	Cimetidine 200mg	**Adults & Peds:** ≥12 yo: 1 tab qd. **Max:** 2 tabs q24h.
Pepcid AC chewable tablets *(Johnson & Johnson/ Merck Consumer)*	Famotidine 10mg	**Adults & Peds:** ≥12 yo: 1 tab qd. **Max:** 2 tabs q24h.
Pepcid AC gelcaps *(Johnson & Johnson/ Merck Consumer)*	Famotidine 10mg	**Adults & Peds:** ≥12 yo: 1 cap qd. **Max:** 2 caps q24h.

BRAND NAME	INGREDIENT/STRENGTH	DOSE
Pepcid AC Maximum Strength tablets *(Johnson & Johnson/ Merck Consumer)*	Famotidine 20mg	**Adults & Peds:** ≥**12 yo:** 1 tab qd. **Max:** 2 tabs q24h.
Pepcid AC tablets *(Johnson & Johnson/Merck Consumer)*	Famotidine 10mg	**Adults & Peds:** ≥**12 yo:** 1 tab qd. **Max:** 2 tabs q24h.
Axid AR tablets *(Wyeth Consumer Healthcare)*	Nizatidine 75mg	**Adults:** 1 tab qd. **Max:** 2 tabs q24h.
Zantac 150 tablets *(Pfizer Consumer Healthcare)*	Ranitidine 150mg	**Adults & Peds:** ≥**12 yo:** 1 tab qd. **Max:** 2 tabs q24h.
Zantac 75 tablets *(Pfizer Consumer Healthcare)*	Ranitidine 75mg	**Adults & Peds:** ≥**12 yo:** 1 tab qd. **Max:** 2 tabs q24h.
H2-ANTAGONIST/ANTACID		
Pepcid Complete chewable tablets *(Johnson & Johnson/ Merck Consumer)*	Famotidine/Calcium Carbonate/ Magnesium Hydroxide 10mg-800mg-165mg	**Adults Peds:** ≥**12 yo:** 1 tab qd. **Max:** 2 tabs q24h.
PROTON-PUMP INHIBITOR		
Prilosec OTC tablets *(Procter & Gamble)*	Omeprazole 20mg	**Adults:** 1 tab qd x 14 days. May repeat 14 day course q 4 months.

Table 2. ANTIDIARRHEALS

BRAND NAME	INGREDIENT/STRENGTH	DOSE
ABSORBENT AGENT		
K-pec *(Hi-tech Pharmacal)*	Attapulgite 750mg/15mL	**Adults:** ≥**12 yo:** 30mL (1500mg) after each loose bowel movement. **Max:** of 9000mg q24h. **Peds: 6-12 yo:** 12mL (600mg) after each loose bowel movement. **Max:** 4200mg q24h. **3-6 yo:** 6mL (300mg) after each loose bowel movement. **Max:** 2100mg q24h.
Equalactin chewable tablets *(Numark Laboratories)*	Calcium Polycarbophil 625mg	**Adults:** >**12 yo:** 2 tabs q30min. prn. **Max:** 6 doses q24h. **Peds: 6-12 yo:** 1 tab q30min. **Max:** 6 doses q24h. **3-6 yo:** 1 tab q30min. **Max:** 3 doses q24h.
Fiberall tablets *(Novartis Consumer Health)*	Calcium Polycarbophil 1250mg	**Adults:** >**12 yo:** 1 tab q30min. prn. **Max:** 6 tabs q24h. **Peds: 6-12 yo:** 1/2 tab q30min. **Max:** 3 doses q24h. **3-6 yo:** 1/2 tab q30min. **Max:** 1.5 tabs q24h.
FiberCon caplets *(Wyeth Consumer Healthcare)*	Calcium Polycarbophil 625mg	**Adults:** >**12 yo:** 2 tabs q30min. prn. **Max:** 6 doses q24h. **Peds: 6-12 yo:** 1 tab q30min. **Max:** 6 doses q24h. **3-6 yo:** 1 tab q30min. **Max:** 3 doses q24h.
Fiber-Lax tablets *(Rugby Laboratories)*	Calcium Polycarbophil 625mg	**Adults:** >**12 yo:** 2 tabs q30min. prn. **Max:** 6 doses q24h. **Peds: 6-12 yo:** 1 tab q30min. **Max:** 6 doses q24h. **3-6 yo:** 1 tab q30min. **Max:** 3 doses q24h.
Konsyl Fiber tablets *(Konsyl Pharmaceuticals)*	Calcium Polycarbophil 625mg	**Adults:** >**12 yo:** 2 tabs q30min. prn. **Max:** 6 doses q24h. **Peds: 6-12 yo:** 1 tab q30min. **Max:** 6 doses q24h. **3-6 yo:** 1 tab q30min. **Max:** 3 doses q24h.
Perdiem tablets *(Novartis Consumer Health)*	Calcium Polycarbophil 625mg	**Adults:** >**12 yo:** 2 tabs q30min. prn. **Max:** 6 doses q24h. **Peds: 6-12 yo:** 1 tab q30min. **Max:** 6 doses q24h. **3-6 yo:** 1 tab q30min. **Max:** 3 doses q24h.
Phillips' Fibercaps *(Bayer Healthcare)*	Calcium Polycarbophil 625mg	**Adults:** >**12 yo:** 2 tabs q30min. prn. **Max:** 6 doses q24h. **Peds: 6-12 yo:** 1 tab q30min. **Max:** 6 doses q24h. **3-6 yo:** 1 tab q30min. **Max:** 3 doses q24h.
Kapectolin *(Consolidated Midland Corp)*	Kaolin/Pectin 90g-2g/30mL	**Adults:** 60-120mL after each loose bowel movement. **Peds:** ≥**12 yo:** 45-60mL after each loose bowel movement. **6-12 yo:** 30-60mL after each loose bowel movement. **3-6 yo:** 15-30mL after each loose bowel movement.
ANTIPERISTALTIC AGENT		
Immodium A-D caplets *(McNeil Consumer)*	Loperimide HCl 2mg	**Adults:** ≥**12 yo:** 2 tabs after first loose stool; 1 tab after each subsequent loose stool. **Max:** 4 tabs q24h. **Peds: 9-11 yo (60-95lbs):** 1 tab after first loose stool; 1/2 tab after each subsequent loose stool. **Max:** 3 tabs q24h. **6-8 yo (48-59lbs):** 1 tab after first loose stool; 1/2 tab after each subsequent loose stool. **Max:** 2 tabs q24h.

BRAND NAME	INGREDIENT/STRENGTH	DOSE
Immodium A-D liquid *(McNeil Consumer)*	Loperimide HCl 1mg/7.5mL	**Adults:** ≥**12 yo:** 30mL after first loose stool; 15mL after each subsequent loose stool. **Max:** 60mL q24h. **Peds: 9-11 yo (60-95 lbs):** 15mL after first loose stool; 7.5mL after each subsequent loose stool. **Max:** 30mL q24h. **6-8 yo (48-59 lbs):** 15mL after first loose stool; 7.5mL after each subsequent loose stool. **Max:** 30mL q24h.

ANTIPERISTALTIC AGENT/ANTIFLATULENT

BRAND NAME	INGREDIENT/STRENGTH	DOSE
Immodium Advanced caplets *(McNeil Consumer)*	Loperimide HCl/Simethicone 2mg-125mg	**Adults:** ≥**12 yo:** 2 tabs after first loose stool; 1 tab after each subsequent loose stool. **Max:** 4 tabs q24h. **Peds: 9-11 yo (60-95 lbs):** 1 tab after first loose stool; 1/2 tab after each subsequent loose stool. **Max:** 3 tabs q24h. **6-8 yo (48-59 lbs):** 1 tab after first loose stool; 1/2 tab after each subsequent loose stool. **Max:** 2 tabs q24h.
Immodium Advanced chewable tablets *(McNeil Consumer)*	Loperimide HCl/Simethicone 2mg-125mg	**Adults:** ≥**12 yo:** 2 tabs after first loose stool; 1 tab after each subsequent loose stool. **Max:** 4 tabs q24h. **Peds: 9-11 yo (60-95 lbs):** 1 tab after first loose stool; 1/2 tab after each subsequent loose stool. **Max:** 3 tabs q24h. **6-8 yo (48-59 lbs):** 1 tab after first loose stool; 1/2 tab after each subsequent loose stool. **Max:** 2 tabs q24h.

BISMUTH SUBSALICYLATE

BRAND NAME	INGREDIENT/STRENGTH	DOSE
Kaopectate caplets *(Pharmacia Consumer Healthcare)*	Bismuth Subsalicylate 262mg caplets	**Adults & Peds:** ≥**12 yo:** 2 tabs q1/2-1h. **Max:** 8 doses q24h.
Kaopectate Extra Strength liquid *(Pharmacia Consumer Healthcare)*	Bismuth Subsalicylate 525mg/15mL	**Adults:** ≥**12 yo:** 2 tbl (30mL). **Peds: 9-12 yo:** 1 tbl (15mL) q1h prn. **6-9 yo:** 2 tsp (10mL) q1h prn. **3-6 yo:** 1 tsp (5mL) q1h prn. **Max:** 8 doses q24h.
Kaopectate liquid *(Pharmacia Consumer Healthcare)*	Bismuth Subsalicylate 262mg/15mL	**Adults:** ≥**12 yo:** 2 tbl (30mL). **Peds: 9-12 yo:** 1 tbl (15mL) q1h prn. **6-9 yo:** 2 tsp (10mL) q1h prn. **3-6 yo:** 1 tsp (5mL) q1h prn. **Max:** 8 doses q24h.
Pepto-Bismol chewable tablets *(Procter & Gamble)*	Bismuth Subsalicylate 262mg	**Adults & Peds:** ≥**12 yo:** 2 tabs q1/2-1h. **Max:** 8 doses q24h.
Pepto-Bismol caplets *(Procter & Gamble)*	Bismuth Subsalicylate 262mg	**Adults & Peds:** ≥**12 yo:** 2 tabs q1/2-1h. **Max:** 8 doses q24h.
Pepto-Bismol liquid *(Procter & Gamble)*	Bismuth Subsalicylate 262mg/15mL	**Adults & Peds:** ≥**12 yo:** 2 tbl (30mL) q1/2-1h. **Max:** 8 doses q24h.
Pepto-Bismol Maximum Strength *(Procter & Gamble)*	Bismuth Subsalicylate 525mg/15mL	**Adults:** ≥**12 yo:** 2 tbl (30mL). **Peds: 9-12 yo:** 1 tbl (15mL) q1h prn. **6-9 yo:** 2 tsp (10mL) q1h prn. **3-6 yo:** 1 tsp (5mL) q1h prn. **Max:** 8 doses q24h.

Table 3. LAXATIVES

BRAND NAME	INGREDIENT/STRENGTH	DOSE
BULK-FORMING		
Equalactin chewable tablets *(Numark Laboratories)*	Calcium Polycarbophil 625mg	**Adults & Peds:** ≥**12 yo:** 2 tabs qd. **Max:** 8 tabs qd.
Fiberall tablets *(Novartis Consumer Health)*	Calcium Polycarbophil 1250mg	**Adults & Peds:** ≥**12 yo:** 1 tabs qd. **Max:** 4 tabs qd.
FiberCon caplets *(Wyeth Consumer Healthcare)*	Calcium Polycarbophil 625mg	**Adults & Peds:** ≥**12 yo:** 2 tabs qd. **Max:** 8 tabs qd.
Fiber-Lax tablets *(Rugby Laboratories)*	Calcium Polycarbophil 625mg	**Adults & Peds:** ≥**12 yo:** 2 tabs qd. **Max:** 8 tabs qd.
Konsyl Fiber tablets *(Konsyl Pharmaceuticals)*	Calcium Polycarbophil 625mg	**Adults & Peds:** ≥**12 yo:** 2 tabs qd. **Max:** 8 tabs qd.
Phillips' Fibercaps *(Bayer Healthcare)*	Calcium Polycarbophil 625mg	**Adults:** ≥**12 yo:** 2 tabs qd. **Max:** 8 tabs qd. **Peds: 6-12 yo:** 1 tab qd. **Max:** 4 tabs qd.
Citrucel powder *(GSK Consumer Healthcare)*	Methylcellulose 2g/tbl	**Adults:** ≥**12 yo:** 1 tbl (11.5g) qd-tid. **Peds: 6-12 yo:** 1/2 tbl (5.75g) qd.
Citrucel caplets *(GSK Consumer Healthcare)*	Methylcellulose 500mg	**Adults:** ≥**12 yo:** 2-4 tabs qd. **Max:** 12 tabs q24h. **Peds: 6-12 yo:** 1 tabs qd. **Max:** 6 tabs q24h.

Brand Name	Ingredient/Strength	Dose
Metamucil capsules *(Procter & Gamble)*	Psyllium 0.52g	**Adults & Peds:** **≥12 yo:** 4 caps qd-tid.
Fiberall powder *(Novartis Consumer Health)*	Psyllium 3.4g/tsp	**Adults:** **≥12 yo:** 1 tsp qd-tid. **Peds:** **6-12 yo:** 1/2 tsp qd-tid.
Konsyl Easy Mix powder *(Konsyl Pharmaceuticals)*	Psyllium 6g/tsp	**Adults:** **≥12 yo:** 1 tsp qd-tid. **Peds:** **6-12 yo:** 1/2 tsp qd-tid.
Konsyl Original powder *(Konsyl Pharmaceuticals)*	Psyllium 6g/tsp	**Adults:** **≥12 yo:** 1 tsp qd-tid. **Peds:** **6-12 yo:** 1/2 tsp qd-tid.
Konsyl-D powder *(Konsyl Pharmaceuticals)*	Psyllium 3.4g/tsp	**Adults:** **≥12 yo:** 1 tsp qd-tid. **Peds:** **6-12 yo:** 1/2 tsp qd-tid.
Metamucil Original Texture powder *(Procter & Gamble)*	Psyllium 3.4g/tsp	**Adults:** **≥12 yo:** 1 tsp qd-tid. **Peds:** **6-11 yo:** 1/2 tsp qd-tid.
Metamucil Smooth Texture powder *(Procter & Gamble)*	Psyllium 3.4g/tsp	**Adults:** **≥12 yo:** 1 tsp qd-tid. **Peds:** **6-11 yo:** 1/2 tsp qd-tid.
Metamucil wafers *(Procter & Gamble)*	Psyllium 1.7g/wafer	**Adults:** **≥12 yo:** 2 wafers qd-tid. **Peds:** **6-12 yo:** 1 wafer qd-tid.

HYPEROSMOTIC

Brand Name	Ingredient/Strength	Dose
Fleet Children's Babylax suppositories *(CB Fleet)*	Glycerin 2.3g	**Peds:** **2-5 yo:** 1 supp. qd.
Fleet Liquid Glycerin Suppositories *(CB Fleet)*	Glycerin 5.6g	**Adults & Peds:** **≥6 yo:** 1 supp. qd.
Fleet Mineral Oil Enema *(CB Fleet)*	Mineral Oil 133mL	**Adults:** **≥12 yo:** 1 bottle (133mL). **Peds:** **2-12 yo:** 1/2 bottle (66.5mL)

SALINE

Brand Name	Ingredient/Strength	Dose
Magnesium Citrate solution *(various)*	Magnesium Citrate 1.75gm/30mL	**Adults:** **≥12 yo:** 300ml. **Peds:** **6-12 yo:** 90-210mL. **2-6 yo:** 60-90mL.
Freelax caplets *(WyethConsumer Healthcare)*	Magnesium Hydroxide 1200mg	**Adults:** **≥12 yo:** 2 tabs qd. **Max:** 4 tabs q24h.
Phillips' Antacid/Laxative chewable tablets *(Bayer Healthcare)*	Magnesium Hydroxide 311mg	**Adults:** **≥12 yo:** 6-8 tabs qd. **Peds:** **6-11 yo:** 3-4 tabs qd. 2-5 yo: 1-2 tabs qd.
Phillips' Milk of Magnesia Concentrated liquid *(Bayer Healthcare)*	Magnesium Hydroxide 800mg/5mL	**Adults:** **≥12 yo:** 15-30mL qd. **Peds:** **6-11 yo:** 7.5-15mL qd. 2-5 yo: 2.5-7.5mL qd.
Phillips' Milk of Magnesia liquid *(Bayer Healthcare)*	Magnesium Hydroxide 400mg/5mL	**Adults:** **≥12 yo:** 30-60mL qd. **Peds:** **6-11 yo:** 15-30mL qd. **2-5 yo:** 5-15mL qd.
Fleet Children's Enema *(CB Fleet)*	Monobasic Sodium Phosphate/ Dibasic Sodium Phosphate 9.5g-3.5g/66mL	**Peds:** **5-11 yo:** 1 bottle (66mL). **2-5 yo:** 1/2 bottle (33mL)
Fleet Enema *(CB Fleet)*	Monobasic Sodium Phosphate/ Dibasic Sodium Phosphate 19g-7g/133mL	**Adults & Peds:** **≥12 yo:** 1 bottle (133mL).
Fleet Phospho-Soda *(CB Fleet)*	Monobasic Sodium Phosphate/ Dibasic Sodium Phosphate 2.4g-0.9g/5mL	**Adults:** **≥12 yo:** 4-9 tsp qd. **Peds:** **10-11 yo:** 2-4 tsp qd. **5-9 yo:** 1-2 tsp qd.

SALINE COMBINATION

Brand Name	Ingredient/Strength	Dose
Dulcolax Milk of Magnesia liquid *(Boehringer Ingelheim Consumer Healthcare)*	Magnesium Hydroxide 400mg/5mL	**Adults:** **≥12 yo:** 30-60mL qd. **Peds:** **6-11 yo:** 15-30mL qd. **2-5 yo:** 5-15mL qd.
Phillips' M-O liquid *(Bayer Healthcare)*	Magnesium Hydroxide/ Mineral Oil 300mg-1.25mL/5mL	**Adults:** **≥12 yo:** 30-60mL qd. **Peds:** **6-11 yo:** 5-15mL qd.

STIMULANT

Brand Name	Ingredient/Strength	Dose
Nature's Remedy caplets *(GSK Consumer Healthcare)*	Aloe/Cascara Sagrada 100mg-150mg	**Adults:** **≥12 yo:** 2 tabs qd-bid. **Max:** 4 tabs bid. **Peds:** **6-12 yo:** 1 tab qd-bid. **Max:** 2 tab bid. **2-6 yo:** 1/2 tab qd-bid. **Max:** 1 tab bid.

BRAND NAME	INGREDIENT/STRENGTH	DOSE
Doxidan capsules (Pharmacia Consumer Healthcare)	Bisacodyl 5mg	**Adults: ≥12 yo:** 1-3 caps (usually 2) qd. **Peds: 6-12 yo:** 1 cap qd.
Dulcolax suppository (Boehringer Ingelheim Consumer Healthcare)	Bisacodyl 10mg	**Adults: ≥12 yo:** 1 supp. qd. **Peds: 6-12 yo:** 1/2 supp. qd
Dulcolax tablets (Boehringer Ingelheim Consumer Healthcare)	Bisacodyl 5mg	**Adults: ≥12 yo:** 1-3 tabs (usually 2) qd. **Peds: 6-12 yo:** 1 tab qd.
Ex-Lax Ultra (Novartis Consumer Health)	Bisacodyl 5mg	**Adults: ≥12 yo:** 1-3 tabs qd. **Peds: 6-12 yo:** 1 tab qd.
Fleet Bisacodyl Suppositories (CB Fleet)	Bisacodyl 10mg	**Adults: ≥12 yo:** 1 supp. qd. **Peds: 6-12 yo:** 1/2 supp. qd.
Fleet Stimulant Laxative tablets (CB Fleet)	Bisacodyl 5mg	**Adults: ≥12 yo:** 1-3 tabs (usually 2) qd. **Peds: 6-12 yo:** 1 tab qd.
Castor Oil (various)	Castor Oil	**Adults: ≥12 yo:** 15-60mL **Peds: 2-12 yo:** 5-15mL.
Ex-Lax Maximum Strength tablets (Novartis Consumer Health)	Sennosides 25mg	**Adults: ≥12 yo:** 2 tabs qd-bid. **Peds: 6-12 yo:** 1 tab qd-bid.
Ex-Lax tablets (Novartis Consumer Health)	Sennosides 15mg	**Adults: ≥12 yo:** 2 tabs qd-bid. **Peds: 6-12 yo:** 1 tab qd-bid.
Perdiem Overnight Relief tablets (Novartis Consumer Health)	Sennosides 15mg	**Adults: ≥12 yo:** 2 tabs qd-bid. **Peds: 6-12 yo:** 1 tab qd-bid.
Senokot tablets (Purdue Products)	Sennosides 8.6mg	**Adults: ≥12 yo:** 2 tabs qd. **Max:** 4 tabs bid. **Peds: 6-12 yo:** 1 tab qd. **Max:** 2 tabs bid. **2-6 yo:** 1/2 tab qd. **Max:** 1 tab bid.
STIMULANT COMBINATION		
Perdiem powder (Novartis Consumer Health)	Senna/Psyllium 0.74g-3.25g/6g	**Adults: ≥12 yo:** 1-2 tsp qd-bid. **Peds: 6-12 yo:** 1 tsp qd-bid.
Peri-Colace tablets (Purdue Products)	Sennosides/Docusate 8.6mg-50mg	**Adults: ≥12 yo:** 2-4 tabs qd. **Peds: 6-12 yo:** 1-2 tabs qd. 2-6 yo: 1 tab qd.
SennaPrompt capsules (Konsyl Pharmaceuticals)	Sennosides/Psyllium 500mg/9mg	**Adults & Peds: ≥12 yo:** 5 caps qd-bid.
Senokot S tablets (Purdue Products)	Sennosides/Docusate 8.6mg-50mg	**Adults: ≥12 yo:** 2 tabs qd. **Max:** 4 tabs bid. **Peds: 6-12 yo:** 1 tab qd. **Max:** 2 tabs bid. **2-6 yo:** 1/2 tab qd. **Max:** 1 tab bid.
SURFACTANT (STOOL SOFTENER)		
Colace capsules (Purdue Products)	Docusate Sodium 100mg	**Adults: ≥12 yo:** 1-3 caps qd. **Peds: 2-12 yo:** 1 cap qd.
Colace capsules (Purdue Products)	Docusate Sodium 50mg	**Adults: ≥12 yo:** 1-6 caps qd. **Peds: 2-12 yo:** 1-3 caps qd.
Colace liquid (Purdue Products)	Docusate Sodium 10mg/mL	**Adults: ≥12 yo:** 5-15mL qd-bid. **Peds: 2-12 yo:** 5-15mL qd.
Colace syrup (Purdue Products)	Docusate Sodium 60mg/15mL	**Adults: ≥12 yo:** 15-90mL qd. **Peds: 2-12 yo:** 5-37.5mL qd.
Dulcolax Stool Softener capsules (Boehringer Ingelheim Consumer Healthcare)	Docusate Sodium 100mg	**Adults ≥12 yo:** 1-3 caps qd. **Peds: 2-12 yo:** 1 cap qd.
Ex-Lax Stool Softener tablets (Novartis Consumer Health)	Docusate Sodium 100mg	**Adults: ≥12 yo:** 1-3 caps qd. **Peds: 2-12 yo:** 1 cap qd.
Fleet Sof-Lax tablets (CB Fleet)	Docusate Sodium 100mg	**Adults: ≥12 yo:** 1-3 caps qd. **Peds: 2-12 yo:** 1 cap qd.
Phillips' Stool Softener capsules (Bayer Healthcare)	Docusate Sodium 100mg	**Adults: ≥12 yo:** 1-3 caps qd. **Peds: 2-12 yo:** 1 cap qd.
Surfak capsules (Pharmacia Consumer Healthcare)	Docusate Sodium 240mg	**Adults & Peds: ≥12 yo:** 1 cap qd until normal bowel movement.
Colace Glycerin Suppositories (Purdue Products)	Glycerin 2.1g; 1.2g	**Adults ≥6 yo:** 2.1g supp. qd. **Peds: 2-6 yo:** 1.2g supp. qd.

Table 4. ALLERGY

Brand Name	Ingredient/Strength	Dose
ANTIHISTAMINE		
Chlor-Trimeton 4-Hour Allergy tablets *(Schering Plough Healthcare)*	Chlorpheniramine Maleate 4mg	**Adults: ≥12 yo:** 1 tab q4-6h. **Max:** 6 tabs q24h. **Peds: 6-12 yo:** 1/2 tab q4-6h. **Max:** 3 tabs q24h.
Tavist Allergy tablets *(Novartis Consumer Health)*	Clemastine Fumarate 1.34mg	**Adults & Peds: ≥12 yo:** 1 tab q12h. **Max:** 2 tabs q24h.
Benadryl Children's Allergy Fastmelt tablets *(Pfizer Consumer Healthcare)*	Diphenhydramine Citrate HCl 19mg	**Adults: ≥12 yo:** 2-4 tabs q4-6h. **Peds: 6-12 yo:** 1-2 tabs q4-6h. **Max:** 6 doses q24h.
Benadryl Allergy capsules *(Pfizer Consumer Healthcare)*	Diphenhydramine HCl 25mg	**Adults: ≥12 yo:** 1-2 caps q4-6h. **Peds: 6-12 yo:** 1 cap q4-6h. **Max:** 6 doses q24h.
Benadryl Allergy chewable tablets *(Pfizer Consumer Healthcare)*	Diphenhydramine HCl 12.5mg	**Adults: ≥12 yo:** 2-4 tabs q4-6h. **Peds: 6-12 yo:** 1-2 tabs q4-6h. **Max:** 6 doses q24h.
Benadryl Allergy liquid *(Pfizer Consumer Healthcare)*	Diphenhydramine HCl 12.5mg/5mL	**Adults: ≥12 yo:** 2-4 tsps (10-20mL) q4-6h. **Peds: 6-12 yo:** 1-2 tsp (5-10mL) q4-6h. **Max:** 6 doses q24h.
Benadryl Allergy Ultratab *(Pfizer Consumer Healthcare)*	Diphenhydramine HCl 25mg	**Adults: ≥12 yo:** 1-2 tabs q4-6h. **Peds: 6-12 yo:** 1 tab q4-6h. **Max:** 6 doses q24h
Alavert 24-Hour Allergy tablets *(Wyeth Consumer Health)*	Loratadine 10mg	**Adults & Peds: ≥6 yo:** 1 tab qd. **Max:** 1 tab q24h.
Claritin 24-Hour Allergy tablets *(Schering Plough Healthcare)*	Loratadine 10mg	**Adults & Peds: ≥6 yo:** 1 tab qd. **Max:** 1 tab q24h.
Claritin Children's syrup *(Schering Plough Healthcare)*	Loratadine 5mg/5mL	**Adults: ≥6 yo:** 2 tsp qd. **Max:** 2 tsp q24h. **Peds: 2-6 yo:** 1 tsp qd. **Max:** 1 tsp q24h.
Claritin RediTabs *(Schering Plough Healthcare)*	Loratadine 10mg	**Adults & Peds: ≥6 yo:** 1 tab qd. **Max:** 1 tab q24h.
Dimetapp ND Children's Allergy liquid *(Wyeth Consumer Health)*	Loratadine 5mg/5mL	**Adults: ≥6 yo:** 2 tsp qd. **Max:** 2 tsp q24h. **Peds: 2-6 yo:** 1 tsp qd. **Max:** 1 tsp q24h.
Dimetapp ND Children's Allergy tablets *(Wyeth Consumer Health)*	Loratadine 10mg	**Adults & Peds: ≥6 yo:** 1 tab qd. **Max:** 1 tab q24h.
Tavist ND 24-Hour Allergy tablets *(Novartis Consumer Health)*	Loratadine 10mg	**Adults & Peds: ≥6 yo:** 1 tab qd. **Max:** 1 tab q24h.
Triaminic Allerchews *(Novartis Consumer Health)*	Loratadine 10mg	**Adults & Peds: ≥6 yo:** 1 tab qd. **Max:** 1 tab q24h.
ANTIHISTAMINE COMBINATION		
Tavist Sinus caplets *(Novartis Consumer Health)*	Acetaminophen/Pseudoephedrine HCl 500mg-30mg	**Adults & Peds: ≥12 yo:** 2 tab q6h. **Max:** 8 tabs q24h.
Sinutab Maximum Strength Sinus Allergy caplets *(Pfizer Consumer Healthcare)*	Chlorpheniramine Maleate/ Acetaminophen/Pseudoephedrine HCl 2mg-500mg-30mg	**Adults & Peds: ≥12 yo:** 2 tabs q6h. **Max:** 8 tabs q24h.
Tylenol Allergy Complete Multi-Symptom Cool Burst caplets *(McNeil Consumer)*	Chlorpheniramine Maleate/ Acetaminophen/ Pseudoephedrine HCl 2mg-500mg-30mg	**Adults & Peds: ≥12 yo:** 2 tabs q6h. **Max:** 8 tabs q24h.
Tylenol Allergy Sinus Day Time caplets *(McNeil Consumer)*	Chlorpheniramine Maleate/ Acetaminophen/ Pseudoephedrine HCl 2mg-500mg-30mg	**Adults & Peds: ≥12 yo:** 2 tabs q4-6h. **Max:** 8 tabs q24h.
Advil Allergy Sinus caplets *(Wyeth Consumer Health)*	Chlorpheniramine Maleate/ Ibuprofen/Pseudoephedrine HCl 2mg-200mg-30mg	**Adults & Peds: ≥12 yo:** 1 tab q4-6h. **Max:** 6 tabs q24h.
Chlor-Trimeton 4-Hour Allergy-D tablets *(Schering Plough Healthcare)*	Chlorpheniramine Maleate/ Pseudoephedrine HCl 4mg-60mg	**Adults: ≥12 yo:** 1 tab q4-6h. **Max:** 4 tabs q24h. **Peds: 6-12 yo:** 1/2 tab q4-6h. **Max:** 2 tabs q24h.

BRAND NAME	INGREDIENT/STRENGTH	DOSE
Sudafed Sinus & Allergy tablets *(Pfizer Consumer Healthcare)*	Chlorpheniramine Maleate/ Pseudoephedrine HCl	**Adults:** ≥12 yo: 1 tab q4-6h. **Peds: 6-12 yo:** 1/2 tab q4-6h. **Max:** 4 doses q24h.
Tavist Allergy/Sinus/Headache caplets *(Novartis Consumer Health)*	Clemastine Fumarate/ Acetaminophen/Pseudoephedrine HCl 0.335mg-500mg-30mg	**Adults & Peds:** ≥12 yo: 2 tab q6h. **Max:** 8 tabs q24h.
Drixoral Allergy Sinus sustained-action tablets *(Schering Plough Healthcare)*	Dexbrompheniramine Maleate/ Acetaminophen/Pseudoephedrine HCl 3mg-500mg-60mg	**Adults & Peds:** ≥12 yo: 2 tabs q12h. **Max:** 4 tabs q24h.
Benadryl-D Allergy & Sinus Fastmelt tablets *(Pfizer Consumer Healthcare)*	Diphenhydramine Citrate/ Pseudoephedrine HCl 19mg-30mg	**Adults & Peds:** ≥12 yo: 2 tabs q4-6h. **Max:** 8 tabs q24h.
Tylenol Severe Allergy caplets *(McNeil Consumer)*	Diphenhydramine HCl/ Acetaminophen 12.5mg-500mg	**Adults & Peds:** ≥12 yo: 2 tabs q4-6h. **Max:** 8 tabs q24h.
Benadryl Allergy & Sinus Headache gelcaps *(Pfizer Consumer Healthcare)*	Diphenhydramine HCl/ Acetaminophen/Pseudoephedrine HCl 12.5mg-500mg-30mg	**Adults & Peds:** ≥12 yo: 2 caps q6h. **Max:** 8 caps q24h.
Benadryl Severe Allergy & Sinus Headache caplets *(Pfizer Consumer Healthcare)*	Diphenhydramine HCl/Acetaminophen/ Pseudoephedrine HCl 25mg-500mg-30mg	**Adults & Peds:** ≥12 yo: 2 tabs q6h. **Max:** 8 tabs q24h.
Tylenol Allergy Complete Nighttime Cool Burst caplets *(McNeil Consumer)*	Diphenhydramine HCl/ Acetaminophen/Pseudoephedrine HCl 25mg-500mg-30mg	**Adults & Peds:** ≥12 yo: 2 tabs q4-6h. **Max:** 8 tabs q24h
Tylenol Allergy Sinus Night Time caplets *(McNeil Consumer)*	Diphenhydramine HCl/ Acetaminophen/Pseudoephedrine HCl 25mg-500mg-30mg	**Adults & Peds:** ≥12 yo: 2 tabs q4-6h. **Max:** 8 tabs q24h.
Benadryl-D Allergy & Sinus liquid *(Pfizer Consumer Healthcare)*	Diphenhydramine HCl/ Pseudoephedrine HCl 12.5mg-30mg/5mL	**Adults:** ≥12 yo: 2 tsp q4-6h. **Peds: 6-12 yo:** 1 tsp q4-6h. **Max:** 4 doses q24h.
Benadryl-D Allergy & Sinus tablets *(Pfizer Consumer Healthcare)*	Diphenhydramine HCl/ Pseudoephedrine HCl 25mg-60mg	**Adults & Peds:** ≥12 yo: 1 tab q4-6h. **Max:** 4 tabs q24h.
Contac Day & Night Allergy/ Sinus Relief caplets *(GSK Consumer Healthcare)*	Diphenhydramine HCl/Acetaminophen/ Pseudoephedrine HCl 50mg-650mg-60mg (Night) Acetaminophen/Pseudoephedrine HCl 650mg-60mg (Day)	**Adults & Peds:** ≥12 yo: 1 tab q6h. **Max:** 4 tabs q24h.
Alavert D-12 Hour Allergy tablets *(Wyeth Consumer Health)*	Loratadine/Pseudoephedrine Sulfate 5mg-120mg	**Adults & Peds:** ≥12 yo: 1 tab q12h. **Max:** 2 tabs q24h.
Claritin-D 12-Hour Allergy & Congestion tablets *(Schering Plough Healthcare)*	Loratadine/Pseudoephedrine Sulfate 5mg-120mg	**Adults & Peds:** ≥12 yo: 1 tab q12h. **Max:** 2 tabs q24h.
Claritin-D 24-Hour Allergy & Congestion tablets *(Schering Plough Healthcare)*	Loratadine/Pseudoephedrine Sulfate 10mg-240mg	**Adults & Peds:** ≥12 yo: 1 tab qd. **Max:** 1 tab q24h.

Table 5. DERMATITIS

BRAND NAME	INGREDIENT/STRENGTH	DOSE
ANTIHISTAMINE		
Benadryl Extra Strength Gel Pump *(Pfizer Consumer Healthcare)*	Diphenhydramine HCl 2%	**Adults & Peds:** ≥12 yo: Apply to affected area tid-qid.
ANTIHISTAMINE COMBINATION		
Benadryl Extra Strength Cream *(Pfizer Consumer Healthcare)*	Diphenhydramine HCl/ Zinc Acetate 2%-0.1%	**Adults & Peds:** ≥12 yo: Apply to affected area tid-qid.
Benadryl Extra Strength Spray *(Pfizer Consumer Healthcare)*	Diphenhydramine HCl/ Zinc Acetate 2%-0.1%	**Adults & Peds:** ≥12 yo: Apply to affected area tid-qid.

Brand Name	Ingredient/Strength	Dose
Benadryl Itch Relief Stick *(Pfizer Consumer Healthcare)*	Diphenhydramine HCl/ Zinc Acetate 2%-0.1%	**Adults & Peds: ≥2 yo:** Apply to affected area tid-qid.
Benadryl Original Cream *(Pfizer Consumer Healthcare)*	Diphenhydramine HCl/ Zinc Acetate 1%-0.1%	**Adults & Peds: ≥2 yo:** Apply to affected area tid-qid.
CalaGel Anti-Itch Gel *(Tec Laboratories)*	Diphenhydramine HCl/ Zinc Acetate/Benzenthonium Chloride 1.8%-0.21%-15%	**Adults & Peds: ≥2 yo:** Apply to affected area qd-tid.
Ivarest Anti-Itch Cream *(Blistex)*	Diphenhydramine HCl/ Calamine 2%-14%	**Adults & Peds: ≥2 yo:** Apply to affrected area tid-qid.
ASTRINGENT		
Domeboro Powder Packets *(Bayer Healthcare)*	Aluminum Acetate/Aluminum Sulfate 938mg-1191mg	**Adults & Peds:** Dissolve 1-2 packets and apply to affected area for 15-30 min. tid.
Ivy-Dry Super Lotion Extra Strength *(Ivy Corporation)*	Zinc Acetate/Benzyl Alcohol 2%-10%	**Adults & Peds: ≥6 yo:** Apply to affected area qd-tid.
ASTRINGENT COMBINATION		
Aveeno Anti-Itch Cream *(Johnson & Johnson Consumer)*	Calamine/Pramoxine HCl/ Camphor 3%-1%-0.47%	**Adults & Peds: ≥2 yo:** Apply to affected area qd-qid.
Aveeno Anti-Itch Lotion *(Johnson & Johnson Consumer)*	Calamine/Pramoxine HCl/ Camphor 3%-1%-0.47%	**Adults & Peds: ≥2 yo:** Apply to affected area qd-qid.
Caladryl Clear Lotion *(Pfizer Consumer Healthcare)*	Zinc Acetate/Pramoxine HCl 0.1%-1% HCl 0.1%-1%	**Adults & Peds: ≥2 yo:** Apply to affected area tid-qid.
Caladryl Lotion *(Pfizer Consumer Healthcare)*	Calamine/Pramoxine HCl 8%-1%	**Adults & Peds: ≥2 yo:** Apply to affected area tid-qid.
Calamine lotion *(Various)*	Calamine/Zinc Oxide HCl 8%-1%	**Adults & Peds:** Apply to affected area prn.
CLEANSER		
Ivy-Dry Scrub *(Ivy Corporation)*	Polyethylene, sodium lauryl sulfoacetate, cetearyl alcohol, nonoxynol-9, camellia sinensis oil, phenoxyethanol, methylparaben, propylparaben, triethanolamine, carbomer, erythorbic acid, aloe barbadensis extract, tocopheryl acetate extract, tetrasodium EDTA	**Adults & Peds:** Wash affected area prn.
IvyStat! Gel/Exfoliant *(Tec Laboratories)*	Hydrocortisone 1% (gel); Cocamidopropylsultaine, PEG-4 laurate, cocamide DEA, polyethylene beads, sodium chloride, benzethonium chloride (cleanser)	**Adults & Peds: ≥2 yo:** Apply to affected area tid-qid.
CORTICOSTEROID		
Aveeno Anti-Itch Cream 1% *(Johnson & Johnson Consumer)*	Hydrocortisone 1%	**Adults & Peds: ≥2 yo:** Apply to affected area tid-qid.
Cortaid Intensive Therapy Cooling Spray *(Pharmacia Consumer)*	Hydrocortisone 1%	**Adults & Peds: ≥2 yo:** Apply to affected area tid-qid.
Cortaid Intensive Therapy Moisturizing Cream *(Pharmacia Consumer)*	Hydrocortisone 1%	**Adults & Peds: ≥2 yo:** Apply to affected area tid-qid.
Cortaid Maximum Strength Cream *(Pharmacia Consumer)*	Hydrocortisone 1%	**Adults & Peds: ≥2 yo:** Apply to affected area tid-qid.
Cortizone-10 Creme *(Pfizer Consumer Healthcare)*	Hydrocortisone 1%	**Adults & Peds: ≥2 yo:** Apply to affected area tid-qid.
Cortizone-10 Maximum Strength Anti-Itch Ointment *(Pfizer Consumer Healthcare)*	Hydrocortisone 1%	**Adults & Peds: ≥2 yo:** Apply to affected area tid-qid.
Cortizone-10 Ointment *(Pfizer Consumer Healthcare)*	Hydrocortisone 1%	**Adults & Peds: ≥2 yo:** Apply to affected area tid-qid.
Cortizone-10 Plus Maximum Strength Creme *(Pfizer Consumer Healthcare)*	Hydrocortisone 1%	**Adults & Peds: ≥2 yo:** Apply to affected area tid-qid.
Cortizone-10 Quick Shot Spray *(Pfizer Consumer Healthcare)*	Hydrocortisone 1%	**Adults & Peds: ≥2 yo:** Apply to affected area tid-qid.

Brand Name	Ingredient/Strength	Dose
Dermarest Eczema Lotion (*Del Laboratories*)	Hydrocortisone 1%	**Adults & Peds: ≥2 yo:** Apply to affected area tid-qid.
COUNTERIRRITANT		
Gold Bond First Aid Quick Spray (*Chattem*)	Menthol/Benzethonium 1%-0.13%	**Adults & Peds: ≥2 yo:** Apply to affected area tid-qid.
Gold Bond Medicated Maximum Strength Anti-Itch Cream (*Chattem*)	Menthol/Pramoxine HCl 1%-1%	**Adults & Peds: ≥2 yo:** Apply to affected area tid-qid.
Ivy Block Lotion (*Enviroderm Pharmaceuticals*)	Bentoquatam 5%	**Adults & Peds: ≥6 yo:** Apply q4h for continued protection.

Table 6. ANALGESICS

Brand Name	Ingredient/Strength	Dose
ACETAMINOPHEN		
Anacin Aspirin Free tablets (Insight Pharmaceuticals)	Acetaminophen 500mg	**Adults & Peds: ≥12 yo:** 2 tabs q6h. **Max:** 8 tabs q24h.
Feverall Childrens' suppositories (Alpharma)	Acetaminophen 120mg	**Peds: 3-6 yo:** 1 supp. q4-6h. max 6 supp. q24h.
Feverall Infants' suppositories (Alpharma)	Acetaminophen 80mg	**Peds: 3-11 months:** 1 supp. q6h. 12-36 months: 1 supp. q4h. **Max:** 6 supp. q24h.
Feverall Jr. Strength suppositories (Alpharma)	Acetaminophen 120mg	**Peds: 6-12 yo:** 1 supp. q4-6h. **Max:** 6 supp. q24h.
Tylenol 8 Hour caplets (McNeil Consumer)	Acetaminophen 650mg	**Adults & Peds: ≥12 yo:** 2 tabs q8h prn. **Max:** 6 tabs q24h.
Tylenol 8 Hour geltabs (McNeil Consumer)	Acetaminophen 650mg	**Adults & Peds: ≥12 yo:** 2 tabs q8h prn. Max: 6 tabs q24h.
Tylenol Arthritis caplets (McNeil Consumer)	Acetaminophen 650mg	**Adults:** 2 tabs q8h prn. **Max:** 6 tabs q24h.
Tylenol Arthritis geltabs (McNeil Consumer)	Acetaminophen 650mg	**Adults:** 2 tabs q8h prn. **Max:** 6 tabs q24h.
Tylenol Children's Meltaways tablets (McNeil Consumer)	Acetaminophen 80mg	**Peds: 2-3 yo (24-35 lbs):** 2 tabs. 4-5 yo (36-47 lbs): 3 tabs. **6-8 yo (48-59 lbs):** 4 tabs. **9-10 yo (60-71 lbs):** 5 tabs. **11 yo (72-95 lbs):** 6 tabs. May repeat q4h. Max: 5 doses q24h.
Tylenol Children's suspension (McNeil Consumer)	Acetaminophen 160mg/5mL	**Peds: 2-3 yo (24-35 lbs):** 1 tsp (5mL). **4-5 yo (36-47 lbs):** 1.5 tsp (7.5mL). **6-8 yo (48-59 lbs):** 2 tsp (10mL). **9-10 yo (60-71 lbs):** 2.5 tsp (12.5mL). **11 yo (72-95 lbs):** 3 tsp (15mL). May repeat q4h. **Max:** 5 doses q24h.
Tylenol Extra Strength caplets (McNeil Consumer)	Acetaminophen 500mg	**Adults & Peds: ≥12 yo:** 2 tabs q4-6h prn. **Max:** 8 tabs q24h.
Tylenol Extra Strength Cool caplets (McNeil Consumer)	Acetaminophen 500mg	**Adults & Peds: ≥12 yo:** 2 tabs q4-6h prn. **Max:** 8 tabs q24h.
Tylenol Extra Strength gelcaps (McNeil Consumer)	Acetaminophen 500mg	**Adults & Peds: ≥12 yo:** 2 caps q4-6h prn. **Max:** 8 caps q24h.
Tylenol Extra Strength geltabs (McNeil Consumer)	Acetaminophen 500mg	**Adults & Peds: ≥12 yo:** 2 tabs q4-6h prn. **Max:** 8 tabs q24h.
Tylenol Extra Strength liquid (McNeil Consumer)	Acetaminophen 1000mg/30mL	**Adults & Peds: ≥12 yo:** 2 tbl (30mL) q4-6h prn. **Max:** 8 tbl (120mL) q24h.
Tylenol Extra Strength tablets (McNeil Consumer)	Acetaminophen 500mg	**Adults & Peds: ≥12 yo:** 2 tabs q4-6h prn. **Max:** 8 tabs q24h.
Tylenol Infants' suspension (McNeil Consumer)	Acetaminophen 80mg/0.8mL	**Peds: 2-3 yo (24-35 lbs):** 1.6 mL q4h prn. **Max:** 5 doses (8mL) q24h.
Tylenol Junior Meltaways tablets (McNeil Consumer)	Acetaminophen 160mg	**Peds: 6-8 yo (48-59 lbs):** 2 tabs. **9-10 yo (60-71 lbs):** 2.5 tabs. **11 yo (72-95 lbs):** 3 tabs. **12 yo (>96 lbs):** 4 tabs. May repeat q4h. **Max:** 5 doses q24h.

BRAND NAME	INGREDIENT/STRENGTH	DOSE
Tylenol Regular Strength tablets *(McNeil Consumer)*	Acetaminophen 325mg	**Adults & Peds: ≥12 yo:** 2 tabs q4-6h prn. **Max:** 12 tabs q24h. **Peds: 6-11 yo:** 1 tab q4-6h. **Max:** 5 tabs q24h.

ACETAMINOPHEN COMBINATION

BRAND NAME	INGREDIENT/STRENGTH	DOSE
Excedrin Extra Strength caplets *(Bristol-Myers Squibb)*	Acetaminophen/Aspirin/ Caffeine 250mg-250mg-65mg	**Adults & Peds: ≥12 yo:** 2 tabs q6h. **Max:** 8 tabs q24h.
Excedrin Extra Strength geltabs *(Bristol-Myers Squibb)*	Acetaminophen/Aspirin/ Caffeine 250mg-250mg-65mg	**Adults & Peds: ≥12 yo:** 2 tabs q6h. **Max:** 8 tabs q24h.
Excedrin Extra Strength tablets *(Bristol-Myers Squibb)*	Acetaminophen/ Aspirin/Caffeine 250mg-250mg-65mg	**Adults & Peds: ≥12 yo:** 2 tabs q6h. **Max:** 8 tabs q24h.
Excedrin Migraine caplets *(Bristol-Myers Squibb)*	Acetaminophen/Aspirin/Caffeine 250mg-250mg-65mg	**Adults:** 2 tabs prn. **Max:** 2 tabs q24h.
Excedrin Migraine geltabs *(Bristol-Myers Squibb)*	Acetaminophen/Aspirin/Caffeine 250mg-250mg-65mg	**Adults:** 2 tabs prn. **Max:** 2 tabs q24h.
Excedrin Migraine tablets *(Bristol-Myers Squibb)*	Acetaminophen/Aspirin/ Caffeine 250mg-250mg-65mg	**Adults:** 2 tabs prn. **Max:** 2 tabs q24h.
Goody's Headache Powders *(GSK Consumer Healthcare)*	Acetaminophen/Aspirin/ Caffeine 260mg-520mg-32.5mg	**Adults & Peds: ≥12 yo:** 1 powder q4-6h. **Max:** 4 powders q24h.
Vanquish caplets *(Bayer Healthcare)*	Acetaminophen/Aspirin/ Caffeine 194mg-227mg-33mg	**Adults & Peds: ≥12 yo:** 2 tabs q6h. **Max:** 8 tabs q24h.
Excedrin Quicktabs tablets *(Bristol-Myers Squibb)*	Acetaminophen/Caffeine 500mg-65mg	**Adults & Peds: ≥12 yo:** 2 tabs q6h. **Max:** 8 tabs q24h.
Excedrin Tension Headache caplets *(Bristol-Myers Squibb)*	Acetaminophen/Caffeine 500mg-65mg	**Adults & Peds: ≥12 yo:** 2 tabs q6h. **Max:** 8 tabs q24h.
Excedrin Tension Headache geltabs *(Bristol-Myers Squibb)*	Acetaminophen/Caffeine 500mg-65mg	**Adults & Peds: ≥12 yo:** 2 tabs q6h. **Max:** 8 tabs q24h.
Midol Menstrual Complete caplets *(Bayer Healthcare)*	Acetaminophen/Caffeine/ Pyrilamine Maleate 500mg-60mg-15mg	**Adults & Peds: ≥12 yo:** 2 tabs q6h. **Max:** 8 tabs q24h.
Midol Menstrual Complete gelcaps *(Bayer Healthcare)*	Acetaminophen/Caffeine/ Pyrilamine Maleate 500mg-60mg-15mg	**Adults & Peds: ≥12 yo:** 2 caps q6h. **Max:** 8 caps q24h.
Midol Teen caplets *(Bayer Healthcare)*	Acetaminophen/Pamabrom 500mg-25mg	**Adults & Peds: ≥12 yo:** 2 tabs q6h. **Max:** 8 tabs q24h.
Tylenol Women's caplets *(McNeil Consumer)*	Acetaminophen/Pamabrom 500mg-25mg	**Adults & Peds: ≥12 yo:** 2 tabs q4-6h. **Max:** 8 tabs q24h.
Midol PMS caplets *(Bayer Healthcare)*	Acetaminophen/Pamabrom/ Pyrilamine Maleate 500mg-25mg-15mg	**Adults & Peds: ≥12 yo:** 2 tabs q6h. **Max:** 8 tabs q24h.
Pamprin Multi-Symptom caplets *(Chattem Consumer Products)*	Acetaminophen/Pamabrom/ Pyrilamine Maleate 500mg-25mg-15mg	**Adults & Peds: ≥12 yo:** 2 tabs q4-6h. **Max:** 8 tabs q24h.
Premsyn PMS caplets *(Chattem Consumer Products)*	Acetaminophen/Pamabrom/ Pyrilamine Maleate 500mg-25mg-15mg	**Adults & Peds: ≥12 yo:** 2 tabs q4-6h. **Max:** 8 tabs q24h.

NSAID

BRAND NAME	INGREDIENT/STRENGTH	DOSE
Advil gelcaps *(Wyeth Consumer Healthcare)*	Ibuprofen 200mg	**Adults & Peds: ≥12 yo:** 1-2 caps q4-6h. Max: 6 caps q24h.
Advil Infants' Drops *(Wyeth Consumer Healthcare)*	Ibuprofen 50mg/1.25mL	**Peds: 6-11 months (12-17 lbs):** 1.25mL. **12-23 months (18-23 lbs):** 1.875mL. May repeat q6-8h. Max: 4 doses q24h.
Advil Junior Strength tablets *(Wyeth Consumer Healthcare)*	Ibuprofen 100mg	**Peds: 6-10 yo (48-71 lbs):** 2 tabs. **11 yo (72-95 lbs):** 3 tabs. May repeat q6-8h. **Max:** 4 doses q24h.
Advil Liqui-gels *(Wyeth Consumer Health)*	Ibuprofen 200mg	**Adults & Peds: >12 yo:** 1-2 caps q4-6h. Max: 6 caps q24h.
Advil Migraine capsules *(Wyeth Consumer Healthcare)*	Ibuprofen 200mg	**Adults:** 2 caps prn. **Max:** 2 caps q24h.

Brand Name	Ingredient/Strength	Dose
Advil tablets *(Wyeth Consumer Health)*	Ibuprofen 200mg	**Adults & Peds: ≥12 yo:** 1-2 tabs q4-6h. **Max:** 6 tabs q24h.
Midol Cramps and Body Aches tablets *(Bayer Healthcare)*	Ibuprofen 200mg	**Adults & Peds: ≥12 yo:** 1-2 tabs q4-6h. **Max:** 6 tabs q24h.
Motrin Children's suspension *(McNeil Consumer)*	Ibuprofen 100mg/5mL	**Peds: 2-3 yo (24-35 lbs):** 1 tsp (5mL). **4-5 yo (36-47 lbs):** 1.5 tsp (7.5mL). **6-8 yo (48-59 lbs):** 2 tsp (10mL). **9-10 yo (60-71 lbs):** 2.5 tsp (12.5mL). **11 yo (72-95 lbs):** 3 tsp (15mL). May repeat q6-8h. **Max:** 4 doses q24h.
Motrin IB caplets *(McNeil Consumer)*	Ibuprofen 200mg	**Adults & Peds: >12 yo:** 1-2 tabs q4-6h. **Max:** 6 tabs q24h.
Motrin Infants' Drops *(McNeil Consumer)*	Ibuprofen 50mg/1.25mL	**Peds: 6-11 months (12-17 lbs):** 1.25mL. **12-23 months (18-23 lbs):** 1.875mL. May repeat q6-8h. **Max:** 4 doses q24h.
Motrin Junior Strength chewable tablets *(McNeil Consumer)*	Ibuprofen 100mg	**Peds: 6-8 yo (48-59 lbs):** 2 tabs. **9-10 yo (60-71 lbs):** 2.5 tabs. **11 yo (72-95 lbs):** 3 tabs. May repeat q6-8h. **Max:** 4 doses q24h.
Nuprin caplets *(Bristol-Myers Squibb)*	Ibuprofen 200mg	**Adults & Peds: ≥12 yo:** 1-2 tabs q4-6h. **Max:** 6 tabs q24h.
Orudis KT tablets *(Wyeth Consumer Healthcare)*	Ketoprofen Magnesium 12.5mg	**Adults:** 1-2 tabs q4-6h. **Max:** 6 tabs q24h.
Aleve caplets *(Bayer Healthcare)*	Naproxen Sodium 220mg	**Adults: ≥65 yo:** 1 tab q12h. **Max:** 2 tabs q24h. **Adults & Peds: ≥12 yo:** 1 tab q8-12h. **Max:** 3 tabs q24h.
Aleve gelcaps *(Bayer Healthcare)*	Naproxen Sodium 220mg	**Adults: ≥65 yo:** 1 cap q12h. **Max:** 2 caps q24h. **Adults & Peds: >12 yo:** 1 cap q8-12h. **Max:** 3 caps q24h.
Aleve tablets *(Bayer Healthcare)*	Naproxen Sodium 220mg	**Adults: ≥65 yo:** 1 tab q12h. **Max:** 2 tabs q24h. **Adults & Peds: ≥12 yo:** 1 tab q8-12h. **Max:** 3 tabs q24h.
Midol Extended Relief caplets *(Bayer Healthcare)*	Naproxen Sodium 220mg	**Adults & Peds: ≥12 yo:** 1 tabs q8-12h. **Max:** 3 tabs q24h.

SALICYLATE

Brand Name	Ingredient/Strength	Dose
Anacin 81 tablets *(Insight Pharmaceuticals)*	Aspirin 81mg	**Adults & Peds: ≥12 yo:** 4-8 tabs q4h. **Max:** 48 tabs q24h.
Aspergum chewable tablets *(Schering Plough Healthcare)*	Aspirin 227mg	**Adults & Peds: ≥12 yo:** 2 tabs q4h. **Max:** 16 tabs q24h.
Bayer Aspirin Extra Strength caplets *(Bayer Healthcare)*	Aspirin 500mg	**Adults & Peds: ≥12 yo:** 1-2 tabs q4-6h. **Max:** 8 tabs q24h.
Bayer Aspirin safety coated caplets *(Bayer Healthcare)*	Aspirin 325mg	**Adults & Peds: ≥12 yo:** 1-2 tabs q4h. **Max:** 12 tabs q24h.
Bayer Children's Aspirin chewable tablets *(Bayer Healthcare)*	Aspirin 81mg	**Adults & Peds: ≥12 yo:** 4-8 tabs q4h. **Max:** 48 tabs q24h.
Bayer Low Dose Aspirin tablets *(Bayer Healthcare)*	Aspirin 81mg	**Adults & Peds: ≥12 yo:** 4-8 tabs q4h. Max: 48 tabs q24h.
Bayer Original Aspirin tablets *(Bayer Healthcare)*	Aspirin 325mg	**Adults & Peds: ≥12 yo:** 1-2 tabs q4h or 3 tabs q6h. **Max:** 12 tabs q24h.
Ecotrin Adult Low Strength tablets *(GSK Consumer Healthcare)*	Aspirin 81mg	**Adults:** 4-8 tabs q4h. **Max:** 48 tabs q24h.
Ecotrin Enteric Low Strength tablets *(GSK Consumer Healthcare)*	Aspirin 81mg	**Adults:** 4-8 tabs q4h. **Max:** 48 tabs q24h.
Ecotrin Enteric Regular Strength tablets *(GSK Consumer Healthcare)*	Aspirin 325mg	**Adults & Peds: ≥12 yo:** 1-2 tabs q4h. **Max:** 12 tabs q24h.
Ecotrin Maximum Strength tablets *(GSK Consumer Healthcare)*	Aspirin 500mg	**Adults & Peds: ≥12 yo:** 2 tabs q6h. **Max:** 8 tabs q24h.

Brand Name	Ingredient/Strength	Dose
Ecotrin Regular Strength tablets (GSK Consumer Healthcare)	Aspirin 325mg	**Adults & Peds:** ≥**12 yo:** 1-2 tabs q4h. **Max:** 12 tabs q24h.
Halfprin 162mg tablets (Kramer Laboratories)	Aspirin 162mg	**Adults & Peds:** ≥**12 yo:** 2-4 tabs q4h. **Max:** 24 tabs q24h.
Halfprin 81mg tablets (Kramer Laboratories)	Aspirin 81mg	**Adults & Peds:** ≥**12 yo:** 4-8 tabs q4h. **Max:** 48 tabs q24h.
St. Joseph Adult Low Strength chewable tablets (McNeil Consumer)	Aspirin 81mg	**Adults & Peds:** ≥**12 yo:** 4-8 tabs q4h. **Max:** 48 tabs q24h.
St. Joseph Adult Low Strength tablets (McNeil Consumer)	Aspirin 81mg	**Adults & Peds:** ≥**12 yo:** 4-8 tabs q4h. **Max:** 48 tabs q24h.
Doan's Extra Strength caplets (Novartis Consumer Health)	Magnesium Salicylate Tetrahydrate 580mg	**Adults & Peds:** ≥**12 yo:** 2 tabs q 6 h; **Max:** 8 tabs q 24 h.
Doan's Regular Strength caplets (Novartis Consumer Health)	Magnesium Salicylate Tetrahydrate 377mg	**Adults & Peds:** ≥**12 yo:** 2 tabs q4h. **Max:** 12 tabs q24h.

SALICYLATE BUFFERED

Brand Name	Ingredient/Strength	Dose
Ascriptin Maximum Strength tablets (Novartis Consumer Health)	Aspirin Buffered with Maalox/ Calcium Carbonate 500mg	**Adults & Peds:** ≥**12 yo:** 2 tabs q4h. **Max:** 8 tabs q24h.
Ascriptin Regular Strength tablets (Novartis Consumer Health)	Aspirin Buffered with Maalox/ Calcium Carbonate 325mg	**Adults & Peds:** ≥**12 yo:** 2 tabs q4h. **Max:** 12 tabs q24h.
Bayer Extra Strength Plus caplets (Bayer Healthcare)	Aspirin Buffered with Calcium Carbonate 500mg	**Adults & Peds:** ≥**12 yo:** 1-2 tabs q4-6h. **Max:** 8 tabs q24h.
Bufferin Extra Strength tablets (Bristol-Myers Squibb)	Aspirin Bufferred with Calcium Carbonate/Magnesium Oxide/ Magnesium Carbonate 500mg	**Adults & Peds:** ≥**12 yo:** 2 tabs q6h. **Max:** 8 tabs q24h.
Bufferin tablets (Bristol-Myers Squibb)	Aspirin Bufferred with Calcium Carbonate/Magnesium Oxide/ Magnesium Carbonate 325mg	**Adults & Peds:** ≥**12 yo:** 2 tabs q4h. **Max:** 12 tabs q24h.

SALICYLATE COMBINATION

Brand Name	Ingredient/Strength	Dose
Alka-Seltzer Morning Relief effervescent tablets (Bayer Healthcare)	Aspirin/Caffeine 500mg-65mg	**Adults & Peds:** ≥**12 yo:** 2 tabs q6h. **Max:** 8 tabs q24h.
Anacin Extra Strength tablets (Insight Pharmaceuticals)	Aspirin/Caffeine 500mg-32mg	**Adults & Peds:** ≥**12 yo:** 2 tabs q6h. **Max:** 8 tabs q24h.
Anacin tablets (Insight Pharmaceuticals)	Aspirin/Caffeine 400mg-32mg	**Adults & Peds:** ≥**12 yo:** 2 tabs q6h. **Max:** 8 tabs q24h.
Bayer Back & Body Pain caplets (Bayer Healthcare)	Aspirin/Caffeine 500mg-32.5mg	**Adults & Peds:** ≥**12 yo:** 2 tabs q6h. **Max:** 8 tabs q24h.
BC Arthritis Strength powders (GSK Consumer Healthcare)	Aspirin/Caffeine/Salicylamide 742mg-38mg-222mg	**Adults & Peds:** ≥**12 yo:** 1 powder q3-4h. **Max:** 4 powders q24h.
BC Original powders (GSK Consumer Healthcare)	Aspirin/Caffeine/Salicylamide 650mg-33.3mg-195mg	**Adults & Peds:** ≥**12 yo:** 1 powder q 3-4 h.
Bayer Women's Aspirin caplets (Bayer Healthcare)	Aspirin/Calcium 81mg-300mg	**Adults & Peds:** ≥**12 yo:** 4 tabs qd. Max: 4 tabs q24h.
Alka-Seltzer effervescent tablets (Bayer Healthcare)	Aspirin/Citric Acid/Sodium Bicarbonate/Sodium 325mg-1000mg-1916mg-567mg	**Adults & Peds:** ≥**12 yo:** 2 tabs q4h. Max: 8 tabs q24h.
Alka-Seltzer Extra Strength effervescent tablets (Bayer Healthcare)	Aspirin/Citric Acid/Sodium Bicarbonate/Sodium 500mg-1000mg-1985mg-588mg	**Adults & Peds:** ≥**12 yo:** 2 tabs q6h. Max: 7 tabs q24h.

Table 7. COUGH, COLD, AND FLU

Brand name	Analgesic	Antihistamine	Decongestant	Cough suppressant	Expectorant	Dose
ANTIHISTAMINE/DECONGESTANT						
Actifed Cold & Allergy caplets *(Pfizer Consumer Healthcare)*		Triprolidine HCl 2.5mg	Pseudoephedrine HCl 60mg			**Adults: ≥12 yo:** 1 tabs q4-6h. **Max:** 4 tabs q24h. **Peds: 3-12 yo:** 1/2 tab q4-6h. **Max:** 2 tabs q24h.
Benadryl Children's Allergy & Cold Fastmelt tablets *(Pfizer Consumer Healthcare)*		Diphenhydramine 19mg	Pseudoephedrine HCl 30mg			**Adults: ≥12 yo:** 2 tabs q4h. **Max:** 8 tabs q24h. **Peds: 6-12 yo:** 1 tab q4h. **Max:** 4 tabs q24h.
Dimetapp Children's Cold & Allergy elixir *(Wyeth Consumer Healthcare)*		Brompheniramine Maleate 1mg/5mL	Pseudoephedrine HCl 15mg/5mL			**Adults ≥12 yo:** 4 tsp (20mL) q4h. **Peds: 6-12 yo:** 2 tsp (10mL) q4h. **Max:** of 4 doses q24h.
Sudafed Sinus Nighttime tablets *(Pfizer Consumer Healthcare)*		Triprolidine HCl 2.5mg	Pseudoephedrine HCl 60mg			**Adults: ≥12 yo:** 1 tabs q4-6h. **Peds: 6-12 yo:** 1/2 tab q4-6h **Max:** 4 doses q24h.
Triaminic Cold & Allergy *(Novartis Consumer Health)*		Chlorpheniramine Maleate 1mg/5mL	Pseudoephedrine HCl 15mg/5mL			**Peds: 6-12 yo:** 2 tsp (10mL) q4-6h. **Max:** 8 tsp (40mL) q24h.
ANTIHISTAMINE/DECONGESTANT/ANALGESIC						
Actifed Cold & Sinus caplets *(Pfizer Consumer Healthcare)*	Acetaminophen 500mg	Chlorpheniramine Maleate 2mg	Pseudoephedrine HCl 30mg			**Adults & Peds: ≥12 yo:** 2 tabs q6h. **Max:** 8 tabs q24h.
Advil Multi-Symptom Cold caplets *(Wyeth Consumer Healthcare)*	Ibuprofen 200mg	Chlorpheniramine Maleate 2mg	Pseudoephedrine HCl 30mg			**Adults & Peds: ≥12 yo:** 1 tab q4-6h. **Max:** 6 tabs q24h.
Alka-Seltzer Plus Cold effervescent tablets *(Bayer Healthcare)*	Acetaminophen 250mg	Chlorpheniramine Maleate 2mg	Phenylephrine HCl 5mg			**Adults & Peds: ≥12 yo:** 2 tabs q4h. **Max:** 8 tabs q24h.
Alka-Seltzer Plus Cold liqui-gels *(Bayer Healthcare)*	Acetaminophen 325mg	Chlorpheniramine Maleate 2mg	Pseudoephedrine HCl 30mg			**Adults: ≥12 yo:** 2 caps q4h. **Peds: 6-12 yo:** 1 cap q4h. **Max:** 4 doses q24h.
Benadryl Children's Allergy & Cold caplets *(Pfizer Consumer Healthcare)*	Acetaminophen 500mg	Diphenhydramine 12.5mg	Pseudoephedrine HCl 30mg			**Adults & Peds: ≥12 yo:** 2 tabs q6h. **Max:** 8 tabs q24h.
Comtrex Acute Head Cold caplets *(Bristol-Myers Squibb)*	Acetaminophen 500mg	Brompheniramine Maleate 2mg	Pseudoephedrine HCl 30mg			**Adults & Peds: ≥12 yo:** 2 tabs q6h. **Max:** 8 tabs q24h.
Comtrex Nighttime Acute Head Cold liquid *(Bristol-Myers Squibb)*	Acetaminophen 1000mg/30mL	Brompheniramine Maleate 4mg/30mL	Pseudoephedrine HCl 60mg/30mL			**Adults & Peds: ≥12 yo:** 2 tbl (30mL) q6h. **Max:** 8 tbl (240mL) q24h.
Coricidin D Cold, Flu & Sinus tablets *(Schering Plough Healthcare)*	Acetaminophen 325mg	Chlorpheniramine Maleate 2mg	Pseudoephedrine Sulfate 30mg			**Adults: ≥12 yo:** 2 tabs q4-6h. **Max:** 8 tabs q24h. **Peds: 6-12 yo:** 1 tab q4h. **Max:** 4 tabs q24h.
Dristan Cold Multi-Symptom tablets *(Wyeth Consumer Healthcare)*	Acetaminophen 325mg	Chlorpheniramine Maleate 2mg	Phenylephrine HCl 5mg			**Adults & Peds: ≥12 yo:** 2 tabs q4. **Max:** 12 caps q24h.
Sudafed Sinus Nighttime Plus Pain Relief caplets *(Pfizer Consumer Healthcare)*	Acetaminophen 500mg	Diphenhydramine HCl 25mg	Pseudoephedrine HCl 30mg			**Adults & Peds: ≥12 yo:** 2 tabs q6h. **Max:** 8 tabs q24h.
Theraflu Flu & Sore Throat packets *(Novartis Consumer Health)*	Acetaminophen 1000mg/packet	Chlorpheniramine Maleate 4mg/packet	Pseudoephedrine HCl 60mg/packet			**Adults & Peds: ≥12 yo:** 1 packet q6h. **Max:** 4 packets q24h.
Tylenol Children's Plus Cold & Allergy liquid *(McNeil Consumer)*	Acetaminophen 160mg/5mL	Diphenhydramine HCl 12.5mg/5mL	Pseudoephedrine HCl 15mg/5mL			**Peds: 6-12 yo (48-95 lbs):** 2 tsp (10mL) q4-6h. **Max:** 8 tsp (40mL) q24h.
Tylenol Children's Plus Cold Nighttime suspension *(McNeil Consumer)*	Acetaminophen 160mg/5mL	Chlorpheniramine Maleate 1mg/5mL	Pseudoephedrine HCl 15mg/5mL			**Peds: 6-12 yo (48-95 lbs):** 2 tsp (10mL) q4-6h. **Max:** 8 tsp (40mL) q24h.
Tylenol Flu Nighttime gelcaps *(McNeil Consumer)*	Acetaminophen 500mg	Diphenhydramine HCl 25mg	Pseudoephedrine HCl 30mg			**Adults & Peds: ≥12 yo:** 2 caps q6h. **Max:** 8 caps q24h.
Tylenol Sinus Nighttime caplets *(McNeil Consumer)*	Acetaminophen 500mg	Doxylamine Succinate 6.25mg	Pseudoephedrine HCl 30mg			**Adults & Peds: ≥12 yo:** 2 tabs q4-6h. **Max:** 8 tabs q24h.
COUGH SUPPRESSANT						
Benylin Adult Formula liquid *(Pfizer Consumer Healthcare)*				Dextromethorphan HBr 15mg/5mL		**Adults: ≥12 yo:** 2 tsp (10mL) q6-8h. **Peds: 6-12 yo:** 1 tsp (5mL) q6-8h. **2-6 yo:** 1/2 tsp (2.5mL) q6-8h. **Max:** 4 doses q24h.
Benylin Pediatric liquid *(Pfizer Consumer Healthcare)*				Dextromethorphan HBr 7.5mg/5mL		**Adults: ≥12 yo:** 4 tsp (20mL) q6-8h. **Peds: 6-12 yo:** 2 tsp (10mL) q6-8h. **2-6 yo:** 1 tsp (5mL) q6-8h. **Max:** 4 doses q24h.

BRAND NAME	ANALGESIC	ANTIHISTAMINE	DECONGESTANT	COUGH SUPPRESSANT	EXPECTORANT	DOSE
Delsym 12 Hour Cough Relief liquid (Celltech Pharmaceuticals)				Dextromethorphan Polistrex 30mg/5mL		**Adults: ≥12 yo:** 2 tsp (10mL) q12h. **Peds: 6-12 yo:** 1 tsp (5mL) q12h. **2-6 yo:** 1/2 tsp (2.5mL) q12h. **Max:** 2 doses q24h.
PediaCare Long-Acting Cough freezer pops (Pharmacia Consumer Healthcare)				Dextromethorphan HBr 7.5mg		**Peds: 6-12 yo:** 2 pops (50mL) q6-8h. **2-6 yo:** 1 pop (25mL) q6-8h. **Max:** 4 doses q24h.
Robitussin Cough Maximum Strength liquid (Wyeth Consumer Healthcare)				Dextromethorphan HBr 15mg/5mL		**Adults & Peds: ≥12 yo:** 2 tsp (10mL) q6-8h. **Max:** 8 tsp (40mL) q24h.
Robitussin CoughGels liqui-gels (Wyeth Consumer Healthcare)				Dextromethorphan HB 15mg		**Adults & Peds: ≥12 yo:** 2 caps q6-8h. **Max:** 8 caps q24h.
Robitussin Honey Cough syrup (Wyeth Consumer Healthcare)				Dextromethorphan HBr 10mg/5mL		**Adults: ≥12 yo:** 3 tsp (15mL) q6-8h. **Peds: 6-12 yo:** 1.5 tsp (7.5mL) q6-8h. **Max:** 4 doses q24h.
Simply Cough liquid (McNeil Consumer)				Dextromethorphan HBr 5mg/5mL		**Peds: 6-12 yo (48-95 lbs):** 2 tsp (10mL) q4h. **2-6 yo (24-47 lbs):** 1 tsp (5mL) q4h. **Max:** 4 doses q24h
Theraflu Long Acting Cough thin-strips (Novartis Consumer Health)				Dextromethorphan 11mg		**Adults & Peds: ≥12 yo:** 2 strips q6-8h. **Max:** 8 strips q24h.
Triaminic Long Acting Cough thin strips (Novartis Consumer Health)				Dextromethorphan 5.5mg		**Peds: 6-12 yo:** 2 strips q6-8h. **Max:** 8 strips q24h.
Vicks 44 liquid (Procter & Gamble)				Dextromethorphan HBr 30mg/15mL		**Adults: ≥12 yo:** 1 tbl (15mL) q6-8h. **Peds: 6-12 yo:** 1.5 tsp (7.5mL) q6-8h. **Max:** 4 doses q24h.
COUGH SUPPRESSANT/ANTIHISTAMINE						
Coricidin HBP Cough & Cold tablets (Schering Plough Healthcare)		Chlorpheniramine Maleate 4mg		Dextromethorphan HBr 30mg		**Adults & Peds: ≥12 yo:** 1 tabs q6h. **Max:** 4 tabs q24h.
Vicks NyQuil Cough liquid (Procter & Gamble)		Doxylamine Succinate 6.25mg/15mL		Dextromethorphan HBr 15mg/15mL		**Adults & Peds: ≥12 yo:** 2 tbl (30mL) q6h. **Max:** 8 tbl (120mL) q24h.
COUGH SUPPRESSANT/ANTIHISTAMINE/ANALGESIC						
Alka-Seltzer Plus Flu effervescent tablets (Bayer Healthcare)	Aspirin 500mg	Chlorpheniramine Maleate 2mg		Dextromethorphan HBr 15mg		**Adults & Peds: ≥12 yo:** 2 tabs q6h. **Max:** 8 tabs q24h.
Coricidin HBP Maximum Strength Flu tablets (Schering Plough Healthcare)	Acetaminophen 500mg	Chlorpheniramine Maleate 2mg		Dextromethorphan HBr 15mg		**Adults & Peds: ≥12 yo:** 2 tabs q6h. **Max:** 8 tabs q24h.
Tylenol Nighttime Cough & Sore Throat Cool Burst liquid (McNeil Consumer)	Acetaminophen 1000mg/30mL	Doxylamine Succinate 12.5mg/30mL		Dextromethorphan HBr 30mg/30mL		**Adults & Peds: ≥12 yo:** 2 tbl (30mL) q6h. **Max:** 8 tbl (120mL) q24h.
COUGH SUPPRESSANT/ANTIHISTAMINE/ANALGESIC/DECONGESTANT						
Alka-Seltzer Plus Cold & Cough liqui-gels (Bayer Healthcare)	Acetaminophen 325mg	Chlorpheniramine Maleate 2mg	Pseudoephedrine HCl 30mg	Dextromethorphan HBr 10mg		**Adults: ≥12 yo:** 2 caps q4h. **Peds: 6-12 yo:** 1 cap q4h. **Max:** 4 doses q24h.
Alka-Seltzer Plus Night-Time liqui-gels (Bayer Healthcare)	Acetaminophen 325mg	Doxylamine 6.25mg	Pseudoephedrine HCl 30mg	Dextromethorphan HBr 10mg		**Adults & Peds: ≥12 yo:** 2 caps q6h. **Max:** 8 caps q24h.
Alka-Seltzer Plus Nose & Throat effervescent tablets (Bayer Healthcare)	Acetaminophen 250mg	Chlorpheniramine Maleate 2mg	Phenylephrine HCl 5mg	Dextromethorphan HBr 10mg		**Adults & Peds: ≥12 yo:** 2 tabs q4h. **Max:** 8 tabs q24h.
Comtrex Cold & Cough Nighttime caplets (Bristol-Myers Squibb)	Acetaminophen 500mg	Chlorpheniramine Maleate 2mg	Pseudoephedrine HCl 30mg	Dextromethorphan HBr 15mg		**Adults & Peds: ≥12 yo:** 2 tabs q6h. **Max:** 8 tabs q24h.
Comtrex Nighttime Cold & Cough liquid (Bristol-Myers Squibb)	Acetaminophen 1000mg/30mL	Chlorpheniramine Maleate 4mg/30mL	Pseudoephedrine HCl 60mg/30mL	Dextromethorphan HBr 30mg/30mL		**Adults & Peds: ≥12 yo:** 2 tbl (30mL) q6h. **Max:** 8 tbl (240mL) q24h.
Contac Cold & Flu Maximum Strength caplets (GSK Consumer Healthcare)	Acetaminophen 500mg	Chlorpheniramine Maleate 2mg	Pseudoephedrine HCl 30mg	Dextromethorphan HBr 15mg		**Adults & Peds: ≥12 yo:** 2 tabs q6h. **Max:** 8 tabs q24h.
Dimetapp Children's Nighttime Flu liquid (Wyeth Consumer Healthcare)	Acetaminophen 160mg/5mL	Brompheniramine Maleate 1mg/5mL	Pseudoephedrine HCl 15mg/5mL	Dextromethorphan HBr 5mg/5mL		**Adults: ≥12 yo:** 4 tsp (20mL) q4h. **Peds: 6-12 yo:** 2 tsp (10mL) q4h. **Max:** 4 doses q24h.
Robitussin Flu liquid (Wyeth Consumer Healthcare)	Acetaminophen 160mg/5mL	Chlorpheniramine Maleate 1mg/5mL	Pseudoephedrine HCl 15mg/5mL	Dextromethorphan HBr 5mg/5mL		**Adults: ≥12 yo:** 4 tsp (20mL) q4h. **Peds: 6-12 yo:** 2 tsp (10mL) q4h. **Max:** 4 doses q24h.

Brand Name	Analgesic	Antihistamine	Decongestant	Cough Suppressant	Expectorant	Dose
Theraflu Cold & Cough packets (Novartis Consumer Health)	Acetaminophen 650mg/packet	Chlorpheniramine Maleate 4mg/packet	Pseudoephedrine HCl 60mg/packet	Dextromethorphan HBr 20mg/packet		**Adults & Peds: ≥12 yo:** 1 packet q4-6h. **Max:** 4 packets q24h.
Theraflu Severe Cold & Cough packets (Novartis Consumer Health)	Acetaminophen 1000mg/packet	Chlorpheniramine Maleate 4mg/packet	Pseudoephedrine HCl 60mg/packet	Dextromethorphan HBr 30mg/packet		**Adults & Peds: ≥12 yo:** 1 packet q6h. **Max:** 4 packets q24h.
Theraflu Severe Cold caplets (Novartis Consumer Health)	Acetaminophen 500mg	Chlorpheniramine Maleate 2mg	Pseudoephedrine HCl 30mg	Dextromethorphan HBr 15mg		**Adults & Peds: ≥12 yo:** 2 tabs q6h. **Max:** 8 tabs q24h.
Theraflu Severe Cold packets (Novartis Consumer Health)	Acetaminophen 1000mg/packet	Chlorpheniramine Maleate 4mg/packet	Pseudoephedrine HCl 60mg/packet	Dextromethorphan HBr 30mg/packet		**Adults & Peds: ≥12 yo:** 1 packet q6h. **Max:** of 4 packets q24h.
Triaminic Flu, Cough, & Fever liquid (Novartis Consumer Health)	Acetaminophen 160mg/5mL	Chlorpheniramine Maleate 1mg/5mL	Pseudoephedrine HCl 15mg/5mL	Dextromethorphan HBr 7.5mg/5mL		**Peds: 6-12 yo:** 2 tsp (10mL) q6h. **Max:** 8 tsp (40mL) q24h.
Tylenol Children's Cold Plus Cough liquid (McNeil Consumer)	Acetaminophen 160mg/5mL	Chlorpheniramine Maleate 1mg/5mL	Pseudoephedrine HCl 15mg/5mL	Dextromethorphan HBr 5mg/5mL		**Peds: 6-12 yo (48-95 lbs):** 2 tsp (10mL) q4-6h. **Max:** 8 tsp (40mL) q24h.
Tylenol Children's Flu liquid (McNeil Consumer)	Acetaminophen 160mg/5mL	Chlorpheniramine Maleate 1mg/5mL	Pseudoephedrine HCl 15mg/5mL	Dextromethorphan HBr 7.5mg/5mL		**Peds: 6-12 yo (48-95 lbs):** 2 tsp (10mL) q6-8h. **Max:** 8 tsp (40mL) q24h.
Tylenol Cold & Flu Severe Nighttime Cool Burst Liquid (McNeil Consumer)	Acetaminophen 1000mg/30mL	Doxylamine Succinate 12.5mg/30mL	Pseudoephedrine HCl 60mg/30mL	Dextromethorphan HBr 30mg/30mL		**Adults & Peds: ≥12 yo:** 2 tbl (30mL) q6h. **Max:** 8 tbl (120mL) q24h.
Tylenol Cold Nighttime Cool Burst caplets (McNeil Consumer)	Acetaminophen 325mg	Chlorpheniramine Maleate 2mg	Pseudoephedrine HCl 30mg	Dextromethorphan HBr 15mg		**Adults & Peds: ≥12 yo:** 2 tabs q6h. **Max:** 8 tabs q24h.
Vicks 44M liquid (Procter & Gamble)	Acetaminophen 162.5mg/5mL	Chlorpheniramine Maleate 1mg/5mL	Pseudoephedrine HCl 15mg/5mL	Dextromethorphan HBr 7.5mg/5mL		**Adults & Peds: ≥12 yo:** 4 tsp (20mL) q6h. **Max:** 16 tsp (80mL) q24h.
Vicks NyQuil liquicaps (Procter & Gamble)	Acetaminophen 325mg	Doxylamine Succinate 6.25mg	Pseudoephedrine HCl 30mg	Dextromethorphan HBr 15mg		**Adults & Peds: ≥12 yo:** 2 caps q6h. **Max:** 8 caps q24h.
Vicks NyQuil liquid (Procter & Gamble)	Acetaminophen 500mg/15mL	Doxylamine Succinate 6.25mg/15mL	Pseudoephedrine HCl 30mg/15mL	Dextromethorphan HBr 15mg/15mL		**Adults & Peds: ≥12 yo:** 2 tbl (30mL) q6h. **Max:** 8 tbl (120mL) q24h.

COUGH SUPPRESSANT/ANTIHISTAMINE/ DECONGESTANT

Brand Name	Analgesic	Antihistamine	Decongestant	Cough Suppressant	Expectorant	Dose
Alka-Seltzer Plus Cold & Cough effervescent tablets (Bayer Healthcare)		Chlorpheniramine Maleate 2mg	Phenylephrine HCl 5mg	Dextromethorphan HBr 10mg		**Adults & Peds: ≥12 yo:** 2 tabs q4h. **Max:** 8 tabs q24h.
Alka-Seltzer Plus Night-Time effervescent tablets (Bayer Healthcare)		Doxylamine 6.25mg	Phenylephrine HCl 5mg	Dextromethorphan HBr 10mg		**Adults & Peds: ≥12 yo:** 2 tabs q4h. **Max:** 8 tabs q24h.
Dimetapp DM Children's Cold & Cough elixir (Wyeth Consumer Healthcare)		Brompheniramine Maleate 1mg/5mL	Pseudoephedrine HCl 15mg/5mL	Dextromethorphan HBr 5mg/5mL		**Adults & Peds: ≥12 yo:** 4 tsp (20mL) q4h. **Peds: 6-12 yo:** 2 tsp (10mL) q4h. **Max:** 4 doses q24h.
PediaCare Multi-Symptom chewable tablets (Pharmacia Consumer Healthcare)		Chlorpheniramine Maleate 1mg	Pseudoephedrine HCl 15mg	Dextromethorphan HBr 5mg		**Peds: 6-12 yo:** 2 tabs q4-6h. **Max:** 8 tabs q24h.
PediaCare Multi-Symptom liquid (Pharmacia Consumer Healthcare)		Chlorpheniramine Maleate 1mg/5mL	Pseudoephedrine HCl 15mg/5mL	Dextromethorphan HBr 5mg/5mL		**Peds: 6-12 yo:** 2 tsp (10mL) q4-6h. **Max:** 8 tsp (40mL) q24h.
PediaCare Night Rest Cough & Cold liquid (Pharmacia Consumer Healthcare)		Chlorpheniramine Maleate 1mg/5mL	Pseudoephedrine HCl 15mg/5mL	Dextromethorphan HBr 7.5mg/5mL		**Peds: 6-12 yo:** 2 tsp (10mL) q6-8h. **Max:** 8 tsp (40mL) q24h.
Robitussin Allergy & Cough liquid (Wyeth Consumer Healthcare)		Brompheniramine Maleate 2mg/5mL	Pseudoephedrine HCl 30mg/5mL	Dextromethorphan HBr 10mg/5mL		**Adults: ≥12 yo:** 2 tsp (10mL) q4h. **Peds: 6-12 yo:** 1 tsp (5mL) q4h. **Max:** 4 doses q24h.
Robitussin Pediatric Night Relief liquid (Wyeth Consumer Healthcare)		Chlorpheniramine Maleate 1mg/5mL	Pseudoephedrine HCl 15mg/5mL	Dextromethorphan HBr 7.5mg/5mL		**Adults & Peds: ≥12 yo (>96 lbs):** 4 tsp (20mL) q6h. **Peds: 6-12 yo (48-95 lbs):** 2 tsp (10mL) q6h. **Max:** 4 doses q24h.
Robitussin PM liquid (Wyeth Consumer Healthcare)		Chlorpheniramine Maleate 1mg/5mL	Pseudoephedrine HCl 15mg/5mL	Dextromethorphan HBr 7.5mg/5mL		**Adults & Peds: ≥12 yo:** 4 tsp (20mL) q6h. **Peds: 6-12 yo:** 2 tsp (10mL) q6h. **Max:** 4 doses q24h.
Triaminic Cold & Cough liquid (Novartis Consumer Health)		Chlorpheniramine Maleate 1mg/5mL	Pseudoephedrine HCl 15mg/5mL	Dextromethorphan HBr 5mg/5mL		**Peds: 6-12 yo:** 2 tsp (10mL) q4-6h. **Max:** 8 tsp (40mL) q24h.
Triaminic Cold & Cough Softchews (Novartis Consumer Health)		Chlorpheniramine Maleate 1mg	Pseudoephedrine HCl 15mg	Dextromethorphan HBr 5mg		**Peds: 6-12 yo:** 2 tabs q4-6h. **Max:** 8 tabs q24h.
Triaminic Night Time Cough & Cold liquid (Novartis Consumer Health)		Chlorpheniramine Maleate 1mg/5mL	Pseudoephedrine HCl 15mg/5mL	Dextromethorphan HBr 7.5mg/5mL		**Peds: 6-12 yo:** 2 tsp (10mL) q6h. **Max:** 8 tsp (40mL) q24h.

BRAND NAME	ANALGESIC	ANTIHISTAMINE	DECONGESTANT	COUGH SUPPRESSANT	EXPECTORANT	DOSE
COUGH SUPPRESSANT/DECONGESTANT						
Dimetapp Children's Infant Decongestant Plus Cough drops *(Wyeth Consumer Healthcare)*			Pseudoephedrine HCl 7.5mg/0.8mL	Dextromethorphan HBr 2.5mg/0.8mL		**Peds: 2-3 yo:** 1.6mL q4-6h. **Max:** 6.4mL q24h.
Dimetapp Children's Long Acting Cough Plus Cold elixir *(Wyeth Consumer Healthcare)*			Pseudoephedrine HCl 15mg/5mL	Dextromethorphan HBr 7.5mg/5mL		**Adults & Peds: ≥12 yo:** 4 tsp (20mL) q6h. **Peds: 6-12 yo:** 2 tsp (10mL) q6h. **2-6 yo:** 1 tsp q6h. **Max:** 4 doses q24h.
PediaCare Decongestant & Cough Infants' drops (Pharmacia Consumer Healthcare)			Pseudoephedrine HCl 7.5mg/0.8mL	Dextromethorphan HBr 2.5mg/0.8mL		**Peds: 2-3 yo:** 1.6mL q4-6h. **Max:** 6.4mL q24h.
PediaCare Long-Acting Cough Plus *(Pharmacia Consumer Healthcare)*			Pseudoephedrine HCl 15mg/5mL	Dextromethorphan HBr 7.5mg/5mL		**Peds: 6-12 yo:** 2 tsp (10mL) q6-8h. **2-6 yo:** 1 tsp (5mL) q6-8h. **Max:** 4 doses q24h.
Robitussin Pediatric Cough & Cold liquid *(Wyeth Consumer Healthcare)*			Pseudoephedrine HCl 15mg/5mL	Dextromethorphan HBr 7.5mg/5mL		**Adults ≥12 yo (>96 lbs):** 4 tsp (20mL) q6h. **Peds: 6-12 yo (48-95 lbs):** 2 tsp (10mL) q6h. **2-6 yo (24-47 lbs):** 1 tsp (5mL) q6h. **Max:** 4 doses q24h.
Sudafed Children's Cold & Cough liquid *(Pfizer Consumer Healthcare)*			Pseudoephedrine HCl 15mg/5mL	Dextromethorphan HBr 5mg/5mL		**Adults & Peds: ≥12 yo:** 4 tsp (20mL) q4h. **Peds: 6-12 yo:** 2 tsp (10mL) q4h. **2-6 yo:** 1 tsp (5mL) q4h. **Max:** 4 doses q24h.
Triaminic Cough & Nasal Congestion liquid *(Novartis Consumer Health)*			Pseudoephedrine HCl 15mg/5mL	Dextromethorphan HBr 7.5mg/5mL		**Peds: 6-12 yo:** 2 tsp (10mL) q6h. **2-6 yo:** 1 tsp (5mL) q6h. **Max:** 4 doses q24h.
Triaminic Cough liquid *(Novartis Consumer Health)*			Pseudoephedrine HCl 15mg/5mL	Dextromethorphan HBr 5mg/5mL		**Peds: 6-12 yo:** 2 tsp (10mL) q4-6h. **2-6 yo:** 1 tsp (5mL) q4-6h. **Max:** 4 doses q24h.
Vicks 44D liquid *(Proctor & Gamble)*			Pseudoephedrine HCl 60mg/15mL	Dextromethorphan HBr 30mg/15mL		**Adults: ≥12 yo:** 1 tbl (15mL) q6h. **Peds: 6-12 yo:** 1.5 tsp (7.5mL) q6h. **Max:** 4 doses q24h.
COUGH SUPPRESSANT/DECONGESTANT/ANALGESIC						
Alka-Seltzer Plus Cold Non-Drowsy effervescent tablets *(Bayer Healthcare)*	Acetaminophen 250mg		Phenylephrine HCl 5mg	Dextromethorphan HBr 10mg		**Adults & Peds: ≥12 yo:** 2 tabs q4h. **Max:** 8 tabs q24h.
Comtrex Cold & Cough caplets *(Bristol-Myers Squibb)*	Acetaminophen 500mg		Pseudoephedrine HCl 30mg	Dextromethorphan HBr 15mg		**Adults & Peds: ≥12 yo:** 2 tabs q6h. **Max:** 8 tabs q24h.
Contac Cold & Flu caplets *(GSK Consumer Healthcare)*	Acetaminophen 325mg		Pseudoephedrine HCl 30mg	Dextromethorphan HBr 15mg		**Adults & Peds: ≥12 yo:** 2 tabs q6h. **Max:** 8 tabs q24h.
Sudafed Severe Cold caplets *(Pfizer Consumer Healthcare)*	Acetaminophen 500mg		Pseudoephedrine HCl 30mg	Dextromethorphan HBr 15mg		**Adults & Peds: ≥12 yo:** 2 tabs q6h. **Max:** 8 tabs q24h.
Theraflu Severe Cold Non-Drowsy caplets *(Novartis Consumer Health)*	Acetaminophen 500mg		Pseudoephedrine HCl 30mg	Dextromethorphan HBr 15mg		**Adults & Peds: ≥12 yo:** 2 tabs q6h. **Max:** 8 tabs q24h.
Theraflu Severe Cold Non-Drowsy packets *(Novartis Consumer Health)*	Acetaminophen 1000mg/packet		Pseudoephedrine HCl 60mg/packet	Dextromethorphan HBr 30mg/packet		**Adults & Peds: ≥12 yo:** 1 packet q6h **Max:** 4 packets q24h.
Triaminic Cough & Sore Throat liquid *(Novartis Consumer Health)*	Acetaminophen 160mg/5mL		Pseudoephedrine HCl 15mg/5mL	Dextromethorphan HBr 7.5mg/5mL		**Peds: 6-12 yo:** 2 tsp (10mL) q6h. **2-6 yo:** 1 tsp (5mL) q6h. **Max:** 4 doses q24h.
Tylenol Cold & Flu Severe Daytime Cool Burst liquid *(McNeil Consumer)*	Acetaminophen 1000mg/30mL		Pseudoephedrine HCl 60mg/30mL	Dextromethorphan HBr 30mg/30mL		**Adults & Peds: ≥12 yo:** 2 tbl (30mL) q6h. **Max:** 8 tbl (120mL) q24h.
Tylenol Cold Daytime Cool Burst caplets *(McNeil Consumer)*	Acetaminophen 325mg		Pseudoephedrine HCl 30mg	Dextromethorphan HBr 15mg		**Adults & Peds: ≥12 yo:** 2 tabs q6h. **Max:** 8 tabs q24h.
Tylenol Cold Daytime gelcaps *(McNeil Consumer)*	Acetaminophen 325mg		Pseudoephedrine HCl 30mg	Dextromethorphan HBr 15mg		**Adults & Peds: ≥12 yo:** 2 caps q6h. **Max:** 8 caps q24h.
Tylenol Cold Plus Cough Infants' drops *(McNeil Consumer)*	Acetaminophen 80mg/0.8mL		Pseudoephedrine HCl 7.5mg/0.8mL	Dextromethorphan HBr 5mg/0.8mL		**Peds: 2-3 yo (24-25 lbs):** 1.6mL q4-6h. **Max:** 6.4mL q24h.
Tylenol Flu Daytime gelcaps *(McNeil Consumer)*	Acetaminophen 500mg		Pseudoephedrine HCl 30mg	Dextromethorphan HBr 15mg		**Adults & Peds: ≥12 yo:** 2 caps q6h. **Max:** 8 caps q24h.
Vicks DayQuil liquicaps *(Procter & Gamble)*	Acetaminophen 325mg		Pseudoephedrine HCl 30mg	Dextromethorphan HBr 15mg		**Adults & Peds: ≥12 yo:** 2 caps q6. **Max:** 8 caps q24h.
Vicks DayQuil liquid *(Procter & Gamble)*	Acetaminophen 325mg/15mL		Pseudoephedrine HCl 30mg/15mL	Dextromethorphan HBr 15mg/15mL		**Adults & Peds: ≥12 yo:** 2 tbl (30mL) q6h. **Max:** 8 tbl (120mL) q24h.

Brand Name	Analgesic	Antihistamine	Decongestant	Cough suppressant	Expectorant	Dose
COUGH SUPPRESSANT/DECONGESTANT/EXPECTORANT						
Robitussin CF liquid (Wyeth Consumer Healthcare)			Pseudoephedrine HCl 30mg/5mL	Dextromethorphan HBr 10mg/5mL	Guaifenesin 100mg/5mL	**Adults: ≥12 yo:** 2 tsp (10mL) q4h. **Peds: 6-12 yo:** q4h. **2-6 yo:** 1/2 tsp (2.5mL) q4h. **Max:** 4 doses q24h.
COUGH SUPPRESSANT/DECONGESTANT/EXPECTORANT/ANALGESIC						
Comtrex Deep Chest Cold capsules (Bristol-Myers Squibb)	Acetaminophen 250mg		Pseudoephedrine HCl 30mg	Dextromethorphan HBr 10mg	Guaifenesin 100mg	**Adults & Peds: ≥12 yo:** 2 caps q4h. **Max:** 12 caps q24h.
Robitussin Multi-Sympton Cold & Flu liqui-gels (Wyeth Consumer Healthcare)	Acetaminophen 250mg		Pseudoephedrine HCl 30mg	Dextromethorphan HBr 10mg	Guaifenesin 100mg	**Adults & Peds: ≥12 yo:** 2 caps q4h. **Max:** 8 caps q24h.
Sudafed Cold & Cough liquid caps (Pfizer Consumer Healthcare)	Acetaminophen 250mg		Pseudoephedrine HCl 30mg	Dextromethorphan HBr 10mg	Guaifenesin 100mg	**Adults & Peds: ≥12 yo:** 2 caps q4h. **Max:** 8 caps q24h.
Theraflu Flu & Chest Congestion packets (Novartis Consumer Health)	Acetaminophen 1000mg/packet		Pseudoephedrine HCl 60mg/packet	Dextromethorphan HBr 30mg/packet	Guaifenesin 400mg/packet	**Adults & Peds: ≥12 yo:** 1 packet q6h. **Max:** 4 packets q24h.
Tylenol Cold Severe Congestion Non-Drowsy caplets (McNeil Consumer)	Acetaminophen 325mg		Pseudoephedrine HCl 30mg	Dextromethorphan HBr 15mg	Guaifenesin 200mg	**Adults & Peds: ≥12 yo:** 2 tabs q6h. **Max:** 8 tabs q24h.
COUGH SUPPRESSANT/EXPECTORANT						
Benylin liquid (Pfizer Consumer Healthcare)				Dextromethorphan HBr 5mg/5mL	Guaifenesin 100mg/5mL	**Adults: ≥12 yo:** 4 tsp (20mL) q4h. **Peds: 6-12 yo:** 2 tsp (10mL) q4h. **2-6 yo:** 1 tsp (5mL) q4h. **Max:** 6 doses q24h.
Coricidin HBP Chest Congestion & Cough softgels (Schering Plough Healthcare)				Dextromethorphan HBr 10mg	Guaifenesin 200mg	**Adults & Peds: ≥12 yo:** 1-2 caps q4h. **Max:** 12 caps q24h.
Mucinex DM extended-release tablets (Adams Respiratory Therapeutics)				Dextromethorphan HBr 30mg	Guaifenesin 600mg	**Adults & Peds: ≥12 yo:** 1-2 tabs q12h. **Max:** 4 tabs q24h.
Robitussin Cough & Congestion liquid (Wyeth Consumer Healthcare)				Dextromethorphan HBr 10mg/5mL	Guaifenesin 200mg/5mL	**Adults: ≥12 yo:** 2 tsp (10mL) q4h. **Peds: 6-12 yo:** 1 tsp (5mL) q4h. **2-6 yo:** 1/2 tsp (2.5mL) q4h. **Max:** 6 doses q24h.
Robitussin DM liquid (Wyeth Consumer Healthcare)				Dextromethorphan HBr 10mg/5mL	Guaifenesin 100mg/5mL	**Adults: ≥12 yo:** 2 tsp (10mL) q4h. **Peds: 6-12 yo:** 1 tsp (5mL) q4h. **2-6 yo:** 1/2 tsp (2.5mL) q4h. **Max:** 6 doses q24h.
Vicks 44E liquid (Procter & Gamble)				Dextromethorphan HBr 20mg/15mL	Guaifenesin 200mg/15mL	**Adults & Peds: ≥12 yo:** 1 tbl (15mL) q4h. **Peds: 6-12 yo:** 1.5 tsp (7.5mL) q4h. **Max:** of 6 doses q24h.
DECONGESTANTS						
Contac Cold timed-release caplets (GSK Consumer Healthcare)			Pseudoephedrine HCl 120mg			**Adults & Peds: ≥12 yo:** 1 tabs q12h. **Max:** 2 tabs q24h.
Dimetapp Children's Infant Decongestant drops (Wyeth Consumer Healthcare)			Pseudoephedrine HCl 7.5mg/0.8mL			**Peds: 2-3 yo:** 1.6mL q4-6h. **Max:** 6.4mL q24h.
Dimetapp Extentabs caplets (Wyeth Consumer Healthcare)			Pseudoephedrine HCl 120mg			**Adults & Peds: ≥12 yo:** 1 tab q12h. **Max:** 2 tabs q24h.
PediaCare Decongestant Infants' drops (Pharmacia Consumer Healthcare)			Pseudoephedrine HCl 7.5mg/0.8mL			**Peds: 2-3 yo:** 1.6mL q4-6h. **Max:** 6.4mL q24h.
Simply Stuffy liquid (McNeil Consumer)			Pseudoephedrine HCl 15mg/5mL			**Peds: 6-12 yo (48-95 lbs):** 2 tsp (10mL) q4-6h. **2-6 yo (24-47 lbs):** 1 tsp (5mL) q4-6h. **Max:** 4 doses q24h.
Sudafed 12 Hour tablets (Pfizer Consumer Healthcare)			Pseudoephedrine HCl 120mg			**Adults & Peds: ≥12 yo:** 1 tab q12h. **Max:** 2 tabs q24h.
Sudafed 24 Hour tablets (Pfizer Consumer Healthcare)			Pseudoephedrine HCl 240mg			**Adults & Peds: ≥12 yo:** 1 tab q24h. **Max:** 1 tab q24h.
Sudafed Children's chewable tablets (Pfizer Consumer Healthcare)			Pseudoephedrine HCl 15mg			**Peds: 6-12 yo:** 2 tabs q4-6h. **Max:** 8 tabs q24h.

BRAND NAME	ANALGESIC	ANTIHISTAMINE	DECONGESTANT	COUGH SUPPRESSANT	EXPECTORANT	DOSE
Sudafed Children's liquid (*Pfizer Consumer Healthcare*)			Pseudoephedrine HCl 15mg/5mL			**Adults:** ≥**12 yo:** 4 tsp (20mL) q4-6h. **Peds: 6-12 yo:** 2 tsp (10mL) q4-6h. **2-6 yo:** 1 tsp (5mL) q4-6h. **Max:** 4 doses q24h.
Sudafed PE tablets (*Pfizer Consumer Healthcare*)			Phenylephrine HCl 10mg			**Adults & Peds:** ≥**12 yo:** 1 tab q4h. **Max:** 6 tabs q24h.
Sudafed tablets (*Pfizer Consumer Healthcare*)			Pseudoephedrine HCl 30mg			**Adults:** ≥**12 yo:** 2 tabs q4-6h. **Peds: 6-12 yo:** 1 tab q4-6h. **Max:** 4 doses q24h.
Theraflu Multi-Symptom thin-strips (*Novartis Consumer Health*)			Diphenhydramine HCl 25mg			**Adults & Peds:** ≥**12 yo:** 1 strip q4h. **Max:** 6 strips q24h.
Triaminic Cough & Runny Nose thin strips (*Novartis Consumer Health*)		Diphenhydramine HCl 12.5mg				**Peds: 6-12 yo:** 1 strip q4h. **Max:** 6 strips q24h.
DECONGESTANT/ANALGESIC						
Advil Children's Cold suspension (*Wyeth Consumer Healthcare*)	Ibuprofen 100mg/5mL		Pseudoephedrine HCl 15mg/5mL			**Peds: 6-12 yo: (48-95 lbs):** 2 tsp (10mL) q6h. **2-6 yo (24-47 lbs):** 1 tsp (5mL) q6h. **Max:** 4 doses q24h.
Advil Cold & Sinus liqui-gels (*Wyeth Consumer Healthcare*)	Ibuprofen 200mg		Pseudoephedrine HCl 30mg			**Adults & Peds:** ≥**12 yo:** 1-2 caps q4-6h. **Max:** 6 caps q24h.
Advil Flu & Body Ache caplets (*Wyeth Consumer Healthcare*)	Ibuprofen 200mg		Pseudoephedrine HCl 30mg			**Adults & Peds:** ≥**12 yo:** 1-2 tabs q4-6h. **Max:** 6 tabs q24h.
Dimetapp Children's Cold and Fever (*Wyeth Consumer Healthcare*)	Ibuprofen 100mg/5mL		Pseudoephedrine HCl 15mg/5mL			**Peds: 6-12 yo: (48-95 lbs):** 2 tsp (10mL) q6h. **2-6 (24-47 lbs):** 1 tsp (5mL) q6h. **Max:** 4 doses q24h.
Dristan Cold capsules (*Wyeth Consumer Healthcare*)	Acetaminophen 500mg		Pseudoephedrine HCl 30mg			**Adults & Peds:** ≥**12 yo:** 2 caps q6h **Max:** 8 caps q24h.
Motrin Children's Cold suspension (*McNeil Consumer*)	Ibuprofen 100mg/5mL		Pseudoephedrine HCl 15mg/5mL			**Peds: 6-12 yo (48-95 lbs):** 2 tsp (10mL) q6h. **2-6 yo (24-47 lbs):** 1 tsp (5mL) q6h. **Max:** 4 doses q24h.
Motrin Cold & Sinus caplets (*McNeil Consumer*)	Ibuprofen 200mg		Pseudoephedrine HCl 30mg			**Adults & Peds:** ≥**12 yo:** 1-2 tabs q4-6h. **Max:** 6 caps q24h.
Sinutab Sinus tablets (*Pfizer Consumer Healthcare*)	Acetaminophen 500mg		Pseudoephedrine HCl 30mg			**Adults & Peds:** ≥**12 yo:** 2 tabs q6h. **Max:** 8 tabs q24h.
Sudafed Sinus and Cold liquid caps (*Bayer Healthcare*)	Acetaminophen 325mg		Pseudoephedrine HCl 30mg			**Adults & Peds:** ≥**12 yo:** 2 caps q4-6h. **Max:** 8 caps q24h.
Tylenol Children's Plus Cold Daytime liquid (*McNeil Consumer*)	Acetaminophen 160mg/5mL		Pseudoephedrine HCl 15mg/5mL			**Peds: 6-12 yo: (48-95 lbs):** 2 tsp (10mL) q4-6h. **2-6 yo (24-47 lbs):** 1 tsp (5mL) q4-6h. **Max:** 4 doses q24h.
Tylenol Cold Infants' drops (*McNeil Consumer*)	Acetaminophen 80mg/0.8mL		Pseudoephedrine HCl 7.5mg/0.8mL			**Peds: 2-3 yo (24-25 lbs):** 1.6mL q4-6h. **Max:** 6.4mL q24h.
Tylenol Sinus Maximum Strength gelcaps (*McNeil Consumer*)	Acetaminophen 500mg		Pseudoephedrine HCl 30mg			**Adults & Peds:** ≥**12 yo:** 2 caps q4-6h. **Max:** 8 caps q24h.
Vicks DayQuil Sinus liquicaps (*Procter & Gamble*)	Acetaminophen 325mg		Pseudoephedrine HCl 30mg			**Adults & Peds:** ≥**12 yo:** 2 caps q6h. **Max:** 8 caps q24h.
DECONGESTANT/EXPECTORANT						
Robitussin PE liquid (*Wyeth Consumer Healthcare*)			Pseudoephedrine HCl 30mg/5mL		Guaifenesin 100mg/5mL	**Adults & Peds:** ≥**12 yo:** 2 tsp (10mL) q4h. **Peds: 6-12 yo:** 1 tsp (5mL) q4h. **2-6 yo:** 1/2 tsp (2.5mL) q4h. **Max:** 4 doses q24h.
Robitussin Severe Congestion liqui-gels (*Wyeth Consumer Healthcare*)			Pseudoephedrine HCl 30mg		Guaifenesin 200mg	**Adults & Peds:** ≥**12 yo:** 2 caps q4h. **Peds: 6-12 yo:** 1 cap q4h. **Max:** 4 doses q24h.
Sudafed Non-Drying Sinus liquid caps (*Pfizer Consumer Healthcare*)			Pseudoephedrine HCl 30mg		Guaifenesin 200mg	**Adults & Peds:** ≥**12 yo:** 2 caps q4h. **Max:** 8 caps q24h.
Triaminic Chest & Nasal Congestion liquid (*Novartis Consumer Health*)			Pseudoephedrine HCl 15mg/5mL		Guaifenesin 50mg/5mL	**Peds: 6-12 yo:** 2 tsp (10mL) q4-6h. **2-6 yo:** 1 tsp (5mL) q4-6h. **Max:** 4 doses q24h.
EXPECTORANT						
Mucinex extended-release tablets (*Adams Respiratory Therapeutics*)					Guaifenesin 600mg	**Adults & Peds:** ≥**12 yo:** 1-2 tabs q12h. **Max:** 4 tabs q24h.
Robitussin liquid (*Wyeth Consumer Healthcare*)					Guaifenesin 100mg/5mL	**Adults:** ≥**12 yo:** 2-4 tsp (10-20mL) q4h. **Peds: 6-12 yo:** 1-2 tsp (5-10mL) q4h. **2-6 yo:** 1/2-1 tsp 2.5-5mL) q4h. **Max:** 6 doses q24h.

PRODUCT IDENTIFICATION GUIDE

For quick identification, this section provides full-color reproductions of product packaging, as well as some actual-sized photographs of tablets and capsules. In all, the section contains over 350 photos.

Products in this section are arranged alphabetically by manufacturer. In some instances, not all dosage forms and sizes are pictured. For more information on any of the products in this section,

please turn to the page indicated above the product's photo or check directly with the product's manufacturer.

While every effort has been made to guarantee faithful reproduction of the photos in this section, changes in size, color, and design are always a possibility. Be sure to confirm a product's identity with the manufacturer or your pharmacist.

MANUFACTURER'S INDEX

ADAMS RESPIRATORY THERAPEUTICS

Adams Respiratory Therapeutics
P. 602

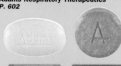

Extended-release/dual-release mechanism. Bi-layer tablets. Available in 20 ct. and 40 ct. bottles

Mucinex®

AKPHARMA INC.

AkPharma Inc.
P. 758

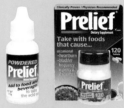

Dietary Supplement Granulate and Tablets

Prelief®

ALPINE PHARMACEUTICALS

Alpine Pharmaceuticals
P. 758

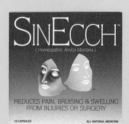

SinEcch™
(Homeopathic Arnica Montana)

BAUSCH & LOMB

Bausch & Lomb Incorporated
P. 604

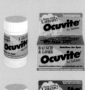

Vitamin and Mineral Supplement

Ocuvite®

Bausch & Lomb Incorporated
P. 604

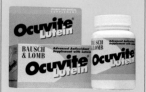

Vitamin and Mineral Supplement

Ocuvite® Lutein

Bausch & Lomb Incorporated
P. 760

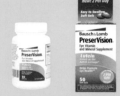

Eye Vitamin and Mineral Supplement

PreserVision® Lutein Soft Gels

Bausch & Lomb Incorporated
P. 760

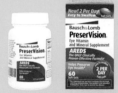

Eye Vitamin and Mineral Supplement

PreserVision® AREDS Soft Gels

Bausch & Lomb Incorporated
P. 605

Eye Vitamin and Mineral Supplement

Original PreserVision™ Tablets

BOEHRINGER INGELHEIM

Boehringer Ingelheim Consumer H.C.
P. 607

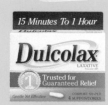

4 Comfort Shaped Suppositories Also available in boxes of 8, 16 and 28 suppositories.

Dulcolax® Laxative

Boehringer Ingelheim Consumer H.C.
P. 608

25 Comfort Coated Tablets Also available in 10, 50 and 100 ct.

Dulcolax® Laxative

Boehringer Ingelheim Consumer H.C.
P. 608

25 Liquid Gels Blister pack of 10 and bottles of 25, 50 or 100 liquid gels

Dulcolax® Stool Softener

CADBURY ADAMS USA LLC

Cadbury Adams USA LLC
P. 611

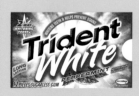

Available in Peppermint, Wintergreen, Spearmint, Cool Rush™, and Cinnamon Tingle™ flavors in a 12-pellet blister foil.

Trident White® Sugarless Gum with Recaldent®

SEEKING AN ALTERNATIVE?

Check the Product Category Index, where you'll find alphabetical listings of all the products in each therapeutic class.

ENIVA

Eniva Corporation
P. 762

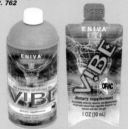

Liquid Antioxidant Multi-Nutrient Supplement 32 fl. oz. bottle and 1 fl. oz. packet

VIBE™

GLAXOSMITHKLINE CONSUMER HEALTHCARE, L. P.

GlaxoSmithKline Consumer Healthcare
P. 612

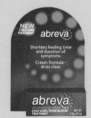

Cold Sore/Fever Blister Treatment Cream

Abreva™

GlaxoSmithKline Consumer Healthcare
P. 613

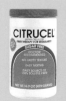

Fiber Therapy for Regularity Sugar Free Orange available in 8.6 oz., 16.9 oz., and 32 oz. containers. Regular Orange available in 16 oz., 30 oz., and 50 oz. containers.

Citrucel®

GlaxoSmithKline Consumer Healthcare
P. 614

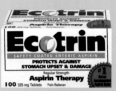

Nasal Decongestant/Antihistamine
Packages of 10 and 20
Maximum Strength Caplets.

Contac® 12 Hour Cold

GlaxoSmithKline Consumer Healthcare
P. 615

Multisymptom Cold & Flu Relief
Maximum Strength Formula in
packages of 16 and 30 caplets.
Non-Drowsy Formula
in packages of 16 caplets.

**Contac® Severe
Cold & Flu**

GlaxoSmithKline Consumer Healthcare
P. 616

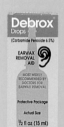

Drops
Available in ½ fl. oz. and 1 fl. oz.

Debrox®

GlaxoSmithKline Consumer Healthcare
P. 616

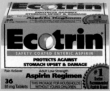

Adult Low Strength Tablets
in Bottles of 36
and 120 tablets.

Ecotrin®

GlaxoSmithKline Consumer Healthcare
P. 616

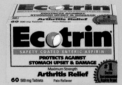

Regular Strength Tablets
in bottles of 100 and 250.

Ecotrin®

GlaxoSmithKline Consumer Healthcare
P. 616

Maximum Strength Tablets
in bottles of 60 and 150.

Ecotrin®

GlaxoSmithKline Consumer Healthcare
P. 764

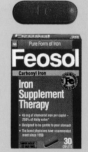

Packages of 30 caplets

Feosol®

GlaxoSmithKline Consumer Healthcare

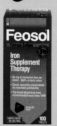

Packages of 100 tablets
Iron Supplement

Feosol®

GlaxoSmithKline Consumer Healthcare
P. 620

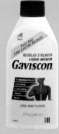

12 fl. oz.

**Gaviscon® Regular
Strength Liquid Antacid**

FACED WITH AN
Rx SIDE EFFECT?

Turn to the
Companion Drug Index
(Green Pages)
for products that provide
symptomatic relief.

GlaxoSmithKline Consumer Healthcare
P. 619

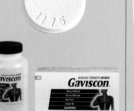

Available in 100-tablet bottles and
30-tablet boxes.

**Gaviscon® Regular
Strength Antacid**

GlaxoSmithKline Consumer Healthcare
P. 620

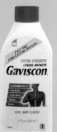

Extra Strength Formula
12 fl. oz.

**Gaviscon® Extra Strength
Liquid Antacid**

GlaxoSmithKline Consumer Healthcare
P. 619

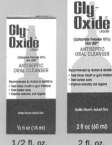

Extra Strength Formula
Available in 100-tablet bottles and
6 and 30-tablet boxes.

**Gaviscon® Extra
Strength Antacid**

GlaxoSmithKline Consumer Healthcare
P. 620

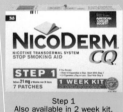

1/2 fl. oz.   2 fl. oz.

Gly-Oxide® Liquid

GlaxoSmithKline Consumer Healthcare
P. 622

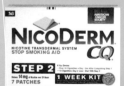

Step 1
Also available in 2 week kit.

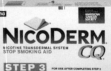

Step 2
Also available in 2 week kit.

Step 3
Also available in 2 week kit.
Includes User's Guide, Audio Tape and
Child Resistant Disposal Tray

Stop Smoking Aid
Nicotine Transdermal System

NicoDerm® CQ™

GlaxoSmithKline Consumer Healthcare
P. 631

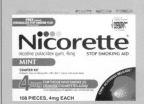

4 mg
Stop Smoking Aid in mint flavor
Nicotine Polacrilex Gum

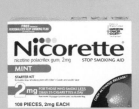

2 mg
Stop Smoking Aid in mint flavor
Nicotine Polacrilex Gum

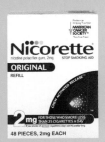

2 mg

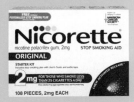

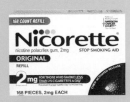

2 mg
Stop Smoking Aid in Original flavor
Nicotine Polacrilex Gum

Nicorette®

GlaxoSmithKline Consumer Healthcare
P. 635

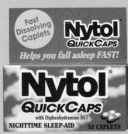

QuickCaps®

Helps you fall asleep FAST!
MAXIMUM STRENGTH
Nytol QUICKGELS
with Diphenhydramine HCl
NIGHTTIME SLEEP-AID
16 SOFTGELS

QuickGels™

Nytol®

GlaxoSmithKline Consumer Healthcare
P. 765

Os-Cal

Calcium Supplement

Os-Cal®

GlaxoSmithKline Consumer Healthcare
P. 635

NEW!
ULTRA STRENGTH
Gas Relief Phazyme
ANTI-GAS/SIMETHICONE
180 mg
FAST RELIEF of:
Pressure
Bloating
Gas Discomfort
EASY TO SWALLOW
12 SOFTGELS (180mg)

180 mg softgels

Gas Relief Phazyme®

GlaxoSmithKline Consumer Healthcare
P. 635

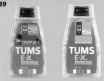

125 mg chewable tablets

**Quick Dissolve
Phazyme®**

GlaxoSmithKline Consumer Healthcare
P. 637

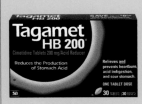

Acid Reducer
Packages of 6, 12, 18,
30, 50, 70 and 80 tablets.

Tagamet HB 200®

GlaxoSmithKline Consumer Healthcare
P. 637

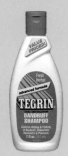

**Tegrin®
Dandruff Shampoo**

GlaxoSmithKline Consumer Healthcare
P. 638

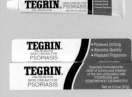

**Tegrin® Skin Cream
for Psoriasis**

GlaxoSmithKline Consumer Healthcare
P. 639

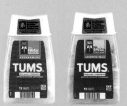

Peppermint and
Assorted flavors

Tums®

GlaxoSmithKline Consumer Healthcare
P. 639

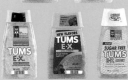

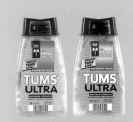

Tropical Fruit, Wintergreen,
Assorted Flavors, Assorted Berry
and SugarFree Orange Cream flavors

Tums E-X®

GlaxoSmithKline Consumer Healthcare
P. 639

Assorted Mint and Fruit Flavors
Also available in Tropical Fruit,
Assorted Berries and
Spearmint flavors.

Tums® Ultra™

GlaxoSmithKline Consumer Healthcare
P. 639

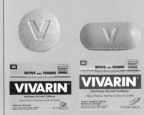

Alertness Aid with Caffeine
Available in tablets and caplets.

Vivarin®

J&J-MERCK CONSUMER

J&J-Merck Consumer
P. 640

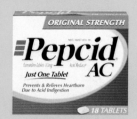

10 mg

Pepcid AC® Tablets
(famotidine)

J&J-Merck Consumer
P. 640

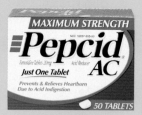

20 mg

**Maximum Strength
Pepcid® AC Tablets**
(famotidine)

J&J-Merck Consumer
P. 640

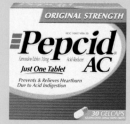

10 mg

Pepcid AC® Gelcaps
(famotidine)

J&J-Merck Consumer
P. 641

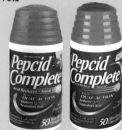
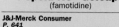

10 mg - 800 mg - 165 mg

**Pepcid® Complete
Chewable Tablets**
(famotidine/calcium carbonate/
magnesium hydroxide)

MANNATECH, INC.

Mannatech, Inc.
P. 768

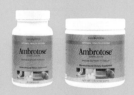

A Glyconutritional Dietary Supplement

Ambrotose®

Mannatech, Inc.
P. 769

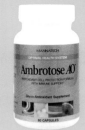

A Glyconutritional Antioxidant
Supplement

Ambrotose AO™

LOOKING FOR
A PARTICULAR
COMPOUND?

In the
Active Ingredients Index
(Yellow Pages),
you'll find all the
brands that contain it.

Mannatech, Inc.
P. 769

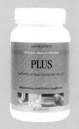

Dietary Supplement

**PLUS with
Ambrotose® complex**

MATRIXX INITIATIVES

Matrixx Initiatives, Inc.

**Zicam®
Cold Remedy**

Matrixx Initiatives, Inc.
P. 642

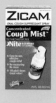

**Zicam® Concentrated
Cough Mist**

Matrixx Initiatives, Inc.

**Zicam® No-Drip
Liquid Nasal Gel
Allergy Relief**

Matrixx Initiatives, Inc.
P. 643

**Zicam® No Drip Nasal
Moisterizer**

SEEKING AN
ALTERNATIVE?

Check the
Product Category Index,
where you'll find
alphabetical listings of
all the products in each
therapeutic class.

MCNEIL

McNeil Consumer
P. 644

Available in 2 and 4 fl. oz. bottles
with a convenient dosage cup, and
caplets in 6's, 12's, 18's, 24's, 48's,
and 72's.

Imodium® A-D

McNeil Consumer
P. 644

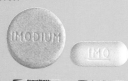

Mint chewable tablets
available in 12's, 18's and
30's. Caplets available
in 12's, 18's and bottles of
30 and 42.

Imodium® Advanced

LOOKING FOR
A PARTICULAR
COMPOUND?

In the
Active Ingredients Index
(Yellow Pages),
you'll find all the
brands that contain it.

Lactaid Inc. Marketed By
McNeil Consumer
P. 770

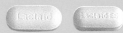

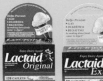

ORIGINAL STRENGTH available
in bottles of 120.

EXTRA STRENGTH available
in bottles of 50.

ULTRA CAPLETS available in
single serve packets of 12, 32,
60 and 90 counts.

ULTRA CHEWABLE TABLETS available
in single serve packets of
32 and 60 counts.

FAST ACT CAPLETS available in
single serve packets of 12, 32,
60 and 90 counts

FAST ACT CHEWABLE tablets are
available in single serve packets of
32 and 60 counts

**Lactaid® Caplets and
Chewable Tablets**

McNeil Consumer
P. 647

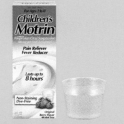

Available in Berry flavor in 4 fl. oz. with
child-resistant safety cap and
convenient dosage cup.

**Children's Motrin®
Non-Staining Dye-Free
Oral Suspension**

FACED WITH AN
Rx SIDE EFFECT?

Turn to the
Companion Drug Index for
products that provide
symptomatic relief.

McNeil Consumer
P. 647

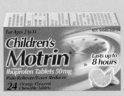

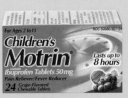

Available in Orange and
Grape-Flavored chewable
tablets of 50 mg.
Available in bottles of 24
with child-resistant safety cap.

**Children's Motrin®
Chewable Tablets**

McNeil Consumer
P. 647

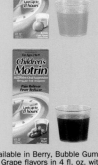

Available in Berry, Bubble Gum and
Grape flavors in 4 fl. oz. with
child-resistant safety cap
and convenient dosage cup.

**Children's Motrin®
Oral Suspension**

McNeil Consumer
P. 648

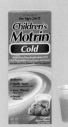

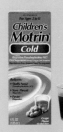

Available in Berry and Grape flavors in
4 fl. oz. with child-resistant safety cap
and convenient dosage cup.

Berry Flavor also available in
Non-Staining Dye-Free.

**Children's Motrin®
Cold Oral Suspension**

McNeil Consumer
P. 647

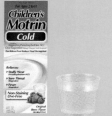

Available in Berry flavor in 4 fl. oz. with child-resistant safety cap and convenient dosage cup.

Children's Motrin® Cold Non-Staining Dye-Free Oral Suspension

McNeil Consumer
P. 647

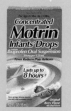

50 mg/1.25 mL
Available in Berry flavor 1/2 fl. oz. bottle.

Infants' Motrin® Concentrated Drops

McNeil Consumer
P. 647

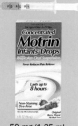

50 mg/1.25 mL
Available in 1/2 fl. oz. and 1 fl. oz. bottle. New Syringe Dosing Device

Infants' Motrin® Non-Staining Dye-Free Concentrated Drops

McNeil Consumer
P. 647

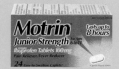

Available in bottles of 24 with child-resistant safety cap.

Junior Strength Motrin® Caplets

McNeil Consumer
P. 647

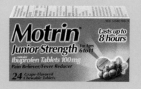

Children's Motrin® Cold Non-Staining Dye-Free Oral Suspension

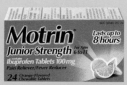

Available in Orange and Grape-flavored chewable tablets of 100 mg.
Available in bottles of 24 with child-resistant safety cap.

Junior Strength Motrin® Chewable Tablets

McNeil Consumer
P. 645

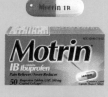

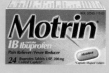

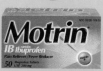

Gelcaps available in tamper evident packaging of 24, 50, and 100. Caplets available in tamper evident packaging of 24, 50, 100, 165, 250 and 300. Tablets available in tamper evident packaging of 24, 50, 100 and 165.

Motrin® IB

McNeil Consumer
P. 646

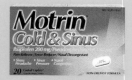

Caplets available in blister packs of 20's and 40's.

Motrin® Cold & Sinus

McNeil Consumer
P. 649

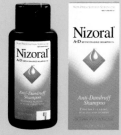

Available in 4 and 7 fl. oz. bottles.

Nizoral® A-D

McNeil Consumer
P. 653

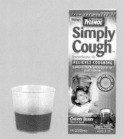

Available in Cherry Berry flavor 4 fl. oz. child-resistant bottles.

Simply Cough™

McNeil Consumer
P. 654

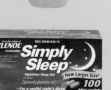

Mini-caplets available in blister packs of 24, 48, 100 and 130.

Simply Sleep™

McNeil Consumer
P. 654

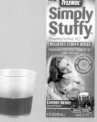

Available in Cherry Berry flavor 4 fl. oz. child-resistant bottles.

Simply Stuffy™

McNeil Consumer
P. 649

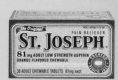

McNeil Consumer
P. 649

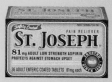

Available in enteric coated tablets and adult chewable tablets.

St. Joseph®

SEEKING AN ALTERNATIVE?

Check the Product Category Index, where you'll find alphabetical listings of all the products in each therapeutic class.

McNeil Consumer
P. 666

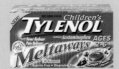

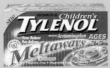

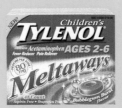

Grape Punch and Wacky Watermelon bottles of 30 with child-resistant safety cap.

Bubblegum Burst bottles of 30 with child resistant safety cap and blister packs of 48.

**Children's TYLENOL®
Meltaways**

LOOKING FOR
A PARTICULAR
COMPOUND?

In the
Active Ingredients Index
(Yellow Pages),
you'll find all the
brands that contain it.

McNeil Consumer
P. 666

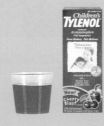

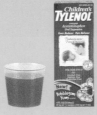

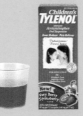

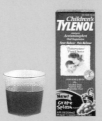

Available in Cherry Blast flavor in 2 and 4 fl. oz. bottles. Bubble Gum Yum, Very Berry Strawberry and Grape Splash flavors in 4 fl. oz. with child-resistant safety cap and convenient dosage cup. Alcohol Free, 80 mg per 1/2 teaspoon.

**Children's TYLENOL®
Suspension Liquid**

McNeil Consumer
P. 667

Available in Bubble Gum flavor in child-resistant 4 fl. oz. bottles.

**Children's TYLENOL®
Plus Cold and
Allergy Suspension Liquid**

McNeil Consumer
P. 668

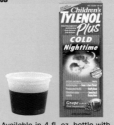

Available in 4 fl. oz. bottle with child-resistant safety cap and convenient dosage cup. Great Grape flavor.

**Children's TYLENOL® Plus
Cold Nighttime
Suspension Liquid**

McNeil Consumer
P. 668

Available in blister pack of 24 chewable tablets. Great Grape flavor.

**Children's TYLENOL® Plus
Cold Chewable Tablets**

McNeil Consumer
P. 668

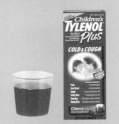

Available in 4 fl. oz. bottle with child-resistant safety cap and convenient dosage cup. Cherry flavor.

**Children's TYLENOL®
Plus Cold & Cough
Suspension Liquid**

McNeil Consumer
P. 668

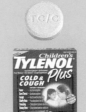

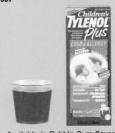

Available in blister pack of 24 chewable tablets. Cherry flavor.

**Children's TYLENOL® Plus
Cold & Cough
Chewable Tablets**

McNeil Consumer
P. 669

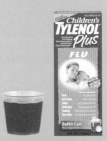

Available in Bubble Gum flavor in child-resistant 4 fl. oz. bottles.

**Children's TYLENOL® Plus
Flu Suspension Liquid**

McNeil Consumer
P. 668

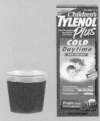

Available in Fruit flavor in child-resistant 4 fl. oz. bottles.

**Children's TYLENOL® Plus
Cold, Daytime
Suspension Liquid**

McNeil Consumer
P. 666

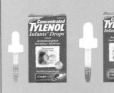

Available in Cherry and Grape flavor 1/2 fl. oz. and 1 fl. oz. bottles with child-resistant safety cap and calibrated droppers. Alcohol Free, 80 mg per 0.8 mL.

**Concentrated TYLENOL®
Infants' Drops**

McNeil Consumer
P. 668

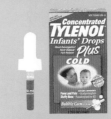

Available in 1/2 fl. oz. bottle with child-resistant safety cap and calibrated dropper. Bubble Gum flavor, Alcohol-free.

**Concentrated TYLENOL®
Infants' Drops Plus Cold**

McNeil Consumer
P. 668

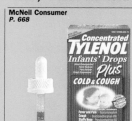

Available in 1/2 fl. oz. bottle with child-resistant safety cap and calibrated dropper. Cherry flavor, Alcohol-free.

**Concentrated TYLENOL®
Infants' Drops Plus
Cold & Cough**

McNeil Consumer
P. 666

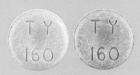

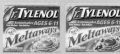

Available in blister pack of 24 chewable tablets. Bubblegum Burst and Grape Punch.

Jr. TYLENOL® Meltaways

McNeil Consumer
P. 655

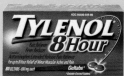

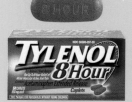

Geltabs available in tamper-evident bottles of 20's, 40's and 80's.
Caplets available in bottles of 24's, 50's, 100's, 150's and 200's.

**TYLENOL® 8 Hour
Extended Release**

McNeil Consumer
P. 655

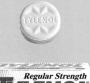

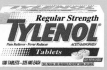

Tablets available in tamper resistant bottles of 50's and 100's.

**Regular Strength
TYLENOL®**

McNeil Consumer
P. 655

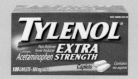

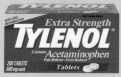

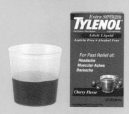

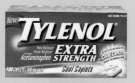

Caplets: tamper-resistant vials of 10 and bottles of 8's, 16's, 24's, 50's, 100's, 150's, 250's and 325's.
Tablets: tamper-resistant vials of 10 and bottles of 30's, 60's, 100's and 200's.
Liquid: tamper-evident 8 fl. oz. bottles.
Cool Caplet: 50's and 100's

Extra Strength TYLENOL®

McNeil Consumer
P. 655

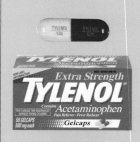

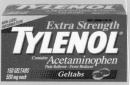

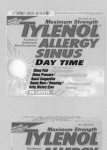

Gelcaps available in tamper-resistant bottles of 16's, 24's, 40's, 50's, 100's, 150's and 225's.

Geltabs available in tamper-resistant bottles of 16's, 24's, 40's, 50's, 100's and 150's.

Extra Strength TYLENOL®

McNeil Consumer
P. 657

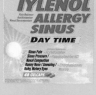

Caplets in blister packs of 24 & 48.
Gelcaps in blister packs of 24 & 48.
Geltabs in blister packs of 24 & 48.

**Maximum Strength
TYLENOL® Allergy Sinus
Day Time**

McNeil Consumer
P. 657

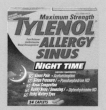

Caplets available in blister packs of 24's.

**TYLENOL® Allergy Sinus
Night Time**

McNeil Consumer
P. 657

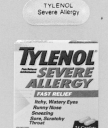

Caplets available in blister packs of 12's and 24's.

TYLENOL® Severe Allergy

McNeil Consumer
P. 655

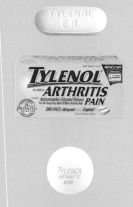

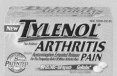

Caplets available in blister packs of 12's and 24's.

Geltabs available in 20's, 40's, and 80's.

**TYLENOL® Arthritis Pain
Extended Release**

McNeil Consumer
P. 659

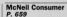

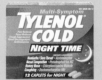

Caplets available in
blister packs of 24.

**TYLENOL® Cold
Night Time**

McNeil Consumer
P. 659

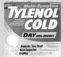
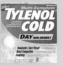

Caplets available in
blister packs of 24.
Gelcaps available in
blister packs of 24.

**TYLENOL®
Cold Day Non-Drowsy**

McNeil Consumer
P. 664

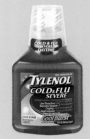

Available in 8 fl. oz. bottles

**TYLENOL® Cold and Flu
Severe Day Time**

McNeil Consumer
P. 664

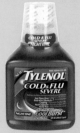

Available in 8 fl. oz. bottles

**TYLENOL® Cold and Flu
Severe Night Time**

McNeil Consumer
P. 664

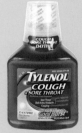

Available in 8 fl. oz. bottles

**TYLENOL® Cough
and Sore Throat Day Time**

McNeil Consumer
P. 664

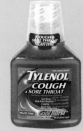

Available in 8 fl. oz. bottles

**TYLENOL® Cough and
Sore Throat Night Time**

McNeil Consumer
P. 660

Available in blister
packs of 24.

**TYLENOL® Cold Severe
Congestion Non-Drowsy**

McNeil Consumer
P. 660

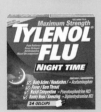

Gelcaps available in
blister packs of 12's and 24's.

TYLENOL® Flu Night Time

McNeil Consumer
P. 660

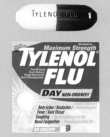

Gelcaps available in blister
packs of 24.

**TYLENOL® Flu Day
Non-Drowsy**

McNeil Consumer
P. 662

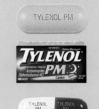

Caplets available in tamper-resistant
bottles of 24, 50, 100, 150 and 225.
Gelcaps available in tamper-resistant
bottles of 24 and 50.
Geltabs available in tamper-resistant
bottles of 24, 50, 100 and 150.
Geltabs, Caplets and Gelcaps
available in bottles of 50 for
households without children.

**Extra Strength
TYLENOL® PM**

McNeil Consumer
P. 663

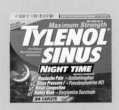

Available in blister packs of 24.

**TYLENOL® Sinus
Night Time**

McNeil Consumer
P. 663

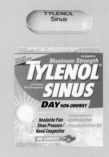

**TYLENOL® Sinus Day
Non-Drowsy**

McNeil Consumer
P. 663

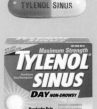

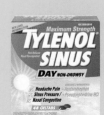

Caplets, Gelcaps and Geltabs
in blister packs of 24 and 48.

**TYLENOL® Sinus Day
Non-Drowsy**

McNeil Consumer
P. 660

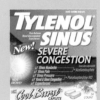

Caplets in blister packs of 12 ct,
24 ct, and 48 ct.

**TYLENOL® Sinus
Severe Congestion**

McNeil Consumer
P. 664

Cherry and Honey Lemon flavors
available in 8 fl. oz.

**Maximum Strength
TYLENOL® Sore Throat**

FACED WITH AN
Rx SIDE EFFECT?

Turn to the
Companion Drug Index
for products that provide
symptomatic relief.

McNeil Consumer
P. 665

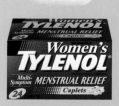

Caplets available in tamper-evident
bottles of 24.

**Women's TYLENOL®
Menstrual Relief**

MEMORY SECRET

Memory Secret
P. 770

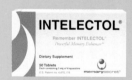

Intelectol®

NOVARTIS CONSUMER HEALTH

Novartis Consumer Health, Inc.
P. 772

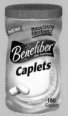

Caplets available in 100 ct.
and 160 ct. bottles.

**Benefiber®
Fiber Supplement
Caplets**

Novartis Consumer Health, Inc.
P. 771

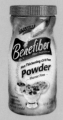

Available in 12 serving, 24 serving,
42 serving, 60 serving and
80 serving (club pack) bottles.

Non-Thickening Powder

**Benefiber®
Fiber Supplement**

Novartis Consumer Health, Inc.
P. 772

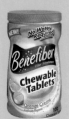

Available in 36 ct. and
100 ct. bottles.

**Benefiber®
Fiber Supplement
Chewable Tablets**

SEEKING AN
ALTERNATIVE?

Check the
Product Category Index,
where you'll find
alphabetical listings of
all the products in each
therapeutic class.

Novartis Consumer Health, Inc.
P. 674

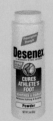

Powder   Spray Powder

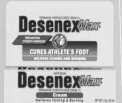

Antifungal Cream
Available in 12 g.

Desenex®

Novartis Consumer Health, Inc.
P. 674

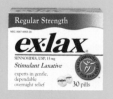

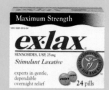

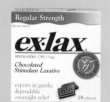

Available in Regular Strength 8's
and 30's, Maximum Strength 24's,
48's, and 90's, and Regular Strength
Chocolated Laxative 18's and 48's.

Ex•Lax®
(senna)

Novartis Consumer Health, Inc.

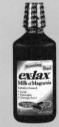

Chocolate Creme
12 fl. oz.
Also available in Mint and
Raspberry Creme flavor.

**Ex•Lax®
Milk of Magnesia**

Novartis Consumer Health, Inc.
P. 675

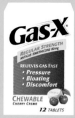

80 mg
Available in Cherry 12 ct.
and 36 ct. and
Peppermint 12 ct. and 36 ct.

Gas-X®
(simethicone)

Novartis Consumer Health, Inc.
P. 675

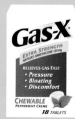

125 mg
Available in Extra Strength Cherry
18 ct. and 48 ct.
Extra Strength Peppermint
18 ct. and 48 ct.

Gas-X®
(simethicone)

Novartis Consumer Health, Inc.
P. 675

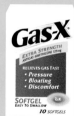

125 mg
Extra Strength Softgels
in cartons of 10's, 30's, 50's,
60's, and 72.

Gas-X®
(simethicone)

Novartis Consumer Health, Inc.
P. 675

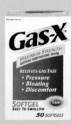

166 mg
Maximum Strength Softgels
in cartons of 50's.

Gas-X®
(simethicone)

Novartis Consumer Health, Inc.
P. 675

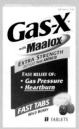

125 mg/500 mg
Available in Extra Strength Wild Berry
8's and 24's and
Extra Strength Orange 8's and 24's.

Gas-X® with Maalox®
(simethicone/calcium carbonate)

Novartis Consumer Health, Inc.
P. 675

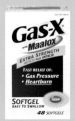

62.5 mg/250 mg
Extra Strength Softgels
in cartons of 24's and 48's.

**Gas-X® with
Maalox® Softgels**
(simethicone/calcium carbonate)

LOOKING FOR
A PARTICULAR
COMPOUND?

In the
Active Ingredients Index
(Yellow Pages),
you'll find all the
brands that contain it.

Novartis Consumer Health, Inc.
P. 676

Novartis Consumer Health, Inc.
P. 676

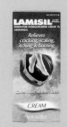

Athlete's Foot Cream available in
12 g and 24 g.
Jock Itch Cream available in 12 g.

LamisilAT® Cream

Novartis Consumer Health, Inc.

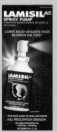

30 mL (1 fl. oz.)

**LamisilAT®
Athlete's Foot
Spray Pump**

Novartis Consumer Health, Inc.

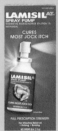

30 mL (1 fl. oz.)

**LamisilAT®
Jock Itch
Spray Pump**

Novartis Consumer Health, Inc.
P. 677

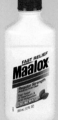

Cooling Mint Liquid
Also available in Smooth Cherry
12 & 26 fl. oz. and
bottles of 5 fl. oz. (Mint Only).

**Maalox® Antacid/Anti-Gas
Regular Strength**

Novartis Consumer Health, Inc.
P. 676

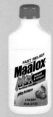

Cherry Liquid
Also available in Cherry and Lemon
(12 & 26 fl. oz.),
Mint, Vanilla Creme, and Wild Berry
(12 fl. oz.).

**Maalox® Antacid/Anti-Gas
Maximum Strength**

Novartis Consumer Health, Inc.
P. 677

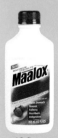

12 fl. oz.
Available in Strawberry & Mint Flavor

**Maalox® TOTAL
Stomach Relief™
Maximum Strength**

Novartis Consumer Health, Inc.
P. 678

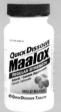

Assorted 85 ct.
Wild Berry 45 ct.
Lemon 85 ct.

**Maalox® Quick Dissolve
Regular Strength Tablets
Antacid/Calcium
Supplement**

Novartis Consumer Health, Inc.
P. 678

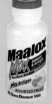

Assorted 35, 65, 90 ct.
Wild Berry 35, 65 ct.
Lemon 35, 65 ct.

**Maalox® Max Quick
Dissolve Maximum
Strength Tablets
Antacid/AntiGas**

Novartis Consumer Health, Inc.
P. 772

Slow Release Iron available
in 30, 60 and 90 ct tablets.
Slow Release Iron & Folic Acid
available in 20 ct tablets.

Slow Fe®

Novartis Consumer Health, Inc.
P. 684

Multi Symptom and Long Acting Cough
Available in 12 ct. cartons.

Theraflu® Thin Strips™

Novartis Consumer Health, Inc.
P. 682

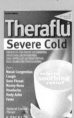

Flu & Chest Congestion Non-Drowsy
Severe Cold & Cough
Flu & Sore Throat
Severe Cold Non-Drowsy
Cold & Sore Throat
Cold & Cough
Available in 6 ct cartons.

TheraFlu®

Novartis Consumer Health, Inc.
P. 679

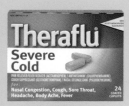

Severe Cold and
Severe Cold Non-Drowsy
Available in 12 ct. and
24 ct. caplets.

**TheraFlu®
Severe Cold**

Novartis Consumer Health, Inc.
P. 689

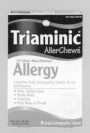

Cough and Runny Nose
and Long Acting Cough
Available in 16 ct. cartons.

Triaminic® Thin Strips™

Novartis Consumer Health, Inc.
P. 684

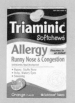

**Triaminic®
AllerChews™
Non-Drowsy Allergy**

Novartis Consumer Health, Inc.
P. 688

Allergy
Runny Nose & Congestion

**Triaminic® Softchews®
Allergy**

Novartis Consumer Health, Inc.
P. 685

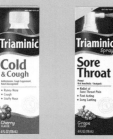

Cold & Cough   Sore Throat Spray

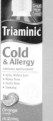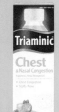

Cold & Allergy   Chest & Nasal
Congestion

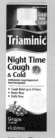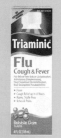

Night Time   Flu,
Cough & Cold   Cough & Fever

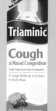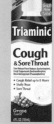

Cough & Nasal   Cough & Sore
Congestion   Throat

Triaminic®

Novartis Consumer Health, Inc.
P. 689

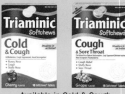

Available in Cold & Cough
and Cough & Sore Throat.

Triaminic® Softchews®

Novartis Consumer Health, Inc.
P. 690

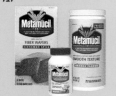

Menthol and
Mentholated Cherry Scents.

Triaminic® Vapor Patch®

PROCTER & GAMBLE

Procter & Gamble
P. 717

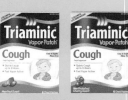

Available in 30, 48, 72, 114 and 180
dose canisters and cartons of 30
one-dose packets.
Also available in sugar free. Capsules
available in 100 ct and 160 ct.
Cinnamon Spice and Apple Crisp
Wafers available in 12-dose cartons.

Metamucil®

Procter & Gamble
P. 718

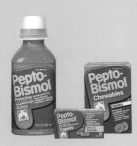

Also available in Maximum Strength
Liquid, Chewable Tablets and
Swallowable Caplets

Pepto-Bismol®

Procter & Gamble
P. 719

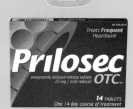

20 mg

Prilosec OTC®
(omeprazole)

Procter & Gamble
P. 720

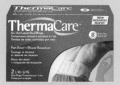

Back/Hip Wrap for Pain Relief
and Muscle Relaxation

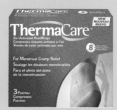

Patches For Menstrual Cramp Relief

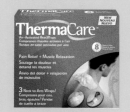

Neck to Arm Wrap for Pain Relief
and Muscle Relaxation

Air-Activated Heat Wraps

ThermaCare®

Procter & Gamble
P. 722

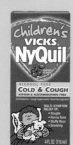

Cherry Flavor
Cold & Cough Relief

**Children's VICKS®
NyQuil®**

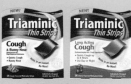

Procter & Gamble
P. 726

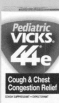

44®e
Cough & Chest Congestion Relief

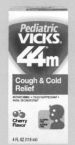

44®m
Cough & Cold Relief

Pediatric Vicks®

Procter & Gamble
P. 725

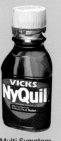

Multi-Symptom
Cold/Flu Relief
Also available as NyQuil LiquiCaps.

**VICKS® NyQuil®
Liquid**

Procter & Gamble
P. 724

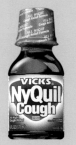

Cough Relief

**VICKS® NyQuil®
Cough**

Procter & Gamble
P. 721

VICKS® 44®
Cough Relief

VICKS® 44®D
Cough & Head Congestion Relief

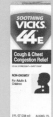

VICKS® 44® E
Cough & Chest Congestion Relief

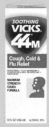

VICKS® 44® M
Cough, Cold & Flu Relief

VICKS®

Procter & Gamble
P. 723

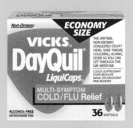

Multi-Symptom
Cold/Flu Relief
Also available as DayQuil Liquid.

**VICKS® DayQuil®
LiquiCaps®**

PURDUE PRODUCTS L.P.

Purdue Products L.P.
P. 728

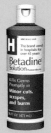

Povidone-iodine Solution

Betadine®

Purdue Products L.P.
P. 729

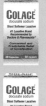

Stool Softener Capsules
Available in capsules, liquid and syrup

Colace®

Purdue Products L.P.
P. 729

Glycerin Suppositories
Available in Adults/Children and
Infants/Children formulations

Colace®

Purdue Products L.P.
P. 730

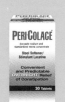

Stool Softener/Stimulant
Laxative Tablets

Peri-Colace® Tablets

Purdue Products L.P.
P. 730

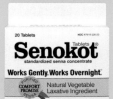

Natural Vegetable Laxative
Ingredient Tablets

Senokot® Tablets

Purdue Products L.P.
P. 730

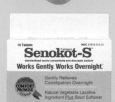

Standardized Senna Concentrate
and Docusate Sodium

Senokot-S® Tablets

Purdue Products L.P.
P. 774

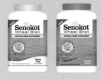

Natural Fiber Supplement

**Senokot™ Brand
Wheat Bran**

Purdue Products L.P.
P. 775

Magnesium Chloride
Dietary Supplement

Slow-Mag® Tablets

REESE PHARMACEUTICAL

Reese Pharmaceutical Company
P. 730

Available in 30 mL. oral suspension
or 24 ct. caplets

**Reese's Pinworm
Treatments**
(pyrantel pamoate)

SCHERING-PLOUGH

Schering-Plough HealthCare Products
P. 731

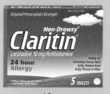

10 mg
Available in 5 ct., 10 ct.,
20 ct. and 30 ct.

Claritin® Tablets
(loratadine)

Schering-Plough HealthCare Products
P. 732

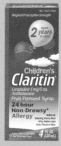

5 mg/5 mL
Available in 2 fl. oz. and 4 fl. oz. bottles.

Children's Claritin® Syrup
(loratadine)

Schering-Plough HealthCare Products
P. 731

5 mg/120 mg
Available in 10 ct., 20 ct. and 30 ct.

10 mg/240 mg
Available in 5 ct., 10 ct. and 15 ct.
Available in 12 hour and
24 hour extended release tablets.

Claritin-D®
(loratadine/pseudoephedrine sulfate)

Schering-Plough HealthCare Products
P. 732

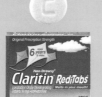

10 mg
Orally Disintegrating Tablets
Available in 4 ct., 10 ct. and 20 ct.

Claritin® RediTabs®
(loratadine)

Schering-Plough HealthCare Products
P. 733

Athlete's Foot Cream

Jock Itch Cream

Lotrimin Ultra®
(butenafine HCl 1%)

SUNPOWER

Sunpower Nutraceutical Inc.
P. 777

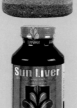

Sun Liver™

TAHITIAN NONI INTERNATIONAL

Tahitian Noni International
P. 777

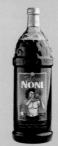

Dietary Supplement

Tahitian Noni® Juice

VEMMA NUTRITION COMPANY

Vemma Nutrition Company
P. 778

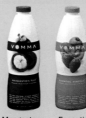

Mangosteen   Essential
Plus™   Minerals®

**Vemma Nutrition
Program™**

NONPRESCRIPTION DRUG INFORMATION

This section presents information on nonprescription drugs, self-testing kits, and other medical products marketed for home use by consumers. It is made possible through the courtesy of the manufacturers whose products appear on the following pages. The information concerning each product has been prepared, edited, and approved by the manufacturer's professional staff.

Pharmaceutical product descriptions in this section must be in compliance with the Code of Federal Regulations' labeling requirements for over-the-counter drugs. The descriptions are designed to provide all information necessary for informed use, including, when applicable, active ingredients, inactive ingredients, indications, actions, warnings, cautions, drug interactions, symptoms and treatment of oral overdosage, dosage and directions for use, professional labeling, and how supplied. In some cases, additional information has been supplied to complement the standard labeling.

In compiling this section, the publisher has emphasized the necessity of describing products comprehensively. The descriptions seen here include all information made available by the manufacturer. The publisher does not warrant or guarantee any product described here, and does not perform any independent analysis of the information provided. Inclusion of a product in this book does not represent an endorsement, and the publisher does not necessarily advocate the use of any product listed.

A.C. Grace Co.
1100 QUITMAN ROAD
P.O. BOX 570
BIG SANDY, TX 75755

Direct Inquiries to:
Inquiries: (903) 636-4368
Orders Only: 800-833-4368
www.acgraceco.com

UNIQUE E®
NATURAL VITAMIN E COMPLEX
MIXED TOCOPHEROL CONCENTRATE

Description:
Established 1962... OUR ONLY PRODUCT.
WHY UNIQUE?
All NATURAL VITAMIN E COMPLEX.
NOT the *dl* SYNTHETIC CHEMICAL
form, *NOT ESTER*IFIED TOCOPH-
ERYL ACETATE (OR SUCCINATE),
NOT the ORDINARY SOY OIL
DILUTED MIXED TOCOPHEROLS OR
ADULTERATED FORMS.

Each soft easy-to-swallow high quality
GEL CAPSULE contains **ALL NATU-
RAL** *UN*ESTERIFIED **VITAMIN E
COMPLEX** providing **400 I.U. ANTI-
THROMBIC** function d-alpha tocoph-
erol with other naturally occuring **AN-
TIOXIDANT** tocopherols, **d-beta, d
GAMMA, d-delta** for maximum protec-
tion against harmful free radical dam-
age and inhibiting peroxynitrites dam-
aging to brain cells.

NO SOY or other OIL FILLER additives
which can turn rancid and cause harmful free radical damage even in sealed
gel capsules.
NO ALLERGY CAUSING PRESERVA-
TIVES, COLORS OR FLAVORINGS.
UNIQUE E® capsule potency is stabilized and Certified by Assay.

Dosage: Up to 6 capsules daily as
directed by your physician according to
individual weight or need, usually 1
capsule per each 40 lbs. of total body
weight. Best results when ENTIRE daily
dose is taken just before or with the
morning meal.

How Supplied:
Bottles of 180 and 90 easy-to-swallow
high quality gel capsules in safety sealed
light protected bottles.

UNKNOWN DRUG?
Consult the
Product Identification Guide
(Gray Pages)
for full-color photos of
leading over-the-counter
medications

Adams Respiratory Therapeutics
425 MAIN STREET
COLONIAL COURT
CHESTER, NJ 07930

Direct Inquiries to:
877-MUCINEX

MUCINEX® 600 mg
**Guaifenesin extended-release bi-layer
tablets**
Expectorant

Drug Facts

Active Ingredient: **Purpose:**
**(in each extended-release
bi-layer tablet)**
Guaifenesin 600 mg .... Expectorant

Uses: Helps loosen phlegm (mucus)
and thin bronchial secretions to rid the
bronchial passageways of bothersome
mucus and make coughs more productive

Warnings:
Do not use
□ for children under 12 years of age
Ask a doctor before use if you have
□ persistent or chronic cough such as occurs with smoking, asthma, chronic
bronchitis, or emphysema
□ cough accompanied by too much
phlegm (mucus)
Stop use and ask a doctor if
□ cough lasts more than 7 days, comes
back, or occurs with fever, rash, or
persistent headache. These could be
signs of a serious illness.
If pregnant or breast-feeding, ask a
health professional before use.
Keep out of reach of children. In case of
overdose, get medical help or contact a
Poison Control Center right away.

Directions:
□ do not crush, chew, or break tablet
□ take with a full glass of water
□ this product can be administered
without regard for the timing of meals
□ adults and children 12 years of age
and over: one or two tablets every 12
hours. Do not exceed 4 tablets in 24
hours.
□ children under 12 years of age: do not
use
Other Information:
• tamper evident: do not use if seal on
bottle printed "SEALED for YOUR
PROTECTION" is broken or missing
• store between 20–25°C (68–77°F)
• see bottom of bottle for lot code and
expiration date

Inactive Ingredients: carbomer 934P,
NF; FD&C blue #1 aluminum lake;
hypromellose, USP; magnesium stearate, NF; microcrystalline cellulose, NF;
sodium starch glycolate, NF

How Supplied:
Bottles of 20 tablets (NDC 63824-008-
20), 40 tablets (NDC 63824-008-40),
sample bottles of 2 tablets (NDC 63824-
008-82), 100 tablets (NDC 63824-008-10)
and 500 tablets (NDC 63824-008-50). A
round bi-layer tablet debossed with "A"

---

on the light blue, marbled layer and
"600" on the white layer. Each tablet
provides 600 mg guaifenesin.
US Patent No. 6,372,252 B1
*Shown in Product Identification
Guide, page 503*

MUCINEX® DM
**600 mg Guaifenesin and 30 mg
Dextromethorphan HBr extended-
release bi-layer tablets**
Expectorant and Cough Suppressant

Drug Facts

Active Ingredients: **Purpose:**
**(in each extended-release
bi-layer tablet)**
Dextromethorphan HBr
 30 mg .... Cough suppressant
Guaifenesin 600 mg .... Expectorant

Uses:
□ helps loosen phlegm (mucus) and thin
bronchial secretions to rid the bronchial passageways of bothersome mucus and make coughs more productive
□ temporarily relieves:
 □ cough due to minor throat and
bronchial irritation as may occur
with the common cold or inhaled
irritants
 □ the intensity of coughing
 □ the impulse to cough to help you get
to sleep

Warnings:
Do not use
□ for children under 12 years of age
□ if you are now taking a prescription
monoamine oxidase inhibitor (MAOI)
(certain drugs for depression, psychiatric or emotional conditions, or Parkinson's disease), or for 2 weeks after
stopping the MAOI drug. If you do not
know if your prescription drug contains a MAOI, ask a doctor or pharmacist before taking this product.
Ask a doctor before use if you have
□ persistent or chronic cough such as occurs with smoking, asthma, chronic
bronchitis, or emphysema
□ cough accompanied by too much
phlegm (mucus)
When using this product
□ do not use more than directed
Stop use and ask a doctor if
□ cough lasts more than 7 days, comes
back, or occurs with fever, rash, or
persistent headache. These could be
signs of a serious illness.
If pregnant or breast-feeding, ask a
health professional before use.
Keep out of reach of children. In case of
overdose, get medical help or contact a
Poison Control Center right away.

Directions:
□ do not crush, chew, or break tablet
□ take with a full glass of water
□ this product can be administered
without regard for timing of meals
□ adults and children 12 years and
older: one or two tablets every 12
hours; not more than 4 tablets in 24
hours
□ children under 12 years of age: do not
use
Other Information:
□ tamper evident: do not use if seal on
bottle printed "SEALED for YOUR
PROTECTION" is broken or missing

□ store at 20–25°C (68–77°F)
□ see bottom of bottle for lot code and expiration date

Inactive Ingredients: carbomer 934P, NF; D&C yellow #10 aluminum lake; hypromellose, USP; magnesium stearate, NF; microcrystalline cellulose, NF; sodium starch glycolate, NF

How Supplied:
Bottles of 20 tablets (NDC 63824-056-20), 40 tablets (NDC 63824-056-40).
A modified oval bi-layer tablet debossed with "Adams" on the yellow layer and "600" on the white layer. Each tablet provides 600 mg guaifenesin and 30 mg dextromethorphan HBr.
US Patent No.6,372,252 B1
Shown in Product Identification Guide, page 503

Alpharma
U.S. Pharmaceuticals Division
**7205 WINDSOR BOULEVARD
BALTIMORE, MD 21244**

For General Inquiries Contact:
Customer Service
800-432-8534

PERMETHRIN LOTION 1%
Lice Treatment

Description:
EACH FLUID OUNCE CONTAINS: Active Ingredient: Permethrin 280 mg (1%). Inactive Ingredients: Balsam fir canada, cetyl alcohol, citric acid, FD&C Yellow No. 6, fragrance, hydrolyzed animal protein, hydroxyethylcellulose, polyoxyethylene 10 cetyl ether, propylene glycol, stearalkonium chloride, water, isopropyl alcohol 5.6 g (20%), methylparaben 56 mg (0.2%), and propylparaben 22 mg (0.08%).
Permethrin Lotion 1% kills lice and their unhatched eggs with usually only one application. Permethrin Lotion 1% protects against head lice reinfestation for 14 days. The creme rinse formula leaves hair manageable and easy to comb.

Indications: For the treatment of head lice. For prophylactic use during head lice epidemics.

Warnings: For external use only. Keep out of eyes when rinsing hair. Adults and children: Close eyes and do not open eyes until product is rinsed out. If product gets into the eyes, immediately flush with water. Do not use near the eyes or permit contact with mucous membranes, such as inside the nose, mouth, or vagina, as irritation may occur. Children: Also protect children's eyes with a washcloth, towel or other suitable material or method. This product should not be used on pediatric patients less than 2 months

of age. Itching, redness, or swelling of the scalp may occur. If skin irritation persists or infection is present or develops, discontinue use and consult a doctor. Consult a doctor if infestation of eyebrows or eyelashes occurs. This product may cause breathing difficulty or an asthmatic episode in susceptible persons. As with any drug, if you are pregnant or nursing a baby, seek the advice of a health professional before using this product. Keep this and all drugs out of the reach of children. In case of accidental ingestion, seek professional assistance or contact a Poison Control Center immediately.

Dosage and Administration:
Treatment: Permethrin Lotion 1% should be used after hair has been washed with patient's regular shampoo, rinsed with water and towel dried. A sufficient amount should be applied to saturate hair and scalp (especially behind the ears and on the nape of the neck). Leave on hair for 10 minutes but not longer. Rinse with water. A single application is usually sufficient. If live lice are observed seven days or more after the first application of this product, a second treatment should be given. For proper head lice management, remove nits with the nit comb provided.

Head lice live on the scalp and lay small white eggs (nits) on the hair shaft close to the scalp. The nits are most easily found on the nape of the neck or behind the ears. All personal headgear, scarfs, coats, and bed linen should be disinfected by machine washing in hot water and drying, using the hot cycle of a dryer for at least 20 minutes. Personal articles of clothing or bedding that cannot be washed may be dry-cleaned, sealed in a plastic bag for a period of about 2 weeks, or sprayed with a product specifically designed for this purpose. Personal combs and brushes may be disinfected by soaking in hot water (above 130°F) for 5 to 10 minutes. Thorough vacuuming of rooms inhabited by infected patients is recommended.

Prophylaxis: Prophylactic use of Permethrin Lotion 1% is only recommended for individuals exposed to head lice epidemics in which at least 20% of the population at an institution are infested and for immediate household members of infested individuals. Casual use is strongly discouraged.

The method of application of Permethrin Lotion 1% for prophylaxis is identical to that described above for treatment of a lice infestation except nit removal is not required.

Directions For Use: One application of Permethrin Lotion 1% has been shown to protect greater than 95% of patients against reinfestation for at least two weeks. In epidemic settings, a second prophylactic application is recommended two weeks after the first because the life cycle of a head louse is approximately four weeks.

How Supplied: Bottles of 2 fl. oz. (59 mL) with nit removal comb and Family Pack of 2 bottles, 2 fl. oz. (59 mL) each, with 2 nit removal combs.
Store at 15° to 25°C (59° to 77°F).
Manufactured by
Alpharma USPD Inc.
Baltimore, MD 21244
FORM NO. 5242   Rev. 9/99
                                     VC1587

Alto Pharmaceuticals, Inc.
**P.O. BOX 271150
TAMPA, FL 33688-1150
12506 CLENDENNING DR.
TAMPA, FL 33618**

Direct Inquiries to:
John J. Cullaro
Customer Service
www.altopharm.com
Tel (800) 330-2891
Fax (813) 968-0527

ZINC-220® CAPSULES
[zĭnk]
(zinc sulfate 220 mg.)

Composition: Each opaque blue and pink capsule contains zinc sulfate 220 mg. delivering 78.5 mg. of elemental zinc. Zinc-220 Capsules do not contain dextrose or glucose. Inactive Ingredients dicalcium phosphate, cellulose, magnesium stearate, magnesium trisilicate and gelatin (capsule shell).

Action and Uses: Zinc-220 Capsules are indicated as a dietary supplement. Normal growth and tissue repair are directly dependent upon an adequate supply of zinc in the diet. Zinc functions as an integral part of a number of enzymes important to protein and carbohydrate metabolism. Zinc-220 Capsules are recommended for deficiencies or the prevention of deficiencies of zinc.

Warnings: Zinc-220 if administered in stat dosages of 2 grams (9 capsules) will cause an emetic effect. This product should not be used by pregnant or lactating women.

Precaution: It is recommended that Zinc-220 Capsules be taken with meals or milk to avoid gastric distress.

Dosage: One capsule daily with milk or meals. One capsule daily provides approximately 523% times the recommended adult requirement for zinc.

How Supplied:

Product	NDC	SIZE
Zinc-220® **Capsules**	0731-0401-06	Unit Dose Boxes… 100 (10×10)
Zinc-220® **Capsules**	0731-0401-01	Bottles 100

ALTO® Pharmaceuticals, Inc.

Bausch & Lomb
1400 NORTH GOODMAN
STREET
ROCHESTER, NY 14609

Direct Inquiries to:
Main Office
(585) 338-6000
Consumer Affairs
1-800-553-5340

OCUVITE®
Antioxidant Vitamin and Mineral Supplement

Description: Each tablet contains:
[See first table above]

Inactive Ingredients: Dibasic calcium phosphate, microcrystalline cellulose, calcium carbonate, crospovidone, hydroxypropyl methylcellulose, titanium dioxide, silicon dioxide, magnesium stearate, stearic acid, FD&C Yellow No. 6, triethyl citrate, polysorbate 80 and sodium lauryl sulfate.

Indications: OCUVITE is specifically formulated to provide nutritional support for the eye, and is recommended for those patients who are already taking a daily multi-vitamin supplement but would like to include Lutein. The Ocuvite formulation contains essential antioxidant vitamins and minerals plus 2 mg of Lutein.

Recommended Intake: Adults. One tablet, one or two times daily or as directed by their doctor.

Current and Former Smokers: Consult your eye care professional about the risks associated with smoking and using Beta-Carotene.

How Supplied: Peach, eye shaped, film coated tablet engraved LL on one side, 04 on the other side.
NDC 24208-387-60—Bottle of 60
NDC 24208-387-62—Bottle of 120
Store at Room Temperature.
MADE IN Germany
Marketed by
Bausch & Lomb
Rochester, NY 14609
Shown in Product Identification Guide, page 503

OCUVITE® EXTRA®
Vitamin and Mineral Supplement

Description: Each tablet contains:
[See second table above]

Inactive Ingredients: dibasic calcium phosphate, microcrystalline cellulose, calcium carbonate, crospovidone, hydroxypropyl methylcellulose, titanium dioxide, silicon dioxide, magnesium stearate, stearic acid, FD&C yellow No. 6, triethyl citrate, polysorbate 80 and sodium lauryl sulfate.

	Source	Amount	% Daily Value
Vitamin A	beta carotene	1000 IU	20%
Vitamin C	ascorbic acid	200 mg	330%
Vitamin E	dl-alpha tocopheryl acetate	60 IU	200%
Zinc	zinc oxide*	40 mg	270%
Selenium	sodium selenate	55 mcg	80%
Copper	cupric oxide	2 mg	100%
Lutein		2 mg	†

* Zinc oxide is the most concentrated form of zinc and contains more elemental zinc than any other zinc salt (ie: zinc sulfate or zinc acetate).
† Daily value not established.

	Source	Amount	% Daily Value
Vitamin A	beta carotene	1000 IU	20%
Vitamin C	ascorbic acid	300 mg	500%
Vitamin E	dl-alpha tocopheryl acetate	100 IU	330%
Riboflavin		3 mg	180%
Niacinamide		40 mg	200%
Zinc	zinc oxide*	40 mg	270%
Selenium	sodium selenate	55 mcg	80%
Copper	cupric oxide	2 mg	100%
Manganese		5 mg	250%
L-Glutathione		5 mg	†
Lutein		2 mg	†

* Zinc oxide is the most concentrated form of zinc and contains more elemental zinc than any other zinc salt (ie: zinc sulfate or zinc acetate).
† Daily value not established.

	Source	Amount	% Daily Value
Vitamin C	**ascorbic acid**	**60 mg**	**100%**
Vitamin E	**dl-alpha tocopheryl acetate**	**30 IU**	**100%**
Zinc	**zinc oxide***	**15 mg**	**100%**
Copper	**cupric oxide**	**2 mg**	**100%**
Lutein		**6 mg**	†

*Zinc oxide is the most concentrated form of zinc and contains more elemental zinc than any other zinc salt (ie: zinc sulfate or zinc acetate)
† Daily value not established

Indications: OCUVITE EXTRA is specifically formulated to provide nutritional support for the eye, and is recommended for those patients who are not taking a daily multi-vitamin supplement. The Ocuvite Extra formulation contains essential antioxidant vitamins and minerals, vitamins B-2 and B-3, plus 2 mg of Lutein.

Recommended Intake: Adults: One tablet, one or two times daily or as directed by their doctor.

Current and Former Smokers: Consult your eye care professional about the risks associated with smoking and using Beta-Carotene.

How Supplied: Orange, eye shaped, film coated tablet engraved OCUVITE on one side, 05 on the other side.
NDC 24208-388-19—Bottle of 50
Store at Room Temperature

MADE IN Germany
Marketed by
Bausch & Lomb
Rochester, NY 14609
Shown in Product Identification Guide, page 503

OCUVITE® LUTEIN
[lu "teen]
Vitamin and Mineral Supplement

Description: Each capsule contains:
[See third table above]

Inactive Ingredients: Lactose monohydrate, Crospovidone, Magnesium Stearate, Silicone dioxide.

• Lutein is a carotenoid found in dark leafy green vegetables such as spinach. Carotenoids are concentrated in the Macula, the part of the eye responsible for central vision. Clinical studies suggest that Lutein plays an essential role in maintaining healthy central vision by protecting against free radical damage and filtering blue light.*

• Lutein levels in your eye are related to the amount in your diet. Ocuvite Lutein contains 6 mg of Lutein per capsule. The leading multi-vitamin contains only a fraction of the amount of lutein used in clinical studies.

• Ocuvite® Lutein helps supplement your diet with antioxidant vitamins and essential minerals that can play an important role in your ocular health.*

Indications: Ocuvite Lutein is an advanced antioxidant supplement formulated to provide nutritional support for the eye. The Ocuvite Lutein formulation contains essential antioxidant vitamins, minerals and 6 mg of Lutein.

Recommended Intake: Adults: One capsule, one or two times daily or as directed by their physician.

*THESE STATEMENTS HAVE NOT BEEN EVALUATED BY THE FOOD AND DRUG ADMINISTRATION. THIS PRODUCT IS NOT INTENDED TO DIAGNOSE, TREAT, CURE OR PREVENT ANY DISEASE.

How Supplied: Yellow capsule with Ocuvite Lutein printed in black. NDC 24208-403-19—Bottle of 36 Store at Room Temperature MADE IN U.S.A. Marketed by Bausch & Lomb Rochester, NY 14609
Shown in Product Identification Guide, page 503

BAUSCH & LOMB PRESERVISION® AREDS High Potency Eye Vitamin and Mineral Supplement† Original, 4 per day tablets

Description: Each tablet contains [See table below]

Other Ingredients: Lactose Monohydrate, Microcrystalline Cellulose, Crospovidone, Stearic Acid, Magnesium Stearate, Silicon Dioxide, Polysorbate 80, Triethyl Citrate, FD&C Yellow #6, FD&C Red #40

• Age-related macular degeneration is the leading cause of vision loss and blindness in people over 55. The National Institutes of Health (NIH) Age Related Eye Disease Study (AREDS) proved that a unique high-potency vitamin and mineral supplement was effective in helping to preserve the sight of certain people most at risk.*

• †Bausch & Lomb **Ocuvite PreserVision** was the one and only eye vitamin and mineral supplement tested and clinically proven effective in the NIH AREDS Study.

• Bausch & Lomb **Ocuvite PreserVision** is a high-potency antioxidant and mineral supplement with the antioxidant vitamins A, C, E and select minerals in amounts well above those in ordinary multivitamins and generally cannot be attained through diet alone.

For a FREE 16-page brochure on Age-Related Macular Degeneration call toll-free 1-886-467-3263 Extension #81 (1-868-HOPE-AMD)

Recommended Intake: To get the high levels proven in the NIH AREDS Study it is important to take 4 tablets per day – 2 in the morning, 2 in the evening taken with meals.

Current and Former Smokers: Consult your eye care professional about the risks associated with smoking and using Beta-Carotene.

Bausch & Lomb Ocuvite PreserVision is the #1 recommended eye vitamin and mineral supplement brand among Retinal Specialists.[1]

* This statement has not been evaluated by the Food and Drug Administration. This product is not intended to diagnose, treat, cure or prevent any disease.

How Supplied: Orange, eye shaped film coated tablet, engraved BL 01 on one side, scored on the other side. Available in bottles of 120 or 240 count tablets Store at room temperature. Made in USA Marketed by Bausch & Lomb Rochester, NY 14609

References: 1. Data on file, Bausch & Lomb, Inc.
© Bausch & Lomb Incorporated. All Rights Reserved.
Bausch & Lomb, Ocuvite and PreserVision are trademarks of Bausch & Lomb

Incorporated or its affiliates. Other brand names are trademarks of their respective owners.
Shown in Product Identification Guide, page 503

Bayer HealthCare LLC Consumer Care Division
36 COLUMBIA ROAD P.O. BOX 1910 MORRISTOWN, NJ 07962-1910

Direct Inquiries to:
Consumer Relations
(800) 331-4536
www.bayercare.com

For Medical Emergency Contact:
Bayer HealthCare LLC
Consumer Care Division
(800) 331-4536

ALEVE® Tablets, Caplets*, Gelcaps**
All Day Strong
naproxen sodium 220 mg
Pain reliever/fever reducer, USP

Active Ingredient: Purpose: (in each tablet/caplet/gelcap)
Naproxen sodium 220 mg Pain reliever/
(naproxen 200 mg) .... fever reducer

Uses: Temporarily relieves minor aches and pains due to:
• headache
• muscular aches
• minor pain of arthritis
• toothache
• backache
• common cold
• menstrual cramps
temporarily reduces fever

Warnings: Allergy alert: Naproxen sodium may cause a severe allergic reaction which may include:
• hives
• facial swelling
• asthma (wheezing)
• shock
Alcohol warning: If you consume 3 or more alcoholic drinks every day, ask your doctor whether you should take naproxen sodium or other pain relievers/fever reducers. Naproxen sodium may cause stomach bleeding.

Do not use if you have ever had an allergic reaction to any other pain reliever/fever reducer

Ask a doctor before use if you have ever had serious side effects from any pain reliever/fever reducer

Contents	Two tablets		Daily Dosage (4 tablets)	
	Amount	% of Daily Value	Amount	% of Daily Value
Vitamin A (Beta-carotene)	14,320 IU	286%	28,640 IU	573%
Vitamin C (ascorbic acid)	226 mg	376%	452 mg	753%
Vitamin E (dl-alpha tocopheryl acetate)	200 IU	666%	400 IU	1333%
Zinc (zinc oxide)	34.8 mg	232%	89.5 mg	484%
Cooper (cupric oxide)	0.8 mg	40%	1.6 mg	80%

Continued on next page

Aleve—Cont.

Ask a doctor or pharmacist before use if you are
- under a doctor's care for any serious condition
- taking other drug
- taking any other product that contains naproxen sodium, or any other pain reliever/fever reducer

Stop use and ask a doctor if
- an allergic reaction occurs. Seek medical help right away.
- pain gets worse or lasts more than 10 days
- fever gets worse or lasts more than 3 days
- you have difficulty swallowing
- it feels like the pill is stuck in your throat
- you develop heartburn
- stomach pain occurs or lasts, even if symptoms are mild
- redness or swelling is present in the painful area
- any new symptoms appear

If pregnant or breast-feeding, ask a health professional before use. It is especially important not to use naproxen sodium during the last 3 months of pregnancy unless definitely directed to do so by a doctor because it may cause problems in the unborn child or complications during delivery.

Keep out of reach of children. In case of overdose, get medical help or contact a Poison Control Center right away.

Directions:
- **do not take more than directed**
- drink a full glass of water with each dose

[See table below]

Other Information:
- **each tablet (caplet, gelcap) contains:** sodium 20 mg
- store at 20–25°C (68–77°F). Avoid high humidity and excessive heat above 40°C (104°F)

Aleve tablets, caplets:

Inactive Ingredients: FD&C blue #2 lake, hypromellose, magnesium stearate, microcrystalline cellulose, polyethylene glycol, povidone, talc, titanium dioxide

Aleve gelcaps:

Inactive Ingredients: D&C yellow #10 aluminum lake, edetate disodium, edible ink, FD&C blue #1, FD&C yellow #6 aluminum lake, gelatin, glycerin, hypromellose, magnesium stearate, microcrystalline cellulose, polyethylene gly-

col, povidone, stearic acid, talc, titanium dioxide

Questions or comments? call **1-800-395-0689** or www.aleve.com

---

* capsule-shaped tablet(s)

** gelatin coated capsule-shaped tablet(s)

How Supplied:

ALEVE® Caplets in boxes of 24, 50, 100, 150, 200.

ALEVE® Gelcaps in boxes of 20, 40, 80.

ALEVE® Tablets in boxes of 24, 50, 100, 150. + 8 count vials

Distributed by
Bayer HealthCare LLC
PO Box 1910
Morristown, NJ 07962-1910 USA
B-R LLC

ASPIRIN REGIMEN BAYER® 81 mg
ASPIRIN REGIMEN BAYER® 325 mg
Delayed Release Enteric Aspirin Adult Low Strength 81 mg Tablets and Regular Strength 325 mg Caplets

Active Ingredient:

(in each tablet)	Purpose:
Aspirin 81 mg	Pain reliever
Aspirin 325 mg	Pain reliever

Uses: For the temporary relief of minor aches and pains or as recommended by your doctor. **Because of its delayed action, this product will not provide fast relief of headaches or other symptoms needing immediate relief.** Ask your doctor about other uses for Bayer safety coated 81mg/325mg aspirin.

Warnings: Reye's syndrome: Children and teenagers should not use this medicine for chicken pox or flu symptoms before a doctor is consulted about Reye's syndrome, a rare but serious illness reported to be associated with aspirin.

Allergy alert: Aspirin may cause a severe allergic reaction which may include:
- hives • facial swelling • asthma (wheezing) • shock

Alcohol warning: If you consume 3 or more alcoholic drinks every day, ask your doctor whether you should take as-

pirin or other pain relievers/fever reducers. Aspirin may cause stomach bleeding.

Do not use if you are allergic to aspirin or any other pain reliever/fever reducer.

Ask a doctor before use if you have
- stomach problems (such as heartburn, upset stomach, or stomach pain) that last or come back
- bleeding problems
- ulcers
- asthma

Ask a doctor or pharmacist before use if you are taking a prescription drug for
- anticoagulation (blood thinning)
- gout
- diabetes
- arthritis

Stop use and ask a doctor if
- an allergic reaction occurs. Seek medical help right away.
- pain gets worse or lasts for more than 10 days
- redness or swelling is present
- new symptoms occur
- ringing in the ears or loss of hearing occurs

If pregnant or breast-feeding, ask a health professional before use. **It is especially important not to use aspirin during the last 3 months of pregnancy unless definitely directed to do so by a doctor because it may cause problems in the unborn child or complications during delivery.**

Keep out of reach of children. In case of overdose, get medical help or contact a Poison Control Center right away.

Directions:

ASPIRIN REGIMEN BAYER® 81 mg:
- drink a full glass of water with each dose
- adults and children 12 years and over: take 4 to 8 tablets every 4 hours not to exceed 48 tablets in 24 hours unless directed by a doctor
- children under 12 years: consult a doctor

ASPIRIN REGIMEN BAYER® 325 mg:
- drink a full glass of water with each dose
- adults and children 12 years and over: take 1 or 2 caplets every 4 hours not to exceed 12 caplets in 24 hours unless directed by a doctor
- children under 12 years: consult a doctor

Other Information:
- save carton for full directions and warnings
- store at room temperature

Inactive Ingredients:

ASPIRIN REGIMEN BAYER® 81 mg:
Black iron oxide, brown iron oxide, carnauba wax, corn starch, D&C yellow #10 aluminum lake, FD&C yellow #6 aluminum lake, hypromellose, methacrylic acid copolymer, polysorbate 80, powdered cellulose, propylene glycol, shellac, sodium lauryl sulfate, talc, titanium dioxide, triacetin, triethyl citrate

ASPIRIN REGIMEN BAYER® 325 mg:
Black iron oxide, brown iron oxide, carnauba wax, corn starch, D&C yellow #10 aluminum lake, FD&C yellow #6 aluminum lake, hypromellose, methacrylic acid copolymer, polysorbate 80, powdered cellulose, propylene glycol, shellac,

Adults and children 12 years and older	• take 1 tablet (caplet, gelcap) every 8 to 12 hours while symptoms last • for the first dose you may take 2 tablets (caplets, gelcaps) within the first hour • the smallest effective dose should be used • do not exceed 2 tablets (caplets, gelcaps) in any 8- to 12-hour period • do not exceed 3 tablets (caplets, gelcaps) in a 24-hour period
Adults over 65 years	• do not take more than 1 tablet (caplet, gelcap) every 12 hours unless directed by a doctor
Children under 12 years	• ask a doctor

sodium lauryl sulfate, titanium dioxide, triacetin, *may contain* talc, triethyl citrate

Questions or comments?
1-800-331-4536 or
www.bayeraspirin.com

How Supplied:
ASPIRIN REGIMEN BAYER® 81 mg: Bottle of 120 tablets delayed release enteric safety coated aspirin.
ASPIRIN REGIMEN BAYER® 325 mg: Bottle of 100 caplets delayed release enteric safety coated aspirin.
Bayer HealthCare LLC
PO Box 1910
Morristown, NJ 07962-1910 USA

Beutlich LP Pharmaceuticals

1541 SHIELDS DRIVE
WAUKEGAN, IL 60085-8304

Direct Inquiries to:
847-473-1100
800-238-8542 in US & Canada
FAX 847–473–1122
www.beutlich.com
e-mail beutlich@beutlich.com

CEO–TWO® Evacuant Laxative Adult Rectal Suppository

NDC #0283-0763-09

Composition: Each suppository contains sodium bicarbonate and potassium bitartrate in a special blend of water-soluble polyethylene glycols.

Indications: For relief of occasional constipation, irregularity or for bowel training programs. CEO-TWO generally produces a bowel movement in 5–30 minutes. The lubrication provided by the emollient base combined with the gentle pressure of the released carbon dioxide slowly distends the rectal ampulla stimulating peristalsis. CEO-TWO does not interfere with normal digestion, is not habit forming, won't cause cramping or irritation or alter the normal peristaltic reflex, and it leaves no residue.

Administration and Dosage: Adults and children over 12 years of age. Rectal dosage is one suppository containing 0.6 gram of sodium bicarbonate and 0.9 gram potassium bitartrate in a single daily dose. For children under 12 years of age: consult a doctor. For most effective results and ease of insertion, moisten a CEO-TWO suppository by placing it under a warm water tap for 30 seconds or in a cup of water for 10 seconds before insertion. Insert rectally past the largest diameter of the suppository. Patient should retain in the rectum as long as possible (usually about 5–30 minutes).

Warnings: For rectal use only. Do not use this product if you are on a low salt diet unless directed by a doctor. (172 milligrams of sodium per suppository) Do not lubricate with mineral oil or petrolatum prior to use. Do not use when abdominal pain, nausea or vomiting are present unless directed by a doctor. Laxative products should not be used for longer than one week unless directed by a doctor. If you have noticed a sudden change of bowel habits that persists over a period of 2 weeks, consult a doctor before using a laxative. Rectal bleeding or failure to have a bowel movement after use of a laxative may indicate a serious problem. Discontinue use and consult your doctor.

How Supplied: In box of 10 individually foil wrapped white opaque suppositories. Keep in cool dry place. **DO NOT REFRIGERATE**

HURRICAINE® TOPICAL ANESTHETIC

Composition: HURRICAINE contains 20% benzocaine in a flavored, water soluble polyethylene glycol base.

Action and Indications: HURRICAINE is a topical anesthetic that provides rapid anesthesia on all accessible mucous membrane in 15 to 30 seconds, short duration of 15 minutes, has virtually no systemic absorption, and tastes good. Hurricaine is used as a lubricant and topical anesthetic to facilitate passage of fiberoptic gastroscopes, laryngoscopes, proctoscopes and sigmoidoscopes. In addition, Hurricaine is effective in suppressing the pharyngeal and tracheal gag reflex during the placement of nasogastric tubes. Hurricaine is used to control pain and discomfort during certain gynecological procedures such as IUD insertion, vaginal speculum placement, and as a preinjection anesthesia prior to LEEP procedures and paracervical blocks. Hurricaine is also effective for the temporary relief of pain due to sore throat, stomatitis and mucositis. It is also effective in controlling various types of pain associated with dental procedures and the temporary relief of minor mouth irritations, canker sores and irritation to the mouth and gums caused by dentures or orthodontic appliances.

Contraindications: Patients with a known hypersensitivity to benzocaine should not use HURRICAINE. True allergic reactions are rare.

Adverse Reactions: Methemoglobinemia has been reported following the use of benzocaine on extremely rare occasions. Intravenous methylene blue is the specific therapy for this condition.

Cautions: DO NOT USE IN THE EYES.
NOT FOR INJECTION.

KEEP THIS AND ALL DRUGS OUT OF THE REACH OF CHILDREN.

Packaging Available
GEL
1 oz. Jar Fresh Mint NDC #0283-0998-31
1 oz. Jar Wild Cherry NDC #0283-0871-31
1 oz. Jar Pina Colada NDC #0283-0886-31
1 oz. Jar Watermelon NDC #0283-0293-31
1/6 oz. Tube Wild Cherry NDC #0283-0871-75
LIQUID
1 fl. oz. Jar Wild Cherry NDC #0283-0569-31
1 fl. oz. Jar Pina Colada NDC #0283-1886-31
.25 ml Dry Handle Swab Wild Cherry 100 Each Per Box NDC #0283-0569-01
.25 ml Dry Handle Swab Wild Cherry 6 Each Per Travel Pack NDC #0283-0569-36
SPRAY
2 oz. Aerosol Wild Cherry NDC #0283-0679-02
SPRAY KIT
2 oz. Aerosol Wild Cherry NDC #0283-0679-60 with 200 Disposable Extension Tubes

---

Boehringer Ingelheim Consumer Healthcare Products Division of Boehringer Ingelheim Pharmceuticals Inc.

900 RIDGEBURY ROAD
P.O. BOX 368
RIDGEFIELD, CT 06877

For Direct Inquiries Contact:
1-888-285-9159

DULCOLAX®
[dul 'cō-Lax]
brand of bisacodyl USP
Tablets of 5 mg
Laxative

Drug Facts
Active Ingredient:
(in each tablet)   **Purpose:**
Bisacodyl USP, 5 mg .... Laxative

Uses:
• Relieves occasional constipation and irregularity.
• This product usually causes bowel movement in 6 to 12 hours.

Warnings:
Do not use • If you cannot swallow without chewing.

Continued on next page

Dulcolax Tablets—Cont.

Ask a doctor before use if you have:
- Stomach pain, nausea or vomiting.
- A sudden change in bowel habits that lasts more than 2 weeks.

When using this product:
- Do not chew or crush tablet.
- Do not use within 1 hour after taking an antacid or milk.
- You may have stomach discomfort, faintness or cramps.

Stop use and ask a doctor if:
- You do not have a bowel movement within 12 hours or if rectal bleeding occurs. These could be signs of a serious condition.
- You need to use a laxative for more than 1 week.

If pregnant or breast-feeding, ask a doctor before use. **Keep out of reach of children.** In case of overdose, get medical help or contact a Poison Control Center right away.

Directions:

Adults and children 12 years and over	Take 1 to 3 tablets (usually 2) daily.
Children 6 to under 12 years	Take 1 tablet daily.
Children under 6 years	Ask a doctor.

Other Information • Store at 20–25°C (68–77°F). Avoid excessive humidity.

Inactive Ingredients: Acacia, acetylated monoglyceride, carnauba wax, cellulose acetate phthalate, corn starch, dibutyl phthalate, docusate sodium, gelatin, glycerin, iron oxides, kaolin, lactose, magnesium stearate, methylparaben, pharmaceutical glaze, polyethylene glycol, povidone, propylparaben, Red No. 30 lake, sodium benzoate, sorbitan monooleate, sucrose, talc, titanium dioxide, white wax, Yellow No. 10 lake.

How Supplied: Boxes of 25 Tablets. Boehringer Ingelheim Consumer Healthcare Products. Division of Boehringer Ingelheim Pharmaceuticals, Inc., Ridgefield, CT 06877 Made in Mexico ©Boehringer Ingelheim Pharmaceuticals, Inc. 2002 **Questions about DULCOLAX?** Call toll-free 1-888-285-9159
Shown in Product Identification Guide, page 503

DULCOLAX®
[dul' co-lax]
brand of bisacodyl USP
Suppositories of 10 mg
Laxative

Drug Facts:

Active Ingredient:
(in each suppository)   **Purpose:**
Bisacodyl USP, 10 mg .... Laxative

Uses:
- Relieves occasional constipation and irregularity.
- This product usually causes bowel movement in 15 minutes to 1 hour.

Warnings:
For rectal use only.
Do not use • When abdominal pain, nausea, or vomiting are present.
Ask a doctor before use if you have:
- Stomach pain, nausea or vomiting.
- A sudden change in bowel habits that lasts more than 2 weeks.

When using this product:
You may have abdominal discomfort, faintness, rectal burning and mild cramps.

Stop use and ask a doctor if:
- Rectal bleeding occurs or you fail to have a bowel movement after using a laxative. This may indicate a serious condition.
- You need to use a laxative for more than 1 week.

If pregnant or breast-feeding, ask a doctor before use. **Keep out of reach of children.** If swallowed, get medical help or contact a Poison Control Center right away.

Directions:

Adults and children 12 years and over	1 suppository once daily. Remove foil. Insert suppository well into rectum, pointed end first. Retain about 15 to 20 minutes.
Children 6 to under 12 years	1/2 suppository once daily.
Children under 6 years	Ask a doctor.

Other Information • Store at controlled room temperature 20–25°C (68–77°F).

Inactive Ingredients: Hydrogenated vegetable oil.

How Supplied: Boxes of 4 Comfort Shaped Suppositories Boehringer Ingelheim Consumer Healthcare Products. Division of Boehringer Ingelheim Pharmaceuticals, Inc., Ridgefield, CT 06877 Made in Italy. ©Boehringer Ingelheim Pharmaceuticals, Inc. 2002 **Questions?** 1-888-285-9159
Shown in Product Identification Guide, page 503

DULCOLAX®

Drug Facts:

Active Ingredient:
(in each softgel)   **Purpose:**
Docusate sodium USP, 100 mg .... Stool Softener

Uses:
- Temporary relief of occasional constipation.
- This product generally produces bowel movement within 12 to 72 hours.

Warnings:
Do not use:
- If abdominal pain, nausea or vomiting are present.
Ask a doctor before use if:
- You have noticed a sudden change in bowel habits that persists over a period of 2 weeks.
- You are presently taking mineral oil.
Stop use and ask a doctor if:
- Rectal bleeding or failure to have a bowel movement occur after use, which may indicate a serious condition.
- You need to use a laxative for more than 1 week.
If pregnant or breast-feeding, ask a health professional before use.
Keep out of reach of children. In case of overdose, get medical help or contact a Poison Control Center immediately.

Directions:

Adults and children 12 years and over.	Take 1 to 3 softgels daily.
Children 2 to under 12 years.	Take 1 softgel daily.
Children under 2 years.	Ask a doctor.

Other Information
- Each softgel contains: sodium, 5 mg
- Store at 15–30°C (59–86°F).
- Protect from excessive moisture.

Inactive Ingredients: FD&C Red #40, FD&C Yellow #6, gelatin, glycerin, polyethylene glycol, propylene glycol, purified water and sorbitol special.

How Supplied: Blister Pack of 10, and bottles of 25, 50, or 100 liquid gels. Boehringer Ingelheim Consumer Healthcare Products. Division of Boehringer Ingelheim Pharmaceuticals, Inc., Ridgefield, CT 06877 ©Boehringer Ingelheim Pharmaceuticals, Inc. 2002 **Questions about DULCOLAX?** Call toll-free 1-888-285-9159
*Among Stool Softener ingredients
Shown in Product Identification Guide, page 503

**FACED WITH AN
Rx SIDE EFFECT?**
Turn to the
Companion Drug Index
for products that
provide symptomatic
relief.

Cadbury Adams USA LLC
**182 TABOR ROAD
MORRIS PLAINS, NJ 07950**

Direct Inquiries to:
1-(800) 524-2854

For Consumer Product Information Call:
1-(800) 524-2854

HALLS FRUIT BREEZERS™
Pectin Throat Drops

Active Ingredient (in each drop):
Pectin 7 mg
Purpose:
Oral Demulcent

Uses: temporarily relieves the following symptoms associated with sore mouth and sore throat:
• minor discomfort
• irritated areas

Warnings:
Sore throat warning: if sore throat is severe, persists for more than 2 days, is accompanied or followed by fever, headache, rash, swelling, nausea, or vomiting, consult a doctor promptly. These may be serious.
Stop use and ask a doctor if
• sore mouth does not improve in 7 days
• irritation, pain, or redness persists or worsens
Keep out of reach of children.

Directions:
• adults and children 5 years and over: dissolve 1 or 2 drops (one at a time) slowly in the mouth. Repeat as needed.
• children under 5 years: ask a doctor
Cool Berry
Inactive Ingredients: FD&C blue no. 2, FD&C red no. 40, flavors, glucose syrup, partially hydrogenated cottonseed oil, sucrose, titanium dioxide, water
Cool Creamy Strawberry
Inactive Ingredients: beta carotene, carboxymethylcellulose sodium, FD&C blue no. 2, FD&C red no. 40, flavors, glucose syrup, sodium chloride, soy lecithin, sucrose, titanium dioxide, water

How Supplied: Halls Fruit Breezers are available in 2 flavors: Cool Berry and Cool Creamy Strawberry in bags of 25 and sticks of 9's.

HALLS MAX™
[hols]
Menthol/Benzocaine Oral Anesthetic

Active Ingredients (in each drop):
Benzocaine 6mg, Menthol 10mg
Purpose: Oral anesthetic

Uses: temporarily relieves occasional:
• minor irritation • sore throat

Warnings: Do not use this product if you have a history of allergy to local anesthetics such as procaine, butacaine, benzocaine or other "caine" anesthetics.
Sore throat warning: if sore throat is severe, persists for more than 2 days, is accompanied or followed by fever, headache, rash, swelling, nausea, or vomiting, consult a doctor promptly. These may be serious.
Stop use and ask a doctor if • sore mouth symptoms do not improve in 7 days • irritation, pain or redness persists or worsens
DO NOT EXCEED RECOMMENDED DOSAGE
Keep out of reach of children. In case of overdose, get medical help or contact a Poison Control Center right away. **If you are pregnant or breast feeding** ask a health professional before use.

Directions: • adults and children 5 years and over: dissolve 1 or 2 drops (one at a time) slowly in the mouth. Repeat every 2 hours as needed. • children under 5 years of age: ask a doctor

Inactive Ingredients: MENTHOL: corn syrup, FD&C blue no. 1, FD&C red no. 40, propylene glycol, sodium bicarbonate, sucrose, water. CHERRY: corn syrup, flavor, propylene glycol, sodium bicarbonate, sucrose, water. HONEY-LEMON: beta carotene, corn syrup, flavors, propylene glycol, sodium bicarbonate, soy lecithin, sucrose, water.

How Supplied: Halls Max™ Menthol/Benzocaine Oral Anesthetic are available in packages of 18. They are available in three flavors: Cherry, Menthol and Honey-Lemon.

HALLS® MENTHO-LYPTUS®
Cough Suppressant/Oral Anesthetic Drops
[Hols]

Active Ingredient: *MENTHO-LYPTUS*®: Menthol 6.5 mg per drop. *CHERRY:* Menthol 7 mg per drop. *HONEY-LEMON:* Menthol 8 mg per drop. *ICE BLUE*™ *PEPPERMINT:* Menthol 10 mg per drop. *SPEARMINT:* Menthol 5.6 mg per drop. *STRAWBERRY:* Menthol 3.1 mg per drop. *TROPICAL FRUIT:* Menthol 3.1 mg per drop.
Purposes: Cough suppressant, Oral anesthetic

Uses: temporarily relieves: • cough due to a cold • occasional minor irritation or sore throat

Warnings:
Sore throat warning: if sore throat is severe, persists for more than 2 days, is accompanied or followed by fever, headache, rash, swelling, nausea, or vomiting, consult a doctor promptly. These may be serious.
Ask a doctor if you have • persistent or chronic cough such as occurs with smoking, asthma, or emphysema • cough accompanied by excessive phlegm (mucus)

Stop use and ask a doctor if • cough persists for more than 1 week, tends to recur, or is accompanied by fever, rash, or persistent headache. These could be signs of a serious condition. • sore mouth does not improve in 7 days • irritation, pain, or redness persists or worsens
Keep out of reach of children.

Directions: *MENTHO-LYPTUS®, CHERRY, HONEY-LEMON, ICE BLUE™ PEPPERMINT and SPEARMINT:* • adults and children 5 years and over: dissolve 1 drop slowly in the mouth. Repeat every 2 hours as needed. • children under 5 years: ask a doctor.
STRAWBERRY and TROPICAL FRUIT: • adults and children 5 years and over: dissolve 2 drops (one at a time) slowly in the mouth. Repeat every 2 hours as needed. • children under 5 years: ask a doctor

Inactive Ingredients: *MENTHO-LYPTUS®:* flavors, glucose syrup, sucrose, water. *CHERRY:* FD&C blue no. 2, FD&C red no. 40, flavors, glucose syrup, sucrose, water. *HONEY-LEMON:* beta carotene, flavors, glucose syrup, honey, soy lecithin, sucrose, water. *ICE BLUE*™ *PEPPERMINT:* FD&C blue no. 1, flavors, glucose syrup, sucrose, water. *SPEARMINT:* beta carotene, FD&C blue no. 1, flavors, glucose syrup, soy lecithin, sucrose, water. *STRAWBERRY:* FD&C red no. 40, flavors, glucose syrup, sucrose, water. *TROPICAL FRUIT:* FD&C red no. 40, flavors, glucose syrup, sucrose, water.

How Supplied: Halls® *Mentho-Lyptus®* Cough Suppressant Drops are available in single sticks of 9 drops each and in bags of 30. They are available in seven flavors: *Regular Mentho-Lyptus®, Cherry, Honey-Lemon, Ice Blue*™ *Peppermint, Spearmint, Strawberry* and *Tropical Fruit.* Regular Mentho-Lyptus®, Cherry, Honey-Lemon, Strawberry flavors are also available in bags of 80 drops. *Mentho-Lyptus®, Cherry,* and *Strawberry* are also available in bags of 200 drops.

HALLS® PLUS
Cough Suppressant/Oral Anesthetic Drops
[Hols]

Active Ingredients: Each drop contains Menthol 10 mg.
Purposes: Cough suppressant, Oral anesthetic

Uses: temporarily relieves: • cough due to a cold • occasional minor irritation or sore throat

Warnings: Sore throat warning: if sore throat is severe, persists for more than 2 days, is accompanied or followed

Continued on next page

Halls Plus—Cont.

by fever, headache, rash, swelling, nausea, or vomiting, consult a doctor promptly. These may be serious.

Ask a doctor before use if you have • persistent or chronic cough such as occurs with smoking, asthma, or emphysema • cough accompanied by excessive phlegm (mucus)

Stop use and ask a doctor if • cough persists for more than 1 week, tends to recur, or is accompanied by fever, rash, or persistent headache. These could be signs of a serious condition. • sore mouth does not improve in 7 days • irritation, pain, or redness persists or worsens

Keep out of reach of children.

Directions: • adults and children 5 years and over: dissolve 1 drop slowly in the mouth. Repeat every 2 hours as needed. • children under 5 years: ask a doctor

Inactive Ingredients: MENTHO-LYPTUS®: carrageenan, flavors, glucose syrup, glycerin, partially hydrogenated cottonseed oil, pectin, soy lecithin, sucrose, water. CHERRY: carrageenan, FD&C blue no. 2, FD&C red no. 40, flavors, glucose syrup, glycerin, partially hydrogenated cottonseed oil, pectin, soy lecithin, sucrose, water. HONEY-LEMON: beta carotene, carrageenan, flavors, glucose syrup, glycerin, honey, partially hydrogenated cottonseed oil, pectin, sucrose, water.

How Supplied: Halls® Plus Cough Suppressant / Throat Drops are available in single sticks of 10 drops each and in bags of 25 drops. They are available in three flavors: Mentho-Lyptus®, Cherry and Honey-Lemon.

HALLS® SUGAR FREE HALLS® SUGAR FREE SQUARES MENTHO-LYPTUS®

Cough Suppressant/Oral Anesthetic Drops

[Hols]

Active Ingredient: Halls® Sugar Free: BLACK CHERRY and CITRUS BLEND™: Menthol 5 mg per drop. MOUNTAIN MENTHOL™: Menthol 5.8 mg per drop. HONEY-LEMON: 7.6 mg per drop. Assorted Mint: Peppermint: 9.4 mg per drop. Freshmint: 5.2 mg per drop. Spearmint: 5.0 mg per drop. Halls® Sugar Free Squares: BLACK CHERRY: Menthol 5.8 mg per drop. MOUNTAIN MENTHOL™: Menthol 6.8 mg per drop.

Purposes: Cough suppressant, Oral anesthetic

Uses: temporarily relieves: • cough due to a cold • occasional minor irritation or sore throat

Warnings:

Sore throat warning: if sore throat is severe, persists for more than 2 days, is accompanied or followed by fever, headache, rash, swelling, nausea, or vomiting, consult a doctor promptly. These may be serious.

Ask a doctor before use if you have • persistent or chronic cough such as occurs with smoking, asthma, or emphysema • cough accompanied by excessive phlegm (mucus)

Stop use and ask a doctor if • cough persists for more than 1 week, tends to recur, or is accompanied by fever, rash or persistent headache. These could be signs of a serious condition. • sore mouth does not improve in 7 days • irritation, pain, or redness persists or worsens

Keep out of reach of children.

Directions: • adults and children 5 years and over: dissolve 1 drop slowly in mouth. Repeat every 2 hours as needed. • children under 5 years: ask a doctor

Additional Information:

Halls® Sugar Free:

Exchange Information*:

1 Drop = Free Exchange

10 Drops = 1 Fruit

*The dietary exchanges are based on the *Exchange Lists for Meal Planning*, Copyright ©1989 by the American Diabetes Association, Inc. and the American Dietetic Association.

Excess consumption may have a laxative effect.

Inactive Ingredients: Halls Sugar Free drops and squares. BLACK CHERRY: acesulfame potassium, aspartame, carboxymethylcellulose sodium, FD&C blue no. 1, FD&C red no. 40, flavors, isomalt, water **Phenylketonurics: Contains Phenylalanine 2 mg Per Drop.** CITRUS BLEND™: acesulfame potassium, aspartame, carboxymethylcellulose sodium, flavors, isomalt, yellow 5 (tartrazine), water **Phenylketonurics: Contains Phenylalanine 2 mg Per Drop.** MOUNTAIN MENTHOL™: acesulfame potassium, aspartame, carboxymethylcellulose sodium, flavors, isomalt, water **Phenylketonurics: Contains Phenylalanine 2 mg Per Drop.** HONEY-LEMON: acesulfame potassium, aspartame, beta carotene, carboxymethylcellulose sodium, flavors, isomalt, water **Phenylketonurics: Contains Phenylalanine 2 mg Per Drop.** ASSORTED MINT: acesulfame potassium, aspartame, beta carotene, FD&C blue 1, flavors, isomalt, sodium carboxymethylcellulose, soy lecithin, water **Phenylketonurics: Contains Phenylalanine 2 mg Per Drop.**

How Supplied: Halls® Sugar Free: Halls® Sugar Free Mentho-Lyptus® Cough Suppressant Drops are available in bags of 25 drops. They are available in four flavors: Black Cherry, Citrus Blend™ and Mountain Menthol™ and Honey-Lemon. Also available in Assorted Mint flavors (Peppermint Spearmint and Freshmint™) Halls® Sugar Free

Squares: Halls® Sugar Free Squares Mentho-Lyptus® Cough Suppressant Drops are available in single sticks of 9 drops each. They are available in two flavors: Black Cherry and Mountain Menthol™.

HALLS DEFENSE® MULTI-BLEND SUPPLEMENT DROPS

Supplement Facts/Ingredients:
Supplement Facts
Serving Size 1 Drop

	Amount Per Drop	% Daily Value*
Calories	15	
Sodium	10 mg	<1%*
Total Carbohydrate	4 g	1%*
Sugars	3 g	†
Vitamin C	60 mg	100%
Zinc	1.5 mg	10%
Standard Echinacea Root Extract	15 mg	†

(Echinacea angustifolia and Echinacea purpurea)

* Percent Daily Values (DV) are based on a 2,000 calorie diet.
† Daily Value (DV) not established.

Other Ingredients: Sugar; Glucose Syrup; Sodium Ascorbate; Citric Acid; Partially Hydrogenated Cottonseed Oil; Natural Flavoring; Ascorbic Acid; Zinc Sulfate; Red 40; Oils of Angelica Root, Anise Star, Ginger, Lemon Grass, Sage and White Thyme; Blue 1.

Description: Halls Defense® Multi-Blend Supplement Drops help you keep going. Each drop provides 100% of the Daily Value of Vitamin C, Zinc to help support your natural resistance system**, plus Echinacea.

** This statement has not been evaluated by the Food & Drug Administration. This product is not intended to diagnose, treat, cure, or prevent any disease.

Indications: Dietary Supplementation

Warnings: Do not use if you have a severe systemic illness such as tuberculosis, leukosis, collagen disease, multiple sclerosis or similar condition. Do not use if you have allergies to the daisy family (Asteraceae). Do not use if you are pregnant or breast-feeding. Keep out of the reach of children.

Suggested Use: As a dietary supplement, take one drop 4 times per day. Not recommended for use for more than 8 weeks consecutively.

How Supplied: Halls Defense® Multi-Blend Supplement Drops are available in Harvest Cherry in bags of 25 drops.

HALLS DEFENSE® Sugarfree Vitamin C Supplement Drops Assorted Citrus

Supplement Facts/Ingredients
Supplement Facts
Serving Size 1 Drop

	Amount Per Drop	% Daily Value*
Calories	5	
Sodium	10 mg	<1 %
Total Carbohydrate	3 g	1%
Sugars	0 g	†
Sugars Alcohols	3 g	†
Vitamin C	60 mg	100%

* Percent Daily Values are based on a 2,000 calorie diet.
† Daily Value not established.

Other Ingredients: ASSORTED CITRUS: Isomalt, Sodium Ascorbate, Citric Acid, Natural Flavoring, Ascorbic Acid, Aspartame, Acesulfame Potassium, Beta Carotene (Color), Red 40, Soy Lecithin.
Phenylketonurics: Contains Phenylalanine Excess consumption may have a laxative effect.

Description: Halls Defense® Sugar Free Vitamin C Supplement Drops help keep you going, because each delicious, fruit-flavored drop delivers 100% of the Daily Value of Vitamin C.

Indications: Dietary Supplementation.

How Supplied: Assorted Citrus Halls Defense® Sugar Free Vitamin C Supplement Drops are available in the following all natural flavors: Lemon, Sweet Grapefruit, and Orange and are available in bags of 25 drops. Assortment in each package may vary.

TRIDENT WHITE®
[Tri-dent White]
Sugarless Gum with Recaldent

Ingredients: *PEPPERMINT*: Sorbitol, Gum Base, Maltitol, Mannitol, Artificial and Natural Flavoring; Less Than 2% of: Acacia, Acesulfame Potassium, Aspartame, BHT (To Maintain Freshness), Calcium Casein Peptone-Calcium Phosphate (Lactose-Free Milk Derivative)**, Candelilla Wax, Sodium Stearate and Titanium Dioxide (Color).
Contains a Milk Derived Ingredient.
Phenylketonurics: Contains Phenylalanine.

Ingredients: *WINTERGREEN:* Sorbitol, Gum Base, Maltitol, Mannitol, Artificial and Natural Flavoring; Less Than 2% of: Acacia, Acesulfame Potassium, Aspartame, BHT (To Maintain Freshness), Calcium Casein Peptone-Calcium Phosphate (Lactose-Free Milk Derivative)**, Candelilla Wax, Glycerin, Sodium Stearate, Soy Lecithin and Titanium Dioxide (Color).
Contains a Milk Derived Ingredient.
Phenylketonurics: Contains Phenylalanine.

Ingredients: *SPEARMINT*: Sorbitol, Gum Base, Maltitol, Mannitol, Artificial and Natural Flavoring; Less Than 2% of: Acacia, Acesulfame Potassium, Aspartame, BHT (To Maintain Freshness), Calcium Casein Peptone-Calcium Phosphate (Lactose-Free Milk Derivative)**, Candelilla Wax, Sodium Stearate, Soy Lecithin and Titanium Dioxide (Color).
Contains a Milk Derived Ingredient.
Phenylketonurics: Contains Phenylalanine.

Ingredients: *COOL RUSH:* Gum Base, Sorbitol, Maltitol, Mannitol, Natural and Artificial Flavoring; Less Than 2% of: Acacia, Acesulfame Potassium, Aspartame, BHT (To Maintain Freshness), Calcium Casein Peptane-Calcium Phosphate (Lactose-Free Milk Derivative)**, Candelilla Wax, Sodium Stearate and Titanium Dioxide (Color).
Contains a Milk Derived Ingredient.
Phenylketonurics: Contains Phenylalanine.

Ingredients: *CINNAMON TINGLE™:* Sorbitol, Gum Base, Maltitol, Natural and Artificial Flavoring, Mannitol, Less than 2% of: Acacia, Acesulfame Potassium, BHT (To Maintain Freshness), Calcium Casein Peptone-Calcium Phosphate (Lactose-Free Milk Derivative)** Candelilla Wax, Sodium Stearate, Soy Lecithin, Sucralose and Titanium Dioxide (Color).
Contains a Milk Derived Ingredient.
RECALDENT**: A patented ingredient derived from casein, a bovine phosphoprotein found in milk. RECALDENT is a trademark of Bonlac Bioscience International PTY LTD.

Description: Trident White® is a whitening gum that uses proprietary surfactant technology to help break up and gently remove stains from teeth. In addition to whitening teeth, chewing Trident White® remineralizes tooth enamel by delivering calcium and phosphate beneath the tooth's surface.

Directions: When used as a part of a daily oral care regimen, Trident White helps gently remove stains caused by common beverages and food items consumed every day.

How Supplied: Trident White® is available in Peppermint, Wintergreen Spearmint, Cool Rush and Cinnamon Tingle™ flavors in a 12-pellet blister foil.
Shown in Product Identification Guide, page 503

Celltech
Pharmaceuticals, Inc.
PO BOX 31766
ROCHESTER, NY 14603

Direct Inquiries to:
Customer Service Department
P.O. Box 31766
Rochester, NY 14603
(585) 274-5300
(888) 963-3382

DELSYM®
(dextromethorphan polistirex)
Extended-Release Suspension
12-Hour Cough Suppressant

DELSYM®
(dextromethorphan polistirex)
Extended-Release Suspension
12 Hour Cough Suppressant for Children

Active Ingredient (in each 5 mL teaspoonful): dextromethorphan polistirex equivalent to 30 mg dextromethorphan hydrobromide.
Purpose: Cough suppressant

Use: Temporarily relieves cough due to minor throat and bronchial irritation as may occur with the common cold or inhaled irritants.

Warnings: Do not use if you are now taking a prescription monoamine oxidase inhibitor (MAOI) (certain drugs for depression, psychiatric or emotional conditions, or Parkinson's disease), or for 2 weeks after stopping the MAOI drug. If you do not know if your prescription drug contains an MAOI, ask a doctor or pharmacist before taking this product.
Ask a doctor before use if you have
• chronic cough that lasts as occurs with smoking, asthma or emphysema
• cough that occurs with too much phlegm (mucus)
Stop use and ask a doctor if cough lasts more than 7 days, cough comes back, or occurs with fever, rash or headache that lasts. These could be signs of a serious condition.
If pregnant or breast-feeding, ask a health professional before use.
Keep out of reach of children. In case of overdose, get medical help or contact a Poison Control Center right away.

Directions:
• shake bottle well before use
• dose as follows or as directed by a doctor

Continued on next page

Delsym—Cont.

adults and children 12 years of age and over	2 teaspoonfuls every 12 hours, not to exceed 4 teaspoonfuls in 24 hours
children 6 to under 12 years of age	1 teaspoonful every 12 hours, not to exceed 2 teaspoonfuls in 24 hours
children 2 to under 6 years of age	½ teaspoonful every 12 hours, not to exceed 1 teaspoonful in 24 hours
children under 2 years of age	consult a doctor

Other Information:
• **each 5 mL teaspoonful contains:** sodium 5 mg
• store at 20°–25°C (68°–77°F)

Inactive Ingredients: alcohol 0.26%, citric acid, ethylcellulose, FD&C Yellow No. 6, flavor, high fructose corn syrup, methylparaben, polyethylene glycol 3350, polysorbate 80, propylene glycol, propylparaben, purified water, sucrose, tragacanth, vegetable oil, xanthan gum.

How Supplied:
89 mL (3 fl oz.) bottles
NDC 53014-842-61
148 ml (5 fl oz.) bottles
NDC 53014-842-56
Celltech Pharmaceuticals, Inc.
Rochester, NY 14623 USA
®Celltech Manufacturing, Inc.

GlaxoSmithKline Consumer Healthcare, L.P.

P.O. BOX 1467
PITTSBURGH, PA 15230

Direct Inquiries to:
Consumer Affairs
1-800-245-1040

For Medical Emergencies Contact:
Consumer Affairs
1-800-245-1040

ABREVA®
Cold Sore/Fever Blister Treatment Cream
Docosanol 10% Cream

Uses:
• Treats cold sore/fever blisters on the face or lips
• Shortens healing time and duration of symptoms: tingling, pain, burning, and/or itching

Active Ingredient: **Purpose:**
Docosanol 10% ... Cold sore/fever blister treatment

Inactive Ingredients: Benzyl alcohol, light mineral oil, propylene glycol, purified water, sucrose distearate, sucrose stearate.

Directions:
• **adults and children 12 years or over:**
  • wash hands before and after applying cream
  • apply to affected area on face or lips at the first sign of cold sore/fever blister (tingle). **Early treatment ensures the best results.**
  • rub in gently but completely
  • use 5 times a day until healed
• **children under 12 years:** ask a doctor

Warnings:
For external use only.
Do not use
• if you are allergic to any ingredient in this product
When using this product
• apply only to affected areas
• do not use in or near the eyes
• avoid applying directly inside your mouth
• do not share this product with anyone. This may spread infection.
Stop use and ask a doctor if
• your cold sore gets worse or the cold sore is not healed within 10 days
• **Keep out of reach of children.** If swallowed, get medical help or contact a poison control center right away.
Other Information:
• store at 20°–25°C (68°–77°F)
• do not freeze

How Supplied: Abreva Cream is supplied in 2.0 g [.07 oz] tubes.
Question? Call 1-877-709-3539 weekdays

Shown in Product Identification Guide, page 503

BC® POWDER
ARTHRITIS STRENGTH BC® POWDER
BC® COLD POWDER LINE

Description: BC® POWDER: **Active Ingredients:** Each powder contains Aspirin 650 mg, Salicylamide 195 mg and Caffeine 33.3 mg. **Inactive Ingredients:** Docusate Sodium, Fumaric Acid, Lactose Monohydrate and Potassium Chloride. ARTHRITIS STRENGTH BC® POWDER: **Active Ingredients:** Each powder contains Aspirin 742 mg, Salicylamide 222 mg and Caffeine 38 mg. **Inactive Ingredients:** Docusate Sodium, Fumaric Acid, Lactose Monohydrate and Potassium Chloride.
BC® ALLERGY SINUS COLD POWDER

Active Ingredients: Aspirin 650 mg, Pseudoephedrine Hydrochloride 60 mg and Chlorpheniramine Maleate 4 mg per powder. **Inactive Ingredients:** Fumaric Acid, Glycine, Lactose, Potassium Chloride, Silica, Sodium Lauryl Sulfate. BC® SINUS COLD POWDER. **Active Ingredients:** Aspirin 650 mg and Pseudoephedrine Hydrochloride 60 mg. per powder. **Inactive Ingredients:** Colloidal Silicon Dioxide, Microcrystalline Cellulose, Povidone, Pregelatinized Starch, Stearic Acid.

Indications: BC Powder is for relief of simple headache; for temporary relief of minor arthritic pain, for relief of muscular aches, discomfort and fever of colds; and for relief of normal menstrual pain and pain of tooth extraction.
Arthritis Strength BC Powder is specially formulated to fight occasional minor pain and inflammation of arthritis. Like Original Formula BC, Arthritis Strength BC provides fast temporary relief of minor arthritis pain and inflammation, relief of muscular aches, discomfort and fever of colds; and pain of tooth extraction.
BC Allergy Sinus Cold Powder is for relief of multiple symptoms such as body aches, fever, nasal congestion, sneezing, running nose, and watery itchy eyes associated with allergy and sinus attacks and the onset of colds. BC Sinus Cold Powder is for relief of such symptoms as body aches, fever, and nasal congestion.

BC Powder®, Arthritis
Strength BC® Powder and BC Cold Powder Line:

Warnings: **Children and teenagers should not use this medicine for chicken pox or flu symptoms before a doctor is consulted about Reye's Syndrome, a rare but serious illness reported to be associated with aspirin. Keep this and all medicines out of children's reach. In case of accidental overdose, contact a physician or poison control center immediately.**
As with any drug, if you are pregnant or nursing a baby seek the advice of a health professional before using this product.
IT IS ESPECIALLY IMPORTANT NOT TO USE ASPIRIN DURING THE LAST 3 MONTHS OF PREGNANCY UNLESS SPECIFICALLY DIRECTED TO DO SO BY A DOCTOR BECAUSE IT MAY CAUSE PROBLEMS IN THE UNBORN CHILD OR COMPLICATIONS DURING DELIVERY.

Alcohol Warning: If you consume 3 or more alcoholic drinks every day, ask your doctor whether you should take aspirin or other pain relievers/fever reducers. Aspirin may cause stomach bleeding.

Allergy Alert: Aspirin may cause a severe allergic reaction which may include hives, facial swelling, shock or asthma (wheezing). **Ask a doctor before use if you have** asthma, ulcers, a bleeding problem, stomach problems that last or come back such as heartburn, upset stomach or pain. **Ask a doctor or pharmacist before use** if you are taking a prescription drug for gout, diabetes, arthritis or anticoagulation (blood thinning). **Stop use and ask a doctor if** an allergic reaction occurs, ringing in ears or loss of hearing occurs, pain gets worse or persists for more than 10 days, fever lasts more than 3 days, redness or swelling is present, or new symptoms occur.

For BC Powder and Arthritis Strength BC Powder:

When using these products limit the use of caffeine containing drugs, foods, or drinks, because too much caffeine may cause nervousness, irritability, sleeplessness, and occasionally, rapid heartbeat. For BC Cold Powder Line:

Do not exceed recommended dosage. If nervousness, dizziness, or sleeplessness occur, discontinue use and consult a doctor. If symptoms do not improve within 7 days, or are accompanied by fever that lasts more than 3 days, or if new symptoms occur, consult a physician before continuing use. Do not take BC if you are sensitive to aspirin, or have heart disease, high blood pressure, thyroid disease, diabetes, asthma, glaucoma, emphysema, chronic pulmonary disease, shortness of breath, difficulty in breathing or difficulty in urination due to enlargement of the prostate gland, or if you are presently taking a prescription antihypertensive or antidepressant drug unless directed by a doctor. *"Drug interaction precaution.* Do not use this product if you are now taking a prescription monoamine oxidase inhibitor (MAOI) (certain drugs for depression, psychiatric or emotional conditions, or Parkinson's disease), or for 2 weeks after stopping the MAOI drug. If you are uncertain whether your prescription drug contains an MAOI, consult a health professional before taking this product." BC Allergy Sinus Cold Powder with antihistamine may cause drowsiness. Avoid alcoholic beverages when taking this product because it may increase drowsiness. Use caution when driving a motor vehicle or operating machinery. May cause excitability, especially in children.

Overdosage: In case of accidental overdosage, contact a physician or poison control center immediately.

Dosage and Administration: BC® Powder, Arthritis Strength BC® Powder, BC® Cold Powder Line:
Place one powder on tongue and follow with liquid. If you prefer, stir powder into glass of water or other liquid.
For BC Powder and Arthritis Strength BC Powder:
Adults and children 12 years and over: Take one powder every 3–4 hours not to exceed 4 powders in 24 hours.
For BC Cold Powder Line:
Adults and children 12 years and over: Take one powder every 6 hours not to exceed 4 powders in 24 hours. For children under 12, consult a physician.

How Supplied: BC Powder: Available in tamper evident overwrapped envelopes of 2 or 6 powders, as well as tamper evident boxes of 24 and 50 powders.
Arthritis Strength BC Powder: Available in tamper evident over wrapped envelopes of 6 powders, and tamper evident overwrapped boxes of 24 and 50 powders.
BC Cold Powder Line:
Available in tamper-evident overwrapped envelopes of 6 powders, as well

as tamper-evident boxes of 12 powders (For BC Allergy Sinus Cold Powder only).

Orange Flavor
CITRUCEL®
[sĭt 'rə-sĕl]
(Methylcellulose)
Bulk-forming Fiber Laxative

Description: Each 19 g adult dose (approximately one heaping measuring tablespoonful) contains Methylcellulose 2 g. Each 9.5 g child's dose (one-half the adult dose) contains Methylcellulose 1 g. Methylcellulose is a nonallergenic fiber. Also contains: Citric Acid, FD&C Yellow No. 6 Lake, Orange Flavors (natural and artificial), Potassium Citrate, Riboflavin, Sucrose, and other ingredients. Each adult dose contains approximately 3 mg of sodium and contributes 60 calories from Sucrose.

Actions: Promotes elimination by providing additional fiber (bulk) to the diet. This product generally produces bowel movement in 12 to 72 hours.

Indications: For relief of constipation (irregularity). May also be used for relief of constipation associated with other bowel disorders such as irritable bowel syndrome, diverticular disease, and hemorrhoids as well as for bowel management during postpartum, postsurgical, and convalescent periods when recommended by a physician.

Contraindications: Intestinal obstruction, fecal impaction, known hypersensitivity to formula ingredients.

Warnings: Patients should be instructed to consult their physician before using any laxative if they have noticed a sudden change in bowel habits which persists for two weeks. Unless directed by a physician, patients should be advised not to use laxative products when abdominal pain, nausea, or vomiting is present. Patients should also be advised to discontinue use and consult a physician if rectal bleeding or failure to have a bowel movement occurs after use of any laxative product. Unless recommended by a physician, patients should not exceed the recommended maximum daily dose. Patients should not use laxative products for a period longer than one week unless directed by a physician.
TAKING THIS PRODUCT WITHOUT ADEQUATE FLUID MAY CAUSE IT TO SWELL AND BLOCK YOUR THROAT OR ESOPHAGUS AND MAY CAUSE CHOKING. DO NOT TAKE THIS PRODUCT IF YOU HAVE DIFFICULTY IN SWALLOWING. IF YOU EXPERIENCE CHEST PAIN, VOMITING, OR DIFFICULTY IN SWALLOWING OR BREATHING AFTER TAKING THIS PRODUCT, SEEK IMMEDIATE MEDICAL ATTENTION. KEEP THIS AND ALL DRUGS OUT OF THE REACH OF CHILDREN.

Dosage and Administration: Adult Dose: dissolve one leveled scoop (one heaping tablespoon – 19g) in 8 ounces of cold water up to three times daily at the first sign of constipation. Children age 6 to 12 years of age: *one-half the adult dose* stirred briskly in 8 ounces of cold water, once daily at the first sign of constipation. The mixture should be administered promptly and drinking another glass of water is highly recommended (see Warnings). Children under 6 years of age: *Use only as directed by a physician.* Continued use for 12 to 72 hours may be necessary for full benefit.
TAKE THIS PRODUCT (CHILD OR ADULT DOSE) WITH AT LEAST 8 OZ. (A FULL GLASS) OF WATER OR OTHER FLUID. TAKING THIS PRODUCT WITHOUT ENOUGH LIQUID MAY CAUSE CHOKING. SEE WARNINGS.

How Supplied: 16 oz., 30 oz., and 50 oz. containers.
Boxes of 20-single-dose packets.
Store below 86°F (30°C). Protect contents from humidity; keep tightly closed.
Shown in Product Identification Guide, page 503

Sugar Free Orange Flavor
CITRUCEL®
[sĭt 'rə-sĕl]
(Methylcellulose)
Bulk-forming Fiber Laxative

Description: Each 10.2 g adult dose (approximately one rounded measuring tablespoonful) contains Methylcellulose 2 g. Each 5.1 g child's dose (one-half the adult dose) contains Methylcellulose 1 g. Methylcellulose is a nonallergenic fiber. Also contains: Aspartame, Dibasic Calcium Phosphate, FD&C Yellow No. 6 Lake, Malic Acid, Maltodextrin, Orange Flavors (natural and artificial), Potassium Citrate, and Riboflavin. Each 10.2 g dose contains approximately 3 mg of sodium and contributes 24 calories from Maltodextrin.

Actions: Promotes elimination by providing additional fiber (bulk) to the diet. This product generally produces bowel movement in 12 to 72 hours.

Indications: For relief of constipation (irregularity). May also be used for relief of constipation associated with other bowel disorders such as irritable bowel syndrome, diverticular disease, and hemorrhoids as well as for bowel management during postpartum, postsurgical, and convalescent periods when recommended by a physician.

Contraindications and Warnings: See entry for "Orange Flavor Citrucel".

Phenylketonurics: CONTAINS PHENYLALANINE 52 mg per adult dose. Individuals with phenylketonuria and other individuals who must restrict their intake of phenylalanine should be

Continued on next page

Citrucel Sugar Free—Cont.

warned that each 10.2 g adult dose contains aspartame which provides 52 mg of phenylalanine.

Dosage and Administration: Adult Dose: dissolve one leveled scoop (one rounded measuring tablespoon – 10.2 g) in 8 ounces of cold water up to three times daily at the first sign of constipation. Children age 6 to 12 years of age: *one-half the adult dose* stirred briskly into at least 8 ounces of cold water, once daily at the first sign of constipation. The mixture should be administered promptly and drinking another glass of water is highly recommended (see Warnings). Children under 6 years of age: *Use only as directed by a physician.* Continued use for 12 to 72 hours may be necessary for full benefit.
TAKE THIS PRODUCT (CHILD OR ADULT DOSE) WITH AT LEAST 8 OZ. (A FULL GLASS) OF WATER OR OTHER FLUID. TAKING THIS PRODUCT WITHOUT ENOUGH LIQUID MAY CAUSE CHOKING. SEE WARNINGS.

How Supplied:
8.6 oz, 16.9 oz, and 32 oz containers. Boxes of 20 single-dose packets. Store below 86°F (30°C). Protect contents from humidity; keep tightly closed.
Shown in Product Identification Guide, page 503

CITRUCEL®
(methylcellulose)
Soluble Fiber Caplet
Bulk-Forming Fiber Laxative

Uses: Helps restore and maintain regularity. Helps relieve constipation. Also useful in treatment of constipation (irregularity) associated with other bowel disorders when recommended by a physician. This product generally produces a bowel movement in 12 to 72 hours.

Active Ingredient: Each caplet contains 500mg Methylcellulose.

Inactive Ingredients: Crospovidone, Dibasic Calcium Phosphate, FD&C Yellow No. 6 Aluminum Lake, Magnesium Stearate, Maltodextrin, Povidone, Sodium Lauryl Sulfate.

Directions: Adult dose: Take two caplets as needed with 8 ounces of liquid, up to six times daily. Children (6–12 years): Take one caplet with 8 ounces of liquid, up to six times per day. The dosage requirement may vary according to the severity of constipation. Children under 6 years: consult a physician. **TAKE THIS PRODUCT (CHILD OR ADULT DOSE) WITH AT LEAST 8 OUNCES (A FULL GLASS) OF WATER OR OTHER FLUID. TAKING THIS PRODUCT WITHOUT ENOUGH LIQUID MAY CAUSE CHOKING. SEE WARNINGS.**

Directions for Use: Take each dose with 8oz. of liquid.

Age	Dose	Daily Maximum
Adults & Children over 12 years	2 Caplets	Up to 6 times daily*
Children (6 to 12 years)	1 Caplet	Up to 6 times daily*
Children under 6 years	Consult a physician	

*Refer to directions below.

Warnings: Consult a physician before using any laxative product if you have noticed a sudden change in bowel habits which persists for two weeks. Unless directed by a physician, do not use laxative products when abdominal pain, nausea, or vomiting are present. Discontinue use and consult a physician if rectal bleeding or failure to produce a bowel movement occurs after use of any laxative product. Unless recommended by a physician, do not exceed recommended maximum daily dose. Laxative products should not be used for a period longer than a week unless directed by a physician. If sensitive to any of the ingredients, do not use. **TAKING THIS PRODUCT WITHOUT ADEQUATE FLUID MAY CAUSE IT TO SWELL AND BLOCK YOUR THROAT OR ESOPHAGUS AND MAY CAUSE CHOKING. DO NOT TAKE THIS PRODUCT IF YOU HAVE DIFFICULTY IN SWALLOWING. IF YOU EXPERIENCE CHEST PAIN, VOMITING, OR DIFFICULTY IN SWALLOWING OR BREATHING AFTER TAKING THIS PRODUCT, SEEK IMMEDIATE MEDICAL ATTENTION. KEEP THIS AND ALL DRUGS OUT OF THE REACH OF CHILDREN.**

Store at room temperature 15–30°C (59–86°F). Protect contents from moisture.

Tamper evident feature: Bottle sealed with printed foil under cap. Do not use if foil is torn or broken.

How Supplied: Bottles of 100 and 164 caplets

Questions or comments?

Call toll-free 1-800-897-6081 weekdays.

Patents Pending

The various Citrucel Logos and design elements of the packaging are Registered Trademarks of GlaxoSmithKline.

©2004 GlaxoSmithKline

Distributed by:

GlaxoSmithKline Consumer Healthcare

GlaxoSmithKline Consumer Healthcare, L.P.

Moon Township, PA 15108, Made in Canada.

CONTAC® Non-Drowsy Decongestant
12 Hour Cold Caplets

Product Information: Each Maximum Strength Contac 12 Hour Cold Caplet provides up to 12 hours of relief. Part of the caplet goes to work right away for fast relief; the rest is released gradually to provide up to 12 hours of prolonged relief. With just one caplet in the morning and one at bedtime, you feel better all day, sleep better at night, breathing freely without congestion or sinus pressure.

Indications: Temporarily relieves nasal congestion due to the common cold, hay fever or other upper respiratory allergies and associated with sinusitis. Helps decongest sinus openings and passages; temporarily relieves sinus congestion and pressure.

Directions: Adults and children over 12 years of age: One caplet every 12 hours, not to exceed 2 caplets in 24 hours, or as directed by a doctor. Children under 12 years of age: consult a doctor.

TAMPER-EVIDENT PACKAGING FEATURES FOR YOUR PROTECTION:
Each caplet is encased in a plastic cell with a foil back; do not use if cell or foil is broken.

Warnings: Do not exceed the recommended dosage. If nervousness, dizziness, or sleeplessness occur, discontinue use and consult a doctor. If symptoms do not improve within 7 days or are accompanied by high fever, consult a doctor. Do not take this product, unless directed by a doctor, if you have heart disease, high blood pressure, thyroid disease, diabetes, glaucoma or difficulty in urination due to enlargement of the prostate gland. KEEP THIS AND ALL DRUGS OUT OF REACH OF CHILDREN. IN CASE OF ACCIDENTAL OVERDOSE, SEEK PROFESSIONAL ASSISTANCE OR CONTACT A POISON CONTROL CENTER IMMEDIATELY. As with any drug, if you are pregnant or nursing a baby, seek the advice of a health professional before using this product.

Drug Interaction Precaution: Do not use this product if you are now taking a prescription monoamine oxidase inhibitor (MAOI) (certain drugs for depression, psychiatric or emotional conditions, or Parkinson's disease), or for 2 weeks after stopping the MAOI drug. If you are uncertain whether your prescription drug contains an MAOI, consult a health professional before taking this product.

Active Ingredient: Pseudoephedrine Hydrochloride 120 mg.

Store at 15° to 25°C (59° to 77°F) in a dry place and protest from light.

Each Caplet Also Contains: Carnauba Wax, Colloidal Silicon Dioxide, Dibasic

Calcium Phosphate, Hypromellose, Magnesium Stearate, Microcrystalline Cellulose, Polyethylene Glycol, Polysorbate 80, Titanium Dioxide.

How Supplied: Consumer packages of 10 and 20 caplets.

Note: There are other CONTAC products. Make sure this is the one you are interested in. See the table below for all of the products in the CONTAC line.

Shown in Product Identification Guide, page 504

CONTAC® Non-Drowsy Timed Release-Maximum Strength 12 Hour Cold Caplets

Indications: For the temporary relief of nasal congestion due to the common cold, hay fever or other upper respiratory allergies, and nasal congestion associated with sinusitis. Promotes nasal and/or sinus drainage; temporarily relieves sinus congestion and pressure. Temporarily restores freer breathing through the nose.

Each Maximum Strength Contac 12-Hour Cold caplet provides up to 12 hours of relief. Part of the caplet goes to work right away for fast relief; the rest is released gradually to provide up to 12 hours of prolonged relief. With just one caplet in the morning and one at bedtime, you feel better all day, sleep better at night, breathing freely without congestion or sinus pressure.

Active Ingredient: Each coated extended-release caplet contains Pseudoephedrine Hydrochloride 120 mg.

Inactive Ingredients: carnauba wax, collodial silicon dioxide, dibasic calcium phosphate, hypromellose, magnesium stearate, microcrystalline cellulose, polyethylene glycol, polysorbate 80, titanium dioxide.

Directions: Adults and children 12 years of age and over – One caplet every 12 hours, not to exceed two caplets in 24 hours. This product is not recommended for children under 12 years of age.

Warnings: Do not exceed recommended dosage. If nervousness, dizziness, or sleeplessness occur, discontinue use and consult a doctor. If symptoms do not improve within 7 days or are accompanied by fever, consult a doctor. Do not take this product if you have heart disease, high blood pressure, thyroid disease, diabetes, or difficulty in urination due to enlargement of the prostate gland unless directed by a doctor. As with any drug, if you are pregnant or nursing a baby, seek the advice of a health professional before using this product.

Drug Interaction Precaution: Do not use this product if you are now taking a prescription monoamine oxidase inhibitor (MAOI) (certain drugs for depression, psychiatric or emotional conditions, or Parkinson's disease), or for 2 weeks after stopping the MAOI drug. If you are uncertain whether your prescription contains an MAOI, consult a health professional before taking this product. **KEEP THIS AND ALL DRUGS OUT OF THE REACH OF CHILDREN.** In case of accidental overdose, seek professional assistance or contact a Poison Control Center immediately.

Store at 15° to 25°C (59° to 77°F) in a dry place and protect from light.

How Supplied: Packets of 10 and 20 Caplets

U.S. Patent No. 5,895,663

Comments or questions?

Call toll-free 1-800-245-1040 weekdays.

CONTAC® Severe Cold and Flu Caplets Maximum Strength Analgesic• Decongestant Antihistamine• Cough Suppressant
CONTAC® Severe Cold and Flu Caplets Non-Drowsy Nasal Decongestant • Analgesic• Cough Suppressant

Active Ingredients: Each *Non-Drowsy Caplet* contains Acetaminophen 325 mg, Psudoephedrine HCl 30 mg and Dextromethorphan Hydrobromide 15 mg.

Each *Maximum Strength Caplet* contains Acetaminophen 500 mg, Dextromethorphan Hydrobromide 15 mg, Pseudoephedrine HCl 30 mg and chlorpheniromine Maleate 2 mg.

Product Information: Two caplets every 6 hours to help relieve the discomforts of severe colds with flu-like symptoms.

Indications: *Non-Drowsy & Maximum Strength Caplets:* Temporarily relieves nasal congestion & coughing due to the common cold. Provides temporary relief of fever, sore throat, headache & minor aches associated with the common cold or the flu.

Maximum Strength Caplets: Temporarily relieves runny nose, sneezing, itchy and watery eyes due to the common cold.

Directions: Adults (12 years and older): Two caplets every 6 hours, not to exceed 8 caplets in any 24-hour period, or as directed by a doctor. Children under 12 years of age: consult a doctor.

TAMPER-EVIDENT PACKAGING FEATURES FOR YOUR PROTECTION:

Caplets are encased in a plastic cell with a foil back; do not use if cell or foil is broken. The letters ND SCF for non-drowsy and SCF for maximum strength appear on each caplet; do not use this product if these letters are missing.

Warnings: For *Non-Drowsy and Maximum Strength Caplets:* Do not exceed recommended dosage. If nervousness, dizziness, or sleeplessness occur, discontinue use and consult a doctor. If symptoms do not improve or are accompanied by fever that lasts for more than 3 days, or if new symptoms occur, consult a doctor. If sore throat is severe, persists for more than 2 days, is accompanied or followed by fever, headache, rash, nausea, or vomiting, consult a doctor promptly. A persistent cough may be a sign of a serious condition. If cough persists for more than 7 days, tends to recur, or is accompanied by rash, persistent headache, fever that lasts for more than 3 days, or if new symptoms occur, consult a doctor. Do not take this product for persistent or chronic cough such as occurs with smoking, asthma, emphysema, or if cough is accompanied by excessive phlegm (mucus) unless directed by a doctor. Do not take this product if you have heart disease, high blood pressure, thyroid disease, diabetes, glaucoma or difficulty in urination due to enlargement of the prostate gland unless directed by a doctor. **Alcohol Warning:** If you consume 3 or more alcoholic drinks every day, ask your doctor whether you should take acetaminophen or other pain relievers/fever reducers. Acetaminophen may cause liver damage. **KEEP THIS AND ALL DRUGS OUT OF THE REACH OF CHILDREN.** Prompt medical attention is critical for adults as well as for children even if you do not notice any signs or symptoms. In case of accidental overdose, seek professional assistance or contact a Poison Control Center immediately. As with any drug, if you are pregnant or nursing a baby, seek the advice of a health professional before using this product.

**Additional Warnings for *Maximum Strength Caplets:* May cause excitability especially in children. Do not take this product, unless directed by a doctor, if you have a breathing problem such as emphysema or chronic bronchitis. May cause marked drowsiness: alcohol, sedatives, and tranquilizers may increase the drowsiness effect. Avoid taking alcoholic beverages while taking this product. Do not take this product if you are taking sedatives or tranquilizers, without first consulting your doctor. Use caution when driving a motor vehicle or operating machinery.

Drug Interaction Precaution: Do not use this product if you are now taking a prescription monoamine oxidase inhibitor (MAOI) (certain drugs for depression, psychiatric or emotional conditions, or Parkinson's disease), or for 2 weeks after stopping the MAOI drug. If you are uncertain whether your prescription drug contains an MAOI, consult a health professional before taking this product.

Inactive Ingredients: Each *Non-Drowsy and Maximum Strength Caplet* contains: Carnauba Wax, Colloidal Silicon Dioxide, Hypromellose, Magnesium stearate, Microcrystalline Cellulose,

Continued on next page

PDR For Nonprescription Drugs

	CONTAC Non-Drowsy 12 Hour Cold Caplets	CONTAC 12 Hour Cold Capsules	CONTAC Severe Cold and Flu Caplets Maximum Strength (each 2 caplet dose)	CONTAC Severe Cold and Flu Non-Drowsy Caplets (each 2 caplet dose)	CONTAC Day & Night Cold & Flu	
					Day Caplets	Night Caplets
Phenylpropanolamine HCl	—	75.0 mg	—	—	—	—
Chlorpheniramine Maleate	—	8.0 mg	4.0 mg	—	—	—
Pseudoephedrine HCl	120 mg	—	60 mg	60.0 mg	60.0 mg	60.0 mg
Acetaminophen	—	—	1000.0 mg	650.0 mg	650.0 mg	650.0 mg
Dextromethorphan Hydrobromide	—	—	30.0 mg	30.0 mg	30.0 mg	—
Diphenhydramine HCl	—	—	—	—	—	50.0 mg

Contac Sev. Cold/Flu—Cont.

Polyethylene Glycol, Polysorbate 80, Starch, Stearic Acid, Titanium Dioxide. Each **Maximum Strength Caplet** also contains: FD&C Blue #1 Al Lake.

Avoid storing at high temperature (greater than 100°F).

How Supplied: Non-Drowsy: Consumer packages of 16. **Maximum Strength:** Consumer packages of 16 & 30.

Product Change: Maximum Strength Caplets now with new decongestant (pseudoephedrine HCl).

Note: There are other CONTAC products. Make sure this is the one you are interested in. See the table below for all of the products in the CONTAC line.
[See table above]
Shown in Product Identification Guide, page 504

DEBROX® Drops
Ear Wax Removal Aid

Active Ingredient: **Purpose:**
Carbamide peroxide
  6.5% non USP* .. Earwax removal aid

Actions: DEBROX®, used as directed, cleanses the ear with sustained microfoam. DEBROX Drops foam on contact with earwax due to the release of oxygen (there may be an associated crackling sound). DEBROX Drops provide a safe, nonirritating method of softening and removing ear wax.

Uses: For occasional use as an aid to soften, loosen, and remove excessive earwax.

Directions: Adults and children over 12 years of age: tilt head sideways and place 5 to 10 drops into ear. Tip of applicator should not enter ear canal. Keep drops in ear for several minutes by keeping head tilted or placing cotton in the ear. Use twice daily for up to four days if needed, or as directed by a doctor. Any wax remaining after treatment may be removed by gently flushing the ear with warm water, using a soft rubber bulb ear syringe. Children under 12 years of age: consult a doctor.

Warnings: FOR USE IN THE EAR ONLY. Do not use if you have ear drainage or discharge, ear pain, irritation or rash in the ear, or are dizzy; consult a doctor. Do not use if you have an injury or perforation (hole) of the eardrum or after ear surgery unless directed by a doctor. Do not use for more than four days. If excessive earwax remains after use of this product, consult a doctor. Avoid contact with the eyes. In case of accidental ingestion, seek professional assistance or contact a poison control center immediately.

Other Information: Avoid exposing bottle to excessive heat and direct sunlight. Keep tip on bottle when not in use. Product foams on contact with earwax due to release of oxygen. There may be an associated "crackling" sound. Keep this and all drugs out of the reach of children.

Inactive Ingredients: citric acid, flavor, glycerin, propylene glycol, sodium lauroyl sarcosinate, sodium stannate, water

How Supplied: DEBROX Drops are available in ½-fl-oz or 1-fl-oz (15 or 30 ml) plastic squeeze bottles with applicator spouts.
Questions or comments? 1-800-245-1040 weekdays.
Shown in Product Identification Guide, page 504

ECOTRIN
Enteric-Coated Aspirin
Antiarthritic, Antiplatelet
COMPREHENSIVE PRESCRIBING INFORMATION

Description: Ecotrin enteric coated aspirin (acetylsalicylic acid) tablets available in 81mg, 325mg and 500 mg tablets for oral administration. The 325 mg and 500 mg tablets contain the following inactive ingredients: Carnuba Wax, Colloidal Silicon Dioxide, FD&C Yellow No. 6, Hypromellose, Methacrylic Acid Copolymer, Microcrystalline Cellulose, Pregelatinized Starch, Propylene Glycol, Simethicone, Sodium Starch Glycolate, Stearic Acid, Talc, Titanium Dioxide, and Triethyl Citrate. The 81 mg tablets contain Carnuba Wax, Corn Starch, D&C Yellow No. 10, FD&C Yellow No. 6, Hypromellose, Methacrylic Acid Copolymer, Microcrystalline Cellulose, Propylene Glycol, Simethicone, Stearic Acid, Talc and Triethyl Citrate.

Aspirin is an odorless white, needle-like crystalline or powdery substance. When exposed to moisture, aspirin hydrolyzes into salicylic and acetic acids, and gives off a vinegary-odor. It is highly lipid soluble and slightly soluble in water.

Clinical Pharmacology: Mechanism of Action: Aspirin is a more potent inhibitor of both prostaglandin synthesis and platelet aggregation than other salicylic acid derivatives. The differences in activity between aspirin and salicylic acid are thought to be due to the acetyl group on the aspirin molecule. This acetyl group is responsible for the inactivation of cyclooxygenase via acetylation.

PHARMACOKINETICS

Absorption: In general, immediate release aspirin is well and completely absorbed from the gastrointestinal (GI) tract. Following absorption, aspirin is hydrolyzed to salicylic acid with peak plasma levels of salicylic acid occurring within 1–2 hours of dosing (see Pharmacokinetics—Metabolism). The rate of absorption from the GI tract is dependent upon the dosage form, the presence or absence of food, gastric pH (the presence or absence of GI antacids or buffering agents), and other physiologic factors. Enteric coated aspirin products are erratically absorbed from the GI tract.

Distribution: Salicylic acid is widely distributed to all tissues and fluids in the body including the central nervous system (CNS), breast milk, and fetal tissues. The highest concentrations are found in the plasma, liver, renal cortex, heart, and lungs. The protein binding of salicylate is concentration-dependent, i.e., non-linear. At low concentrations (< 100 mcg/mL) approximately 90 percent of plasma salicylate is bound to albumin while at higher concentrations (> 400 mcg/mL), only about 75 percent is bound. The early signs of salicylic overdose (salicylism), including tinnitus (ringing in the ears), occur at plasma concentrations approximating 200 mcg/mL. Severe toxic effects are associated with levels > 400 mcg/mL (See Adverse Reactions and Overdosage.)

Metabolism: Aspirin is rapidly hydrolyzed in the plasma to salicylic acid such that plasma levels of aspirin are essentially undetectable 1–2 hours after dosing. Salicylic acid is primarily conjugated in the liver to form salicyluric acid, a phenolic glucuronide, an acyl glucuronide, and a number of minor metabolites. Salicylic acid has a plasma half-life of approximately 6 hours. Salicylate metabolism is saturable and total body clearance decreases at higher serum concentrations due to the limited ability of the liver to form both salicyluric acid and phenolic glucuronide. Following toxic doses (10–20 grams (g)), the plasma half-life may be increased to over 20 hours.

Elimination: The elimination of salicylic acid follows zero order pharmacokinetics; (i.e., the rate of drug elimination is constant in relation to plasma concentration). Renal excretion of unchanged drug depends upon urine pH. As urinary pH rises above 6.5, the renal clearance of free salicylate increases from < 5 percent to > 80 percent. Alkalinization of the urine is a key concept in the management of salicylate overdose. (See Overdosage.) Following therapeutic doses, approximately 10 percent is found excreted in the urine as salicylic acid, 75 percent as salicyluric acid, and 10 percent phenolic and 5 percent acyl glucuronides of salicylic acid.

Pharmacodynamics: Aspirin affects platelet aggregation by irreversibly inhibiting prostaglandin cyclo-oxygenase. This effect lasts for the life of the platelet and prevents the formation of the platelet aggregating factor thromboxane A2. Non-acetylated salicylates do not inhibit this enzyme and have no effect on platelet aggregation. At somewhat higher doses, aspirin reversibly inhibits the formation of prostaglandin 1_2 (prostacyclin), which is an arterial vasodilator and inhibits platelet aggregation.

At higher doses aspirin is an effective anti-inflammatory agent, partially due to inhibition of inflammatory mediators via cyclooxygenase inhibition in peripheral tissues. In vitro studies suggest that other mediators of inflammation may also be suppressed by aspirin administration, although the precise mechanism of action has not been elucidated. It is this non-specific suppression of cyclooxygenase activity in peripheral tissues following large doses that leads to its primary side effect of gastric irritation. (See Adverse Reactions.)

Clinical Studies: Ischemic Stroke and Transient Ischemic Attack (TIA): In clinical trials of subjects with TIA's due to fibrin platelet emboli or ischemic stroke, aspirin has been shown to significantly reduce the risk of the combined endpoint of stroke or death and the combined endpoint of TIA, stroke, or death by about 13–18 percent.

Suspect Acute Myocardial Infarction (MI): In a large, multi-center study of aspirin, streptokinase, and the combination of aspirin and streptokinase in 17,187 patients with suspected acute MI, aspirin treatment produced a 23-percent reduction in the risk of vascular mortality. Aspirin was also shown to have an additional benefit in patients given a thrombolytic agent.

Prevention of Recurrent MI and Unstable Angina Pectoris: These indications are supported by the results of six large, randomized, multi-center, placebo-controlled trials of predominantly male post-MI subjects and one randomized placebo-controlled study of men with unstable angina pectoris. Aspirin therapy in MI subjects was associated with a significant reduction (about 20 percent) in the risk of the combination endpoint of subsequent death and/or nonfatal reinfarction in these patients. In aspirin-treated unstable angina patients the event rate was reduced to 5 percent from the 10 percent rate in the placebo group.

Chronic Stable Angina Pectoris: In a randomized, multi-center, double-blind trial designed to assess the role of aspirin for prevention of MI in patients with chronic stable angina pectoris, aspirin significantly reduced the primary combined endpoint of nonfatal MI, fatal MI, and sudden death by 34 percent. The secondary endpoint for vascular events (first occurrence of MI, stroke, or vascular death) was also significantly reduced (32 percent).

Revascularization Procedures: Most patients who undergo coronary artery revascularization procedures have already had symptomatic coronary artery disease for which aspirin is indicated. Similarly, patients with lesions of the carotid bifurcation sufficient to require carotid endarterectomy are likely to have had a precedent event. Aspirin is recommended for patients who undergo revascularization procedures if there is a pre-existing condition for which aspirin is already indicated.

Rheumatologic Diseases: In clinical studies in patients with rheumatoid arthritis, juvenile rheumatoid arthritis, ankylosing spondylitis and osteoarthritis, aspirin has been shown to be effective in controlling various indices of clinical disease activity.

Animal Toxicology: The acute oral 50 percent lethal dose in rats is about 1.5 g/kg and in mice 1.1 g/kg. Renal papillary necrosis and decreased urinary concentrating ability occur in rodents chronically administered high doses. Dose-dependent gastric mucosal injury occurs in rats and humans. Mammals may develop aspirin toxicosis associated with GI symptoms, circulatory effects, and central nervous system depression. (See Overdosage.)

Indications and Usage: Vascular Indications (Ischemic Stroke, TIA, Acute MI, Prevention of Recurrent MI, Unstable Angina Pectoris, and Chronic Stable Angina Pectoris): Aspirin is indicated to: (1) Reduce the combined risk of death and nonfatal stroke in patients who have had ischemic stroke or transient ischemia of the brain due to fibrin platelet emboli, (2) reduce the risk of vascular mortality in patients with a suspected acute MI, (3) reduce the combined risk of death and nonfatal MI in patients with a previous MI or unstable angina pectoris, and (4) reduce the combined risk of MI and sudden death in patients with chronic stable angina pectoris.

Revascularization Procedures (Coronary Artery Bypass Graft (CABG), Percutaneous Transluminal Coronary Angioplasty (PTCA), and Carotid Endarterectomy): Aspirin is indicated in patients who have undergone revascularization procedures (i.e., CABG, PTCA, or carotid endarterectomy) when there is a pre-existing condition for which aspirin is already indicated.

Rheumatologic Disease Indications (Rheumatoid Arthritis, Juvenile Rheumatoid Arthritis, Spondyloarthropathies, Osteoarthritis, and the Arthritis and Pleurisy of Systemic Lupus Erythematosus (SLE)): Aspirin is indicated for the relief of the signs and symptoms of rheumatoid arthritis, juvenile rheumatoid arthritis, osteoarthritis, spondyloarthropathies, and arthritis and pleurisy associated with SLE.

Contraindications: Allergy: Aspirin is contraindicated in patients with known allergy to nonsteroidal anti-inflammatory drug products and in patients with the syndrome of asthma, rhinitis, and nasal polyps. Aspirin may cause severe urticaria, angioedema, or bronchospasm (asthma).

Reye's Syndrome: Aspirin should not be used in children or teenagers for viral infections, with or without fever, because of the risk of Reye's syndrome with concomitant use of aspirin in certain viral illnesses.

Warnings: Alcohol Warning: Patients who consume three or more alcoholic drinks every day should be counseled about the bleeding risks involved with chronic, heavy alcohol use while taking aspirin.

Coagulation Abnormalities: Even low doses of aspirin can inhibit platelet function leading to an increase in bleeding time. This can adversely affect patients with inherited (hemophilia) or acquired (liver disease or vitamin K deficiency) bleeding disorders.

GI Side Effects: GI side effects include stomach pain, heartburn, nausea, vomiting, and gross GI bleeding. Although mi-

Continued on next page

Ecotrin—Cont.

nor upper GI symptoms, such as dyspepsia, are common and can occur anytime during therapy, physicians should remain alert for signs of ulceration and bleeding, even in the absence of previous GI symptoms. Physicians should inform patients about the signs and symptoms of GI side effects and what steps to take if they occur.

Peptic Ulcer Disease: Patients with a history of active peptic ulcer disease should avoid using aspirin, which can cause gastric mucosal irritation and bleeding.

Precautions
General

Renal Failure: Avoid aspirin in patients with severe renal failure (glomerular filtration rate less than 10 mL/minute).

Hepatic Insufficiency: Avoid aspirin in patients with severe hepatic insufficiency.

Sodium Restricted Diets: Patients with sodium-retaining states, such as congestive heart failure or renal failure, should avoid sodium-containing buffered aspirin preparations because of their high sodium content.

Laboratory Tests: Aspirin has been associated with elevated hepatic enzymes, blood urea nitrogen and serum creatinine, hyperkalemia, proteinuria, and prolonged bleeding time.

Drug Interactions

Angiotensin Converting Enzyme (ACE) Inhibitors: The hyponatremic and hypotensive effects of ACE inhibitors may be diminished by the concomitant administration of aspirin due to its direct effect on the renin-angiotensin conversion pathway.

Acetazolamide: Concurrent use of aspirin and acetazolamide can lead to high serum concentrations of acetazolamide (and toxicity) due to competition at the renal tubule for secretion.

Anticoagulant Therapy (Heparin and Warfarin): Patients on anticoagulation therapy are at increased risk for bleeding because of drug-drug interactions and the effect on platelets. Aspirin can displace warfarin from protein binding sites, leading to prolongation of both the prothrombin time and the bleeding time. Aspirin can increase the anticoagulant activity of heparin, increasing bleeding risk.

Anticonvulsants: Salicylate can displace protein-bound phenytoin and valproic acid, leading to a decrease in the total concentration of phenytoin and an increase in serum valproic acid levels.

Beta Blockers: The hypotensive effects of beta blockers may be diminished by the concomitant administration of aspirin due to inhibition of renal prostaglandins, leading to decreased renal blood flow, and salt and fluid retention.

Diuretics: The effectiveness of diuretics in patients with underlying renal or cardiovascular disease may be diminished by the concomitant administration of aspirin due to inhibition of renal prostaglandins, leading to decreased renal blood flow and salt and fluid retention.

Methotrexate: Salicylate can inhibit renal clearance of methotrexate, leading to bone marrow toxicity, especially in the elderly or renal impaired.

Nonsteroidal Anti-inflammatory Drugs (NSAID's): The concurrent use of aspirin with other NSAID's should be avoided because this may increase bleeding or lead to decreased renal function.

Oral Hypoglycemics: Moderate doses of aspirin may increase the effectiveness of oral hypoglycemic drugs, leading to hypoglycemia.

Uricosuric Agents (Probenecid and Sulfinpyrazone): Salicylates antagonize the uricosuric action of uricosuric agents.

Carcinogenesis, Mutagenesis, Impairment of Fertility: Administration of aspirin for 68 weeks at 0.5 percent in the feed of rats was not carcinogenic. In the Ames Salmonella assay, aspirin was not mutagenic; however, aspirin did induce chromosome aberrations in cultured human fibroblasts. Aspirin inhibits ovulation in rats. (See Pregnancy.)

Pregnancy: Pregnant women should only take aspirin if clearly needed. Because of the known effects of NSAID's on the fetal cardiovascular system (closure of the ductus arteriosus), use during the third trimester of pregnancy should be avoided. Salicylate products have also been associated with alterations in maternal and neonatal hemostasis mechanisms, decreased birth weight, and with perinatal mortality.

Labor and Delivery: Aspirin should be avoided 1 week prior to and during labor and delivery because it can result in excessive blood loss at delivery. Prolonged gestation and prolonged labor due to prostaglandin inhibition have been reported.

Nursing Mothers: Nursing mothers should avoid using aspirin because salicylate is excreted in breast milk. Use of high doses may lead to rashes, platelet abnormalities, and bleeding in nursing infants.

Pediatric Use: Pediatric dosing recommendations for juvenile rheumatoid arthritis are based on well-controlled clinical studies. An initial dose of 90–130 mg/kg/day in divided doses, with an increase as needed for anti-inflammatory efficacy (target plasma salicylate levels of 150–300 mcg/mL) are effective. At high doses (i.e., plasma levels of greater than 200 mg/mL), the incidence of toxicity increases.

Adverse Reactions: Many adverse reactions due to aspirin ingestion are dose-related. The following is a list of adverse reactions that have been reported in the literature. (See Warnings.)

Body as a Whole: Fever, hypothermia, thirst.

Cardiovascular: Dysrhythmias, hypotension, tachycardia.

Central Nervous System: Agitation, cerebral edema, coma, confusion, dizziness, headache, subdural or intracranial hemorrhage, lethargy, seizures.

Fluid and Electrolyte: Dehydration, hyperkalemia, metabolic acidosis, respiratory alkalosis.

Gastrointestinal: Dyspepsia, GI bleeding, ulceration and perforation, nausea, vomiting, transient elevations of hepatic enzymes, hepatitis, Reye's Syndrome, pancreatitis.

Hematologic: Prolongation of the prothrombin time, disseminated intravascular coagulation, coagulopathy, thrombocytopenia.

Hypersensitivity: Acute anaphylaxis, angioedema, asthma, bronchospasm, laryngeal edema, urticaria.

Musculoskeletal: Rhabdomyolysis.

Metabolism: Hypoglycemia (in children), hyperglycemia.

Reproductive: Prolonged pregnancy and labor, stillbirths, lower birth weight infants, antepartum and postpartum bleeding.

Respiratory: Hyperpnea, pulmonary edema, tachypnea.

Special Senses: Hearing loss, tinnitus. Patients with high frequency hearing loss may have difficulty perceiving tinnitus. In these patients, tinnitus cannot be used as a clinical indicator of salicylism.

Urogenital: Interstitial nephritis, papillary necrosis, proteinuria, renal insufficiency and failure.

Drug Abuse and Dependence: Aspirin is non-narcotic. There is no known potential for addiction associated with the use of aspirin.

Overdosage: Salicylate toxicity may result from acute ingestion (overdose) or chronic intoxication. The early signs of salicylic overdose (salicylism), including tinnitus (ringing in the ears), occur at plasma concentrations approaching 200 mcg/mL. Plasma concentrations of aspirin above 300 mcg/mL are clearly toxic. Severe toxic effects are associated with levels above 400 mcg/mL. (See Clinical Pharmacology.) A single lethal dose of aspirin in adults is not known with certainty but death may be expected at 30 g. For real or suspected overdose, a Poison Control Center should be contacted immediately. Careful medical management is essential.

Signs and Symptoms: In acute overdose, severe acid-base and electrolyte disturbances may occur and are complicated by hyperthermia and dehydration. Respiratory alkalosis occurs early while hyperventilation is present, but is quickly followed by metabolic acidosis.

Treatment: Treatment consists primarily of supporting vital functions, increasing salicylate elimination, and correcting the acid-base disturbance. Gastric emptying and/or lavage is recommended as soon as possible after ingestion, even if the patient has vomited spontaneously. After lavage and/or emesis, administration of activated charcoal, as a slurry, is beneficial, if less than 3 hours have passed since ingestion. Charcoal adsorption should not be employed prior to emesis and lavage.

Severity of aspirin intoxication is determined by measuring the blood salicylate level. Acid-base status should be closely followed with serial blood gas and serum pH measurements. Fluid and electrolyte balance should be maintained.

In severe cases, hyperthermia and hypovolemia are the major immediate threats to life. Children should be sponged with tepid water. Replacement fluid should be administered intravenously and augmented with correction of acidosis. Plasma electrolytes and pH should be monitored to promote alkaline diuresis of salicylate if renal function is normal. Infusion of glucose may be required to control hypoglycemia.

Hemodialysis and peritoneal dialysis can be performed to reduce the body drug content. In patients with renal insufficiency or in cases of life-threatening intoxication, dialysis is usually required. Exchange transfusion may be indicated in infants and young children.

Dosage and Administration: Each dose of aspirin should be taken with a full glass of water unless patient is fluid restricted. Anti-inflammatory and analgesic dosages should be individualized. When aspirin is used in high doses, the development of tinnitus may be used as a clinical sign of elevated plasma salicylate levels except in patients with high frequency hearing loss.

Ischemic Stroke and TIA: 50–325 mg once a day. Continue therapy indefinitely.

Suspected Acute MI: The initial dose of 160–162.5 mg is administered as soon as an MI is suspected. The maintenance dose of 160–162.5 mg a day is continued for 30 days post infarction. After 30 days, consider further therapy based on dosage and administration for prevention of recurrent MI.

Prevention of Recurrent MI: 75–325 mg once a day. Continue therapy indefinitely.

Unstable Angina Pectoris: 75–325 mg once a day. Continue therapy indefinitely.

Chronic Stable Angina Pectoris: 75–325 mg once a day. Continue therapy indefinitely.

CABG: 325 mg daily starting 6 hours post-procedure. Continue therapy for 1 year post-procedure.

PTCA: The initial dose of 325 mg should be given 2 hours pre-surgery. Maintenance dose is 160–325 mg daily. Continue therapy indefinitely.

Carotid Endarterectomy: Doses of 80 mg once daily to 650 mg twice daily, started presurgery, are recommended. Continue therapy indefinitely.

Rheumatoid Arthritis: The initial dose is 3 g a day in divided doses. Increase as needed for anti-inflammatory efficacy with target plasma salicylate levels of 150–300 mcg/mL. At high doses (i.e.,

plasma levels of greater than 200 mg/mL), the incidence of toxicity increases. Juvenile Rheumatoid Arthritis: Initial dose is 90–130 mg/kg/day in divided doses. Increase as needed for anti-inflammatory efficacy with target plasma salicylate levels of 150–300 mcg/mL. At high doses (i.e., plasma levels of greater than 200 mg/mL), the incidence of toxicity increases.

Spondyloarthropathies: Up to 4 g per day in divided doses.

Osteoarthritis: Up to 3 g per day in divided doses.

Arthritis and Pleurisy of SLE: The initial dose is 3 g a day in divided doses. Increase as needed for anti-inflammatory efficacy with target plasma salicylate levels of 150–300 mcg/mL. At high doses (i.e., plasma levels of greater than 200 mg/mL), the incidence of toxicity increases.

How Supplied: 81 mg convex orange film coated tablet with ECOTRIN LOW printed in black ink on one side of the tablet. Available as follows
NDC 0108-0117-82 Bottle of 36 tablets
NDC 0108-0117-83 Bottle of 120 tablets
325 mg convex orange film coated tablet with ECOTRIN REG printed in black ink on one side of the tablet. Available as follows:
NDC 0108-0014-26 Bottle of 100 tablets
NDC 0108-0014-29 Bottle of 250 tablets
500 mg convex orange film coated tablet with ECOTRIN MAX printed in black ink on one side of the tablet. Available as follows:
NDC 0108-0016-23 Bottle of 60 tablets
NDC 0108-0016-27 Bottle of 150 tablets
Store in a tight container at 25°C (77° F); excursions permitted to 15–30°C (59–86°F).

Shown in Product Identification Guide, page 504

GAVISCON® Regular Strength Antacid Tablets
[găv 'ĭs-kŏn]

Composition: Each chewable tablet contains the following active ingredients:
Aluminum hydroxide dried gel... 80 mg
Magnesium trisilicate .... 20 mg
and the following inactive ingredients: alginic acid, calcium stearate, flavor, sodium bicarbonate, starch (may contain corn starch), and sucrose.

Actions: Unique formulation produces soothing foam which floats on stomach contents. Foam containing antacid precedes stomach contents into the esophagus when reflux occurs to help protect the sensitive mucosa from further irritation. GAVISCON® acts locally without neutralizing entire stomach contents to help maintain integrity of the digestive process. Endoscopic studies indicate that GAVISCON Antacid Tablets are equally as effective in the erect or supine patient.

Indications: GAVISCON is specifically formulated for the temporary relief

of heartburn (acid indigestion) due to acid reflux. GAVISCON is not indicated for the treatment of peptic ulcers.

Directions: Chew 2 to 4 tablets four times a day or as directed by a physician. Tablets should be taken after meals and at bedtime or as needed. For best results follow by a half glass of water or other liquid. DO NOT SWALLOW WHOLE.

Warnings: Do not take more than 16 tablets in a 24-hour period or 16 tablets daily for more than 2 weeks, except under the advice and supervision of a physician. Do not use this product except under the advice and supervision of a physician if you are on a sodium-restricted diet. Each GAVISCON Tablet contains approximately 19 mg of sodium.

Drug Interaction Precaution: Antacids may interact with certain prescription drugs. If you are presently taking a prescription drug, do not take this product without checking with your physician or other health professional.

Store at a controlled room temperature in a dry place.

Keep this and all drugs out of the reach of children. In case of accidental overdose, seek professional assistance or contact a poison control center immediately.

How Supplied: Bottles of 100 tablets and in foil-wrapped 2s in boxes of 30 tablets.

Shown in Product Identification Guide, page 504

GAVISCON® EXTRA STRENGTH Antacid Tablets
[găv 'ĭs-kŏn]

Composition: Each chewable tablet contains the following active ingredients:
Aluminum hydroxide .... 160 mg
Magnesium carbonate .... 105 mg
and the following inactive ingredients: alginic acid, calcium stearate, flavor, sodium bicarbonate, and sucrose. May contain stearic acid. Contains sorbitol or mannitol. May contain starch.

Actions: Gavison's unique antacid foam barrier neutralizes stomach acid.

Indications: For the relief of heartburn, sour stomach, acid indigestion and upset stomach associated with these conditions.

Directions: Chew 2 to 4 tablets four times a day or as directed by a physician. Tablets should be taken after meals and at bedtime or as needed. For best results follow by a half glass of water or other liquid. DO NOT SWALLOW WHOLE.

Warnings: Do not take more than 16 tablets in a 24-hour period or 16 tablets daily for more than 2 weeks, except under the advice and supervision of a physician. Do not use this product except under the advice and supervision of a

Continued on next page

Gaviscon Tab. Ex. Str.—Cont.

physician if you are on a sodium-restricted diet. Each Extra Strength Gaviscon tablet contains approximately 19 mg of sodium.

Drug Interaction Precaution: Antacids may interact with certain prescription drugs. If you are presently taking a prescription drug, do not take this product without checking with your physician or other health professional.

Store at a controlled room temperature in a dry place.

Keep this and all drugs out of the reach of children. In case of accidental overdose, seek professional assistance or contact a poison control center immediately.

How Supplied: Bottles of 100 tablets and in foil-wrapped 2s in boxes of 6 and 30 tablets.

Shown in Product Identification Guide, page 504

GAVISCON® Regular Strength
Liquid Antacid
[găv 'ĭs-kŏn]

Composition: Each tablespoonful (15 ml) contains the following active ingredients:

Aluminum hydroxide .... 95 mg
Magnesium carbonate .... 358 mg
and the following inactive ingredients: Benzyl alcohol, D&C Yellow #10, edetate disodium, FD&C Blue #1, flavor, glycerin, saccharin sodium, sodium alginate, sorbitol solution, water, and xanthan gum.

Actions: Gaviscon's unique antacid foam barrier neutralizes stomach acid.

Indications: For the relief of heartburn, sour stomach, acid indigestion and upset stomach associated with these conditions.

Directions: SHAKE WELL BEFORE USING. Take 1 or 2 tablespoonfuls four times a day or as directed by a physician. GAVISCON Regular Strength Liquid should be taken after meals and at bedtime. Dispense product only by spoon or other measuring device.

Warnings: Except under the advice and supervision of a physician, do not take more than 8 tablespoonfuls in a 24-hour period or 8 tablespoonfuls daily for more than 2 weeks. May have laxative effect. Do not use this product if you have a kidney disease. Do not use this product if you are on a sodium-restricted diet except under the advice and supervision of a physician. Each tablespoonful of GAVISCON Regular Strength Liquid contains approximately 1.7 mEq sodium.

Keep this and all drugs out of the reach of children. In case of accidental overdose, seek professional assistance or contact a poison control center immediately.

Drug Interaction Precaution: Antacids may interact with certain prescription drugs. If you are presently taking a prescription drug, do not take this product without checking with your physician or other health professional.

Keep tightly closed. Avoid freezing. Store at a controlled room temperature.

How Supplied: 12 fluid oz (355 ml) bottles.

Shown in Product Identification Guide, page 504

GAVISCON® EXTRA STRENGTH
Liquid Antacid
[găv 'ĭs-kŏn]

Composition: Each 2 teaspoonfuls (10 mL) contains the following active ingredients:

Aluminum hydroxide .... 508 mg
Magnesium carbonate .... 475 mg
and the following inactive ingredients: Benzyl alcohol, edetate disodium, flavor, glycerin, saccharin sodium, simethicone emulsion, sodium alginate, sorbitol solution, water, and xanthan gum.

Actions: Gaviscon's unique antacid foam barrier neutralizes stomach acid.

Indications: For the relief of heartburn, sour stomach, acid indigestion and upset stomach associated with these conditions.

Directions: SHAKE WELL BEFORE USING. Take 2 to 4 teaspoonfuls four times a day or as directed by a physician. GAVISCON Extra Strength Liquid should be taken after meals and at bedtime. Dispense product only by spoon or other measuring device.

Warnings: Except under the advice and supervision of a physician, do not take more than 16 teaspoonfuls in a 24-hour period or 16 teaspoonfuls daily for more than 2 weeks. May have laxative effect. Do not use this product if you have a kidney disease. Do not use this product if you are on a sodium-restricted diet except under the advice and supervision of a physician. Each teaspoonful contains approximately 0.9 mEq sodium.

Keep this and all drugs out of the reach of children. In case of accidental overdose, seek professional assistance or contact a poison control center immediately.

Drug Interaction Precaution: Antacids may interact with certain prescription drugs. If you are presently taking a prescription drug, do not take this product without checking with your physician or other health professional.

Keep tightly closed. Avoid freezing. Store at a controlled room temperature.

How Supplied: 12 fl oz (355 mL) bottles.

Shown in Product Identification Guide, page 504

GLY–OXIDE® Liquid

Description/Active Ingredient: GLY-OXIDE® Liquid contains carbamide peroxide 10%.

Actions: Gly-Oxide is specially formulated to release peroxide and oxygen bubbles in your mouth. The peroxide and oxygen-rich microfoam help:
- gently remove unhealthy tissue, then cleanse and soothe canker sores and minor wounds and inflammations so natural healing can better occur.
- kill odor-forming germs.
- foam and flush out food particles ordinary brushing can miss.
- clean stains from orthodontics/dentures/bridgework/etc. better than brushing alone.

Indications For Temporary Use: Gly-Oxide liquid is for temporary use in cleansing canker sores and minor wound or gum inflammation resulting from minor dental procedures, dentures, orthodontic appliances, accidental injury, or other irritations of the mouth and gums. Gly-Oxide can also be used to guard against the risk of infections in the mouth and gums.

Everyday Uses: Gly-Oxide may be used routinely to improve oral hygiene as an aid to regular brushing or when regular brushing is inadequate or impossible such as total care geriatrics, etc. Gly-Oxide kills germs to reduce mouth odors and/or odors on dental appliances. Gly-Oxide penetrates between teeth and other areas of the mouth to flush out food particles ordinary brushing can miss. This can be especially useful when brushing is made more difficult by the presence of orthodontics or other dental appliances. Plus, Gly-Oxide helps remove stains on dental appliances to improve appearance.

Directions For Temporary Use: Do not dilute. Replace tip on bottle when not in use. **Adults and children 2 years of age and older:** Apply several drops directly from bottle onto affected area; spit out after 2 to 3 minutes. Use up to four times daily after meals and at bedtime or as directed by dentist or doctor. OR place 10 drops on tongue, mix with saliva, swish for several minutes, and then spit out. Use by children under 12 years of age should be supervised. **Children under 2 years of age:** Consult a dentist or doctor.

Directions For Everyday Use: The product may be used following the temporary use directions above. OR apply Gly-Oxide to the toothbrush (it will sink into the brush), cover with toothpaste, brush normally, and spit out.

Warnings: Severe or persistent oral inflammation, denture irritation, or gingivitis may be serious. If sore mouth symptoms do not improve in 7 days, or if irritation, pain, or redness persists or worsens, or if swelling, rash, or fever develops, discontinue use of product and see your dentist or doctor promptly. Avoid contact with eyes. **KEEP THIS AND ALL**

DRUGS OUT OF THE REACH OF CHILDREN. In case of accidental overdose, seek professional assistance or contact a poison control center immediately.

Inactive Ingredients: Citric Acid, Flavor, Glycerin, Propylene Glycol, Sodium Stannate, Water, and Other Ingredients.
Protect from excessive heat and direct sunlight.

How Supplied: GLY-OXIDE® Liquid is available in ½-fl-oz and 2-fl-oz plastic squeeze bottles with applicator spouts.
Comments or Questions? Call Toll-free 1-800-245-1040 Weekdays
GlaxoSmithKline Consumer Healthcare, L.P.
Moon Township, PA 15108
Made in U.S.A.
Shown in Product Identification Guide, page 504

GOODY'S®
Body Pain Formula Powder

Indications: For temporary relief of minor body aches & pains due to muscular aches, arthritis & headaches.

Directions: Adults: Place one powder on tongue and follow with liquid, or stir powder into a glass of water or other liquid. May be repeated in 4 to 6 hours. Do not take more than 4 powders in any 24-hour period. Children under 12 years of age: Consult a doctor.

Warnings: Children and teenagers should not use this medicine for chicken pox or flu symptoms before a doctor is consulted about Reye's Syndrome, a rare but serious illness reported to be associated with aspirin. Do not use with any other product containing acetaminophen. **Ask a doctor before use if you have** asthma, ulcers, a bleeding problem, stomach problems that last or come back such as heartburn, upset stomach or pain. **Ask a doctor or pharmacist before use** if you are taking a prescription drug for gout, diabetes, arthritis or anticoagulation (blood thinning). **Stop use and ask a doctor if** an allergic reaction occurs, ringing in ears or loss of hearing occurs, pain gets worse or persists for more than 10 days, fever lasts more than 3 days, redness or swelling is present, or new symptoms occur. As with any drug, if you are pregnant, or nursing a baby, seek the advice of a health professional before using this product.
IT IS ESPECIALLY IMPORTANT NOT TO USE ASPIRIN DURING THE LAST 3 MONTHS OF PREGNANCY UNLESS SPECIFICALLY DIRECTED TO DO SO BY A DOCTOR BECAUSE IT MAY CAUSE PROBLEMS IN THE UNBORN CHILD OR COMPLICATIONS DURING DELIVERY.
Alcohol Warning: If you consume 3 or more alcoholic drinks every day, ask your doctor whether you should take acetaminophen and aspirin or other pain relievers/fever reducers. Acetaminophen and aspirin may cause liver damage and stomach bleeding.
Keep this and all medicines out of the reach of children. Overdose warning: Taking more than the recommended dose can cause serious health problems. In case of overdose, contact a doctor or poison control center immediately.

Active Ingredients: Each powder contains: 500 mg. aspirin and 325 mg. acetaminophen.

Inactive Ingredients: Each powder contains: Lactose Monohydrate and Potassium Chloride.

GOODY'S®
Extra Strength Headache Powder

Indications: For Temporary Relief of Minor Aches & Pains Due to Headaches, Arthritis, Colds & Fever

Directions: Adults: Place one powder on tongue and follow with liquid or stir powder into a glass of water or other liquid. May be repeated in 4 to 6 hours. Do not take more than 4 powders in any 24-hour period. Children under 12 years of age: Consult a doctor.

Warnings: Children and teenagers should not use this medicine for chicken pox or flu symptoms before a doctor is consulted about Reye's Syndrome, a rare but serious illness reported to be associated with aspirin. Do not use with any other product containing acetaminophen. **Ask a doctor before use if you have** asthma, ulcers, a bleeding problem, stomach problems that last or come back such as heartburn, upset stomach or pain. **Ask a doctor or pharmacist before use** if you are taking a prescription drug for gout, diabetes, arthritis or anticoagulation (blood thinning). **When using this product** limit the use of caffeine containing drugs, foods, or drinks, because too much caffeine may cause nervousness, irritability, sleeplessness, and occasionally, rapid heartbeat. **Stop use and ask a doctor if** an allergic reaction occurs, ringing in ears or loss of hearing occurs, pain gets worse or persists for more than 10 days, fever lasts for more than 3 days, redness or swelling is present, or new symptoms occur. As with any drug, if you are pregnant, or nursing a baby, seek the advice of a health professional before using this product.
IT IS ESPECIALLY IMPORTANT NOT TO USE ASPIRIN DURING THE LAST 3 MONTHS OF PREGNANCY UNLESS SPECIFICALLY DIRECTED TO DO SO BY A DOCTOR BECAUSE IT MAY CAUSE PROBLEMS IN THE UNBORN CHILD OR COMPLICATIONS DURING DELIVERY.
Alcohol Warning: If you consume 3 or more alcoholic drinks every day, ask your doctor whether you should take acetaminophen and aspirin or other pain relievers/fever reducers. Acetaminophen and aspirin may cause liver damage and stomach bleeding.
Keep this and all medicines out of the reach of children. Overdose warning: Taking more than the recommended dose can cause serious health problems. In case of overdose, contact a doctor or poison control center immediately.

Active Ingredients: Each powder contains: 500 mg. aspirin and 325 mg. acetaminophen.

Inactive Ingredients: Each powder contains: Lactose Monohydrate and Potassium Chloride.

GOODY'S®
Extra Strength Pain Relief Tablets

Indications: Goody's EXTRA STRENGTH tablets are a specially developed pain reliever that provide fast & effective temporary relief from minor aches & pain due to headaches, arthritis, colds or "flu," muscle strain, backache & menstrual discomfort. It is recommended for temporary relief of toothaches and to reduce fever.

Dosage: Adults: Two tablets with water or other liquid. May be repeated in 4 to 6 hours. Do not take more than 8 tablets in any 24-hour period. Children under 12 years of age: Consult a doctor.

Warnings: Children and teenagers should not use this medicine for chicken pox or flu symptoms before a doctor is consulted about Reye's Syndrome, a rare but serious illness reported to be associated with aspirin. Do not use with any other product containing acetaminophen. **Ask a doctor before use if you have** asthma, ulcers, a bleeding problem, stomach problems that last or come back such as heartburn, upset stomach or pain. **Ask a doctor or pharmacist before use** if you are taking a prescription drug for gout, diabetes, arthritis or anticoagulation (blood thinning) **When using this product** limit the use of caffeine containing drugs, foods, or drinks, because too much caffeine may cause nervousness, irritability, sleeplessness, and occasionally, rapid heartbeat. **Stop use and ask a doctor if** an allergic reaction occurs, ringing in ears or loss of hearing occurs, pain gets worse or persists for more than 10 days, fever lasts more than 3 days, redness or swelling is present, or new symptoms occur.
As with any drug, if you are pregnant, or nursing a baby, seek the advice of a health professional before using this product. IT IS ESPECIALLY IMPORTANT NOT TO USE ASPIRIN DURING THE LAST 3 MONTHS OF PREGNANCY UNLESS SPECIFICALLY DIRECTED TO DO SO BY A DOCTOR BECAUSE IT MAY CAUSE PROBLEMS

and aspirin may cause liver damage and stomach bleeding. **Keep this and all medicines out of the reach of children. Overdose warning:** Taking more than the recommended dose can cause serious health problems. In case of overdose, contact a doctor or poison control center immediately.

Active Ingredients: Each Powder contains 520 mg. aspirin in combination with 260 mg. acetaminophen and 32.5 mg. caffeine.

Inactive Ingredients: Lactose Monohydrate and Potassium Chloride.

Continued on next page

Goody's Pain Relief—Cont.

IN THE UNBORN CHILD OR COMPLI-CATIONS DURING DELIVERY. **Alcohol Warning:** If you consume 3 or more alcoholic drinks every day, ask your doctor whether you should take acetaminophen and aspirin or other pain relievers/fever reducers. Acetaminophen and aspirin may cause liver damage and stomach bleeding. **Keep this and all medicines out of the reach of children. Overdose warning:** Taking more than the recommended dose can cause serious health problems. In case of overdose, contact a doctor or poison control center immediately.

Active Ingredients: Each tablet contains 260 mg. aspirin in combination with 130 mg. acetaminophen and 16.25 mg. caffeine. **Inactive Ingredients:** Corn Starch, Crospovidone, Povidone, Pregelatinized Starch and Stearic Acid.

GOODY'S PM® POWDER
For Pain with Sleeplessness

Indications: For temporary relief of occasional headaches and minor aches and pains with accompanying sleeplessness.

Directions: Adults and children 12 years of age and older: One dose (2 powders). Take both powders at bedtime, if needed, or as directed by a doctor. Place powders on tongue and follow with liquid. If you prefer, stir powders into glass of water or other liquid.

Warnings: Keep this and all medicines out of the reach of children. Overdose Warning: Taking more than the recommended dose can cause serious health problems. In case of accidental overdose, contact a doctor or poison control center immediately. Prompt medical attention is critical for adults as well as for children even if you do not notice any signs or symptoms.
As with any drug, if you are pregnant or nursing a baby, seek the advice of a health professional before using this product. Do not give this product to children under 12 years of age. Do not use for more than 10 days or for fever for more than 3 days unless directed by a doctor. Consult your doctor if redness or swelling is present, symptoms persist or get worse or new ones occur. If sleeplessness persists continuously for more than 2 weeks consult your doctor. Insomnia may be a symptom of serious underlying medical illness. Do not take this product, unless directed by a doctor, if you have a breathing problem such as emphysema or chronic bronchitis or if you have glaucoma or difficulty in urination due to enlargement of the prostate gland. **Do Not Use** with any other product containing diphenhydramine, including one applied topically, or with any other product containing acetaminophen. Avoid alcoholic beverages while taking this product. Do not use this product if you are taking sedatives or tranquilizers without first consulting your doctor. **Alcohol Warning:** If you consume 3 or more alcoholic drinks every day, ask your doctor whether you should take acetaminophen or other pain relievers/fever reducers. Acetaminophen may cause liver damage.

Caution: This product will cause drowsiness. Do not drive a motor vehicle or operate machinery after use.

Active Ingredients: Each powder contains 500 mg. Acetaminophen and 38 mg. Diphenhydramine Citrate.

Inactive Ingredients: Citric Acid, Docusate Sodium, Fumaric Acid, Glycine, Lactose Monohydrate, Magnesium Stearate, Potassium Chloride, Silica Gel, Sodium Citrate Dihydrate.

MASSENGILL®
[mas 'sen-gil]
Baby Powder Scent Soft Cloth Towelette

Ingredients: Purified Water, Octoxynol-9, Lactic Acid, Disodium Edta, Fragrance, Potassium Sorbate, Cetylpyridinium Chloride, and Sodium Bicarbonate.

Indications: For cleansing and refreshing the external vaginal area.

Actions: Massengill Baby Powder Scent Soft Cloth Towelette safely cleanse the external vaginal area. The towelette delivery system makes the application soft and gentle.

Directions: Remove towelette from foil packet, unfold, and gently wipe from front to back. After towelette has been used once, return towelette to foil packet and throw it away. Safe to use daily as often as needed. For external use only.

How Supplied: 50 individually sealed soft cloth towelettes per carton.
Comments, questions or for information about STD's and vaginal health, call toll free 1-800-245-1040 weekdays.

MASSENGILL Feminine Cleansing Wash, Floral
[mas 'sen-gil]

Ingredients: Purified Water, sodium laureth sulfate, magnesium laureth sulfate, sodium laureth-8 sulfate, magnesium laureth-8 sulfate, sodium oleth sulfate, magnesium oleth sulfate, lauramidopropyl betaine, myristamine oxide, lactic acid, PEG-120 methyl glucose dioleate, fragrance, sodium methylparaben, sodium ethylparaben, sodium propylparaben, methylchloroisothiazolinone, methylisothiazolinone, D&C Red #33.

Indications: For cleansing and refreshing of external vaginal area.

Actions: Massengill feminine cleansing wash safely and gently cleanses the external vaginal area.

Directions: Pour small amount into palm of hand or wash cloth and lather into wet skin. Rinse clean. Safe to use daily. For external use only.

How Supplied: 8 fl. oz plastic flip-top bottle.

NICODERM® CQ®
Nicotine Transdermal System/Stop Smoking Aid

Formerly available only by prescription Available as:

Step 1 - 21 mg/24 hours
Step 2 - 14 mg/24 hours
Step 3 - 7 mg/24 hours

If you smoke:
More than 10 Cigarettes per Day: Start with Step 1
10 Cigarettes a Day or Less: Start with Step 2
WHAT IS THE NICODERM CQ PATCH AND HOW IS IT USED?
NicoDerm CQ is a small, nicotine containing patch. When you put on a NicoDerm CQ patch, nicotine passes through the skin and into your body. NicoDerm CQ is very thin and uses special material to control how fast nicotine passes through the skin. Unlike the sudden jolts of nicotine delivered by cigarettes, the amount of nicotine you receive remains relatively smooth throughout the 24 or 16 hours period you wear the NicoDerm CQ patch. This helps to reduce cravings you may have for nicotine.

Active Ingredient: Nicotine

Purpose: Stop Smoking Aid

Use: reduces withdrawal symptoms, including nicotine craving, associated with quitting smoking

Directions:
• if you are under 18 years of age, ask a doctor before use

- before using this product, read the enclosed user's guide for complete directions and other information
- stop smoking completely when you begin using the patch
- **if you smoke more than 10 cigarettes per day,** use according to the following 10 week schedule:

STEP 1	STEP 2	STEP 3
Use one 21 mg patch/day	Use one 14 mg patch/day	Use one 7 mg patch/day
Weeks 1–6	Weeks 7–8	Weeks 9–10

- if you smoke **10 or less cigarettes per day,** do not use **STEP 1 (21 mg)**. Start with **STEP 2 (14 mg)** for 6 weeks, then **STEP 3 (7 mg)** for two weeks and then stop.
- steps 2 and 3 allow you to gradually reduce your level of nicotine. Completing the full program will increase your chances of quitting successfully.
- apply one new patch every 24 hours on skin that is dry, clean and hairless
- remove backing from patch and immediately press onto skin. Hold for 10 seconds.
- wash hands after applying or removing patch. Throw away the patch in the enclosed disposal tray. See enclosed user's guide for safety and handling.
- you may wear the patch for 16 or 24 hours
- if you crave cigarettes when you wake up, wear the patch for 24 hours
- if you have vivid dreams or other sleep disturbances, you may remove the patch at bedtime and apply a new one in the morning
- the used patch should be removed and a new one applied to a different skin site at the same time each day
- do not wear more than one patch at a time
- do not cut patch in half or into smaller pieces
- do not leave patch on for more than 24 hours because it may irritate your skin and loses strength after 24 hours
- stop using the patch at the end of 10 weeks. If you started with **STEP 2**, stop using the patch at the end of 8 weeks. If you still feel the need to use the patch talk to your doctor.

Warnings:

If you are pregnant or breast-feeding, only use this medicine on the advice of your health care provider. Smoking can seriously harm your child. Try to stop smoking without using any nicotine replacement medicine. This medicine is believed to be safer than smoking. However, the risks to your child from this medicine are not fully known.

Do Not Use

- if you continue to smoke, chew tobacco, use snuff, or use a nicotine gum or other nicotine containing products

Ask a doctor before use if you have

- heart disease, recent heart attack, or irregular heartbeat. Nicotine can increase your heart rate.
- high blood pressure not controlled with medication. Nicotine can increase your blood pressure.
- an allergy to adhesive tape or skin problems because you are more likely to get rashes

Ask a doctor or pharmacist before use if you are

- using a non-nicotine stop smoking drug
- taking a prescription medication for depression or asthma. Your prescription dose may need to be adjusted.

When using this product

- do not smoke even when not wearing the patch. The nicotine in your skin will still be entering your blood stream for several hours after you take off the patch.
- if you have vivid dreams or other sleep disturbances remove this patch at bedtime

Stop use and ask a doctor if

- skin redness caused by the patch does not go away after four days, or if skin swells, or you get a rash
- irregular heartbeat or palpitations occur
- you get symptoms of nicotine overdose such as nausea, vomiting, dizziness, weakness and rapid heartbeat

Keep out of reach of children and pets. Used patches have enough nicotine to poison children and pets. If swallowed, get medical help or contact a Poison Control Center right away. Dispose of the used patches by folding sticky ends together and inserting in disposal tray in this box.

READ THE LABEL

Read the carton and the User's Guide before using this product. Keep the carton and User's Guide. They contain important information.

Inactive Ingredients: Ethylene vinyl acetate-copolymer, polyisobutylene and high density polyethylene between pigmented and clear polyester backings. Store at 20–25°C (68–77°F).

TO INCREASE YOUR SUCCESS IN QUITTING:

1. You must be motivated to quit.
2. Complete the full treatment program, applying a new patch every day.
3. Use with a support program as described in the Users Guide.

NicoDerm CQ User's Guide
KEYS TO SUCCESS

1) You must really want to quit smoking for **NicoDerm® CQ®** to help you.
2) Complete the full program, applying a new patch every day.
3) **NicoDerm CQ** works best when used together with a support program: See page 3 for details.
4) If you have trouble using **NicoDerm CQ**, ask your doctor or pharmacist or call GlaxoSmithKline 1-800-834-5895 weekdays (10:00 am 4:30 pm EST).

SO, YOU'VE DECIDED TO QUIT.

Congratulations. Your decision to stop smoking is one of the most important things you can do to improve your health. Quitting smoking is a two-part process that involves:
1) overcoming your physical need for nicotine, and
2) breaking your smoking habit.
NicoDerm CQ helps smokers quit by reducing nicotine withdrawal symptoms.
Many NicoDerm CQ users will be able to stop smoking for a few days but often will start smoking again. Most smokers have to try to quit several times before they completely stop.

Your own chances of quitting smoking depend on how strongly you are addicted to nicotine, how much you want to quit, and how closely you follow a quitting plan like the one that comes with NicoDerm CQ.

QUITTING SMOKING IS HARD!

If you find you cannot stop or if you start smoking again after using NicoDerm CQ please talk to a health care professional who can help you find a program that may work better for you. Breaking this addiction doesn't happen overnight.
Because NicoDerm CQ provides some nicotine, the NicoDerm CQ patch will help you stop smoking by reducing nicotine withdrawal symptoms such as nicotine craving, nervousness and irritability.
This User's Guide will give you support as you become a non-smoker. It will answer common questions about NicoDerm CQ and give tips to help you stop smoking, and should be referred to often.

WHERE TO GET HELP.

You are more likely to stop smoking by using NicoDerm CQ with a support program that helps you break your smoking habit. There may be support groups in your area for people trying to quit. Call your local chapter of the American Lung Association, American Cancer Society or American Heart Association for further information. Toll free phone numbers are printed on the wallet card on the back cover of this User's Guide.
If you find you cannot stop smoking or if you start smoking again after using NicoDerm CQ, remember breaking this addiction doesn't happen overnight. You may want to talk to a health care professional who can help you improve your chances of quitting the next time you try NicoDerm CQ or another method.

LET'S GET ORGANIZED.

Your reason for quitting may be a combination of concerns about health, the effect of smoking on your appearance, and pressure from your family and friends to stop smoking. Or maybe you're concerned about the dangerous effect of second-hand smoke on the people you care about.
All of these are good reasons. You probably have others. Decide your most important reasons, and write them down on the wallet card inside the back cover of this User's Guide. Carry this card with you. In difficult moments, when you want to smoke, the card will remind you why you are quitting.

WHAT YOU'RE UP AGAINST.

Smoking is addictive in two ways. Your need for nicotine has become both physical and mental. You must overcome both addictions to stop smoking. So while NicoDerm CQ will lessen your body's craving for nicotine, you've got to want to quit smoking to overcome the mental dependence on cigarettes. Once you've decided that you're going to quit, it's time to get started. But first, there are some important cautions you should consider.

Continued on next page

NicoDerm CQ—Cont.

SOME IMPORTANT WARNINGS.
This product is only for those who want to stop smoking.

If you are pregnant or breast-feeding, only use this medicine on the advice of your health care provider. Smoking can seriously harm your child. Try to stop smoking without using any nicotine replacement medicine. This medicine is believed to be safer than smoking. However, the risks to your child from this medicine are not fully known.

Do not use
- if you continue to smoke, chew tobacco, use snuff or use a nicotine gum or other nicotine products.

Ask a doctor before use if you have:
- heart disease, recent heart attack, or irregular heartbeat, Nicotine can increase your heart rate.
- high blood pressure not controlled with medication. Nicotine can increase your blood pressure.
- an allergy to adhesive tape or have skin problems because you are more likely to get rashes.

Ask a doctor or pharmacist before use if you are
- using a non-nicotine stop smoking drug
- taking a prescription medication for asthma or depression. Your prescription dose may need to be adjusted.

When using this product:
- do not smoke even when not wearing the patch. The nicotine in your skin will still be entering your bloodstream for several hours after you take off the patch.
- you have vivid dreams or other sleep disturbances remove this patch at bedtime.

Stop use and ask a doctor if:
- skin redness caused by the patch does not go away after four days, or if your skin swells or you get a rash.
- irregular heartbeat or palpitations occur
- you get symptoms of nicotine overdose, such as nausea, vomiting, dizziness, weakness and rapid heartbeat.

Keep out of reach of children and pets. Used patches have enough nicotine to poison children and pets. If swallowed, get medical help or contact a Poison Control Center right away. Dispose of the used patches by folding sticky ends together and inserting in the disposal tray in this box.

LET'S GET STARTED.
If you are under 18 years of age, ask a doctor before use.

Becoming a non-smoker starts today. Your first step is to read through this entire User's Guide carefully.

First, check that you bought the right starting dose.

If you smoke more than 10 cigarettes a day, begin with Step 1 (21 mg). As the carton indicates, people who smoke 10 or less cigarettes per day should not use Step 1 (21 mg). They should start with Step 2 (14 mg). Throughout this User's Guide we will give specific instructions for people who smoke 10 or less cigarettes per day.

Next, set your personalized quitting schedule.

Take out a calendar that you can use to track your progress. Pick a quit date, and mark this on your calendar using the stickers in the middle of this User's Guide, as described below.

DIRECTIONS: FOR PEOPLE WHO SMOKE MORE THAN 10 CIGARETTES PER DAY
STEP 1. (Weeks 1–6). Your quit date (and the day you'll start using NicoDerm CQ patch).

Choose your quit date (it should be soon).

This is the day you will quit smoking cigarettes entirely and begin using NicoDerm CQ to reduce your cravings for nicotine. Place the Step 1 sticker on this date. For the first six weeks, you'll use the highest-strength (21 mg) NicoDerm CQ patches. Be sure to follow the directions on page 10.

Completing the full program will increase your chances of quitting successfully. This is done by changing over to the Step 2 (14mg) patch for 2 weeks followed by a final 2 weeks with the Step 3 (7mg) patch. The Step 2 and Step 3 treatment periods allow you to gradually reduce the amount of nicotine you get, rather than stopping suddenly, and will increase your chances of quitting.

STEP 2. (Weeks 7–8). The day you'll start reducing your use of NicoDerm CQ patch.

Switching to Step 2 (14mg) patches after 6 weeks begins to gradually reduce your nicotine usage. Place the Step 2 sticker on this date (the first day of week seven). Use the 14mg patches for two weeks.

STEP 3. (Weeks 9–10). The day you'll further start reducing your use of Nico-Derm CQ patch.

After eight weeks, nicotine intake is further reduced by moving down to Step 3 (7mg) patches. Place the Step 3 sticker on this date (the first day of week nine). Use the 7 mg patches for two weeks.

THE NICODERM CQ PROGRAM

STEP 1	STEP 2	STEP 3
Use one	Use one	Use one
21 mg	14 mg	7 mg
patch/day	patch/day	patch/day
Weeks 1–6	Weeks 7–8	Weeks 9–10

STOP USING NICODERM CQ AT THE END OF WEEK 10. If you still feel the need to use the patch after Week 10, talk with your doctor or health professional.

DIRECTIONS: FOR PEOPLE WHO SMOKE 10 OR LESS CIGARETTES PER DAY
Do not use Step 1 (21 mg).

Begin with STEP 2 – Initial Treatment Period (Weeks 1–6): 14mg patches.

Choose our quit date (it should be soon). This is the Day you will quit smoking cigarettes entirely and begin using NicoDerm CQ to reduce your cravings for nicotine. Place the Step 2 sticker on this date. For the first six weeks, you'll use the Step 2 (14mg) NicoDerm CQ patches. Be sure to follow the directions on page 10.

Continue with STEP 3 – Step Down Treatment Period (Weeks 7–8): 7mg patches.

Completing the full program will increase your chances of quitting successfully. This is done by changing over to the Step 3 (7mg) patches for 2 weeks. The two week step down treatment period allows you to gradually reduce the amount of nicotine you get, rather than stopping suddenly, and will increase your chances of quitting. Place the Step 3 sticker on the first day of week seven. Use the 7mg patches for two weeks.

People who smoke 10 or less cigarettes per day should not use NicoDerm CQ for longer than 8 weeks. If you still feel the need to use NicoDerm CQ after 8 weeks, talk with your doctor.

PLAN AHEAD.
Because smoking is an addiction, it is not easy to stop. After you've given up nicotine, you may still have a strong urge to smoke. Plan ahead NOW for these times, so you're not tempted to start smoking again in a moment of weakness. The following tips may help:
- Keep the phone numbers of supportive friends and family members handy.
- Keep a record of your quitting process. In the event that you slip, immediately stop smoking and resume your quit attempt with the NicoDerm CQ patch. If you smoke at all, write down what you think caused the slip.
- Put together an Emergency Kit that includes items that will help take your mind off occasional urges to smoke. You might include cinnamon gum or lemon drops to suck on, a relaxing cassette tape, and something for your hands to play with, like a smooth rock, rubber band or small metal balls.
- Set aside some small rewards, like a new magazine or a gift certificate from your favorite store, which you'll "give" yourself after passing difficult hurdles.
- Think now about the times when you most often want a cigarette, and then plan what else you might do instead of smoking. For instance, you might plan to take your coffee break in a new location, or take a walk right after dinner, so you won't be tempted to smoke.

HOW NICODERM CQ WORKS.
NicoDerm CQ patches provide nicotine to your system. They work as a temporary aid to help you quit smoking by reducing nicotine withdrawal symptoms, including nicotine craving. NicoDerm CQ provides a lower level of nicotine to your blood than cigarettes, and allows you to gradually do away with your body's need for nicotine.

Because NicoDerm CQ does not contain the tar or carbon monoxide of cigarette smoke, it does not have the same health dangers as tobacco. However, it still delivers nicotine, the addictive part of cigarette smoke. Nicotine can cause side effects such as headache, nausea, upset stomach, and dizziness.

HOW TO USE NICODERM CQ PATCHES.
Read all the following instructions, and the instructions on the outer carton, before using NicoDerm CQ. Refer to them

often to make sure you're using Nico-Derm CQ correctly. Please refer to the CD for additional help.

1) Stop smoking completely before you start using NicoDerm CQ.

2) To reduce nicotine craving and other withdrawal symptoms, use NicoDerm CQ according to the directions on pages 6–8.

3) Insert used NicoDerm CQ patches in the child resistant disposal tray provided in the box – safely away from children and pets.

When to apply and remove NicoDerm CQ patches.

Each day apply a new patch to a different place on skin that is dry, clean and hairless. **You can wear a NicoDerm CQ patch for either 16 or 24 hours.** If you crave cigarettes when you wake up, wear the patch for 24 hours. If you begin to have vivid dreams or other disruptions of your sleep while wearing the patch 24 hours, try taking the patch off at bedtime (after about 16 hours) and putting on a new one when you get up the next day.

PLACE THESE STICKERS ON YOUR CALENDAR

STEP 1	STEP 2
A new 21 mg patch every day AT THE BEGINNING OF WEEK #1 (QUIT DAY)	A new 14 mg patch every day AT THE BEGINNING OF WEEK #7

For people who smoke 10 or less cigarettes per day: Do not use STEP 1 (21 mg). Use STEP 2 (14 mg) at the beginning of week #1 and STEP 3 (7 mg) at the beginning of week #7.

PLACE THESE STICKERS ON YOUR CALENDAR

STEP 3	EX-SMOKER
A new 7 mg patch every day AT THE BEGINNING OF WEEK #9	WHEN YOU HAVE COMPLETED YOUR QUITTING PROGRAM

Do not smoke even when you are not wearing the patch.

Remove the used patch and put on a new patch at the same time every day. Applying the patch at about the same time each day (first thing in the morning, for instance) will help you remember when to put on a new patch. Do not leave the same NicoDerm CQ patch on for more than 24 hours because it may irritate your skin and because it loses strength after 24 hours.

Do not use NicoDerm CQ continuously for more than 10 weeks (8 weeks for people who smoke 10 or less cigarettes per day).

How to apply a NicoDerm CQ patch.

1. Do not remove the NicoDerm CQ patch from its sealed protective pouch until you are ready to use it. NicoDerm CQ patches will lose nicotine to the air if you store them out of the pouch.

2. Choose a non-hairy, clean, dry area of skin. Do not put a NicoDerm CQ patch on skin that is burned, broken out, cut, or irritated in any way. Make sure your skin is free of lotion and soap before applying a patch.

3. A clear, protective liner covers the sticky back side of the NicoDerm CQ patch—the side that will be put on your skin. The liner has a slit down the middle to help you remove it from the patch. With the sticky back side facing you, pull half the liner away from the NicoDerm CQ patch starting at the middle slit, as shown in the illustration above. Hold the NicoDerm CQ patch at one of the outside edges (touch the sticky side as little as possible), and pull off the other half of the protective liner.

Place this liner in the slot in the disposable tray provided in the NicoDerm CQ package where it will be out of reach of children and pets.

4. Immediately apply the sticky side of the NicoDerm CQ patch to your skin. **Press the patch firmly on your skin with the heel of your hand for at least 10 seconds.** Make sure it sticks well to your skin, especially around the edges.

5. Wash your hands when you have finished applying the NicoDerm CQ patch. Nicotine on your hands could get into your eyes and nose, and cause stinging, redness, or more serious problems.

6. After 24 or 16 hours, remove the patch you have been wearing. Fold the used NicoDerm CQ patch in half with the sticky side together. Carefully dispose of the used patch in the slot of the disposal tray provided in the NicoDerm CQ package where it will be out of the reach of children and pets. Even used patches have enough nicotine to poison children and pets. Wash your hands.

7. Chose a different place on your skin to apply the next NicoDerm CQ patch and repeat Steps 1 to 6. Do not apply a new patch to a previously used skin site for at least one week.

If your NicoDerm CQ patch gets wet during wearing.

Water will not harm the NicoDerm CQ patch you are wearing if applied properly. You can bathe, swim, or shower for short periods while you are wearing the NicoDerm CQ patch.

If your NicoDerm CQ patch comes off while wearing.

NicoDerm CQ patches generally stick well to most people's skin. However, a patch may occasionally come off. If your NicoDerm CQ patch falls off during the day, put on a new patch, making sure you select a non-hairy, non-irritated area of the skin that is clean and dry.

If the soap you use has lanolin or moisturizers, the patch may not stick well. Using a different soap may help. Body creams, lotions and sunscreens can also cause problems with keeping your patch on. Do not apply creams or lotions to the place on your skin where you will put the patch.

If you have followed the directions and the patch still does not stick to you, try using medical adhesive tape over the patch.

Disposing of NicoDerm CQ patches.

Fold the used patch in half with the sticky side together.

Carefully dispose of the patch in the disposal slot of the tray provided in the NicoDerm CQ package where it will be out of the reach of children and pets. Small amounts of nicotine, even from a used patch, can poison children and pets. **Keep all nicotine patches away from children and pets.** Wash your hands after disposing of the patch.

If your skin reacts to the NicoDerm CQ patch.

When you first put on a NicoDerm CQ patch, mild itching, burning, or tingling is normal and should go away within an hour. After you remove a NicoDerm CQ patch, the skin under the patch might be somewhat red. Your skin should not stay red for more than a day after removing the patch. **Stop use and ask a doctor if skin redness caused by the patch does not go away after four days, or if your skin swells, or you get a rash. Do not put on a new patch.**

Storage Instructions

Keep each NicoDerm CQ patch in its protective pouch, unopened, until you are ready to use it, because the patch will lose nicotine to the air if it's outside the pouch.

Store NicoDerm CQ patches at 20–25 C (68–77 F) because they are sensitive to heat. Remember, the inside of your car can reach temperatures much higher than this. A slight yellowing of the sticky side of the patch is normal. Do not use NicoDerm CQ patches stored in pouches that are open or torn.

TIPS TO MAKE QUITTING EASIER.

Within the first few weeks of giving up smoking, you may be tempted to smoke for pleasure, particularly after completing a difficult task, or at a party or bar. Hear are some tips to help get you through the important first stages of becoming a nonsmoker:

On Your Quit Date:

- Ask your family, friends and co-workers to support you in your efforts to stop smoking.
- Throw away all your cigarettes, matches, lighters, ashtrays, etc.
- Keep busy on your quit day. Exercise. Go to a movie. Take a walk. Get together with friends.
- Figure out how much money you'll save by not smoking. Most ex-smokers can save more than $1,000 a year on the price of cigarettes alone.
- Write down what you will do with the money you save.
- Know your high risk situations and plan ahead how you will deal with them.
- Visit your dentist and have your teeth cleaned to get rid of the tobacco stains.

Right after Quitting:

- During the first few days after you've stopped smoking, spend as much time as possible at places where smoking is not allowed.
- Drink large quantities of water and fruit juices.
- Try to avoid alcohol, coffee and other beverages you associate with smoking.
- Remember that temporary urges to smoke will pass, even if you don't smoke a cigarette.

Continued on next page

NicoDerm CQ—Cont.

- Keep your hands busy with something like a pencil or a paper clip.
- Find other activities that help you relax without cigarettes. Swim, jog, take a walk, play basketball.
- Don't worry too much about gaining weight. Watch what you eat, take time for daily exercise, and change your eating habits if you need to.
- Laughter helps. Watch or read something funny

WHAT TO EXPECT.

The First Few Days.

Your body is now coming back to balance. During the first few days after you stop smoking, you might feel edgy and nervous and have trouble concentrating. You might get headaches, feel dizzy and a little out of sorts, feel sweaty or have stomach upsets. You might even have trouble sleeping at first. These are typical nicotine withdrawal symptoms that will go away with time. Your smoker's cough will get worse before it gets better. But don't worry, that's a good sign. Coughing helps clear the tar deposits out of your lungs.

After A Week Or Two.

By now you should be feeling more confident that you can handle those smoking urges. Many of your nicotine withdrawal symptoms have left by now, and you should be noticing some positive signs: less coughing, better breathing and an improved sense of taste and smell, to name a few.

After A Month.

You probably have the urge to smoke much less often now. But urges may still occur, and when they do, they are likely to be powerful ones that come out of nowhere. Don't let them catch you off guard. Plan ahead for these difficult times.

Concentrate on the ways non-smokers are more attractive than smokers. Their skin is less likely to wrinkle. Their teeth are whiter, cleaner. Their breath is fresher.

Their hair and clothes smell better. That cough that seems to make even a laugh sound more like a rattle is a thing of the past. Their children and others around them are healthier, too.

What To Do About Relapse.

What should you do if you slip and start smoking again? The answer is simple. A lapse of one or two or even a few cigarettes should not spoil your efforts! Throw away your cigarettes, forgive yourself and continue with the program. Listen to the Compact Disc again and re-read the User's Guide to ensure that you're using NicoDerm CQ correctly and following the other important tips for dealing with the mental and social dependence on nicotine. Your doctor, pharmacist or other health professional can also provide useful counseling on the importance of stopping smoking. You should consider them partners in your quit attempt.

What To Do About Relapse After a Successful Quit Attempt.

If you have taken up regular smoking again, don't be discouraged. Research shows that the best thing you can do is try again, since several quitting attempts may be needed before you're successful. And your chances of quitting successfully increase with each quit attempt.

The important thing is to learn from your last attempt.

- Admit that you've slipped, but don't treat yourself as a failure.
- Try to identify the "trigger" that caused you to slip, and prepare a better plan for dealing with this problem next time.
- Talk positively to yourself – tell yourself that you have learned something from this experience.
- Make sure you used NicoDerm CQ patches correctly
- Remember that it takes practice to do anything, and quitting smoking is no exception.

WHEN THE STRUGGLE IS OVER.

Once you've stopped smoking, take a second and pat yourself on your back. Now do it again. You deserve it. Remember now why you decided to stop smoking in the first place. Look at your list of reasons. Read them again. And smile.

Now think about all the money you are saving and what you'll do with it. All the non-smoking places you can go, and what you might do there. All those years you may have added to your life, and what you'll do with them. Remember that temptation may not be gone forever. However, the hard part is behind you so look forward with a positive attitude, and enjoy your new life as a non-smoker.

QUESTIONS & ANSWERS

1. How will I feel when I stop smoking and start using NicoDerm CQ?

You'll need to prepare yourself for some nicotine withdrawal symptoms. These begin almost immediately after you stop smoking, and are usually at their worst during the first three or four days. Understand that any of the following is possible:

- craving for nicotine
- anxiety, irritability, restlessness, mood changes, nervousness
- disruptions of your sleep
- drowsiness
- trouble concentrating
- increased appetite and weight gain
- headaches, muscular pain, constipation, fatigue.

NicoDerm CQ reduces nicotine withdrawal symptoms such as irritability and nervousness, as well as the craving for nicotine you used to satisfy by having a cigarette.

2. Is NicoDerm CQ just substituting one form of nicotine for another?

NicoDerm CQ does contain nicotine. The purpose of NicoDerm CQ is to provide you with enough nicotine to reduce the physical withdrawal symptoms so you can deal with the mental aspects of quitting.

3. Can I be hurt by using NicoDerm CQ?

For most adults, the amount of nicotine delivered from the patch is less than

from smoking. If you believe you may be sensitive to even this amount of nicotine, you should not use this product without advice from your doctor. There are also some important warnings in this User's Guide (See page 4).

4. Will I gain weight?

Many people do tend to gain a few pounds the first 8–10 weeks after they stop smoking. This is a very small price to pay for the enormous gains that you will make in your overall health and attractiveness. If you continue to gain weight after the first two months, try to analyze what you're doing differently. Reduce your fat intake, choose healthy snacks, and increase your physical activity to burn off the extra calories. Drink lots of water. This is good for your body and skin, and also helps to reduce the amount you eat.

5. Is NicoDerm CQ more expensive than smoking?

The total cost of NicoDerm CQ program is similar to what a person who smokes one and a half packs of cigarettes a day would spend on cigarettes for the same period of time. Also, use of NicoDerm CQ is only a short-term cost, while the cost of smoking is a long-term cost, including the health problems smoking causes.

6. What if I slip up?

Discard your cigarettes, forgive yourself and then get back on track. Don't consider yourself a failure or punish yourself. In fact, people who have already tried to quit are more likely to be successful the next time.

GOOD LUCK!

WALLET CARD

My most important reasons to quit smoking are:

WALLET CARD

Where to call for Help:

American Lung Association	American Cancer Society	American Heart Association
800-586-4872	800-227-2345	800-242-8721

For people who smoke more than 10 cigarettes per day:

STEP 1	STEP 2	STEP 3
Use one 21 mg patch/day Weeks 1–6	Use one 14 mg patch/day Weeks 7–8	Use one 7 mg patch/day Weeks 9–10

People who smoke 10 or less cigarettes per day. Do not use STEP 1 (21 mg). Use STEP 2 (14 mg) for six weeks and STEP 3 (7 mg) for two weeks and then stop.

Copyright © 2002 GlaxoSmithKline

For your family's protection, NicoDerm CQ patches are supplied in child resistant pouches. Do not use if individual pouch is open or torn. Manufactured by ALZA Corporation, Mountain View, CA 94043 for GlaxoSmithKline Consumer Healthcare, L.P. Comments or Questions? Call 1–800–834–5895 Weekdays. (10 a.m.–4:30 p.m. EST).

- **Not for sale to those under 18 years of age.**
- **Proof of age required.**

- Not for sale in vending machines or from any source where proof of age cannot be verified.

Available as

NicoDerm CQ Step 1 (21 mg/24 hours)–7 Patches*

NicoDerm CQ Step 1 (21 mg/24 hours)–14 Patches*

NicoDerm CQ Step 2 (14 mg/24 hours)–14 Patches*

NicoDerm CQ Step 3 (7 mg/24 hours)–14 Patches**

NicoDerm CQ Clear Step 1 (21 mg/24 hours)–7 Patches*

NicoDerm CQ Clear Step 1 (21 mg/24 hours)–14 Patches*

NicoDerm CQ Clear Step 1 (21 mg/24 hours)–21 Patches*

NicoDerm CQ Clear Step 2 (14 mg/24 hours)–14 Patches*

NicoDerm CQ Clear Step 3 (7 mg/24 hours)–14 Patches**

* User's Guide, CD & Child Resistant Disposal Tray

** User's Guide, & Child Resistant Disposal Tray

Shown in Product Identification Guide, page 505

NICODERM® CQ® CLEAR
Nicotine Transdermal System/Stop Smoking Aid

Formerly available only by prescription
Available as:

Step 1 - 21 mg/24 hours
Step 2 - 14 mg/24 hours
Step 3 - 7 mg/24 hours

If you smoke:
More than 10 Cigarettes per Day:
Start with Step 1
10 Cigarettes a Day or Less:
Start with Step 2

WHAT IS THE NICODERM CQ PATCH AND HOW IS IT USED?
NicoDerm CQ is a small, nicotine containing patch. When you put on a NicoDerm CQ patch, nicotine passes through the skin and into your body. NicoDerm CQ is very thin and uses special material to control how fast nicotine passes through the skin. Unlike the sudden jolts of nicotine delivered by cigarettes, the amount of nicotine you receive remains relatively smooth throughout the 24 or 16 hours period you wear the NicoDerm CQ patch. This helps to reduce cravings you may have for nicotine.

Active Ingredient: Nicotine

Purpose: Stop Smoking Aid

Use: reduces withdrawal symptoms, including nicotine craving, associated with quitting smoking

Directions:
- if you are under 18 years of age, ask a doctor before use
- before using this product, read the enclosed user's guide for complete directions and other information
- stop smoking completely when you begin using the patch
- **if you smoke more than 10 cigarettes per day,** use according to the following 10 week schedule:

STEP 1	STEP 2	STEP 3
Use one 21 mg patch/day	Use one 14 mg patch/day	Use one 7 mg patch/day
Weeks 1–6	Weeks 7–8	Weeks 9–10

- if you smoke **10 or less cigarettes per day,** do not use **STEP 1 (21 mg).** Start with **STEP 2 (14 mg)** for 6 weeks, then **STEP 3 (7 mg)** for two weeks and then stop.
- steps 2 and 3 allow you to gradually reduce your level of nicotine. Completing the full program will increase your chances of quitting successfully.
- apply one new patch every 24 hours on skin that is dry, clean and hairless
- remove backing from patch and immediately press onto skin. Hold for 10 seconds.
- wash hands after applying or removing patch. Throw away the patch in the enclosed disposal tray. See enclosed user's guide for safety and handling.
- you may wear the patch for 16 or 24 hours
- if you crave cigarettes when you wake up, wear the patch for 24 hours
- if you have vivid dreams or other sleep disturbances, you may remove the patch at bedtime and apply a new one in the morning
- the used patch should be removed and a new one applied to a different skin site at the same time each day
- do not wear more than one patch at a time
- do not cut patch in half or into smaller pieces
- do not leave patch on for more than 24 hours because it may irritate your skin and loses strength after 24 hours
- stop using the patch at the end of 10 weeks. If you started with **STEP 2,** stop using the patch at the end of 8 weeks. If you still feel the need to use the patch talk to your doctor.

Warnings:
If you are pregnant or breast-feeding, only use this medicine on the advice of your health care provider. Smoking can seriously harm your child. Try to stop smoking without using any nicotine replacement medicine. This medicine is believed to be safer than smoking. However, the risks to your child from this medicine are not fully known.

Do Not Use
- if you continue to smoke, chew tobacco, use snuff, or use a nicotine gum or other nicotine containing products

Ask a doctor before use if you have
- heart disease, recent heart attack, or irregular heartbeat. Nicotine can increase your heart rate.
- high blood pressure not controlled with medication. Nicotine can increase your blood pressure.
- an allergy to adhesive tape or skin problems because you are more likely to get rashes

Ask a doctor or pharmacist before use if you are
- using a non-nicotine stop smoking drug
- taking a prescription medication for depression or asthma. Your prescription dose may need to be adjusted.

When using this product
- do not smoke even when not wearing the patch. The nicotine in your skin will still be entering your blood stream for several hours after you take off the patch.
- if you have vivid dreams or other sleep disturbances remove this patch at bedtime

Stop use and ask a doctor if
- skin redness caused by the patch does not go away after four days, or if skin swells, or you get a rash
- irregular heartbeat or palpitations occur
- you get symptoms of nicotine overdose such as nausea, vomiting, dizziness, weakness and rapid heartbeat

Keep out of reach of children and pets. Used patches have enough nicotine to poison children and pets. If swallowed, get medical help or contact a Poison Control Center right away. Dispose of the used patches by folding sticky ends together and inserting in disposal tray in this box.

READ THE LABEL
Read the carton and the User's Guide before using this product. Keep the carton and User's Guide. They contain important information.

Inactive Ingredients: Ethylene vinyl acetate-copolymer, polyisobutylene and high density polyethylene between clear polyester backings.

Store at 20–25°C (68–77°F)

TO INCREASE YOUR SUCCESS IN QUITTING:
1. You must be motivated to quit.
2. Complete the full treatment program, applying a new patch every day.
3. Use with a support program as described in the Users Guide.

NicoDerm CQ User's Guide
KEYS TO SUCCESS
1) You must really want to quit smoking for **NicoDerm® CQ®** to help you.
2) Complete the full program, applying a new patch every day.
3) **NicoDerm CQ** works best when used together with a support program: See page 3 for details.
4) If you have trouble using **NicoDerm CQ,** ask your doctor or pharmacist or call GlaxoSmithKline 1-800-834-5895 weekdays (10:00 am 4:30 pm EST).

SO, YOU'VE DECIDED TO QUIT.
Congratulations. Your decision to stop smoking is one of the most important things you can do to improve your health. Quitting smoking is a two-part process that involves:
1) overcoming your physical need for nicotine, and
2) breaking your smoking habit.

NicoDerm CQ helps smokers quit by reducing nicotine withdrawal symptoms.

Many NicoDerm CQ users will be able to stop smoking for a few days but often will start smoking again. Most smokers have to try to quit several times before they completely stop.

Your own chances of quitting smoking depend on how strongly you are addicted to nicotine, how much you want to quit,

Continued on next page

NicoDerm CQ—Cont.

and how closely you follow a quitting plan like the one that comes with NicoDerm CQ.

QUITTING SMOKING IS HARD!

If you find you cannot stop or if you start smoking again after using NicoDerm CQ please talk to a health care professional who can help you find a program that may work better for you. Breaking this addiction doesn't happen overnight.

Because NicoDerm CQ provides some nicotine, the NicoDerm CQ patch will help you stop smoking by reducing nicotine withdrawal symptoms such as nicotine craving, nervousness and irritability.

This User's Guide will give you support as you become a non-smoker. It will answer common questions about NicoDerm CQ and give tips to help you stop smoking, and should be referred to often.

WHERE TO GET HELP.

You are more likely to stop smoking by using NicoDerm CQ with a support program that helps you break your smoking habit. There may be support groups in your area for people trying to quit. Call your local chapter of the American Lung Association, American Cancer Society or American Heart Association for further information. Toll free phone numbers are printed on the wallet card on the back cover of this User's Guide.

If you find you cannot stop smoking or if you start smoking again after using NicoDerm CQ, remember breaking this addiction doesn't happen overnight. You may want to talk to a health care professional who can help you improve your chances of quitting the next time you try NicoDerm CQ or another method.

LET'S GET ORGANIZED.

Your reason for quitting may be a combination of concerns about health, the effect of smoking on your appearance, and pressure from your family and friends to stop smoking. Or maybe you're concerned about the dangerous effect of second-hand smoke on the people you care about.

All of these are good reasons. You probably have others. Decide your most important reasons, and write them down on the wallet card inside the back cover of this User's Guide. Carry this card with you. In difficult moments, when you want to smoke, the card will remind you why you are quitting.

WHAT YOU'RE UP AGAINST.

Smoking is addictive in two ways. Your need for nicotine has become both physical and mental. You must overcome both addictions to stop smoking. So while NicoDerm CQ will lessen your body's craving for nicotine, you've got to want to quit smoking to overcome the mental dependence on cigarettes. Once you've decided that you're going to quit, it's time to get started. But first, there are some important cautions you should consider.

SOME IMPORTANT WARNINGS.

This product is only for those who want to stop smoking.

If you are pregnant or breast-feeding, only use this medicine on the advice of your health care provider. Smoking can seriously harm your child. Try to stop smoking without using any nicotine replacement medicine. This medicine is believed to be safer than smoking. However, the risks to your child from this medicine are not fully known.

Do not use
- if you continue to smoke, chew tobacco, use snuff or use a nicotine gum or other nicotine products.

Ask a doctor before use if you have:
- heart disease, recent heart attack, or irregular heartbeat. Nicotine can increase your heart rate.
- high blood pressure not controlled with medication. Nicotine can increase your blood pressure.
- an allergy to adhesive tape or have skin problems because you are more likely to get rashes.

Ask a doctor or pharmacist before use if you are
- using a non-nicotine stop smoking drug
- taking a prescription medication for asthma or depression. Your prescription dose may need to be adjusted.

When using this product:
- do not smoke even when not wearing the patch. The nicotine in your skin will still be entering your bloodstream for several hours after you take off the patch.
- you have vivid dreams or other sleep disturbances remove this patch at bedtime.

Stop use and ask a doctor if:
- skin redness caused by the patch does not go away after four days, or if your skin swells or you get a rash.
- irregular heartbeat or palpitations occur
- you get symptoms of nicotine overdose, such as nausea, vomiting, dizziness, weakness and rapid heartbeat.

Keep out of reach of children and pets. Used patches have enough nicotine to poison children and pets. If swallowed, get medical help or contact a Poison Control Center right away. Dispose of the used patches by folding sticky ends together and inserting in the disposal tray in this box.

LET'S GET STARTED.

If you are under 18 years of age, ask a doctor before use.

Becoming a non-smoker starts today. Your first step is to read through this entire User's Guide carefully.

First, check that you bought the right starting dose.

If you smoke more than 10 cigarettes a day, begin with Step 1 (21 mg). As the carton indicates, people who smoke 10 or less cigarettes per day should not use Step 1 (21 mg). They should start with Step 2 (14 mg). Throughout this User's Guide we will give specific instructions for people who smoke 10 or less cigarettes per day.

Next, set your personalized quitting schedule.

Take out a calendar that you can use to track your progress. Pick a quit date, and mark this on your calendar using the stickers in the middle of this User's Guide, as described below.

DIRECTIONS: FOR PEOPLE WHO SMOKE MORE THAN 10 CIGARETTES PER DAY

STEP 1. (Weeks 1–6). Your quit date (and the day you'll start using NicoDerm CQ patch).

Choose your quit date (it should be soon).

This is the day you will quit smoking cigarettes entirely and begin using NicoDerm CQ to reduce your cravings for nicotine. Place the Step 1 sticker on this date. For the first six weeks, you'll use the highest-strength (21 mg) NicoDerm CQ patches. Be sure to follow the directions on page 10.

Completing the full program will increase your chances of quitting successfully. This is done by changing over to the Step 2 (14mg) patch for 2 weeks followed by a final 2 weeks with the Step 3 (7mg) patch. The Step 2 and Step 3 treatment periods allow you to gradually reduce the amount of nicotine you get, rather than stopping suddenly, and will increase your chances of quitting.

STEP 2. (Weeks 7–8). The day you'll start reducing your use of NicoDerm CQ patch.

Switching to Step 2 (14mg) patches after 6 weeks begins to gradually reduce your nicotine usage. Place the Step 2 sticker on this date (the first day of week seven). Use the 14mg patches for two weeks.

STEP 3. (Weeks 9–10). The day you'll further start reducing your use of NicoDerm CQ patch.

After eight weeks, nicotine intake is further reduced by moving down to Step 3 (7mg) patches. Place the Step 3 sticker on this date (the first day of week nine). Use the 7 mg patches for two weeks.

THE NICODERM CQ PROGRAM

STEP 1	STEP 2	STEP 3
Use one	Use one	Use one
21 mg	14 mg	7 mg
patch/day	patch/day	patch/day
Weeks 1–6	Weeks 7–8	Weeks 9–10

STOP USING NICODERM CQ AT THE END OF WEEK 10. If you still feel the need to use the patch after Week 10, talk with your doctor or health professional.

DIRECTIONS: FOR PEOPLE WHO SMOKE 10 OR LESS CIGARETTES PER DAY

Do not use Step 1 (21 mg).

Begin with STEP 2 – Initial Treatment Period (Weeks 1–6): 14mg patches.

Choose our quit date (it should be soon). This is the Day you will quit smoking cigarettes entirely and begin using NicoDerm CQ to reduce your cravings for nicotine. Place the Step 2 sticker on this date. For the first six weeks, you'll use the Step 2 (14mg) NicoDerm CQ patches. Be sure to follow the directions on page 10.

Continue with STEP 3 – Step Down Treatment Period (Weeks 7–8): 7mg patches.

Completing the full program will increase your chances of quitting successfully. This is done by changing over to the Step 3 (7mg) patches for 2 weeks. The two week step down treatment period allows you to gradually reduce the amount of nicotine you get, rather than stopping suddenly, and will increase your chances of quitting. Place the Step 3 sticker on the first day of week seven. Use the 7mg patches for two weeks.

People who smoke 10 or less cigarettes per day should not use NicoDerm CQ for longer than 8 weeks. If you still feel the need to use NicoDerm CQ after 8 weeks, talk with your doctor.

PLAN AHEAD.

Because smoking is an addiction, it is not easy to stop. After you've given up nicotine, you may still have a strong urge to smoke. Plan ahead NOW for these times, so you're not tempted to start smoking again in a moment of weakness. The following tips may help:

- Keep the phone numbers of supportive friends and family members handy.
- Keep a record of your quitting process. In the event that you slip, immediately stop smoking and resume your quit attempt with the NicoDerm CQ patch. If you smoke at all, write down what you think caused the slip.
- Put together an Emergency Kit that includes items that will help take your mind off occasional urges to smoke. You might include cinnamon gum or lemon drops to suck on, a relaxing cassette tape, and something for your hands to play with, like a smooth rock, rubber band or small metal balls.
- Set aside some small rewards, like a new magazine or a gift certificate from your favorite store, which you'll "give" yourself after passing difficult hurdles.
- Think now about the times when you most often want a cigarette, and then plan what else you might do instead of smoking. For instance, you might plan to take your coffee break in a new location, or take a walk right after dinner, so you won't be tempted to smoke.

HOW NICODERM CQ WORKS.

NicoDerm CQ patches provide nicotine to your system. They work as a temporary aid to help you quit smoking by reducing nicotine withdrawal symptoms, including nicotine craving. NicoDerm CQ provides a lower level of nicotine to your blood than cigarettes, and allows you to gradually do away with your body's need for nicotine.

Because NicoDerm CQ does not contain the tar or carbon monoxide of cigarette smoke, it does not have the same health dangers as tobacco. However, it still delivers nicotine, the addictive part of cigarette smoke. Nicotine can cause side effects such as headache, nausea, upset stomach, and dizziness.

HOW TO USE NICODERM CQ PATCHES.

Read all the following instructions, and the instructions on the outer carton, before using NicoDerm CQ. Refer to them often to make sure you're using NicoDerm CQ correctly. Please refer to the CD for additional help.

1) Stop smoking completely before you start using NicoDerm CQ.
2) To reduce nicotine craving and other withdrawal symptoms, use NicoDerm CQ according to the directions on pages 6–8.
3) Insert used NicoDerm CQ patches in the child resistant disposal tray provided in the box – safely away from children and pets.

When to apply and remove NicoDerm CQ patches.

Each day apply a new patch to a different place on skin that is dry, clean and hairless. **You can wear a NicoDerm CQ patch for either 16 or 24 hours.** If you crave cigarettes when you wake up, wear the patch for 24 hours. If you begin to have vivid dreams or other disruptions of your sleep while wearing the patch 24 hours, try taking the patch off at bedtime (after about 16 hours) and putting on a new one when you get up the next day.

PLACE THESE STICKERS ON YOUR CALENDAR

STEP 1	STEP 2
A new 21 mg patch every day AT THE BEGINNING OF WEEK #1 (QUIT DAY)	A new 14 mg patch every day AT THE BEGINNING OF WEEK #7

For people who smoke 10 or less cigarettes per day: Do not use STEP 1 (21 mg). Use STEP 2 (14 mg) at the beginning of week #1 and STEP 3 (7 mg) at the beginning of week #7.

PLACE THESE STICKERS ON YOUR CALENDAR

STEP 3	EX-SMOKER
A new 7 mg patch every day AT THE BEGINNING OF WEEK #9	WHEN YOU HAVE COMPLETED YOUR QUITTING PROGRAM

Do not smoke even when you are not wearing the patch.

Remove the used patch and put on a new patch at the same time every day. Applying the patch at about the same time each day (first thing in the morning, for instance) will help you remember when to put on a new patch. Do not leave the same NicoDerm CQ patch on for more than 24 hours because it may irritate your skin and because it loses strength after 24 hours.

Do not use NicoDerm CQ continuously for more than 10 weeks (8 weeks for people who smoke 10 or less cigarettes per day).

How to apply a NicoDerm CQ patch.

1. Do not remove the NicoDerm CQ patch from its sealed protective pouch until you are ready to use it. NicoDerm CQ patches will lose nicotine to the air if you store them out of the pouch.
2. Choose a non-hairy, clean, dry area of skin. Do not put a NicoDerm CQ patch on skin that is burned, broken out, cut, or irritated in any way. Make sure your skin is free of lotion and soap before applying a patch.
3. A clear, protective liner covers the sticky back side of the NicoDerm CQ patch—the side that will be put on your skin. The liner has a slit down the middle to help you remove it from the patch. With the sticky back side facing you, pull half the liner away from the NicoDerm CQ patch starting at the middle slit, as shown in the illustration above. Hold the NicoDerm CQ patch at one of the outside edges (touch the sticky side as little as possible), and pull off the other half of the protective liner.

Place this liner in the slot in the disposable tray provided in the NicoDerm CQ package where it will be out of reach of children and pets.

4. Immediately apply the sticky side of the NicoDerm CQ patch to your skin. **Press the patch firmly on your skin with the heel of your hand for at least 10 seconds.** Make sure it sticks well to your skin, especially around the edges.
5. Wash your hands when you have finished applying the NicoDerm CQ patch. Nicotine on your hands could get into your eyes and nose, and cause stinging, redness, or more serious problems.
6. After 24 or 16 hours, remove the patch you have been wearing. Fold the used NicoDerm CQ patch in half with the sticky side together. Carefully dispose of the used patch in the slot of the disposal tray provided in the NicoDerm CQ package where it will be out of the reach of children and pets. Even used patches have enough nicotine to poison children and pets. Wash your hands.
7. Chose a different place on your skin to apply the next NicoDerm CQ patch and repeat Steps 1 to 6. Do not apply a new patch to a previously used skin site for at least one week.

If your NicoDerm CQ patch gets wet during wearing.

Water will not harm the NicoDerm CQ patch you are wearing if applied properly. You can bathe, swim, or shower for short periods while you are wearing the NicoDerm CQ patch.

If your NicoDerm CQ patch comes off while wearing.

NicoDerm CQ patches generally stick well to most people's skin. However, a patch may occasionally come off. If your NicoDerm CQ patch falls off during the day, put on a new patch, making sure you select a non-hairy, non-irritated area of the skin that is clean and dry.

If the soap you use has lanolin or moisturizers, the patch may not stick well. Using a different soap may help. Body creams, lotions and sunscreens can also cause problems with keeping your patch on. Do not apply creams or lotions to the place on your skin where you will put the patch.

If you have followed the directions and the patch still does not stick to you, try using medical adhesive tape over the patch.

Disposing of NicoDerm CQ patches.

Fold the used patch in half with the sticky side together.

Continued on next page

NicoDerm CQ—Cont.

Carefully dispose of the patch in the disposal slot of the tray provided in the NicoDerm CQ package where it will be out of the reach of children and pets. Small amounts of nicotine, even from a used patch, can poison children and pets. **Keep all nicotine patches away from children and pets.** Wash your hands after disposing of the patch.

If your skin reacts to the NicoDerm CQ patch.

When you first put on a NicoDerm CQ patch, mild itching, burning, or tingling is normal and should go away within an hour. After you remove a NicoDerm CQ patch, the skin under the patch might be somewhat red. Your skin should not stay red for more than a day after removing the patch. **Stop use and ask a doctor if skin redness caused by the patch does not go away after four days, or if your skin swells, or you get a rash. Do not put on a new patch.**

Storage Instructions

Keep each NicoDerm CQ patch in its protective pouch, unopened, until you are ready to use it, because the patch will lose nicotine to the air if it's outside the pouch.

Store NicoDerm CQ patches at 20–25 C (68–77 F) because they are sensitive to heat. Remember, the inside of your car can reach temperatures much higher than this. A slight yellowing of the sticky side of the patch is normal. Do not use NicoDerm CQ patches stored in pouches that are open or torn.

TIPS TO MAKE QUITTING EASIER.

Within the first few weeks of giving up smoking, you may be tempted to smoke for pleasure, particularly after completing a difficult task, or at a party or bar. Hear are some tips to help get you through the important first stages of becoming a nonsmoker:

On Your Quit Date:
- Ask your family, friends and co-workers to support you in your efforts to stop smoking.
- Throw away all your cigarettes, matches, lighters, ashtrays, etc.
- Keep busy on your quit day. Exercise. Go to a movie. Take a walk. Get together with friends.
- Figure out how much money you'll save by not smoking. Most ex-smokers can save more than $1,000 a year on the price of cigarettes alone.
- Write down what you will do with the money you save.
- Know your high risk situations and plan ahead how you will deal with them.
- Visit your dentist and have your teeth cleaned to get rid of the tobacco stains.

Right after Quitting:
- During the first few days after you've stopped smoking, spend as much time as possible at places where smoking is not allowed.
- Drink large quantities of water and fruit juices.
- Try to avoid alcohol, coffee and other beverages you associate with smoking.

- Remember that temporary urges to smoke will pass, even if you don't smoke a cigarette.
- Keep your hands busy with something like a pencil or a paper clip.
- Find other activities that help you relax without cigarettes. Swim, jog, take a walk, play basketball.
- Don't worry too much about gaining weight. Watch what you eat, take time for daily exercise, and change your eating habits if you need to.
- Laughter helps. Watch or read something funny

WHAT TO EXPECT.

The First Few Days.

Your body is now coming back into balance. During the first few days after you stop smoking, you might feel edgy and nervous and have trouble concentrating. You might get headaches, feel dizzy and a little out of sorts, feel sweaty or have stomach upsets. You might even have trouble sleeping at first. These are typical nicotine withdrawal symptoms that will go away with time. Your smoker's cough will get worse before it gets better. But don't worry, that's a good sign. Coughing helps clear the tar deposits out of your lungs.

After A Week Or Two.

By now you should be feeling more confident that you can handle those smoking urges. Many of your nicotine withdrawal symptoms have left by now, and you should be noticing some positive signs: less coughing, better breathing and an improved sense of taste and smell, to name a few.

After A Month.

You probably have the urge to smoke much less often now. But urges may still occur, and when they do, they are likely to be powerful ones that come out of nowhere. Don't let them catch you off guard. Plan ahead for these difficult times.

Concentrate on the ways non-smokers are more attractive than smokers. Their skin is less likely to wrinkle. Their teeth are whiter, cleaner. Their breath is fresher.

Their hair and clothes smell better. That cough that seems to make even a laugh sound more like a rattle is a thing of the past. Their children and others around them are healthier, too.

What To Do About Relapse.

What should you do if you slip and start smoking again? The answer is simple. A lapse of one or two or even a few cigarettes should not spoil your efforts! Throw away your cigarettes, forgive yourself and continue with the program. Listen to the Compact Disc again and re-read the User's Guide to ensure that you're using NicoDerm CQ correctly and following the other important tips for dealing with the mental and social dependence on nicotine. Your doctor, pharmacist or other health professional can also provide useful counseling on the importance of stopping smoking. You should consider them partners in your quit attempt.

What To Do About Relapse After a Successful Quit Attempt.

If you have taken up regular smoking again, don't be discouraged. Research shows that the best thing you can do is try again, since several quitting attempts may be needed before you're successful. And your chances of quitting successfully increase with each quit attempt.

The important thing is to learn from your last attempt.
- Admit that you've slipped, but don't treat yourself as a failure.
- Try to identify the "trigger" that caused you to slip, and prepare a better plan for dealing with this problem next time.
- Talk positively to yourself – tell yourself that you have learned something from this experience.
- Make sure you used NicoDerm CQ patches correctly
- Remember that it takes practice to do anything, and quitting smoking is no exception.

WHEN THE STRUGGLE IS OVER.

Once you've stopped smoking, take a second and pat yourself on your back. Now do it again. You deserve it. Remember now why you decided to stop smoking in the first place. Look at your list of reasons. Read them again. And smile.

Now think about all the money you are saving and what you'll do with it. All the non-smoking places you can go, and what you might do there. All those years you may have added to your life, and what you'll do with them. Remember that temptation may not be gone forever. However, the hard part is behind you so look forward with a positive attitude, and enjoy your new life as a non-smoker.

QUESTIONS & ANSWERS

1. How will I feel when I stop smoking and start using NicoDerm CQ?

You'll need to prepare yourself for some nicotine withdrawal symptoms. These begin almost immediately after you stop smoking, and are usually at their worst during the first three or four days. Understand that any of the following is possible:
- craving for nicotine
- anxiety, irritability, restlessness, mood changes, nervousness
- disruptions of your sleep
- drowsiness
- trouble concentrating
- increased appetite and weight gain
- headaches, muscular pain, constipation, fatigue

NicoDerm CQ reduces nicotine withdrawal symptoms such as irritability and nervousness, as well as the craving for nicotine you used to satisfy by having a cigarette.

2. Is NicoDerm CQ just substituting one form of nicotine for another?

NicoDerm CQ does contain nicotine. The purpose of NicoDerm CQ is to provide you with enough nicotine to reduce the physical withdrawal symptoms so you can deal with the mental aspects of quitting.

3. Can I be hurt by using NicoDerm CQ?

For most adults, the amount of nicotine delivered from the patch is less than from smoking. If you believe you may be sensitive to even this amount of nicotine, you should not use this product without advice from your doctor. There are also some important warnings in this User's Guide (See page 4).

4. Will I gain weight?
Many people do tend to gain a few pounds the first 8–10 weeks after they stop smoking. This is a very small price to pay for the enormous gains that you will make in your overall health and attractiveness. If you continue to gain weight after the first two months, try to analyze what you're doing differently. Reduce your fat intake, choose healthy snacks, and increase your physical activity to burn off the extra calories. Drink lots of water. This is good for your body and skin, and also helps to reduce the amount you eat.

5. Is NicoDerm CQ more expensive than smoking?
The total cost of NicoDerm CQ program is similar to what a person who smokes one and a half packs of cigarettes a day would spend on cigarettes for the same period of time. Also, use of NicoDerm CQ is only a short-term cost, while the cost of smoking is a long-term cost, including the health problems smoking causes.

6. What if I slip up?
Discard your cigarettes, forgive yourself and then get back on track. Don't consider yourself a failure or punish yourself. In fact, people who have already tried to quit are more likely to be successful the next time.
GOOD LUCK!
WALLET CARD
My most important reasons to quit smoking are:
WALLET CARD
Where to call for Help:

| American Lung Association 800-586-4872 | American Cancer Society 800-227-2345 | American Heart Association 800-242-8721 |

For people who smoke more than 10 cigarettes per day:

STEP 1	STEP 2	STEP 3
Use one 21 mg patch/day Weeks 1–6	Use one 14 mg patch/day Weeks 7–8	Use one 7 mg patch/day Weeks 9–10

People who smoke 10 or less cigarettes per day. Do not use STEP 1 (21 mg). Use STEP 2 (14 mg) for six weeks and STEP 3 (7 mg) for two weeks and then stop.
Copyright © 2004 GlaxoSmithKline
For your family's protection, NicoDerm CQ patches are supplied in child resistant pouches. Do not use if individual pouch is open or torn.
Manufactured by ALZA Corporation, Mountain View, CA 94043 for GlaxoSmithKline Consumer Healthcare, L.P. Comments or Questions? Call 1–800–834–5895 Weekdays. (10 a.m.–4:30 p.m. EST).
• **Not for sale to those under 18 years of age.**

• **Proof of age required.**
• **Not for sale in vending machines or from any source where proof of age cannot be verified.**
Available as
NicoDerm CQ Step 1 (21 mg/24 hours)– 7 Patches*
NicoDerm CQ Step 1 (21 mg/24 hours)– 14 Patches*
NicoDerm CQ Step 2 (14 mg/24 hours)– 14 Patches*
NicoDerm CQ Step 3 (7 mg/24 hours)– 14 Patches**
NicoDerm CQ Clear Step 1 (21 mg/24 hours)–7 patches*
NicoDerm CQ Clear Step 1 (21 mg/24 hours)–14 patches*
NicoDerm CQ Clear Step 1 (21 mg/24 hours)–21 patches*
NicoDerm CQ Clear Step 2 (14 mg/24 hours)–14 patches*
NicoDerm CQ Clear Step 3 (7 mg/24 hours)–14 patches**
* User's Guide, CD & Child Resistant Disposal Tray
** User's Guide, & Child Resistant Disposal Tray
Shown in Product Identification Guide, page 504

NICORETTE®
Nicotine Polacrilex Gum/Stop Smoking Aid
Available in Original 2mg and 4mg Strengths,
Mint 2mg and 4mg Strengths and Orange 2mg and 4mg Strengths

IF YOU SMOKE LESS THAN 25 CIGARETTES A DAY: Use 2 mg
IF YOU SMOKE 25 OR MORE CIGARETTES A DAY: Use 4 mg

Action: Stop Smoking Aid

Drug Facts:

| **Active Ingredient:** (In each chewing piece) Nicotine polacrilex, 2 or 4 mg .... | **Purpose:** Stop smoking aid |

Use:
• reduces withdrawal symptoms, including nicotine craving, associated with quitting smoking

Warnings:
If you are pregnant or breast-feeding, only use this medicine on the advice of your health care provider. Smoking can seriously harm your child. Try to stop smoking without using any nicotine replacement medicine. This medicine is believed to be safer than smoking. However, the risks to your child from this medicine are not fully known.
Do not use:
• if you continue to smoke, chew tobacco, use snuff, or use a nicotine patch or other nicotine containing products

Ask a doctor before use if you have:
• heart disease, recent heart attack, or irregular heartbeat. Nicotine can increase your heart rate.
• high blood pressure not controlled with medication. Nicotine can increase blood pressure.
• stomach ulcer or diabetes
Ask a doctor or pharmacist before use if you are:
• using a non-nicotine stop smoking drug
• taking prescription medicine for depression or asthma. Your prescription dose may need to be adjusted.
Stop use and ask a doctor if:
• mouth, teeth or jaw problems occur
• irregular heartbeat or palpitations occur
• you get symptoms of nicotine overdose such as nausea, vomiting, dizziness, diarrhea, weakness and rapid heartbeat
Keep out of reach of children and pets. Pieces of nicotine gum may have enough nicotine to make children and pets sick. Wrap used pieces of gum in paper and throw away in the trash. In case of overdose, get medical help or contact a Poison Control Center right away.

Directions:
• if you are under 18 years of age, ask a doctor before use
• before using this product, read the enclosed User's Guide for complete directions and other important information
• stop smoking completely when you begin using the gum
• **if you smoke 25 or more cigarettes a day; use 4 mg nicotine gum**
• **if you smoke less than 25 cigarettes a day; use 2 mg nicotine gum**
Use according to the following 12 week schedule:
[See table below]
• nicotine gum is a medicine and must be used a certain way to get the best results
• chew the gum slowly until it tingles. Then park it between your cheek and gum. When the tingle is gone, begin chewing again, until the tingle returns.
• repeat this process until most of the tingle is gone (about 30 minutes)
• do not eat or drink for 15 minutes before chewing the nicotine gum, or while chewing a piece
• to improve your chances of quitting, use at least 9 pieces per day for the first 6 weeks
• if you experience strong or frequent cravings, you may use a second piece within the hour. However, do not continuously use one piece after another since this may cause you hiccups, heartburn, nausea or other side effects.
• do not use more than 24 pieces a day
• stop using the nicotine gum at the end of 12 weeks. If you still feel the need to use nicotine gum, talk to your doctor.

Continued on next page

Weeks 1 to 6	Weeks 7 to 9	Weeks 10 to 12
1 piece every 1 to 2 hours	1 piece every 2 to 4 hours	1 piece every 4 to 8 hours

Nicorette—Cont.

Other Information:
- store at 20–25°C (68–77°F)
- protect from light

Inactive Ingredients:

Original [2 mg] Inactive Ingredients: Flavors, glycerin, gum base, sodium carbonate, sorbitol, sodium bicarbonate.

Original [4 mg] Inactive Ingredients: Flavors, glycerin, gum base, sodium carbonate, sorbitol, D&C Yellow 10.

Mint [2 mg] Inactive Ingredients: Gum base, magnesium oxide, menthol, peppermint oil, sodium bicarbonate, sodium carbonate, xylitol.

Mint [4 mg] Inactive Ingredients: Gum base, magnesium oxide, menthol, peppermint oil, sodium carbonate, xylitol, D&C yellow #10 Al. lake.

Orange [2 mg] Inactive Ingredients: Flavor, gum base, magnesium oxide, sodium bicarbonate, sodium carbonate, xylitol

Orange [4 mg] Inactive Ingredients: Flavor, gum base, magnesium oxide, sodium carbonate, xylitol, D&C Yellow #10 Al. lake.

TO INCREASE YOUR SUCCESS IN QUITTING:

1. You must be motivated to quit.
2. **Use Enough**—Chew **at least 9 pieces** of Nicorette per day during the first six weeks.
3. **Use Long Enough**—Use Nicorette for the full 12 weeks.
4. **Use with a support program** as directed in the enclosed User's Guide.*

*The American Cancer Society supports the use of a stop smoking aid and counseling as effective tools when quitting smoking but does not endorse any specific product. GlaxoSmithKline pays a fee to the American Cancer Society for the use of its logo.

To remove the gum, tear off single unit.

Peel off backing starting at corner with loose edge.

Push gum through foil.

Blister packaged for your protection. **Do not use if individual seals are open or torn.**

- **not for sale to those under 18 years of age**
- **proof of age required**
- **not for sale in vending machines or from any source where proof of age cannot be verified**

READ THE LABEL

Read the carton and the User's Guide before taking this product. Do not discard carton or User's Guide. They contain important information.

How Supplied: Nicorette Original and Mint are available in:

2 mg or 4 mg Starter kit*—110 pieces
2 mg or 4 mg Refill—48 pieces, 168 pieces or 192 pieces
Nicorette Orange is available in:
2 mg or 4 mg Starter kit*—110 pieces
2 mg or 4 mg Refill—48 pieces
*User's Guide and CD included in kit
Questions or comments? call **1-800-419-4766** weekdays (10:00 a.m.– 4:30 p.m. EST)
Manufactured by Pharmacia AB, Stockholm, Sweden for
GlaxoSmithKline Consumer Healthcare, L.P.
Moon Township, PA 15108

USER'S GUIDE:

HOW TO USE NICORETTE TO HELP YOU QUIT SMOKING

KEYS TO SUCCESS:

1) You must really want to quit smoking for **Nicorette**® to help you.
2) You can greatly increase your chances for success by using at least 9 to 12 pieces every day when you start using **Nicorette**.
3) You should continue to use **Nicorette** as explained in the User's Guide for 12 full weeks.
4) **Nicorette** works best when used together with a support program.
5) If you have trouble using **Nicorette**, ask your doctor or pharmacist or call GlaxoSmithKline at 1-800-419-4766 weekdays (10:00am–4:30pm EST).

SO YOU DECIDED TO QUIT

Congratulations. Your decision to stop smoking is an important one. That's why you've made the right choice in choosing **Nicorette** gum. Your own chances of quitting smoking depend on how much you want to quit, how strongly you are addicted to tobacco, and how closely you follow a quitting program like the one that comes with **Nicorette**.

QUITTING SMOKING IS HARD!

If you've tried to quit before and haven't succeeded, don't be discouraged! Quitting isn't easy. It takes time, and most people try a few times before they are successful. The important thing is to try again until you succeed. This User's Guide will give you support as you become a non-smoker. It will answer common questions about **Nicorette** and give tips to help you stop smoking, and should be referred to often.

WHERE TO GET HELP

You are more likely to stop smoking by using **Nicorette** with a support program that helps you break your smoking habit. There may be support groups in your area for people trying to quit. Call your local chapter of the American Lung Association (1-800-586-4872), American Cancer Society (1-800-227-2345) or American Heart Association (1-800-242-8721) for further information. If you find you cannot stop smoking or if you start smoking again after using **Nicorette**, remember breaking this addiction doesn't happen overnight. You may want to talk to a health care professional who can help you improve your chances of quitting the next time you try **Nicorette** or another method.

LET'S GET ORGANIZED

Your reason for quitting may be a combination of concerns about health, the effect of smoking on your appearance, and pressure from your family and friends to stop smoking. Or maybe you're concerned about the dangerous effect of second-hand smoke on the people you care about. All of these are good reasons. You probably have others. Decide your most important reasons, and write them down on the wallet card inside the back cover of the User's Guide. Carry this card with you. In difficult moments, when you want to smoke, the card will remind you why you are quitting.

WHAT YOU'RE UP AGAINST

Smoking is addictive in two ways. Your need for nicotine has become both physical and mental. You must overcome both addictions to stop smoking. So while **Nicorette** will lessen your body's physical addition to nicotine, you've got to want to quit smoking to overcome the mental dependence on cigarettes. Once you've decided that you're going to quit, it's time to get started. But first, there are some important cautions you should consider.

SOME IMPORTANT WARNINGS. This product is only for those who want to stop smoking.

If you are pregnant or breast-feeding, only use this medicine on the advice of your health care provider. Smoking can seriously harm your child. Try to stop smoking without using any nicotine replacement medicine. This medicine is believed to be safer than smoking. However, the risks to your child from this medicine are not fully known.

Do not use

- if you continue to smoke, chew tobacco, use snuff, or use a nicotine patch or other nicotine containing products.

Ask a doctor before use if you have

- heart disease, recent heart attack, or irregular heartbeat. Nicotine can increase your heart rate.
- high blood pressure not controlled with medication. Nicotine can increase your blood pressure.
- stomach ulcer or diabetes

Ask a doctor or pharmacist before use if you are

- using a non-nicotine stop smoking drug
- taking a prescription medicine for depression or asthma. Your prescription dose may need to be adjusted.

Stop use and ask a doctor if

- mouth, teeth or jaw problems occur
- irregular heartbeat or palpitations occur
- you get symptoms of nicotine overdose such as nausea, vomiting, dizziness, diarrhea, weakness and rapid heartbeat

Keep out of reach of children and pets. Pieces of nicotine gum may have enough nicotine to make children and pets sick. Wrap used pieces of gum in paper and throw away in the trash. In case of overdose, get medical help or contact a Poison Control Center right away.

LET'S GET STARTED

Becoming a non-smoker starts today. First, check that you bought the right starting dose. **If you smoke 25 or more cigarettes a day**, use 4 mg nicotine gum. **If you smoke less than 25 cigarettes a day**, use 2 mg nicotine gum. Next read through the entire User's Guide carefully. Then, set your personalized quitting schedule. Take out a calendar that you can use to track your progress, and identify four dates, using the stickers in the User's Guide.

STEP 1: (Weeks 1–6) Your quit date (and the day you'll start using Nicorette gum). Choose your quit date (it should be soon). This is the day you will quit smoking cigarettes entirely and begin using **Nicorette** to satisfy your cravings for nicotine. For the first six weeks, you'll use a piece of **Nicorette** every hour or two. Be sure to follow the directions starting on pages 9 and 11 of the User's Guide. Place the Step 1 sticker on this date.

STEP 2: (Weeks 7–9) The day you'll start reducing your use of Nicorette. After six weeks, you'll begin gradually reducing your **Nicorette** usage to one piece every two to four hours. Place the Step 2 sticker on this date (the first day of week seven).

STEP 3: (Weeks 10–12) The day you'll further reduce your use of Nicorette. Nine weeks after you begin using **Nicorette**, you will further reduce your nicotine intake by using one piece every four to eight hours. Place the Step 3 sticker on this date (the first day of week ten). For the next three weeks, you'll use a piece of **Nicorette** every four to eight hours. **End of treatment: The day you'll complete Nicorette therapy.**

The following chart lists the recommended usage schedule for **Nicorette**e:

Weeks 1 through 6	Weeks 7 through 9	Weeks 10 through 12
1 piece every 1 to 2 hours	1 piece every 2 to 4 hours	1 piece every 4 to 8 hours

DO NOT USE MORE THAN 24 PIECES PER DAY.

Nicorette should not be used for longer than twelve weeks. Identify the date thirteen weeks after the date you chose in Step 1 and place the "EX-Smoker" sticker on your calendar.

PLAN AHEAD

Because smoking is an addiction, it is not easy to stop. After you've given up cigarettes, you will still have a strong urge to smoke. Plan ahead NOW for these times, so you're not defeated in a moment of weakness. The following tips may help:

- Keep the phone numbers of supportive friends and family members handy.
- Keep a record of your quitting process. Track the number of **Nicorette** pieces you use each day, and whether you feel a craving for cigarettes. In the event that you slip, immediately stop smoking and resume your quit attempt with **Nicorette**.
- Put together an Emergency Kit that includes items that will help take your mind off occasional urges to smoke. Include cinnamon gum or lemon drops to suck on, a relaxing cassette tape and something for your hands to play with, like a smooth rock, rubber band or small metal balls.
- Set aside some small rewards, like a new magazine or a gift certificate from your favorite store, which you'll 'give' yourself after passing difficult hurdles.
- Think about the times when you most often want a cigarette, and then plan what else you might do instead of smoking. For instance, you might plan to take your coffee break in a new location, or take a walk right after dinner, so you won't be tempted to smoke.

HOW NICORETTE GUM WORKS

Nicorette's sugar-free chewing pieces provide nicotine to your system—they work as a temporary aid to help you quit smoking by reducing nicotine withdrawal symptoms. **Nicorette** provides a lower level of nicotine to your blood than cigarettes, and allows you to gradually do away with your body's need for nicotine. Because **Nicorette** does not contain the tar or carbon monoxide of cigarette smoke, it does not have the same health dangers as tobacco. However, it still delivers nicotine, the addictive part of cigarette smoke. Nicotine can cause side effects such as headache, nausea, upset stomach and dizziness.

HOW TO USE NICORETTE GUM

If you are under 18 years of age, ask a doctor before use.

Before you can use **Nicorette** correctly, you have to practice! That sounds silly, but it isn't.

Nicorette isn't like ordinary chewing gum. It's a medicine, and must be chewed a certain way to work right. Chewed like ordinary gum, **Nicorette**

won't work well and can cause side effects. An overdose can occur if you chew more than one piece of **Nicorette** at the same time, or if you chew many pieces one after another. Read all the following instructions before using **Nicorette**. Refer to them often to make sure you're using **Nicorette** gum correctly. If you chew too fast, or do not chew correctly, you may get hiccups, heartburn, or other stomach problems. Don't eat or drink for 15 minutes before using **Nicorette**, or while chewing a piece. The effectiveness of **Nicorette** may be reduced by some foods and drinks, such as coffee, juices, wine or soft drinks.

1. Stop smoking completely before you start using **Nicorette**.
2. To reduce craving and other withdrawal symptoms, use **Nicorette** according to the dosage schedule on page 11 of the User's Guide.
3. Chew each **Nicorette** piece <u>very slowly several times</u>.
4. Stop chewing when you notice a peppery taste, or a slight tingling in your mouth. (This usually happens after about 15 chews, but may vary from person to person.)
5. "PARK" the **Nicorette** piece between your cheek and gum and leave it there.
6. When the peppery taste or tingle is almost gone (in about a minute), start to chew a few times slowly again. When the taste or tingle returns, stop again.
7. Park the **Nicorette** piece again (in a different place in your mouth).
8. Repeat steps 3 to 7 (chew, chew, park) until most of the nicotine is gone from the **Nicorette** piece (usually happens in about half an hour; the peppery taste or tingle won't return).
9. Wrap the used **Nicorette** in paper and throw away in the trash.

See the chart in the **"DIRECTIONS"** section above for the recommended usage schedule for **Nicorette**.

[See table above]

To improve your chances of quitting, use at least 9 pieces of **Nicorette** a day. If you experience strong or frequent cravings you may use a second piece within the hour. However, do not continuously use one piece after another, since this may cause you hiccups, heartburn, nausea or other side effects.

HOW TO REDUCE YOUR NICORETTE USAGE

The goal of using **Nicorette** is to slowly reduce your dependence on nicotine. The schedule for using **Nicorette** will help you reduce your nicotine craving gradually. Here are some tips to help you cut back during each step:

- After a while, start chewing each **Nicorette** piece for only 10 to 15 minutes, instead of half an hour. Then gradually begin to reduce the number of pieces used.

Continued on next page

- Or, try chewing each piece for longer than half an hour, but reduce the number of pieces you use each day.
- Substitute ordinary chewing gum for some of the **Nicorette** pieces you would normally use. Increase the number of pieces of ordinary gum as you cut back on the **Nicorette** pieces.

STOP USING NICORETTE AT THE END OF WEEK 12. If you still feel the need to use **Nicorette** after Week 12, talk with your doctor.

TIPS TO MAKE QUITTING EASIER

Within the first few weeks of giving up smoking, you may be tempted to smoke for pleasure, particularly after completing a difficult task, or at a party or bar. Here are some tips to help get you through the important first stages of becoming a non-smoker:

On your Quit Date:
- Ask your family, friends, and co-workers to support you in your efforts to stop smoking.
- Throw away all your cigarettes, matches, lighters, ashtrays, etc.
- Keep busy on your quit day. Exercise. Go to a movie. Take a walk. Get together with friends.
- Figure out how much money you'll save by not smoking. Most ex-smokers can save more than $1,000 a year.
- Write down what you will do with the money you save.
- Know your high risk situations and plan ahead how you will deal with them.
- Keep **Nicorette** gum near your bed, so you'll be prepared for any nicotine cravings when you wake up in the morning.
- Visit your dentist and have your teeth cleaned to get rid of the tobacco stains.

Right after Quitting:
- During the first few days after you've stopped smoking, spend as much time as possible at places where smoking is not allowed.
- Drink large quantities of water and fruit juices.
- Try to avoid alcohol, coffee and other beverages you associate with smoking.
- Remember that temporary urges to smoke will pass, even if you don't smoke a cigarette.
- Keep your hands busy with something like a pencil or a paper clip.
- Find other activities which help you relax without cigarettes. Swim, jog, take a walk, play basketball.
- Don't worry too much about gaining weight. Watch what you eat, take time for daily exercise, and change your eating habits if you need to.
- Laughter helps. Watch or read something funny.

WHAT TO EXPECT

Your body is now coming back into balance. During the first few days after you stop smoking, you might feel edgy and nervous and have trouble concentrating. You might get headaches, feel dizzy and a little out of sorts, feel sweaty or have stomach upsets. You might even have trouble sleeping at first. These are typical withdrawal symptoms that will go away with time. Your smoker's cough will get worse before it gets better. But don't worry, that's a good sign. Coughing

helps clear the tar deposits out of your lungs.

After a Week or Two.

By now you should be feeling more confident that you can handle those smoking urges. Many of your withdrawal symptoms have left by now, and you should be noticing some positive signs: less coughing, better breathing and an improved sense of taste and smell, to name a few.

After a Month.

You probably have the urge to smoke much less often now. But urges may still occur, and when they do, they are likely to be powerful ones that come out of nowhere. Don't let them catch you off guard. Plan ahead for these difficult times. Concentrate on the ways non-smokers are more attractive than smokers. Their skin is less likely to wrinkle. Their teeth are whiter, cleaner. Their breath is fresher. Their hair and clothes smell better. That cough seems to make even a laugh sound more like a rattle is a thing of the past. Their children and others around them are healthier, too.

What To Do About Relapse.

What should you do if you slip and start smoking again? The answer is simple. A lapse of one or two or even a few cigarettes has not spoiled your efforts! Discard your cigarettes, forgive yourself and try again. If you start smoking again, keep your box of **Nicorette** for your next quit attempt. If you have taken up regular smoking again, don't be discouraged. Research shows that the best thing you can do is to try again. The important thing is to learn from your last attempt.

- Admit that you've slipped, but don't treat yourself as a failure.
- Try to identify the 'trigger' that caused you to slip, and prepare a better plan for dealing with this problem next time.
- Talk positively to yourself—tell yourself that you have learned something from this experience.
- Make sure you used **Nicorette** gum correctly over the full 12 weeks to reduce your craving for nicotine.
- Remember that it takes practice to do anything, and quitting smoking is no exception.

WHEN THE STRUGGLE IS OVER

Once you've stopped smoking, take a second and pat yourself on the back. Now do it again. You deserve it. Remember now why you decided to stop smoking in the first place. Look at your list of reasons. Read them again. And smile. Now think about all the money you are saving and what you'll do with it. All the non-smoking places you can go, and what you might do there. All those years you may have added to your life, and what you'll do with them. Remember that temptation may not be gone forever. However, the hard part is behind you, so look forward with a positive attitude and enjoy your new life as a non-smoker.

QUESTIONS & ANSWERS

1. How will I feel when I stop smoking and start using Nicorette? You'll need to prepare yourself for some nicotine withdrawal symptoms. These begin almost immediately after you stop smoking, and are usually at their worst during the first three to four days. Understand that any of the following is possible:
- craving for cigarettes
- anxiety, irritability, restlessness, mood changes, nervousness
- drowsiness
- trouble concentrating
- increased appetite and weight gain
- headaches, muscular pain, constipation, fatigue.

Nicorette can help provide relief from withdrawal symptoms such as irritability and nervousness, as well as the craving for nicotine you used to satisfy by having a cigarette.

2. Is Nicorette just substituting one form of nicotine for another? **Nicorette** does contain nicotine. The purpose of **Nicorette** is to provide you with enough nicotine to help control the physical withdrawal symptoms so you can deal with the mental aspects of quitting. During the 12 week program, you will gradually reduce your nicotine intake by switching to fewer pieces each day. Remember, don't use **Nicorette** together with nicotine patches or other nicotine containing products.

3. Can I be hurt by using Nicorette? For most adults, the amount of nicotine in the gum is less than from smoking. Some people will be sensitive to even this amount of nicotine and should not use this product without advice from their doctor (see page 4 of User's Guide). Because **Nicorette** is a gum-based product, chewing it can cause dental fillings to loosen and aggravate other mouth, tooth and jaw problems. **Nicorette** can also cause hiccups, heartburn and other stomach problems especially if chewed too quickly or not chewed correctly.

4. Will I gain weight? Many people do tend to gain a few pounds in the first 8–10 weeks after they stop smoking. This is a very small price to pay for the enormous gains that you will make in your overall health and attractiveness. If you continue to gain weight after the first two months, try to analyze what you're doing differently. Reduce your fat intake, choose healthy snacks, and increase your physical activity to burn off the extra calories.

5. Is Nicorette more expensive than smoking? The total cost of **Nicorette** for the twelve week program is about equal to what a person who smokes one and a half packs of cigarettes a day would spend on cigarettes for the same period of time. Also use of **Nicorette** is only a short-term cost, while the cost of smoking is a long-term cost, because of the health problems smoking causes.

6. What if I slip up? Discard your cigarettes, forgive yourself and then get back on track. Don't consider yourself a failure or punish yourself. In fact, people who have already tried to quit are more likely to be successful the next time.
GOOD LUCK!
[End User's Guide]
Copyright © 2004 **GlaxoSmithKline** Consumer Healthcare, L.P.

Shown in Product Identification Guide, page 505

Maximum Strength
NYTOL® QUICKGELS® SOFTGELS

Indication: For relief of occasional sleeplessness.

Directions: Adults and children 12 years of age and over: oral dosage is one softgel (50 mg) at bedtime if needed, or as directed by a doctor.

Warnings: Do not give to children under 12 years of age. If sleeplessness persists continuously for more than two weeks, consult your doctor. Insomnia may be a symptom of serious underlying medical illness. **Do not take this product, unless directed by a doctor, if you have a breathing problem such as emphysema or chronic bronchitis, or if you have glaucoma or difficulty in urination due to enlargement of the prostate gland. Do not use** with any other product containing diphenhydramine, including one applied topically. Avoid alcoholic beverages while taking this product. Do not take this product if you are taking sedatives or tranquilizers, without first consulting your doctor. In case of accidental overdose, seek professional assistance or contact a Poison Control Center immediately. As with any drug, if you are pregnant or nursing a baby, seek the advice of a health professional before using this product. Keep out of reach of children.

Drug Interactions: Alcohol and other drugs which cause CNS depression will heighten the depressant effect of this product. Monoamine oxidase (MAO) inhibitors will prolong and intensify the anticholinergic effects of antihistamines.

Symptoms and Treatment of Oral Overdosage: In adults overdose may cause CNS depression resulting in hypnosis and coma. In children CNS hyperexcitability may follow sedation; the stimulant phase may bring tremor, delirium and convulsions. Gastrointestinal reactions may include dry mouth, appetite loss, nausea and/or vomiting. Respiratory distress and cardiovascular complications (hypotension) may be evident. Treatment includes inducing emesis and controlling symptoms.

Active Ingredient: Diphenhydramine Hydrochloride 50 mg per softgel.

Inactive Ingredients: Edible Ink, Gelatin, Glycerin, Polyethylene Glycol, Purified Water, Sorbitol.

How Supplied: Available in packages of 8 and 16 softgels.

Shown in Product Identification Guide, page 505

NYTOL® QUICKCAPS® CAPLETS

Indication: For relief of occasional sleeplessness.

Directions: Adults and children 12 years of age and over: oral dosage is two caplets (50 mg) at bedtime if needed, or as directed by a doctor.

Warnings: Do not give to children under 12 years of age. If sleeplessness persists continuously for more than two weeks, consult your doctor. Insomnia may be a symptom of serious underlying medical illness. **Do not take this product, unless directed by a doctor, if you have a breathing problem such as emphysema or chronic bronchitis, or if you have glaucoma or difficulty in urination due to enlargement of the prostate gland. Do not use** with any other product containing diphenhydramine, including one applied topically. Avoid alcoholic beverages while taking this product. Do not take this product if you are taking sedatives or tranquilizers, without first consulting your doctor. In case of accidental overdose, seek professional assistance or contact a Poison Control Center immediately. As with any drug, if you are pregnant or nursing a baby, seek the advice of a health professional before using this product. Keep out of reach of children.

Drug Interactions: Alcohol and other drugs which cause CNS depression will heighten the depressant effect of this product. Monoamine oxidase (MAO) inhibitors will prolong and intensify the anticholinergic effects of antihistamines.

Symptoms and Treatment of Oral Overdosage: In adults, overdose may cause CNS depression resulting in hypnosis and coma. In children, CNS hyperexcitability may follow sedation; the stimulant phase may bring tremor, delirium and convulsions. Gastrointestinal reactions may include dry mouth, appetite loss, nausea and/or vomiting. Respiratory distress and cardiovascular complications (hypotension) may be evident. Treatment includes inducing emesis and controlling symptoms.

Active Ingredient: Diphenhydramine Hydrochloride 25 mg per caplet.

Inactive Ingredients: Corn Starch, Lactose, Microcrystalline Cellulose, Silica, Stearic Acid.

How Supplied: Available in tamper-evident packages of 16, 32 and 72 caplets.

Shown in Product Identification Guide, page 505

Quick Dissolve
PHAZYME®–125 MG Chewable Tablets
[fay-zime]

Description: A great tasting, smooth cool mint chewable tablet containing simethicone, an antiflatulent to alleviate or relieve the symptoms referred to as gas. Uniquely formulated to dissolve quickly and completely in your mouth. It has no known side effects or drug interactions.

Active Ingredient: Each tablet contains simethicone 125 mg.

Inactive Ingredients: Aspartame, citricacid, colloidal silicon dioxide, crospovidone, dextrates, maltodextrin, mannitol, peppermint flavor, pregelatinized starch, sodium bicarbonate, sorbitol, talc, tribasic calcium phosphate.

Actions: Simethicone minimizes gas formation and relieves gas entrapment in both the stomach and the lower G.I. tract. This action combats the distress due to gastrointestinal gas.

Other Information: Each tablet contains sodium 8 mg. Phenylketonurics: contains phenylalanine 0.4 mg per tablet.

Indication: Relieves pressure, bloating or fullness commonly referred to as gas.

Warnings: Keep this and all drugs out of the reach of children. If condition persists, consult your physician.

Store at room temperature 59°–86°F (15°–30°C).

Dosage: Directions: Chew one or two tablets thoroughly, as needed after a meal. Do not exceed four tablets per day except under the advice and supervision of a physician.

How Supplied: White, bevel-edged tablets imprinted with "Phazyme 125" in 18 count and 48 count bottles.

Shown in Product Identification Guide, page 505

Ultra Strength
PHAZYME®–180 MG Softgels
[fay-zime]

Description: An orange, easy to swallow softgel, containing simethicone, an antiflatulent to alleviate or relieve the symptoms referred to as gas. It has no known side effects or drug interactions.

Active Ingredient: Each softgel contains simethicone 180 mg.

Inactive Ingredients: FD&C Yellow No. 6, gelatin, glycerin, and white edible ink.

Actions: Simethicone minimizes gas formation and relieves gas entrapment in both the stomach and the lower G.I. tract. This action combats the distress due to gastrointestinal gas.

Indication: Relieves pressure, bloating or fullness commonly referred to as gas.

Warnings: Keep this and all drugs out of the reach of children. If condition persists, consult your physician.

Store at room temperature 59°–86°F (15°–30°C).

Dosage: Directions: Swallow one or two softgels as needed after a meal. Do not exceed two softgels per day except under the advice and supervision of a physician.

Continued on next page

Phazyme—Cont.

How Supplied: Orange softgel imprinted with "PZ 180" in 12 count and 36 count blister pack, 60 count and 100 count bottles.

SENSODYNE® FRESH MINT
SENSODYNE® FRESH IMPACT
SENSODYNE® COOL GEL
SENSODYNE® WITH BAKING SODA
SENSODYNE® TARTAR CONTROL
SENSODYNE® TARTAR CONTROL PLUS WHITENING
SENSODYNE® ORIGINAL FLAVOR
SENSODYNE® EXTRA WHITENING
Anticavity toothpaste for sensitive teeth

Active Ingredients: "Fresh Impact" Potassium Nitrate 5% Sodium Fluoride 0.15% w/v fluoride ion 5% Potassium Nitrate and 0.15% w/v Sodium Monofluorophosphate (Extra Whitening) or Sodium Fluoride (Fresh Mint, 0.15% w/v; Baking Soda, 0.15% w/v; Cool Gel, 0.13% w/v; Tartar Control, 0.13% w/v; Tartar Control Plus Whitening 0.145% w/v; Original Flavor, 0.13% w/v), or Sodium Fluoride 0.15% w/v fluoride ion (Fresh Impact). Sensodyne Fresh Mint, Sensodyne Fresh Impact, Sensodyne Cool Gel, Sensodyne with Baking Soda, Sensodyne Tartar Control, Sensodyne Tartar Control Plus Whitening, Sensodyne Original Flavor and Sensodyne Extra Whitening contain fluoride for cavity prevention and Potassium Nitrate clinically proven to reduce pain sensitivity for relief of dentinal hypersensitivity resulting from the exposure of tooth dentin due to periodontal surgery, cervical (gum line) erosion, abrasion or recession which causes pain on contact with hot, cold, or tactile stimuli.

Inactive Ingredients: *Baking Soda:* Flavor, Glycerin, Hydrated Silica, Hydroxyethylcellulose, Methylparaben, Propylparaben, Silica, Sodium Bicarbonate, Sodium Lauryl Sulfate, Sodium Saccharin, Titanium Dioxide, Water.
Extra Whitening: Calcium Peroxide, Flavor, Glycerin, Hydrated Silica, PEG-12, PEG-75, Silica, Sodium Carbonate, Sodium Lauryl Sulfate, Sodium Saccharin, Titanium Dioxide, Water.
Tartar Control: Cellulose Gum, Cocamidopropyl Betaine, Flavor, Glycerin, Hydrated Silica, Silica, Sodium Bicarbonate, Sodium Saccharin, Tetrapotassium Pyrophosphate, Titanium Dioxide, Water.
Tartar Control Plus Whitening: Cellulose Gum, Flavor, Glycerin, Polyethylene Glycol, Silica, Sodium Lauryl Sulfate, Sodium Saccharin, Tetrapotassium Pyrophosphate, Titanium Dioxide, Water.
Cool Gel: Cellulose Gum, FD&C Blue #1, Flavor, Glycerin, Hydrated Silica, Silica, Sodium Methyl Cocoyl Taurate, Sodium Saccharin, Sorbitol, Trisodium Phosphate, Water. *Fresh Impact:* D&C yellow #10 lake, FD&C blue #1 lake, flavor, glycerin, hydrated silica, sodium benzoate, sodium hydroxide, sodium lauryl sulfate, sodium saccharin, sorbitol, titanium dioxide, water, xanthan gum
Fresh Mint: Inactive Ingredients: Carbomer, cellulose gum, D&C yellow #10, FD&C blue #1, flavor, glycerin, hydrated silica, octadecene/MA copolymer, poloxamer 407, potassium hydroxide, sodium lauroyl sarcosinate, sodium saccharin, sorbitol, titanium dioxide, water, xanthan gum.
Original Flavor: Cellulose Gum, D&C Red No. 28, Glycerin, Hydrated Silica, Peppermint Oil, Silica, Sodium Methyl Cocoyl Taurate, Sodium Saccharin, Sorbitol, Titanium Dioxide, Trisodium Phosphate, Water.

Actions: All Sensodyne Formulas significantly reduce tooth hypersensitivity, with response to therapy evident after two weeks of use. Controlled double-blind clinical studies provide substantial evidence of the safety and effectiveness of Potassium Nitrate. The current theory on mechanism of action is that potassium nitrate has an effect on neural transmission, interrupting the signal which would result in the sensation of pain. Fluorides are anticariogenic, forming fluoroapatite in the outer surface of the dental enamel which is resistant to acids and caries.

Warnings: Sensitive teeth may indicate a serious problem that may need prompt care by a dentist. See your dentist if the problem persists or worsens. Do not use this product longer than 4 weeks unless recommended by a dentist or physician. Keep this and all drugs out of the reach of children. If you accidentally swallow more than used for brushing, seek professional assistance or contact a Poison Control Center immediately.

Dosage and Administration: Adults and children 12 years of age and older: Apply a 1-inch strip of the product onto a soft bristle toothbrush. Brush teeth thoroughly for at least 1 minute twice a day (morning and evening) or as recommended by a dentist or physician. Make sure to brush all sensitive areas of the teeth. Children under 12 years of age: consult a dentist or physician.

How Supplied: All Sensodyne formulas are supplied in 2.1 oz. (60g), 4.0 oz. (113g) and 6.0 oz. (170g) tubes. Sensodyne Cool Gel is supplied in 4.0 oz. and 6.0 oz. tubes. Sensodyne Baking Soda is supplied in 4.0 oz and 6.0 oz. only.

SINGLET® For Adults
Nasal Decongestant/Antihistamine/ Analgesic (pain reliever)/Antipyretic (fever reducer)

Indications: For temporary relief of nasal congestion and sinus and headache pain associated with sinusitis or due to a cold, hay fever or other upper respiratory allergies. Also temporarily relieves nasal congestion, sinus headache, runny nose, sneezing, itching of the nose or throat, and itchy, watery eyes due to hay fever or other upper respiratory allergies. Also temporarily relieves fever due to the common cold.

Directions: Adults (12 years and older): 1 caplet every 4 to 6 hours, **not to exceed 4 caplets in any 24-hour period,** or as directed by a doctor. Children under 12 years of age: Consult a doctor.

Warnings: Do not exceed recommended dosage. If nervousness, dizziness, or sleeplessness occur, discontinue use and consult a doctor. Do not take this product for more than 10 days. If symptoms do not improve or are accompanied by fever that lasts for more than 3 days, or if new symptoms occur, consult a doctor. Do not take this product, unless directed by a doctor, if you have a breathing problem such as emphysema or chronic bronchitis, or if you have heart disease, high blood pressure, thyroid disease, diabetes, glaucoma or difficulty in urination due to enlargement of the prostate gland. May cause excitability especially in children. May cause drowsiness; alcohol, sedatives, and tranquilizers may increase the drowsiness effect. Avoid alcoholic beverages while taking this product. Do not take this product if you are taking sedatives or tranquilizers, without first consulting your doctor. Use caution when driving a motor vehicle or operating machinery. **KEEP THIS AND ALL DRUGS OUT OF THE REACH OF CHILDREN.** Prompt medical attention is critical for adults as well as for children even if you do not notice any signs or symptoms. In case of accidental overdose, seek professional assistance or contact a Poison Control Center immediately. As with any drug, if you are pregnant or nursing a baby, seek the advice of a health professional before using this product.

Alcohol Warning: If you consume 3 or more alcoholic drinks every day, ask your doctor whether you should take acetaminophen or other pain reliever/fever reducers. Acetaminophen may cause liver damage.

Drug Interaction Precaution: Do not use this product if you are now taking a prescription monoamine oxidase inhibitor (MAOI) (certain drugs for depression, psychiatric or emotional conditions, or Parkinson's disease), or for 2 weeks after stopping the MAOI drug. If you are uncertain whether your prescription drug contains an MAOI, consult a health professional before taking this product.

Active Ingredients: Each caplet contains: Pseudoephedrine Hydrochloride 60 mg, Chlorpheniramine Maleate 4 mg, Acetaminophen 650 mg.

Inactive Ingredients: D&C Red 27, D&C Yellow 10, FD&C Blue 1, Hydroxypropyl Cellulose, Hypromellose, Magnesium Stearate, Microcrystalline Cellulose, Polyethylene Glycol, Pregelatinized Corn Starch, Sodium Starch Glycolate, Sucrose and Titanium Dioxide.

Store at room temperature (59°–86°F). Avoid excessive heat and humidity.

Comments or Questions? Call toll-free 1-800-245-1040 weekdays

Distributed by: GlaxoSmithKline Consumer Healthcare, L.P.

Moon Township, PA 15108. Made in U.S.A.

SOMINEX Original Formula Nighttime Sleep Aid
Doctor-preferred sleep ingredient

Indications: Helps to reduce difficulty falling asleep.

Directions: Adults and children 12 years and over: Take 2 tablets at bedtime if needed, or as directed by a doctor. For best results, take recommended dose. This will provide approximately six to eight hours of restful sleep.

Warnings: Do not give to children under 12 years of age. If sleeplessness persists continually for more than 2 weeks, consult your doctor. Insomnia may be a symptom of serious underlying medical illness. Do not take this product, unless directed by a doctor, if you have a breathing problem such as emphysema or chronic bronchitis, or if you have glaucoma or difficulty in urination due to enlargement of the prostate gland. Avoid alcoholic beverages while taking this product. Do not take this product if you are taking sedatives or tranquilizers, without first consulting your doctor. As with any drug, if you are pregnant or nursing a baby, seek the advice of a health professional before using this product. **Keep this and all drugs out of the reach of children.** In case of accidental overdose, seek professional assistance or contact a poison control center immediately.

Active Ingredients: Each tablet contains 25 mg Diphenhydramine HCl.

Inactive Ingredients: Dibasic Calcium Phosphate, FD&C Blue #1, Magnesium Stearate, Microcrystalline Cellulose, Silicon Dioxide, Starch.

Tamper Evident Feature: Individually sealed in foil for your protection. Do not use if foil or plastic bubble is torn or punctured.

Store at room temperature, avoid excessive heat (greater than 100°F) or humidity.

How Supplied: Consumer Packages of 16, 32 and 72 tablets

Also Available in Maximum Strength Formula.

Comments or Questions? Call Toll-Free 1-800-245-1040 Weekdays.

GlaxoSmithKline Consumer Healthcare, L.P.

Moon Township, PA 15108. Made in U.S.A.

TAGAMET HB® 200
Cimetidine Tablets 200 mg/ Acid Reducer

Tagamet HB® 200 relieves and prevents heartburn, acid indigestion and sour stomach when used as directed. It contains the same ingredient found in prescription strength Tagamet. Tagamet HB 200 reduces the production of stomach acid.

Active Ingredient: Cimetidine, 200 mg.

Inactive Ingredients: Cellulose, cornstarch, hypromellose, magnesium stearate, polyethylene glycol, polysorbate 80, povidone, sodium lauryl sulfate, sodium starch glycolate, titanium dioxide.

Uses:
- For relief of heartburn associated with acid indigestion and sour stomach.
- For prevention of heartburn associated with acid indigestion and sour stomach brought on by eating or drinking certain food and beverages.

Directions:
- For **relief** of symptoms, swallow 1 tablet with a glass of water.
- For **prevention** of symptoms, swallow 1 tablet with a glass of water **right before or anytime up to 30 minutes before** eating food or drinking beverages that cause heartburn.
- Tagamet HB 200 can be used up to twice daily (up to 2 tablets in 24 hours).
- This product should not be given to children under 12 years old unless directed by a doctor.

Warnings:

Allergy Warning: Do not use if you are allergic to Tagamet HB 200 (cimetidine) or other acid reducers.

Ask a Doctor Before Use If You are Taking:
- theophylline (oral asthma medicine)
- warfarin (blood thinning medicine)
- phenytoin (seizure medicine)

If you are not sure whether your medication contains one of these drugs or have any other questions about medicines you are taking, call our consumer affairs specialist at 1-800-482-4394.

- Do not take the maximum daily dosage for more than 2 weeks continuously except under the advice and supervision of a doctor.
- If you have trouble swallowing, or persistent abdominal pain, see your doctor promptly. You may have a serious condition that may need a different treatment.
- As with any drug, if you are pregnant or nursing a baby, seek the advice of a health professional before using this product.
- Keep this and all medications out of the reach of children.
- In case of accidental overdose, seek professional assistance or contact a poison control center immediately.

READ THE LABEL
Read the directions and warnings before taking this medication.

Store at 15°–30°C (59°–86°F).

Comments or questions? Call Toll-Free 1-800-482-4394 weekdays.

PHARMACOKINETIC INTERACTIONS

Cimetidine at prescription doses is known to inhibit various P450 metabolizing isoenzymes, which could affect metabolism of other drugs and increase their blood concentration. Investigation of pharmacokinetic interactions at the recommended OTC doses of cimetidine have thus far shown only small effects. A pharmacokinetic study conducted in 26 normal male subjects (mean age, 38 years) at steady state using the maximum recommended OTC dose level (200 mg twice a day), showed that Tagamet HB 200, on average, increased the 24 hour AUC of theophylline by 14% and increased peak theophylline levels by 15%. This interaction should be borne in mind in advising patients on the use of Tagamet HB 200. At the prescription doses of cimetidine, clinically significant pharmacokinetic interactions between cimetidine and warfarin, phenytoin, and theophylline have been reported. At prescription doses, pharmacokinetic interactions have been reported for a number of other drugs as well, such as with dihydropyridine calcium channel blockers or some short acting benzodiazepines. At the maximum recommended OTC dose level (200 mg twice a day), a pharmacokinetic study conducted in 21 normal male subjects (mean age, 38 years) showed that Tagamet HB 200, on average, increased the total AUC of triazolam by 26–28% and increased peak triazolam levels by 11–23%. Tagamet HB 200 did not alter the apparent terminal elimination half-life of triazolam.

How Supplied: Tagamet HB 200 (Cimetidine Tablets 200 mg) is available in boxes of blister packs in 6, 30, 50, & 70 tablet sizes.

Shown in Product Identification Guide, page 505

TEGRIN® DANDRUFF SHAMPOO – EXTRA CONDITIONING

Description: Tegrin® Dandruff Shampoo contains 7% w/w Coal Tar Solution, USP, equivalent to 0.7% w/w coal tar, in a pleasantly scented, high-foaming, cleansing shampoo base with emollients, conditioners and other formula components.

Active Ingredients:	Purpose:
7% w/w Coal tar solution, USP equivalent to 0.7% w/w Coal tar	Anti Dandruff Anti Seborrheic Dermatitis Anti Psoriasis

Use: controls the flaking and itching of the scalp associated with dandruff, seborrheic dermatitis, and psoriasis.

Continued on next page

Tegrin—Cont.

Warnings: For external use only. Ask a doctor before use if you have psoriasis or seborrheic dermatitis that covers a large area of the body. **Ask a doctor or pharmacist if you are** using other forms of psoriasis therapy such as ultraviolet radiation or prescription drugs. **When using this product** • do not use for prolonged periods • avoid contact with eyes. If contact occurs, rinse eyes thoroughly with water. • use caution in exposing skin to sunlight after application. It may increase your tendency to sunburn for up to 24 hours after application. **Stop use and ask a doctor if** condition worsens or does not improve after regular use of this product as directed. **Keep out of reach of children.** If swallowed, get medical help or contact a Poison Control Center right away.

Directions: Shake well. Wet hair, lather, rinse, repeat. For best results use at least twice a week or as directed by a doctor.

Other Information:
Store at 20°–25°C (68°–77°F)

Inactive Ingredients:
Alcohol (7.0%), Ammonium Lauryl Sulfate, Citric Acid, FD&C Blue #1, Fragrance, Glycol Stearate (and) Sodium Laureth Sulfate (and) Hexylene Glycol, Guar Hydroxypropyltrimonium Chloride, Hydroxypropyl Methylcellulose, Lauramide DEA, Methylparaben, Propylparaben, Sodium Lauryl Sulfate, Water.

How Supplied: Tegrin® Dandruff Shampoo is available in Extra Conditioning and Fresh Herbal formulas and supplied in 7 fl. oz. (207 ml) plastic bottles.

Coal Tar is obtained in the destructive distillation of bituminous coal and is a highly effective agent for controlling the flaking and itching of the scalp associated with dandruff, seborrheic dermatitis, and psoriasis. The action of coal tar is believed to be keratolytic, antiseptic, antipruritic, and astringent. The coal tar solution used in Tegrin® Dandruff Shampoo is prepared in such a way as to reduce the itch and other irritant components found in crude coal tar without reduction in therapeutic potency.

Coal Tar Solution has been used clinically for many years as a remedy for dandruff and for scaling associated with scalp disorders such as seborrhea and psoriasis. Its mechanism of action has not been fully established, but it is believed to retard the rate of turnover of epidermal cells with regular use. A number of clinical studies have demonstrated the performance attributes of Tegrin® Dandruff Shampoo against dandruff and seborrheic dermatitis. In addition to relieving the above symptoms, Tegrin® Dandruff Shampoo, used regularly, maintains scalp and hair cleanliness and leaves the hair lustrous and manageable.

TEGRIN® DANDRUFF SHAMPOO-FRESH HERBAL

Description: Tegrin® Dandruff Shampoo contains 7% w/w Coal Tar Solution, USP, equivalent to 0.7% w/w coal tar, in a pleasantly scented, high-foaming, cleansing shampoo base with emollients, conditioners and other formula components.

Active Ingredients: **Purpose:**
7% w/w Coal tar
    solution, USP .... Anti Dandruff
equivalent to 0.7%
    w/w Coal tar .... Anti Seborrheic
           Dermatitis Anti Psoriasis

Use: controls the flaking and itching of the scalp associated with dandruff, seborrheic dermatitis, and psoriasis.

Warnings:
For external use only
Ask a doctor before use if you have psoriasis or seborrheic dermatitis that covers a large area of the body
Ask a doctor or pharmacist if you are using other forms of psoriasis therapy such as ultraviolet radiation or prescription drugs
When using this product • do not use for prolonged periods
• avoid contact with eyes. If contact occurs, rinse eyes thoroughly with water.
• use caution in exposing skin to sunlight after application. It may increase your tendency to sunburn for up to 24 hours after application.
Stop use and ask a doctor if condition worsens or does not improve after regular use of this product as directed.
Keep out of reach of children. If swallowed, get medical help or contact a Poison Control center right away.

Directions: Shake well. Wet hair. Lather, rinse, repeat. For best results use at least twice a week or as directed by a doctor.

Other Information:
Store at 20°–25°C (68°–77°F)

Inactive Ingredients:
Alcohol (7.0%), Citric Acid, Cocamide DEA, FD&C Blue #1, Fragrance, Glycol Stearate (and) Sodium Laureth Sulfate (and) Hexylene Glycol, Hydroxypropyl Methylcellulose, Methylparaben, Propylparaben, Sodium Lauryl Sulfate, Water.

How Supplied: Tegrin® Dandruff Shampoo is available in Extra Conditioning and Fresh Herbal formulas and supplied in 7 fl. oz. (207 ml) plastic bottles.

Coal Tar is obtained in the destructive distillation of bituminous coal and is a highly effective agent for controlling the flaking and itching of the scalp associated with dandruff, seborrheic dermatitis and psoriasis. The action of coal tar is believed to be keratolytic, antiseptic, antipruritic, and astringent. The coal tar solution used in Tegrin® Dandruff Shampoo is prepared in such a way as to reduce the pitch and other irritant components found in crude coal tar without reduction in therapeutic potency.

Coal Tar Solution has been used clinically for many years as a remedy for dandruff and for scaling associated with scalp disorders such as seborrhea and psoriasis. Its mechanism of action has not been fully established, but it is believed to retard the rate of turnover of epidermal cells with regular use. A number of clinical studies have demonstrated the performance attributes of Tegrin® Dandruff Shampoo against dandruff and seborrheic dermatitis. In addition to relieving the above symptoms, Tegrin® Dandruff Shampoo, used regularly, maintains scalp and hair cleanliness and leaves the hair lustrous and manageable.

Shown in Product Identification Guide, page 505

TEGRIN® SKIN CREAM FOR PSORIASIS

Description: Tegrin® Skin Cream for Psoriasis contains 5% Coal Tar Solution, USP, equivalent to 0.8% Coal Tar and alcohol of 4.7%.

Active Ingredient: 5% Coal Tar Solution, USP, equivalent to 0.8% Coal Tar.

Use: relieves itching, flaking and irritation of the skin associated with psoriasis and seborrheic dermatitis.

Directions: Apply to affected areas one to four times daily or as directed by a doctor.

Warnings:
For external use only
Ask a doctor before use if you have psoriasis or seborrheic dermatitis that covers a large area of the body
Ask a doctor or pharmacist before use if you are using other forms of psoriasis therapy such as ultraviolet radiation or prescription drugs
When using this product
• avoid contact with eyes. If contact occurs, rinse eyes thoroughly with water.
• use caution in exposing skin to sunlight after application. It may increase tendency to sunburn for up to 24 hours after application.
• do not use for prolonged periods
• do not use in or around the rectum or in the genital area or groin
Stop use and ask a doctor if condition worsens or does not improve after regular use

Warning: This product contains a chemical known to the State of California to cause cancer.

Keep out of reach of children. If swallowed, get medical help or contact a Poison Control Center right away.

Inactive Ingredients: Acetylated Lanolin Alcohol, Alcohol (4.7%), Carbomer-934P, Ceteth-2, Ceteth-16, Cetyl Acetate, Cetyl Alcohol, D&C Red No. 28, Fragrance, Glyceryl Tribehenate, Laneth-16, Lanolin Alcohol, Laureth-23, Methyl Gluceth-20, Methylchloroisothiazolinone, Methylisothiazolinone, Mineral

Oil, Octyldodecanol, Oleth-16, Petrolatum, Potassium Hydroxide, Purified Water, Steareth-16, Stearyl Alcohol, Titanium Dioxide.

How Supplied: Tegrin® Skin Cream for Psoriasis is available in a 2 oz (57g) tube.

Shown in Product Identification Guide, page 505

TUMS® Regular Antacid/Calcium Supplement Tablets
TUMS E–X® and TUMS E–X® Sugar Free Antacid/Calcium Supplement Tablets
TUMS ULTRA® Antacid/Calcium Supplement Tablets

Professional Labeling: Indicated for the symptomatic relief of hyperacidity associated with the diagnosis of peptic ulcer, gastritis, peptic esophagitis, gastric hyperacidity, and hiatal hernia.

Indications: For fast relief of acid indigestion, heartburn, sour stomach, and upset stomach associated with these symptoms.

Active Ingredient:
Tums, Calcium Carbonate 500 mg
Tums E-X, Calcium Carbonate 750 mg
Tums ULTRA, Calcium Carbonate 1000 mg

Actions: Tums provides rapid neutralization of stomach acid. Each Tums tablet has an acid-neutralizing capacity (ANC) of 10 mEq. Each Tums E-X tablet has an ANC of 15 mEq and each Tums ULTRA tablet, an ANC of 20 mEq. This high neutralization capacity makes Tums tablets an ideal antacid for management of conditions associated with hyperacidity. It effectively neutralizes free acid yet does not cause systemic alkalosis in the presence of normal renal function. A double-blind placebo-controlled clinical study demonstrated that calcium carbonate taken at a dosage of 16 Tums tablets daily for a two-week period was non-constipating/non-laxative.

Warnings: Tums: Do not take more than 15 tablets in a 24-hour period or use the maximum dosage of this product for more than 2 weeks, except under the advice and supervision of a physician. If symptoms persist for 2 weeks, stop using this product and see a physician. Keep this and all drugs out of the reach of children.
Tums E-X: Do not take more than 10 tablets in a 24-hour period or use the maximum dosage of this product for more than two weeks, except under the advice and supervision of a physician. If symptoms persist for two weeks, stop using this product and see a physician. Keep this and all drugs out of the reach of children.
Additionally, for Tums Ex Sugar Free: Phenylketonurics: Contains phenylalanine, less than 1 mg per tablet.

Supplement Facts

Serving Size	Tums 2 Tablets	Tums E-X 2 Tablets	Tums E-X Sugar Free 2 Tablets	Tums Ultra 2 Tablets
Amount Per Serving				
Calories	5	10	5	10
Sorbitol (g)	—	—	1	—
Sugars (g)	1	2	—	3
Calcium (mg)	400	600	600	800
% Daily Value	40	60	60	80
Sodium (mg)		5		10
% Daily Value	—	<1%	—	<1%

Tums ULTRA: Do not take more than 7 tablets in 24-hour period or use the maximum dosage of this product for more than two weeks, except under the advice and supervision of a physician. If symptoms persist for two weeks, stop using and see a physician. Keep this and all drugs out of the reach of children.

Drug Interaction Precaution: Antacids may interact with certain prescription drugs. If you are presently taking a prescription drug, do not take this product without checking with your physician or other health professional.

Dosage and Administration:
Tums: Chew 2-4 tablets as symptoms occur. Repeat hourly if symptoms return, or as directed by physician.
Tums E-X: Chew 2-4 tablets as symptoms occur. Repeat hourly if symptoms return, or as directed by a physician.
Tums ULTRA: Chew 2-3 tablets as symptoms occur. Repeat hourly if symptoms return, or as directed by a physician.

AS A DIETARY SUPPLEMENT: Calcium Supplement Directions
Tums, Tums E-X, & Tums ULTRA:
USES: As a daily source of extra calcium. Tums is recommended by the National Osteoporosis Foundation.

IMPORTANT INFORMATION ON OSTEOPOROSIS: Research shows that certain ethnic, age and other groups are at higher risk for developing osteoporosis, including Caucasian and Asian teen and young adult women, menopausal women, older persons and those persons with a family history of fragile bones. **A balanced diet with enough calcium and regular exercise throughout life will help you to build and maintain healthy bones and may reduce your risk of developing osteoporosis.** Adequate calcium intake is important, but daily intakes above 2,000 mg are not likely to provide any additional benefit.
DIRECTIONS: Chew 2 tablets twice daily.
[See table above]

Ingredients (all variants except sugar free): Sucrose, Corn Starch, Talc, Mineral Oil, Flavors (natural and/or artificial), Sodium Polyphosphate. May also contain 1% or less of Adipic Acid, Blue 1 Lake, Yellow 6 Lake, Yellow 5 Lake, Red 40 Lake.

Ingredients (Sugar Free): Sorbitol, Acacia, Natural and Artificial Flavors,

Calcium Stearate, Adipic Acid, Yellow 6 Lake, Aspartame.

How Supplied:
Tums: Peppermint flavor is available in 12-tablet rolls, 3-roll wraps, and bottles of 75, 150, and 180. **Assorted Flavors** (Cherry, Lemon, Orange, and Lime), are available in 12-tablet rolls, 3-roll wraps, and bottles of 75, 150, and 320.
Tums E-X: Wintergreen 3-roll wraps and bottles of 48, 96, and 116.
Tums E-X: Assorted Fruit, Assorted Tropical Fruit, and Assorted Berries, Fresh Blend 8 tablet rolls, 3-roll wraps, 6-roll wraps, and bottles of 48, 96, and 116. Assorted Tropical Fruit and Assorted Berries are also available in bottles of 200 tablets.
Tums EX Sugar Free: Orange Cream; bottles of 48 and 80 tablets.
Tums ULTRA: Assorted Berries, and **Spearmint** bottles of 160 tablets. **Assorted Fruit** and **Assorted Mint** bottles of 36, 72, and 86 tablets. Assorted Fruit also available in bottles of 160 tablets. **Tropical Fruit** bottles of 160 tablets.

Shown in Product Identification Guide, page 505

VIVARIN Tablets & Caplets
Alertness Aid with Caffeine Maximum Strength

Each Tablet or Caplet Contains 200 mg. Caffeine, Equal to About Two Cups of Coffee
Take Vivarin for a safe, fast pick up anytime you feel drowsy and need to be alert. The caffeine in Vivarin is less irritating to your stomach than coffee, according to a government appointed panel of experts.

FDA APPROVED USES: Helps restore mental alertness or wakefulness when experiencing fatigue or drowsiness.

Active Ingredients: Caffeine 200 mg.

Inactive Ingredients: Tablet: Colloidal Silicon Dioxide, D&C Yellow #10 Al. Lake, Dextrose, FD&C Yellow #6 Al. Lake, Magnesium Stearate, Microcrystalline Cellulose, Starch.

Continued on next page

Vivarin—Cont.

Caplet: Carnauba Wax, Colloidal Silicon Dioxide, D&C Yellow #10 Al Lake, Dextrose, FD&C Yellow #6 Al Lake, Hypromellose, Magnesium Stearate, Microcrystalline Cellulose, Polyethylene Glycol, Polysorbate 80, Starch, Titanium Dioxide.

Directions: Adults and children 12 years and over: Take 1 tablet (200 mg) not more often than every 3 to 4 hours.

Warnings: The recommended dose of this product contains about as much caffeine as two cups of coffee. Limit the use of caffeine containing medications, foods, or beverages while taking this product because too much caffeine may cause nervousness, irritability, sleeplessness, and occasionally, rapid heartbeat. For occasional use only. Not intended for use as a substitute for sleep. If fatigue or drowsiness persists or continues to recur, consult a doctor. Do not give to children under 12 years of age. As with any drug, if you are pregnant or nursing a baby, seek the advice of a health professional before using this product. In case of accidental overdose, seek professional assistance or contact a poison control center immediately. Keep this and all drugs out of the reach of children.

Tamper Evident Feature: Individually sealed in foil for your protection. Do not use if foil or plastic bubble is torn or punctured.

Store at room temperature, avoid excessive heat (greater than 100°F) or humidity.

How Supplied:
Tablets: Consumer packages of 16, 40 and 80 tablets
Caplets: Consumer packages of 24 and 48 caplets
Comments or Questions? Call Toll-Free 1-800-245-1040 Weekdays.
GlaxoSmithKline Consumer Healthcare, L.P.
Moon Township, PA 15108. Made in U.S.A.
©2004 GlaxoSmithKline, L.P.
Shown in Product Identification Guide, page 505

UNKNOWN DRUG?
Consult the
Product Identification Guide
(Gray Pages)
for full-color photos of
leading over-the-counter
medications

Hyland's, Inc.
See Standard Homeopathic Company

Johnson & Johnson • MERCK
**Consumer Pharmaceuticals Co.
7050 CAMP HILL ROAD
FORT WASHINGTON, PA 19034**

Direct Inquiries to:
Consumer Relationship Center
Fort Washington, PA 19034
(800) 775-4008

**PEPCID AC®
TABLETS, CHEWABLE TABLETS AND GELCAPS
Maximum Strength PEPCID AC Tablets
Acid reducer**

Description: (PEPCID AC)
Each Pepcid AC Tablet, Chewable tablet, and gelcap contain famotidine 10 mg as an active ingredient.

Each Maximum Strength Pepcid AC Tablet contains famotidine 20 mg as an active ingredient.

Inactive Ingredients:
TABLETS: Hydroxypropyl cellulose, hypromellose, red iron oxide, magnesium stearate, microcrystalline cellulose red iron oxide, starch, talc, titanium dioxide.
CHEWABLE TABLETS: aspartame, cellulose acetate, flavors, hydroxypropyl cellulose, hypromellose, lactose, magnesium stearate, mannitol, microcrystalline cellulose, red ferric oxide.
GELCAPS: benzyl alcohol, black iron oxide, butylparaben, castor oil, edetate calcium disodium, FD&C red #40, gelatin, hypromellose, magnesium stearate, methylparaben, microcrystalline cellulose, pregelatinized corn starch, propylene glycol, propylparaben, sodium lauryl sulfate, sodium propionate, talc, titanium dioxide.

Inactive Ingredients: (Max. Strength Pepcid AC.)
carnauba wax, hydroxypropyl cellulose, hypromellose, magnesium stearate, microcrystalline cellulose, pregelatinized starch, talc, titanium dioxide.

Product Benefits:
• **1 Tablet, Chewable Tablet or Gelcap** relieves heartburn associated with acid indigestion and sour stomach.
• prevents heartburn associated with acid indigestion and sour stomach brought on by eating or drinking certain food and beverages.
It contains famotidine, a prescription-proven medicine.
The ingredient in PEPCID AC and Maximum Strength Pepcid AC, famotidine, has been prescribed by doctors for years to treat millions of patients safely and

effectively. The active ingredient in PEPCID AC and Maximum Strength Pepcid AC has been taken safely with many frequently prescribed medications.

Action:
It is normal for the stomach to produce acid, especially after consuming food and beverages. However, acid in the wrong place (the esophagus), or too much acid, can cause burning pain and discomfort that interfere with everyday activities.
• **Heartburn—Caused by acid in the esophagus**

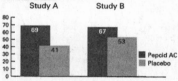

In clinical studies, PEPCID AC and Maximum Strength Pepcid AC film-coated tablets were significantly better than placebo tablet (tablets without the medicine) in relieving and preventing heartburn. Pepcid AC and Maximum Strength Pepcid AC chewables contain the same active ingredient.

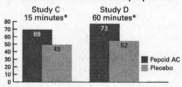

*Time taken before eating a meal that is expected to cause symptoms.

• **Relieves** heartburn, associated with acid indigestion and sour stomach;
• **Prevents** of heartburn associated with acid indigestion and sour stomach brought on by eating or drinking certain food and beverages.

Tips for Managing Heartburn:
• Do not lie flat or bend over soon after eating.
• Do not eat late at night, or just before bedtime.
• Certain foods or drinks are more likely to cause heartburn, such as rich, spicy, fatty, and fried foods, chocolate, caffeine, alcohol, and even some fruits and vegetables.
• Eat slowly and do not eat big meals.
• If you are overweight, lose weight.
• If you smoke, quit smoking.
• Raise the head of your bed.
• Wear loose fitting clothing around your stomach.

Warnings:

Allergy alert Do not use if you are allergic to famotidine or other acid reducers

Do not use:
- if you have trouble swallowing
- with other acid reducers
- if you have kidney disease, except under the advice and supervision of a doctor (for Maximum Strength Pepcid AC)

Stop use and ask a doctor if:
- stomach pain continues
- you need to take this product for more than 14 days

If pregnant or breast-feeding, ask a health professional before use.

Keep out of reach of children. In case of overdose, get medical help or contact a Poison Control Center right away.

Directions:

Pepcid AC:
- Adults and children 12 years and over:
- Tablet: To **relieve** symptoms, swallow 1 tablet with a glass of water.
  Chewable Tablet: **Do not swallow tablet whole: chew completely.** To **relieve** symptoms, **chew** one tablet before swallowing.
  Gelcap: To **relieve** symptoms, swallow one gelcap with a glass of water.
  Tablet & Gelcap: To **prevent** symptoms, swallow 1 tablet or gelcap with a glass of water at any time from **15 to 60 minutes before** eating food or drinking beverages that cause heartburn.
- Chewable Tablet: To **prevent** symptoms, **chew** one chewable tablet with a glass of water at any time from **15 to 60 minutes before** eating food or drinking beverages that cause heartburn.
- Do not use more than 2 tablets, chewable tablets or gelcaps in 24 hours.
- Children under 12 years: ask a doctor.

Maximum Strength Pepcid AC:
- adults and children 12 years and over:
  - to **relieve** symptoms, swallow 1 tablet with a glass of water
  - to **prevent** symptoms, swallow 1 tablet with a glass of water at any time from **15 to 60 minutes before** eating food or drinking beverages that cause heartburn.
  - do not use more than 2 tablets in 24 hours
- children under 12 years: ask a doctor

Other Information:
- read the directions and warnings before use
- store at 25°–30°C (77°–86°F)
- keep the carton and package insert. They contain important information
- protect from moisture
in addition to the above the following also applies to the chewable tablet
- phenylketonurics: Contains Phenylalanine 1.4 mg per chewable tablet

How Supplied:

Pepcid AC Tablet is available as a rose-colored tablet identified as 'PEPCID AC'. NDC 16837-872

Pepcid AC Gelcap is available as a rose and white gelatin coated, capsule shaped tablet identified as 'PEPCID AC'. NDC 16837-856

Pepcid AC Chewable Tablet is available as a rose-colored chewable tablet identified as 'PEPCID AC'. NDC 16837-873

Maximum Strength Pepcid AC Tablet is a white, "D" shaped, film coated tablet identifed as "PAC 20." NDC 16837 855
Shown in Product Identification Guide, page 506

PEPCID® COMPLETE
Acid Reducer + Antacid
with DUAL ACTION
Reduces and Neutralizes Acid

Description:

Active Ingredients (in each chewablet tablet):	Purpose:
famotidine 10mg	Acid Reducer
calcium carbonate 800 mg	Antacid
magnesium hydroxide 165 mg	Antacid

Inactive Ingredients:
Mint flavor: cellulose acetate, corn starch, dextrates, flavors, hydroxypropyl cellulose, hypromellose, lactose, magnesium stearate, pregelatinized starch, red iron oxide, sodium lauryl sulfate, sugar
Berry flavor: cellulose acetate, corn starch, D&C red #7, dextrates, FD&C blue #1, FD&C red #40, flavors, hydropropyl cellulose, hypromellose, lactose, magnesium stearate, pregelatinized starch, sodium lauryl sulfate, sugar

Sodium Content:
Each chewable tablet contains 0.5 mg of sodium.

Acid Neutralizing Capacity:
Each chewable tablet contains 21.7 mEq of acid neutralizing capacity.

Product Benefits: Pepcid Complete combines an acid reducer (famotidine) with antacids (calcium carbonate and magnesium hydroxide) to relieve heartburn in two different ways: Acid reducers decrease the production of new stomach acid; antacids neutralize acid that is already in the stomach. The active ingredients in PEPCID COMPLETE have been used for years to treat acid-related problems in millions of people safely and effectively.

Uses: Relives heartburn associated with acid indigestion and sour stomach.

Action: It is normal for the stomach to produce acid, especially after consuming food and beverages. However, acid in the stomach may move up into the wrong place (the esophagus), causing burning pain and discomfort that interfere with everyday activities.

Heartburn—Caused by acid in the esophagus
- Burning pain/discomfort in esophagus
- A valve-like muscle called the lower esophageal sphincter (LES) is relaxed in an open position
- Acid moves up from stomach

Tips For Managing Heartburn
- Do not lie flat or bend over soon after eating.
- Do not eat late at night, or just before bedtime.
- Certain foods or drinks are more likely to cause heartburn, such as rich, spicy, fatty, and fried foods, chocolate, caffeine, alcohol, and even some fruits and vegetables.
- Eat slowly and do not eat big meals.
- If you are overweight, lose weight.
- If you smoke, quit smoking.
- Raise the head of your bed.
- Wear loose fitting clothing around your stomach.

PROVEN EFFECTIVE IN CLINICAL STUDIES
[See graphic below]

Warnings:
- **Allergy alert:** Do not use if you are allergic to famotidine or other acid reducers.
- **Do not use:** if you have trouble swallowing.
- With other famotidine products or acid reducers.
- **Ask a doctor or pharmacist before use if you are presently** taking a prescription drug. Antacids may interact with certain prescription drugs.
- **Stop use and ask a doctor if** stomach pain continues
- You need to take this product for more than 14 days.
- **If pregnant or breast-feeding,** ask a health professional before use.
- **Keep out of reach of children.** In case of overdose, get medical help or contact a Poison Control Center right away.

Directions:
- Adults and children 12 years and over:
  - **do not swallow tablet whole; chew completely.**
  - to relieve symptoms, **chew** 1 tablet before swallowing.
  - do not use more than 2 chewable tablets in 24 hours.
- Children under 12 years: ask a doctor.

Other Information:
- read the directions and warnings before use.

Continued on next page

In clinical studies, PEPCID COMPLETE was significantly better than placebo pills tablets (without medicine) in relieving heartburn.

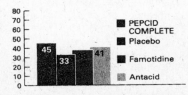

Onset of Relief
Percent of heartburn episodes relieved within 30 minutes

Legend: ■ PEPCID COMPLETE, ■ Placebo, ■ Famotidine, ▨ Antacid

Values: 45, 33, 41

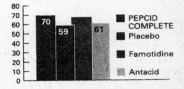

Duration of Relief
Percent of heartburn episodes relieved for at least 7 hours from the time of dosing

Legend: ■ PEPCID COMPLETE, ■ Placebo, ■ Famotidine, ▨ Antacid

Values: 70, 59, 58, 61

Pepcid Complete—Cont.

- keep the carton and package insert booklet. They contain important information.
- store at 25°–30°C (77–86 F).
- protect from moisture.

How Supplied:
Pepcid Complete is available as a rose-colored chewable tablet identified by 'P'.
NDC 16837-888 – Mint flavor
Pepcid Complete Berry flavor
NDC 16837-291

Shown in Product Identification Guide, page 506

Matrixx Initiatives, Inc.
**4742 NORTH 24TH STREET
SUITE 455
PHOENIX, AZ 85016**

Direct Inquiries:
Phone: 602-385-8888
Fax: 602-385-8850
Web Site: www.zicam.com

ZICAM® Concentrated Cough Mist - Honey Lemon & Cool Cherry
[zī'kăm]
Oral Cough Suppressant Spray

Drug Facts

**Active Ingredient
(in each spray):** **Purpose:**
Dextromethorphan .... Cough
HBr 3.3 mg Suppressant

Uses: temporarily relieves
- cough due to minor throat and bronchial irritation associated with a cold

Warnings:
Do not use if you are now taking a prescription monoamine oxidase inhibitor (MAOI) (certain drugs for depression, psychiatric or emotional conditions, or Parkinson's disease), or for 2 weeks after stopping the MAOI drug. If you do not know if your prescription drug contains an MAOI, ask a doctor or pharmacist before taking this product.
Ask a doctor before use if you have
- cough accompanied by excessive phlegm (mucus)
- persistent or chronic cough such as occurs with smoking, asthma, or emphysema
Stop use and ask a doctor if
- cough lasts more than 7 days, comes back, or occurs with fever, rash, or headache that lasts. These could be signs of a serious condition.
If pregnant or breast-feeding, ask a health professional before use.
Keep out of reach of children. In case of overdose, get medical help or contact a Poison Control Center right away.

Directions:
- Remove safety cap.
- Prime pump by spraying into a tissue.

- Hold close to mouth and depress sprayer fully. Swallow.
  12 yrs & older .... 3 sprays (10.0 mg Dextromethorphan HBr)
  6–11 yrs .... 2 sprays (6.7 mg Dextromethorphan HBr)
  Under 6 yrs .... consult a doctor
- Repeat every 4 hours, not to exceed 6 doses per day.
- May be followed by water or liquids if desired.

Inactive Ingredients: citric acid, fructose, hydroxylated lecithin, menthol, natural flavors, polyethylene glycol, polysorbate 60, potassium sorbate, purified water, sucralose

Other Information:
Store at room temperature 15°C–29°C (59°F–84°F)

Questions? Comments?
call 877-942-2626 toll-free or visit us on the web at www.zicam.com

How Supplied: .75 fl oz bottle in Cool Cherry and Honey Lemon flavors
Shown in Product Identification Guide, page 506

ZICAM® Concentrated Cough Mist Nite-Cool Cherry
[zī 'kăm]
Oral Cough Suppressant Spray

Drug Facts

**Active Ingredient
(in each spray):** **Purpose:**
Dextromethorphan HBr
6.0 mg .... Cough Suppressant

Uses: temporarily relieves
- cough due to minor throat and bronchial irritation associated with a cold

Warnings:
Do not use if you are now taking a prescription monoamine oxidase inhibitor (MAOI) (certain drugs for depression, psychiatric or emotional conditions, or Parkinson's disease), or for 2 weeks after stopping the MAOI drug. If you do not know if your prescription drug contains an MAOI, ask a doctor or pharmacist before taking this product.
Ask a doctor before use if you have
- cough accompanied by excessive phlegm (mucus)
- persistent or chronic cough such as occurs with smoking, asthma, or emphysema
Stop use and ask a doctor if
- cough lasts more than 7 days, comes back, or occurs with fever, rash, or headache that lasts. These could be signs of a serious condition.
If pregnant or breast-feeding, ask a health professional before use. **Keep out of reach of children.** In case of overdose, get medical help or contact a Poison Control Center right away.

Directions:
- Remove safety cap.
- Prime pump by spraying into a tissue.
- Hold close to mouth and depress sprayer fully. Swallow.

12 yrs & older .... 5 sprays (30.0 mg Dextromethorphan HBr)
Under 12 yrs .... consult a doctor
- Repeat every 6–8 hours, not to exceed 4 doses per day.
- May be followed by water or liquids if desired.

Inactive Ingredients: alcohol, benzyl alcohol, glycerin, lecithin, menthol, natural flavors, polyethylene glycol, polysorbate 60, potassium sorbate, purified water, sucralose

Other Information:
Store at room temperature 15°C–29°C (59°F–84°F)

Questions? Comments?
call 877-942-2626 toll-free or visit us on the web at www.zicam.com

How Supplied: .75 fl oz bottle in Cool Cherry flavor
Shown in Product Identification Guide, page 506

ZICAM® CONCENTRATED COUGH MIST PLUS D
[zī-kăm]
**Oral Cough Suppressant
Spray/Nasal Decongestant**

Drug Facts

**Active Ingredients
(in each spray):** **Purpose:**
Dextromethorphan HBr
3.3 mg .... Cough Suppressant
Phenylephrine HCl
3.3 mg .... Nasal Decongestant

Uses: temporarily relieves
- cough due to minor throat and bronchial irritation associated with a cold
- nasal decongestion due to the common cold

Warnings: **Do not use** if you are now taking a prescription monoamine oxidase inhibitor (MAOI) (certain drugs for depression, psychiatric or emotional conditions, or Parkinson's disease), or for 2 weeks after stopping the MAOI drug. If you do not know if your prescription drug contains an MAOI, ask a doctor or pharmacist before taking this product.
Ask a doctor before use if you have
- heart disease
- high blood pressure
- thyroid disease
- diabetes
- trouble urinating due to an enlarged prostate gland
- cough accompanied by excessive phlegm (mucus)
- persistent or chronic cough such as occurs with smoking, asthma, or emphysema
When using this product do not use more than directed.
Stop use and ask a doctor if
- you get nervous, dizzy, or sleepless
- symptoms do not get better within 7 days or are accompanied by fever
- cough lasts more than 7 days, comes back, or occurs with fever, rash, or headache that lasts. These could be signs of a serious condition.
If pregnant or breast-feeding, ask a health professional before use.

Keep out of reach of children. In case of overdose, get medical help or contact a Poison Control Center right away.

Directions:
- Remove safety cap.
- Prime pump by spraying into a tissue.
- Hold close to mouth and depress sprayer fully. Swallow.
  12 yrs & older .... 3 sprays (10.0 mg Dextromethorphan HBr); 10.0 Phenylephrine HCl)
  Under 12 yrs .... consult a doctor
- Repeat every 4 hours, not to exceed 6 doses per day.
- May be followed water or liquids if desired.

Inactive Ingredients: citric acid, fructose, hydroxylated lecithin, menthol, natural flavors, polyethylene glycol, polysorbate 60, potassium sorbate, purified water, sucralose

Other Information:
Store at room temperature 15°C–29°C (59°F–84°F)

Questions? Comments?
call 877-942-2626 toll-free or visit us on the web at www.zicam.com

How Supplied: .75 fl oz bottle in Cool Cherry Flavor
Shown in Product Identification Guide, page 506

ZICAM® CONCENTRATED COUGH MIST FOR KIDS
[zĭ 'kăm]
Oral Cough Suppressant Spray

Drug Facts

Active Ingredient
(in each spray): **Purpose:**
Dextromethorphan HBr
  2.5 mg .... Cough Suppressant

Uses: temporarily relieves
- cough due to minor throat and bronchial irritation associated with a cold

Warnings:
Do not use in a child who is taking a prescription monoamine oxidase inhibitor (MAOI) (certain drugs for depression, psychiatric or emotional conditions, or Parkinson's disease), or for 2 weeks after stopping the MAOI drug. If you do not know if your child's prescription drug contains an MAOI, as a doctor or pharmacist before giving this product.
Ask a doctor before use if the child has
- cough accompanied by excessive phlegm (mucus)
- persistent or chronic cough such as occurs with asthma
Stop use and ask a doctor if
- cough lasts more than 7 days, comes back, or occurs with fever, rash, or headache that lasts. These could be signs of a serious condition.
Keep out of reach of children. In case of overdose, get medical help or contact a Poison Control Center right away.

Directions:
- Remove safety cap.
- Prime pump by spraying into a tissue.
- Hold close to mouth and depress sprayer fully. Swallow.

6–11 yrs .... 4 sprays (10.0 mg Dextromethorphan HBr)
2–5 yrs .... 2 sprays (5.0 mg Dextromethorphan HBr)
Under 2 yrs .... consult a doctor
- Repeat every 4 hours, not to exceed 6 doses per day.
- May be followed by water or liquids if desired.

Inactive Ingredients: citric acid, fructose, hydroxylated lecithin, natural flavors, polysorbate 60, potassium sorbate, purified water, sucralose
Other Information:
Store at room temperature 15°C–29°C (59°F–84°F)
Questions? Comments?
call 877-942-2626 toll-free or visit us on the web at www.zicam.com
How Supplied: .75 fl oz bottle in Cool Cherry flavor
Shown in Product Identification Guide, page 506

ZICAM® CONCENTRATED COUGH MIST PLUS D FOR KIDS
[zĭ 'kăm]
Oral Cough Suppressant Spray/Nasal Decongestant

Drug Facts

Active Ingredients
(in each spray): **Purpose:**
Dextromethorphan HBr
  2.5 mg .... Cough Suppressant
Phenylephrine HCl
  1.25 mg .... Nasal Decongestant
Uses: temporarily relieves
- cough due to minor throat and bronchial irritation associated with a cold
- nasal congestion due to the common cold
Warnings:
Do not use in a child who is taking a prescription monoamine oxidase inhibitor (MAOI) (certain drugs for depression, psychiatric or emotional conditions, or Parkinson's disease), or for 2 weeks after stopping the MAOI drug. If you do not know if your child's prescription drug contains an MAOI, ask a doctor or pharmacist before giving this product.
Ask a doctor before use if the child has
- heart disease • high blood pressure
- thyroid disease • diabetes
- cough accompanied by excessive phlegm (mucus)
- persistent or chronic cough such as occurs with asthma
When using this product do not use more than directed.
Stop use and ask a doctor if
- the child gets nervous, dizzy, or sleepless
- symptoms do not get better within 7 days or are accompanied by fever
- cough lasts more than 7 days, comes back, or occurs with fever, rash, or headache that lasts. These could be signs of a serious condition.
Keep out of reach of children. In case of overdose, get medical help or contact a Poison Control Center right away.

Directions:
- Remove safety cap.
- Prime pump by spraying into a tissue.

- Hold close to mouth and depress sprayer fully. Swallow.
  6–11 yrs ...... 4 sprays (10.0 mg Dextromethorphan HBr, 5.0 mg Phenylephrine HCl)
  2–5 yrs ...... 2 sprays (5.0 mg Dextromethorphan HBr, 2.5 mg Phenylephrine HCl)
  Under 2 yrs ...... consult a doctor
- Repeat every 4 hours, not to exceed 6 doses per day.
- May be followed by water or liquids if desired.

Inactive Ingredients: citric acid, fructose, hydroxylated lecithin, natural flavors, polysorbate 60, potassium sorbate, purified water, sucralose
Other Information:
Store at room temperature 15°C–29°C (59°F–84°F)
Questions? Comments?
call 877-942-2626 toll-free or visit us on the web at www.zicam.com
How Supplied: .75 fl oz bottle in Cool Cherry flavor.
Shown in Product Identification Guide, page 506

ZICAM® NO-DRIP NASAL MOISTURIZER
[zĭ 'kăm]

Description: Soothes and moisturizes dry nasal passages due to colds, allergies, sinusitis, low humidity, overuse of decongestant sprays/drops, air pollution, smoke, air travel.

Caution:
For nasal use only.
Keep out of reach of children. Use of this container by more than one person may spread infection.

Directions:
- Remove cap and safety clip (also see illustrations on side of carton and insert).
- Hold with thumb at bottom of bottle and nozzle between fingers.
- Before using the first time, prime pump by depressing several times.
- Pump once into each nostril without tilting your head.
- Sniff deeply. Use as often as needed. Wipe clean after use.
Contains: purified water, hydroxyethylcellulose, glycerin, sodium phosphate (monohydrate), disodium phosphate (heptahydrate), alkoxylated diester, aloe barbadensis gel, hydrolyzed algin, chlorella vulgaris extract, sea water, benzalkonium chloride, benzyl alcohol, disodium EDTA, hydroxylated lecithin, tocopherol, polysorbate 80
Other Information:
Store at room temperature 15°C–29°C (59°F–84°F)
Questions? Comments?
call 877-942-2626 toll-free or visit us on the web at www.zicam.com

How Supplied: 0.50 Fl. Oz. bottle
Shown in Product Identification Guide, page 506

McNeil Consumer & Specialty Pharmaceuticals

Division of McNeil-PPC, Inc.
FORT WASHINGTON, PA 19034

Direct Inquiries to:
Consumer Relationship Center
Fort Washington, PA 19034
(800) 962-5357

IMODIUM® A–D LIQUID AND CAPLETS
(loperamide hydrochloride)

Description: Each 7.5 mL (1½ teaspoonful) of *IMODIUM® A-D* liquid contains loperamide hydrochloride 1 mg. *IMODIUM® A-D* liquid is stable, and has a mint flavor.
Each caplet of *IMODIUM® A-D* contains 2 mg of loperamide hydrochloride and is scored and colored green.

Actions: *IMODIUM® A-D* contains a clinically proven antidiarrheal medication. Loperamide HCl acts by slowing intestinal motility and by affecting water and electrolyte movement through the bowel.

Uses: controls symptoms of diarrhea, including Travelers' Diarrhea.

Directions:
Imodium A-D Caplets
- **drink plenty of clear fluids to help prevent dehydration caused by diarrhea**
- find right dose on chart. If possible, use weight to dose; otherwise, use age

adults and children 12 years and over	2 caplets after the first loose stool; 1 caplet after each subsequent loose stool; but no more than 4 caplets in 24 hours
children 9–11 years (60–95 lbs)	1 caplet after first loose stool; ½ caplet after each subsequent loose stool; but no more than 3 caplets in 24 hours
children 6–8 years (48–59 lbs)	1 caplet after first loose stool; ½ caplet after each subsequent loose stool; but no more than 2 caplets in 24 hours
children under 6 years (up to 47 lbs)	ask a doctor

Imodium A-D Liquid
- **drink plenty of clear fluids to help prevent dehydration caused by diarrhea**
- find right dose on chart. If possible, use weight to dose; otherwise use age.
- shake well before using
- only use attached measuring cup to dose product

adults and children 12 years and over	30 mL (6 tsp) after the first loose stool; 15 mL (3 tsp) after each subsequent loose stool; but no more than 60 mL (12 tsp) in 24 hours
children 9–11 years (60–95 lbs)	15 mL (3 tsp) after first loose stool; 7.5 mL (1½ tsp) after each subsequent loose stool; but no more than 45 mL (9 tsp) in 24 hours
children 6–8 years (48–59 lbs)	15 mL (3 tsp) after first loose stool; 7.5 mL (1½ tsp) after each subsequent loose stool; but no more than 30 mL (6 tsp) in 24 hours
children under 6 years (up to 47 lbs)	ask a doctor

Imodium A-D Liquid Professional Dosage Schedule for children 2–5 years old (24–47 lbs): 1½ teaspoonful after first loose bowel movement, followed by 1½ teaspoonful after each subsequent loose bowel movement. Do not exceed 4½ teaspoonful a day.

Warnings:
Allergy alert: Do not use if you have ever had a rash or other allergic reaction to loperamide HCl
Do not use if you have bloody or black stool
Ask a doctor before use if you have
- fever • mucus in the stool • a history of liver disease
Ask a doctor or pharmacist before use if you are taking antibiotics
When using this product tiredness, drowsiness or dizziness may occur. Be careful when driving or operating machinery
Stop use and ask a doctor if
- symptoms get worse • diarrhea lasts for more than 2 days
- you get abdominal swelling or bulging. These may be signs of a serious condition
If pregnant or breast feeding, ask a health professional before use. **Keep out of reach of children.** In case of overdose, get medical help or contact a Poison Control Center right away.
Other Information:

Liquid:
- **4oz and 2oz: do not use if printed plastic neck wrap is broken or missing**
  4oz and 2oz label: do not use if printed plastic neck wrap is broken or missing
- each 30 mL (6 tsp) contains: sodium 10 mg
- store between 20–25°C (68–77°F)

Caplets:
- store between 20–25°C (68–77°F)

- **Carton: do not use if carton or blister unit is open or torn**
- Pouch: do not use if pouch is opened
- see bottom panel for lot and expiration date

Professional Information:

Overdosage Information
Overdosage of loperamide HCl in man may result in constipation, CNS depression and nausea. A slurry of activated charcoal administered promptly after ingestion of loperamide hydrochloride can reduce the amount of drug which is absorbed. If vomiting occurs spontaneously upon ingestion, a slurry of 100 grams of activated charcoal should be administered orally as soon as fluids can be retained. If vomiting has not occurred, and CNS depression is evident, gastric lavage should be performed followed by administration of 100 gms of the activated charcoal slurry through the gastric tube. In the event of overdosage, patients should be monitored for signs of CNS depression for at least 24 hours. Children may be more sensitive to central nervous system effects than adults. If CNS depression is observed, naloxone may be administered. If responsive to naloxone, vital signs must be monitored carefully for recurrence of symptoms of drug overdose for at least 24 hours after the last dose of naloxone.

Inactive Ingredients:
Liquid: cellulose, citric acid, D&C yellow #10, FD&C blue #1, glycerin, flavor, propylene glycol, simethicone, sodium benzoate, sucralose, titanium dioxide, xanthan gum
Caplets: colloidal silicon dioxide, D&C yellow no. 10, dibasic calcium phosphate, FD&C blue no. 1, magnesium stearate, microcrystalline cellulose.

How Supplied:
Liquid: Mint flavored liquid 2 fl. oz. and 4 fl. oz. tamper evident bottles with child resistant safety caps and special dosage cups.
Caplets: Green scored caplets in 6s, 12s, 18s, 24s, 48s and 72s blister packaging which is tamper evident and child resistant.

Shown in Product Identification Guide, page 507

IMODIUM® ADVANCED
(loperamide HCl/simethicone)
Caplets & Chewable Tablets

Description: Each easy to swallow caplet and mint-flavored chewable tablet of *Imodium® Advanced* contains loperamide HCl 2 mg/simethicone 125 mg.

Actions: *Imodium® Advanced* combines original prescription strength Imodium® to control the symptoms of diarrhea plus simethicone to relieve bloat-

PRODUCT INFORMATION

ing, pressure and cramps commonly referred to as gas. Loperamide HCl acts by slowing intestinal motility and by affecting water and electrolyte movement through the bowel. Simethicone acts in the stomach and intestines by altering the surface tension of gas bubbles enabling them to coalesce, thereby freeing and eliminating the gas more easily by belching or passing flatus.

Use: Controls symptoms of diarrhea plus bloating, pressure, and cramps commonly referred to as gas.

Directions:
- **drink plenty of clear fluids to help prevent dehydration caused by diarrhea**
- find right dose on chart. If possible, use weight to dose; otherwise use age

adults and children 12 years and over	swallow 2 caplets or chew 2 tablets and take with water (for chewables) after the first loose stool; 1 caplet/tablet and take with water (for chewables) after each subsequent loose stool; but no more than 4 caplets/tablets in 24 hours
children 9–11 years (60–95 lbs)	swallow 1 caplet or chew 1 tablet and take with water (for chewables) after the first loose stool; ½ caplet/tablet and take with water (for chewables) after each subsequent loose stool; but no more than 3 caplets/tablets in 24 hours
children 6–8 years (48–59 lbs)	swallow 1 caplet or chew 1 tablet and take with water (for chewables) after the first loose stool; ½ caplet/tablet and take with water (for chewables) after each subsequent loose stool; but no more than 2 caplets/tablets in 24 hours
children under 6 years (up to 47 lbs)	ask a doctor

Warnings:
Allergy alert: Do not use if you have ever had a rash or other allergic reaction to loperamide HCl
Do not use if you have bloody or black stool
Ask a doctor before use if you have • fever • mucus in the stool • a history of liver disease
Ask a doctor or pharmacist before use if you are taking antibiotics

When using this product tiredness, drowsiness, or dizziness may occur. Be careful when driving or operating machinery
Stop use and ask a doctor if • symptoms get worse • diarrhea lasts for more than 2 days • you get abdominal swelling or bulging. These may be signs of a serious condition.
If pregnant or breast-feeding, ask a health professional before use.
Keep out of reach of children. In case of overdose, get medical help or contact a Poison Control Center right away.
Other Information:
Caplets:
- store between 20–25°C (68–77°F)
- protect from light
- see side panel for expiration date and lot number
Blister statement:
- Carton: do not use if carton is open or if blister unit is open or torn
- Pouch: do not us if pouch is opened
Bottle statement:
- do not use if carton if open or if printed foil seal under bottle cap is open or torn
Chewable Tablets:
- Carton: do not use if carton is opened or if blister unit is broken
- Pouch: do not use if pouch is opened
- store between 20–25°C (68–77°F)
- protect from light
- see side panel for expiration date and lot number

Professional Information:
Overdosage Information:
Overdosage of loperamide HCl in man may result in constipation, CNS depression and nausea. A slurry of activated charcoal administered promptly after ingestion of loperamide hydrochloride can reduce the amount of drug which is absorbed. If vomiting occurs spontaneously upon ingestion, a slurry of 100 grams of activated charcoal should be administered orally as soon as fluids can be retained. If vomiting has not occurred, and CNS depression is evident, gastric lavage should be performed followed by administration of 100 gms of the activated charcoal slurry through the gastric tube. In the event of overdosage, patients should be monitored for signs of CNS depression for at least 24 hours. Children may be more sensitive to central nervous system effects than adults. If CNS depression is observed, naloxone may be administered. If responsive to naloxone, vital signs must be monitored carefully for recurrence of symptoms of drug overdose for at least 24 hours after the last dose of naloxone. No treatment is necessary for the simethicone ingestion in this circumstance.

Inactive Ingredients:
Caplets: acesulfame K, cellulose, dibasic calcium phosphate, flavor, sodium starch glycolate, stearic acid **Chewable Tablets:** cellulose acetate, corn starch, D&C Yellow No. 10, dextrates, FD&C Blue No. 1, flavors, microcrystalline cellulose, polymethacrylates, saccharin sodium, sorbitol, stearic acid, sucrose, tribasic calcium phosphate.

How Supplied: Mint Chewable Tablets in 6's, 12's, 18's, 30's, and blister packaging which is tamper evident and child resistant. Each Imodium® Advanced tablet is round, light green in color and has "IMODIUM" embossed on one side and "2/125" on the other side. Imodium Advanced Caplets are available in blister packs of 12's and 18's and bottles of 30's and 42's. Each Imodium® Advanced Caplet is oval, white color and has "IMO" embossed on one side and "2/125" on the other side.
Shown in Product Identification Guide, page 507

MOTRIN® IB Ibuprofen
Pain Reliever/
Fever Reducer
Tablets, Caplets and Gelcaps

Description: Each *MOTRIN® IB Tablet, Caplet and Gelcap* contains ibuprofen 200 mg.

Uses: Temporarily relieves minor aches and pains due to:
- headache • muscular aches • minor pain of arthritis • toothache • backache • the common cold • menstrual cramps
Temporarily reduces fever

Directions:
- **do not take more than directed**

| adults and children 12 years and older | • take 1 tablet, caplet, or gelcap every 4 to 6 hours while symptoms persist • if pain or fever does not respond to 1 tablet, caplet or gelcap, 2 tablets, caplets or gelcaps may be used, • do not exceed 6 tablets, caplets or gelcaps in 24 hours, unless directed by a doctor • the smallest effective dose should be used |
| children under 12 years | • ask a doctor |

Warnings: Allergy alert: Ibuprofen may cause a severe allergic reaction which may include:
- hives • facial swelling
- asthma (wheezing) • shock
Stomach bleeding warning: Taking more than recommended may cause stomach bleeding.
Alcohol Warning: If you consume 3 or more alcoholic drinks every day, ask your doctor whether you should take ibuprofen or other pain relievers/fever reducers. Ibuprofen may cause stomach bleeding.
Do not use if you have ever had an allergic reaction to any other pain reliever/fever reducer.

Continued on next page

Motrin IB—Cont.

Ask a doctor before use if you have
- problems or serious side effects from taking pain relievers or fever reducers
- stomach problems that last or come back, such as heartburn, upset stomach, or pain
- ulcers
- bleeding problems
- high blood pressure, heart or kidney disease, are taking a diuretic, or are over 65 years of age.

Ask a doctor or pharmacist before use if you are
- under a doctor's care for any serious condition
- taking any other product that contains ibuprofen, or any other pain reliever/fever reducer
- taking a prescription drug for anticoagulation (blood thinning)
- taking any other drug

When using this product take with food or milk if stomach upset occurs.

Stop use and ask a doctor if
- an allergic reaction occurs. Seek medical help right away.
- pain gets worse or lasts more than 10 days
- fever gets worse or lasts more than 3 days
- stomach pain or upset gets worse or lasts
- redness or swelling is present in the painful area
- any new symptoms appear.

If pregnant or breast-feeding, ask a health professional before use. It is especially important not to use ibuprofen during the last 3 months of pregnancy unless definitely directed to do so by a doctor because it may cause problems in the unborn child or complications during delivery.

Keep out of reach of children. In case of overdose, get medical help or contact a Poison Control Center right away.

Other Information:
- Do not use if neck wrap or foil inner seal imprinted "Safety Seal®" is broken or missing.
- Store at 20°–25°C (68°–77°F) (applies to gelcaps only)
- avoid high humidity and excessive heat above 40°C (104°F) (applies to gelcaps only)

Professional Information:
Overdosage Information for Adult Motrin®
IBUPROFEN

The *toxicity of ibuprofen* overdose is dependent upon the amount of drug ingested and the time elapsed since ingestion, though individual response may vary, which makes it necessary to evaluate each case individually. Although uncommon, serious toxicity and death have been reported in the medical literature with ibuprofen overdosage. The most frequently reported symptoms of ibuprofen overdose include abdominal pain, nausea, vomiting, lethargy and drowsiness. Other central nervous system symptoms include headache, tinnitus, CNS depression and seizures. Metabolic acidosis, coma, acute renal failure and apnea (primarily in very young children) may

rarely occur. Cardiovascular toxicity, including hypotension, bradycardia, tachycardia and atrial fibrillation, also have been reported. The *treatment of acute ibuprofen overdose* is primarily supportive. Management of hypotension, acidosis and gastrointestinal bleeding may be necessary. In cases of acute overdose, the stomach should be emptied through ipecac-induced emesis or lavage. Emesis is most effective if initiated within 30 minutes of ingestion. Orally administered activated charcoal may help in reducing the absorption and reabsorption of ibuprofen. In children, the estimated amount of ibuprofen ingested per body weight may be helpful to predict the potential for development of toxicity although each case must be evaluated. Ingestion of less than 100 mg/kg is unlikely to produce toxicity. Children ingesting 100 to 200 mg/kg may be managed with induced emesis and a minimal observation time of four hours. Children ingesting 200 to 400 mg/kg of ibuprofen should have immediate gastric emptying and at least four hours observation in a health care facility. Children ingesting greater than 400 mg/kg require immediate medical referral, careful observation and appropriate supportive therapy. Ipecac-induced emesis is not recommended in overdoses greater than 400 mg/kg because of the risk of convulsions and the potential for aspiration of gastric contents. In adult patients the history of the dose reportedly ingested does not appear to be predictive of toxicity. The need for referral and follow-up must be judged by the circumstances at the time of the overdose ingestion. Symptomatic adults should be admitted to a health care facility for observation.

Our Adult MOTRIN® combination products contain pseudoephedrine in addition to ibuprofen. For basic overdose information regarding pseudoephedrine, please see below. For additional emergency information, please contact your local poison control center.
PSEUDOEPHEDRINE
Symptoms from pseudoephedrine overdose consist most often of mild anxiety, tachycardia and/or mild hypertension. Symptoms usually appear within 4 to 8 hours and are transient, usually requiring no treatment.

Inactive Ingredients:
Tablets and Caplets: carnauba wax, corn starch, FD&C Yellow #6, hypromellose, iron oxide, polydextrose, polyethylene glycol, silicon dioxide, stearic acid, titanium dioxide.
Gelcaps: benzyl alcohol, butylparaben, castor oil, cellulose, corn starch, edetate calcium disodium, FD&C Yellow No. 6, gelatin, hypromellose, iron oxide, methylparaben, povidone, propylparaben, silicon dioxide, sodium lauryl sulfate, sodium propionate, sodium starch glycolate, titanium dioxide.

How Supplied:
Tablets: (orange, printed "MOTRIN IB" in black) in tamper evident packaging of 24, 50, 100, and 165.

Caplets: (orange, printed "MOTRIN IB" in black) in tamper evident packaging of 24, 50, 100, 165, 250, 300 and
Gelcaps: (colored orange and white, printed "MOTRIN IB" in black) in tamper evident packaging of 24, 50 and 100.

Shown in Product Identification Guide, page 508

MOTRIN® COLD & SINUS CAPLETS

Description: Each MOTRIN® Cold & Sinus Caplet contains ibuprofen 200 mg and pseudoephedrine HCl 30 mg.

Uses: temporarily relieves these symptoms associated with the common cold, sinusitis, and flu:
- headache • nasal congestion
- fever • minor body aches and pains

Directions:

Adults and children 12 years of age and older	• take 1 caplet every 4 to 6 hours while symptoms persist • If symptoms do not respond to 1 caplet, 2 caplets may be used. • do not use more than 6 caplets in any 24-hour period unless directed by a doctor • the smallest effective dose should be used
Children under 12 years of age	Consult a doctor

Warnings: Allergy alert: Ibuprofen may cause a severe allergic reaction which may include:
- hives • facial swelling
- asthma (wheezing) • shock

Alcohol warning: If you consume 3 or more alcoholic drinks every day, ask your doctor whether you should take ibuprofen or other pain relievers/fever reducers. Ibuprofen may cause stomach bleeding.

Do not use if you
- have ever had an allergic reaction to any other pain reliever/fever reducer
- are now taking a prescription monoamine oxidase inhibitor (MAOI) (certain drugs for depression, psychiatric or emotional conditions, or Parkinson's disease), or for 2 weeks after stopping the MAOI drug. If you do not know if your prescription drug contains an MAOI, ask a doctor or pharmacist before taking this product.

Ask a doctor before use if you have
- heart disease • high blood pressure
- thyroid disease • diabetes
- trouble urinating due to an enlarged prostate gland
- problems or serious side effects from taking any pain reliever/fever reducers.

Ask a doctor or pharmacist before use if you are
- taking any other product that contains ibuprofen or pseudoephedrine.
- taking any other pain reliever/fever reducer or nasal decongestant
- under a doctor's care for any continuing medical condition
- taking other drugs on a regular basis

When using this product
- do not use more than directed
- give with food or milk if stomach upset occurs

Stop use and ask a doctor if
- an allergic reaction occurs. Seek medical help right away
- you get nervous, dizzy, or sleepless
- nasal congestion lasts for more than 7 days
- fever lasts for more than 3 days
- symptoms continue or get worse
- new or unexpected symptoms occur
- stomach pain occurs with use of this product or even if mild symptoms persist

If pregnant or breast-feeding, ask a health professional before use. It is especially important not to use this product during the last 3 months of pregnancy unless definitely directed to do so by a doctor because it may cause problems in the unborn child or complications during delivery.

Keep out of reach of children. In case of overdose, get medical help or contact a Poison Control Center right away.

Other Information:
Carton:
- Pouch: do not use if packet is opened
- Dispensit: do not use if packet is opened
- **do not use if blister unit is broken or open**
- store between 20–25°C (68–77°F).
- avoid excessive heat
- read all warnings and directions before use. Keep carton.

Professional Information:
Overdosage Information:
For overdosage information, please refer to pg. 646.

Inactive Ingredients:
Caplets: carnauba wax, cellulose, corn starch, FD&C Red #40, hypromellose, silicon dioxide, sodium lauryl sulfate, sodium starch glycolate, stearic acid, titanium dioxide, triacetin.

How Supplied:
Caplets: (white, printed "Cold & Sinus" in red) in blister packs of 20.
Shown in Product Identification Guide, page 508

Infants' MOTRIN® ibuprofen Concentrated Drops

Children's MOTRIN® ibuprofen Oral Suspension and Chewable Tablets

Junior Strength MOTRIN® ibuprofen Caplets and Chewable Tablets

Product information for all dosages of Children's MOTRIN have been combined under this heading

Description: *Infants' MOTRIN® Concentrated Drops* are available in an alcohol-free, berry-flavored suspension and a non-staining, dye-free, berry-flavored suspension. Each 1.25 mL contains ibuprofen 50 mg. *Children's MOTRIN® Oral Suspension* is available as an alcohol-free, berry, dye-free berry, bubblegum or grape-flavored suspension. Each 5 mL (teaspoon) of *Children's MOTRIN® Oral Suspension* contains ibuprofen 100 mg. Each *Children's MOTRIN® Chewable Tablet* contains 50 mg of ibuprofen and is available as orange or grape-flavored chewable tablets. *Junior Strength MOTRIN® Chewable Tablets* and *Junior Strength MOTRIN® Caplets* contain ibuprofen 100 mg. *Junior Strength MOTRIN® Chewable Tablets* are available in orange or grape flavors. *Junior Strength MOTRIN® Caplets* are available as easy-to-swallow caplets (capsule-shaped tablet).

Uses: temporarily:
- reduces fever
- relieves minor aches and pains due to the common cold, flu, sore throat, headaches and toothaches

Directions: See Table 2: Children's Motrin Dosing Chart on pg. 650.

Warnings:
Allergy alert: Ibuprofen may cause a severe allergic reaction which may include:
- hives • facial swelling
- asthma (wheezing) • shock

Sore throat warning: Severe or persistent sore throat or sore throat accompanied by high fever, headache, nausea, and vomiting may be serious. Consult doctor promptly. Do not use more than 2 days or administer to children under 3 years of age unless directed by doctor.

Do not use if the child has never had an allergic reaction to any other fever reducer/pain reliever

Ask a doctor before use if the child has
- not been drinking fluids
- lost a lot of fluid due to continued vomiting or diarrhea
- stomach pain
- problems or serious side effects from taking fever reducers or pain relievers

Ask a doctor or pharmacist before use if the child is:
- under a doctor's care for any serious condition
- taking any other drug
- taking any other product that contains ibuprofen, or any other fever reducer/pain reliever

When using this product
- mouth or throat burning may occur; give with food or water (*Children's MOTRIN® Chewable Tablets and Junior Strength MOTRIN® Chewable Tablets only*)
- give with food or milk if stomach upset occurs

Stop use and ask a doctor if
- an allergic reaction occurs. Seek medical help right away.
- fever or pain gets worse or lasts more than 3 days
- the child does not get any relief within first day (24 hours) of treatment
- stomach pain or upset gets worse or lasts

- redness or swelling is present in the painful area
- any new symptoms appear

Keep out of reach of children. In case of overdose, get medical help or contact a Poison Control Center right away.

Other Information: *Infants', Children's and Junior Strength MOTRIN® products:*
- Store at 20–25°C (68–77°F)

Infants' MOTRIN® Concentrated Drops:
- do not use if plastic carton wrap or bottle wrap imprinted "Safety Seal®" and "Use with Enclosed Dosage Device" is broken or missing.

Children's MOTRIN® Suspension Liquid:
- do not use if plastic carton wrap or bottle wrap imprinted "Safety Seal®" is broken or missing

Children's MOTRIN® Chewable Tablets:
- Phenylketonurics: Contains phenylalanine 1.4 mg per tablet
- do not use if neck wrap or foil inner seal imprinted "Safety Seal®" is broken or missing

Junior Strength MOTRIN® Caplets and Chewable Tablets:
- do not use if neck wrap or foil inner seal imprinted "Safety Seal®" is broken or missing

Junior Strength MOTRIN® Chewable Tablets:
- phenylketonurics: contains phenylalanine 2.8 mg per tablet (tablet only)
- see end panel for lot and expiration date

Professional Information:
Overdosage Information for all Infants', Children's & Junior Strength Motrin® Products

IBUPROFEN: The *toxicity of ibuprofen* overdose is dependent upon the amount of drug ingested and the time elapsed since ingestion, though individual response may vary, which makes it necessary to evaluate each case individually. Although uncommon, serious toxicity and death have been reported in the medical literature with ibuprofen overdosage. The most frequently reported symptoms of ibuprofen overdose include abdominal pain, nausea, vomiting, lethargy and drowsiness. Other central nervous system symptoms include headache, tinnitus, CNS depression and seizures. Metabolic acidosis, coma, acute renal failure and apnea (primarily in very young children) may rarely occur. Cardiovascular toxicity, including hypotension, bradycardia, tachycardia and atrial fibrillation, also have been reported.

The *treatment of acute ibuprofen overdose* is primarily supportive. Management of hypotension, acidosis and gastrointestinal bleeding may be necessary. In cases of acute overdose, the stomach should be emptied through ipecac-induced emesis or lavage. Emesis is most effective if initiated within 30 minutes of ingestion. Orally administered activated charcoal may help in reducing the absorption and reabsorption of ibuprofen. In children, the estimated amount of

Continued on next page

Motrin Infants'—Cont.

ibuprofen ingested per body weight may be helpful to predict the potential for development of toxicity although each case must be evaluated. Ingestion of less than 100 mg/kg is unlikely to produce toxicity. Children ingesting 100 to 200 mg/kg may be managed with induced emesis and a minimal observation time of four hours. Children ingesting 200 to 400 mg/kg of ibuprofen should have immediate gastric emptying and at least four hours observation in a health care facility. Children ingesting greater than 400 mg/kg require immediate medical referral, careful observation and appropriate supportive therapy. Ipecac-induced emesis is not recommended in overdoses greater than 400 mg/kg because of the risk of convulsions and the potential for aspiration of gastric contents.

In adult patients the history of the dose reportedly ingested does not appear to be predictive of toxicity. The need for referral and follow-up must be judged by the circumstances at the time of the overdose ingestion. Symptomatic adults should be admitted to a health care facility for observation.

Our Children's MOTRIN® Cold products contain pseudoephedrine in addition to ibuprofen. The following is basic overdose information regarding pseudoephedrine.

PSEUDOEPHEDRINE: Symptoms from pseudoephedrine overdose consist most often of mild anxiety, tachycardia and/or mild hypertension. Symptoms usually appear within 4 to 8 hours of ingestion and are transient, usually requiring no treatment.

For additional emergency information, please contact your local poison control center.

Inactive Ingredients:
Infants' MOTRIN® Concentrated Drops:
Berry-Flavored: citric acid, corn starch, FD&C Red #40, flavors, glycerin, polysorbate 80, purified water, sodium benzoate, sorbitol, sucrose, xanthan gum.
Dye-Free Berry-Flavored: artificial flavors, citric acid, corn starch, glycerin, polysorbate 80, purified water, sodium benzoate, sorbitol, sucrose, xanthan gum.
Children's MOTRIN® Oral Suspension:
Berry-Flavored: acesulfame potassium, citric acid, corn starch, D&C Yellow #10, FD&C Red #40, glycerin, natural and artificial flavors, polysorbate 80, purified water, sodium benzoate, sucrose, xanthan gum. **Dye-Free Berry-Flavored:** acesulfame potassium, citric acid, corn starch, glycerin, natural and artificial flavors, polysorbate 80, purified water, sodium benzoate, sucrose, xanthan gum.
Bubble Gum-Flavored: acesulfame potassium, citric acid, corn starch, FD&C Red #40, glycerin, natural and artificial flavors, polysorbate 80, purified water, sodium benzoate, sucrose, xanthan gum.
Grape-Flavored: acesulfame potassium,

citric acid, corn starch, D&C Red #33, FD&C Blue #1, FD&C Red #40 flavors, glycerin, natural and artificial flavors, polysorbate 80, purified water, sodium benzoate, sucrose, xanthan gum.
Children's MOTRIN® Chewable Tablets:
Orange-Flavored: acesulfame K, aspartame, cellulose, citric acid, FD&C Yellow #6, flavor, fumaric acid, hydroxyethyl cellulose, hypromellose, magnesium stearate, mannitol, povidone, sodium lauryl sulfate, sodium starch glycolate.
Grape-Flavored: acesulfame K, aspartame, cellulose, citric acid, FD&C Red #7, D&C Red #30, FD&C Blue #1, flavor, fumaric acid, hydroxyethyl cellulose, hypromellose, magnesium stearate, mannitol, povidone, sodium lauryl sulfate, sodium starch glycolate.
Junior Strength MOTRIN® Chewable Tablets: **Orange-Flavored:** acesulfame K, aspartame, cellulose, citric acid, FD&C yellow #6, flavor, fumaric acid, hydroxyethyl cellulose, hypromellose, magnesium stearate, mannitol, povidone, sodium lauryl sulfate, sodium starch glycolate. **Grape-Flavored:** acesulfame K, aspartame, cellulose, citric acid, D&C Red #7, D&C Red #30, FD&C Blue #1, flavor, fumaric acid, hydroxyethyl cellulose, hypromellose, magnesium stearate, mannitol, povidone, sodium lauryl sulfate, sodium starch glycolate. **Easy-To-Swallow Caplets:** carnauba wax, cellulose, corn starch, D&C Yellow #10, FD&C Yellow #6, hypromellose, polydextrose, polyethylene glycol, propylene glycol, silicon dioxide, sodium starch glycolate, titanium dioxide, triacetin.

How Supplied:
Infants' MOTRIN® Concentrated Drops: Berry-flavored, pink-colored liquid and Berry-Flavored, Dye-Free, white-colored liquid in ½ fl. oz. bottles w/calibrated plastic syringe. Dye-Free Berry also available in 1 oz. size
Children's MOTRIN® Oral Suspension: Berry-flavored, pink-colored; (2 and 4 fl. oz) Berry-Flavored, Dye-Free white-colored, Bubble Gum-flavored, pink-colored and Grape-flavored, purple-colored liquid in tamper evident bottles (4 fl. oz.)
Children's MOTRIN® Chewable Tablets: Orange-flavored, orange-colored and Grape-flavored, purple-colored chewable tablets in 24 count bottles.
Junior Strength MOTRIN® Chewable Tablets: Orange-flavored, orange-colored chewable tablets or Grape-flavored, purple-colored chewable tablets in 24 count bottles.
Junior Strength MOTRIN® Caplets: Easy-to-swallow
caplets (capsule shaped tablets) in 24 count bottles.

Shown in Product Identification Guide, page 507 & 508

Children's MOTRIN® Cold ibuprofen/pseudoephedrine HCl Oral Suspension

Description: *Children's MOTRIN® Cold Oral Suspension* is an alcohol-free

berry, dye-free berry, or grape-flavored suspension. Each 5 mL (teaspoonful) contains the pain reliever/fever reducer ibuprofen 100 mg and the nasal decongestant pseudoephedrine HCl 15 mg.

Uses: temporarily relieves these cold, sinus and flu symptoms:
• nasal and sinus congestion
• stuffy nose • headache • sore throat
• minor body aches and pains • fever

Directions: See Table 2: Children's Motrin Dosing Chart on pg. 650.

Warnings: Allergy alert: Ibuprofen may cause a severe allergic reaction which may include:
• hives • facial swelling
• asthma (wheezing) • shock
Sore throat warning: Severe or persistent sore throat or sore throat accompanied by high fever, headache, nausea, and vomiting may be serious. Consult a doctor promptly. Do not use more than 2 days or administer to children under 3 years of age unless directed by doctor.
Do not use
• if the child has ever had an allergic reaction to any other pain reliever/fever reducer and/or nasal decongestant
• in a child who is taking a prescription monoamine oxidase inhibitor [MAOI] (certain drugs for depression, psychiatric or emotional conditions, or Parkinson's disease), or for 2 weeks after stopping the MAOI drug. If you do not know if your child's prescription drug contains an MAOI, ask a doctor or pharmacist before giving this product.
Ask a doctor before use if the child has
• not been drinking fluids
• lost a lot of fluid due to continued vomiting or diarrhea
• problems or serious side effects from taking pain relievers, fever reducers or nasal decongestants
• stomach pain
• heart disease
• high blood pressure
• thyroid disease
• diabetes
Ask a doctor or pharmacist before use if the child is
• under a doctor's care for any continuing medical condition
• taking any other drug
• taking any other product that contains ibuprofen or pseudoephedrine
• taking any other pain reliever/fever reducer and/or nasal decongestant
When using this product
• do not exceed recommended dosage
• give with food or milk if stomach upset occurs
Stop use and ask a doctor if
• an allergic reaction occurs. Seek medical help right away.
• the child does not get any relief within first day (24 hours) of treatment
• fever, pain or nasal congestion gets worse, or lasts for more than 3 days
• stomach pain or upset gets worse or lasts
• symptoms continue or get worse
• redness or swelling is present in the painful area
• the child gets nervous, dizzy, sleepless or sleepy
• any new symptoms appear

Keep out of reach of children. In case of overdose, get medical help or contact a Poison Control Center right away.

Other Information:
- **do not use if plastic carton wrap or bottle wrap imprinted "Safety Seal®" is broken or missing.**
- Store at 20–25°C (68–77°F)
- see bottom of box for lot number and expiration date

Professional Information:
Overdosage Information
For overdosage information, please refer to pgs. 647–648.

Inactive Ingredients:
Berry Flavor: acesulfame potassium, citric acid, corn starch, D&C Yellow #10, FD&C Red #40, flavors, glycerin, polysorbate 80, purified water, sodium benzoate, sucrose, xanthan gum. **Dye-Free Berry Flavor:** acesulfame potassium, citric acid, corn starch, flavors, glycerin, polysorbate 80, purified water, sodium benzoate, sucrose, xanthan gum. **Grape Flavor:** acesulfame potassium, citric acid, corn starch, D&C Red #33, FD&C Blue #1, FD&C Red #40, flavors, glycerin, polysorbate 80, purified water, sodium benzoate, sucrose, xanthan gum.

How Supplied:
Berry-flavored, pink-colored; Grape-flavored, purple-colored, and Dye-Free Berry-flavored, white-colored liquid in child resistant tamper-evident bottles of 1 fl. oz. and 4 fl. oz.

Shown in Product Identification Guide, page 507 & 508

Children's Motrin® Dosing Chart
[See table on next page]

NIZORAL® A-D
KETOCONAZOLE SHAMPOO 1%

Description: *Nizoral® A-D (Ketoconazole Shampoo 1%) Anti-Dandruff Shampoo* is a light-blue liquid for topical application, containing the broad spectrum synthetic antifungal agent Ketoconazole in a concentration of 1%.

Use: Controls flaking, scaling and itching associated with dandruff.

Directions:

Adults and children 12 years and over:	• wet hair thoroughly • apply shampoo, generously lather, rinse thoroughly. Repeat. • use every 3–4 days for up to 8 weeks or as directed by a doctor. Then use only as needed to control dandruff.
children under 12 years	• ask a doctor

Warnings:
- **For external use only**

Do Not Use
- on scalp that is broken or inflamed
- if you are allergic to ingredients in this product

When Using This Product
- avoid contact with eyes
- if product gets into eyes, rinse thoroughly with water

Stop use and ask a doctor if
- rash appears
- condition worsens or does not improve in 2–4 weeks

If pregnant or breast-feeding, ask a doctor before use.

Keep out of the reach of children. If swallowed get medical help or contact a Poison Control Center right away.

Other Information
- store between 35° and 86°F (2° and 30°C)
- protect from light • protect from freezing
- see bottom panel for lot number and expiration date

Professional Information:
Overdosage Information *Nizoral® A-D (Ketoconazole) 1% Shampoo* is intended for external use only. In the event of accidental ingestion, supportive measures should be employed. Induced emesis and gastric lavage should usually be avoided.

Inactive Ingredients: acrylic acid polymer (carbomer 1342), butylated hydroxytoluene, cocamide MEA, FD&C Blue #1, fragrance, glycol distearate, polyquaternium-7, quaternium-15, sodium chloride, sodium cocoyl sarcosinate, sodium hydroxide and/or hydrochloric acid, sodium laureth sulfate, tetrasodium EDTA, water.

How Supplied: Available in 4 and 7 fl oz bottles

Shown in Product Identification Guide, page 508

ST. JOSEPH® 81 mg Aspirin
ST. JOSEPH 81 mg Adult Low Strength Aspirin Chewable & Enteric Coated Tablets

Description: Each St. Joseph Adult Low Strength Aspirin tablet contains 81 mg of aspirin.

Uses:
- temporarily relieves minor aches and pains or as recommended by your doctor
- ask your doctor about other uses for St. Joseph Adult 81 mg Aspirin

Directions:
- drink a full glass of water with each dose
- **adults and children 12 years and over:**
  - take 4 to 8 tablets every 4 hours while symptoms persist
  - do not exceed 48 tablets in 24 hours or as directed by a doctor

- **children under 12:**
  - do not use unless directed by a doctor

Warnings:
Reye's syndrome: Children and teenagers should not use this drug for chicken pox or flu symptoms before a doctor is consulted about Reye's syndrome, a rare but serious illness reported to be associated with aspirin.

Allergy alert: Aspirin may cause a severe allergic reaction which may include:
- hives
- facial swelling
- asthma (wheezing)
- shock

Alcohol warning: If you consume 3 or more alcoholic drinks every day, ask your doctor whether you should take aspirin or other pain relievers/fever reducers. Aspirin may cause stomach bleeding.

Do not use
- if you have ever had an allergic reaction to any other pain reliever/fever reducer
- for at least 7 days after tonsillectomy or oral surgery unless directed by a doctor (*chewable tablet formulation only*)

Ask a doctor before use if you have
- asthma
- ulcers
- bleeding problems
- stomach problems that last or come back such as heartburn, upset stomach or pain

Ask a doctor or pharmacist before use if you are taking a prescription for:
- anticoagulation (blood thinning)
- gout
- diabetes
- arthritis

Stop use and ask a doctor if
- allergic reaction occurs. Seek medical help right away.
- ringing in the ears or loss of hearing occurs
- pain gets worse or lasts more than 10 days
- new symptoms occur
- redness or swelling is present

If pregnant or breast-feeding, ask a health professional before use. It is especially important not to use aspirin during the last three months of pregnancy unless definitely directed to do so by a doctor because it may cause problems in the unborn child or complications during delivery.

Keep out of reach of children. In case of overdose, get medical help or contact a Poison Control Center right away.

Other Information:
- **do not use if carton is opened or neck wrap or foil inner seal imprinted with "Safety Seal®" is broken**
- store at room temperature. Avoid high humidity and excessive heat (40° C).
- see end panel for lot number and expiration date

Inactive Ingredients: *St. Joseph 81 mg Adult Low Strength Aspirin Chewable Tablets:* corn starch, FD&C yellow #6 aluminum lake, flavor, mannitol, saccharin, silicon dioxide, stearic acid. *Enteric Coated Tablets:* cellulose, corn starch, FD&C Red #40, FD&C Yel-

Continued on page 651

Table 2. Children's Motrin Dosing Chart

PRODUCT FORM	INGREDIENTS	0-5 mos* (6-11 lbs)	6-11 mos (12-17 lbs)	12-23 mos (18-23 lbs)	2-3 yrs (24-35 lbs)	4-5 yrs (36-47 lbs)	6-8 yrs (48-59 lbs)	9-10 yrs (60-71 lbs)	11 yrs (72-95 lbs)	Maximum doses/ 24 hrs
AGE GROUP* / **WEIGHT** (if possible use weight to dose; otherwise use age)	Dose to be administered based on weight or age†									
Infants' Drops Per 1.25 mL										
Infants' Motrin Concentrated Drops	Ibuprofen 50 mg	—	1.25 mL	1.875 mL	—	—	—	—	—	4 times in 24 hrs
Children's Liquid Per 5 mL teaspoonful (TSP)										
Children's Motrin Suspension	Ibuprofen 100 mg	—	—	—	1 TSP	1½ TSP	2 TSP	2½ TSP	3 TSP	4 times in 24 hrs
Children's Motrin Cold Suspension Liquid†	Ibuprofen 100 mg Pseudoephedrine HCl 15 mg	—	—	—	1 TSP	1 TSP	2 TSP	2 TSP	2 TSP	4 times in 24 hrs
Children's Tablets & Caplets Per tablet/caplet										
Children's Motrin Chewable Tablets	Ibuprofen 50 mg	—	—	—	2 tablets	3 tablets	4 tablets	5 tablets	6 tablets	4 times in 24 hrs
Junior Strength Motrin Chewable Tablets	Ibuprofen 100 mg	—	—	—	—	—	2 tablets	2½ tablets	3 tablets	4 times in 24 hrs
Junior Strength Motrin Caplets	Ibuprofen 100 mg	—	—	—	—	—	2 caplets	2½ caplets	3 caplets	4 times in 24 hrs

†Do not give, take or chew more than directed. If needed, repeat dose every 6-8 hours; except for Children's Motrin Cold which is every 6 hours, shake well before using.
* Under 6 years, call a doctor.
• Infant drops: dispense liquid slowly into the child's mouth, toward the inner cheek.
• Infants' Motrin Drops are more concentrated than Children's Motrin Liquids. The Infants' Concentrated Drops have been specifically designed for use only with enclosed dosing device. Do not use any other dosing device with this product.
• Children's Motrin Liquids are less concentrated than Infants' Motrin Drops. The Children's Motrin Liquids have been specifically designed for use with the enclosed measuring cup. Use only enclosed measuring cup to dose this product.
• Children's Motrin Suspensions (including cold)—replace original bottle cap to maintain child resistance
• Children's Motrin Chewable Tablets are not the same concentration as Junior Strength Motrin Chewable Tablets.
• Junior Strength Motrin Chewable Tablets contain twice as much medicine as Children's Motrin Chewable Tablets.

low #6, glyceryl monostearate, iron oxide, methacrylic acid, silicon dioxide, simethicone, stearic acid, triethyl citrate.

How Supplied: *St. Joseph 81 mg Adult Low Strength Chewable Aspirin Tablets:* tamper evident bottles of 36 108 (Tri-Pack). *Enteric Coated Tablets:* tamper evident bottles of 36 100, 180, 300 and 395.

Comprehensive Prescribing Information

Description: St. Joseph Adult Low Strength Aspirin Chewable & Enteric Coated Tablets (acetylsalicylic acid) are available in 81 mg for oral administration. *St. Joseph 81 mg Adult Low Strength Aspirin Chewable Tablets* contain the following inactive ingredients: corn starch, FD&C yellow #6 aluminum lake, flavor, mannitol, saccharin, silicon dioxide, stearic acid. *St. Joseph 81 mg Adult Low Strength Aspirin Enteric Coated Tablets* contain the following inactive ingredients: cellulose, corn starch, FD&C Red #40, FD&C Yellow #6, glyceryl monostearate, iron oxide, methacrylic acid, silicon dioxide, simethicone, stearic acid, triethyl citrate. Aspirin is an odorless white, needle-like crystalline or powdery substance. When exposed to moisture, aspirin hydrolyzes into salicylic and acetic acids, and gives off a vinegary-odor. It is highly lipid soluble and slightly soluble in water.

Clinical Pharmacology:

Mechanism of Action: Aspirin is a more potent inhibitor of both prostaglandin synthesis and platelet aggregation than other salicylic acid derivatives. The differences in activity between aspirin and salicylic acid are thought to be due to the acetyl group on the aspirin molecule. This acetyl group is responsible for the inactivation of cyclo-oxygenase via acetylation.

Pharmacokinetics: Absorption: In general, immediate release aspirin is well and completely absorbed from the gastrointestinal (GI) tract. Following absorption, aspirin is hydrolyzed to salicylic acid with peak plasma levels of salicylic acid occurring within 1–2 hours of dosing (see Pharmacokinetics—Metabolism). The rate of absorption from the GI tract is dependent upon the dosage form, the presence or absence of food, gastric pH (the presence or absence of GI antacids or buffering agents), and other physiologic factors. Enteric coated aspirin products are erratically absorbed from the GI tract.

Distribution: Salicylic acid is widely distributed to all tissues and fluids in the body including the central nervous system (CNS), breast milk, and fetal tissues. The highest concentrations are found in the plasma, liver, renal cortex, heart, and lungs. The protein binding of salicylate is concentration-dependent, i.e., nonlinear. At low concentrations (<100 micrograms/milliliter µg/mL), approximately 90 percent of plasma salicylate is bound to albumin while at

higher concentrations (400 µg/mL), only about 75 percent is bound. The early signs of salicylic overdose (salicylism), including tinnitus (ringing in the ears), occur at plasma concentrations approximating 200 µg/mL. Severe toxic effects are associated with levels 400 µg/mL. (See Adverse Reactions and Overdosage.)

Metabolism: Aspirin is rapidly hydrolyzed in the plasma to salicylic acid such that plasma levels of aspirin are essentially undetectable 1–2 hours after dosing. Salicylic acid is primarily conjugated in the liver to form salicyluric acid, a phenolic glucuronide, an acyl glucuronide, and a number of minor metabolites. Salicylic acid has a plasma half-life of approximately 6 hours. Salicylate metabolism is saturable and total body clearance decreases at higher serum concentrations due to the limited ability of the liver to form both salicyluric acid and phenolic glucuronide. Following toxic doses (10–20 grams (g)), the plasma half-life may be increased to over 20 hours.

Elimination: The elimination of salicylic acid follows zero order pharmacokinetics; (i.e., the rate of drug elimination is constant in relation to plasma concentration). Renal excretion of unchanged drug depends upon urine pH. As urinary pH rises above 6.5, the renal clearance of free salicylate increases from <5 percent to 80 percent. Alkalinization of the urine is a key concept in the management of salicylate overdose. (See Overdosage.) Following therapeutic doses, approximately 10 percent is found excreted in the urine as salicylic acid, 75 percent as salicyluric acid, and 10 percent phenolic and 5 percent acyl glucuronides of salicylic acid.

Pharmacodynamics: Aspirin affects platelet aggregation by irreversibly inhibiting prostaglandin cyclo-oxygenase. The effect lasts for the life of the platelet and prevents the formation of the platelet aggregating factor thromboxane A2. Nonacetylated salicylates do not inhibit this enzyme and have no effect on platelet aggregation. At somewhat higher doses, aspirin reversibly inhibits the formation of prostaglandin I2 (prostacyclin), which is an arterial vasodilator and inhibits platelet aggregation.

At higher doses, aspirin is an effective anti-inflammatory agent, partially due to inhibition of inflammatory mediators via cyclo-oxygenase inhibition in peripheral tissues. In vitro studies suggest that other mediators of inflammation may also be suppressed by aspirin administration, although the precise mechanism of action has not been elucidated. It is this nonspecific suppression of cyclo-oxygenase activity in peripheral tissues following large doses that leads to its primary side effect of gastric irritation. (See Adverse Reactions.)

Clinical Studies: Ischemic Stroke and Transient Ischemic Attack (TIA): In clinical trials of subjects with TIA's due to fibrin platelet emboli or ischemic stroke,

aspirin has been shown to significantly reduce the risk of the combined endpoint of stroke or death and the combined endpoint of TIA, stroke, or death by about 13–18 percent.

Suspected Acute Myocardial Infarction (MI): In a large, multi-center study of aspirin, streptokinase, and the combination of aspirin and streptokinase in 17,187 patients with suspected acute MI, aspirin treatment produced a 23-percent reduction in the risk of vascular mortality. Aspirin was also shown to have an additional benefit in patients given a thrombolytic agent.

Prevention of Recurrent MI and Unstable Angina Pectoris: These indications are supported by the results of six large, randomized, multi-center, placebo-controlled trials of predominantly male post-MI subjects and one randomized placebo-controlled study of men with unstable angina pectoris. Aspirin therapy in MI subjects was associated with a significant reduction (about 20 percent) in the risk of the combined endpoint of subsequent death and/or nonfatal reinfarction in these patients. In aspirin-treated unstable angina patients, the event rate was reduced to 5 percent from the 10 percent rate in the placebo group.

Chronic Stable Angina Pectoris: In a randomized, multi-center, double-blind trial designed to assess the role of aspirin for prevention of MI in patients with chronic stable angina pectoris, aspirin significantly reduced the primary combined endpoint of nonfatal MI, fatal MI, and sudden death by 34 percent. The secondary endpoint for vascular events (first occurrence of MI, stroke, or vascular death) was also significantly reduced (32 percent).

Revascularization Procedures: Most patients who undergo coronary artery revascularization procedures have already had symptomatic coronary artery disease for which aspirin is indicated. Similarly, patients with lesions of the carotid bifurcation sufficient to require carotid endarterectomy are likely to have had a precedent event. Aspirin is recommended for patients who undergo revascularization procedures if there is a preexisting condition for which aspirin is already indicated.

Rheumatologic Diseases: In clinical studies in patients with rheumatoid arthritis, juvenile rheumatoid arthritis, ankylosing spondylitis and osteoarthritis, aspirin has been shown to be effective in controlling various indices of clinical disease activity.

Animal Toxicology: The acute oral 50 percent lethal dose in rats is about 1.5 g/kilogram (kg) and in mice 1.1 g/kg. Renal papillary necrosis and decreased urinary concentrating ability occur in rodents chronically administered high doses. Dose-dependent gastric mucosal injury occurs in rats and humans. Mammals may develop aspirin toxicosis asso-

Continued on next page

St. Joseph Aspirin—Cont.

ciated with GI symptoms, circulatory effects, and central nervous system depression. (See Overdosage.)

Indications and Usage: Vascular Indications (Ischemic Stroke, TIA, Acute MI, Prevention of Recurrent MI, Unstable Angina Pectoris, and Chronic Stable Angina Pectoris): Aspirin is indicated to: (1) Reduce the combined risk of death and nonfatal stroke in patients who have had ischemic stroke or transient ischemia of the brain due to fibrin platelet emboli, (2) reduce the risk of vascular mortality in patients with a suspected acute MI, (3) reduce the combined risk of death and nonfatal MI in patients with a previous MI or unstable angina pectoris, and (4) reduce the combined risk of MI and sudden death in patients with chronic stable angina pectoris.
Revascularization Procedures (Coronary Artery Bypass Graft (CABG), Percutaneous Transminase Coronary Angioplasty (PTCA), and Carotid Endarterectomy): Aspirin is indicated in patients who have undergone revascularization procedures (i.e., CABG, PTCA, or carotid endarterectomy) when there is a preexisting condition for which aspirin is already indicated.
Rheumatologic Disease Indications (Rheumatoid Arthritis, Juvenile Rheumatoid Arthritis, Spondyloarthropathies, Osteoarthritis, and the Arthritis and Pleurisy of Systemic Lupus Erythematosus (SLE)): Aspirin is indicated for the relief of the signs and symptoms of rheumatoid arthritis, juvenile rheumatoid arthritis, osteoarthritis, spondyloarthropathies, and arthritis and pleurisy associated with SLE.

Contraindications: Allergy: Aspirin is contraindicated in patients with known allergy to nonsteroidal anti-inflammatory drug products and in patients with the syndrome of asthma, rhinitis, and nasal polyps. Aspirin may cause severe urticaria, angioedema, or bronchospasm (asthma).
Reye's Syndrome: Aspirin should not be used in children or teenagers for viral infections, with or without fever, because of the risk of Reye's syndrome with concomitant use of aspirin in certain viral illnesses.

Warnings: Alcohol Warning: Patients who consume three or more alcoholic drinks every day should be counseled about the bleeding risks involved with chronic, heavy alcohol use while taking aspirin.
Coagulation Abnormalities: Even low doses of aspirin can inhibit platelet function leading to an increase in bleeding time. This can adversely affect patients with inherited (hemophilia) or acquired (liver disease or vitamin K deficiency) bleeding disorders.
GI Side Effects: GI side effects include stomach pain, heartburn, nausea, vomiting, and gross GI bleeding. Although mi-

nor upper GI symptoms, such as dyspepsia, are common and can occur anytime during therapy, physicians should remain alert for signs of ulceration and bleeding, even in the absence of previous GI symptoms. Physicians should inform patients about the signs and symptoms of GI side effects and what steps to take if they occur.
Peptic Ulcer Disease: Patients with a history of active peptic ulcer disease should avoid using aspirin, which can cause gastric mucosal irritation and bleeding.

Precautions:

General: Renal Failure: Avoid aspirin in patients with severe renal failure (glomerular filtration rate less than 10 mL/minute)
Hepatic Insufficiency: Avoid aspirin in patients with severe hepatic insufficiency.
Sodium Restricted Diets: Patients with sodium-retaining states, such as congestive heart failure or renal failure, should avoid sodium-containing buffered aspirin preparations because of their high sodium content.
Laboratory Tests: Aspirin has been associated with elevated hepatic enzymes, blood urea nitrogen and serum creatinine, hyperkalemia, proteinuria, and prolonged bleeding time.
Drug Interactions: Angiotensin Converting Enzyme (ACE) Inhibitors: The hyponatremic and hypotensive effects of ACE inhibitors may be diminished by the concomitant administration of aspirin due to its indirect effect on the renin-angiotensin conversion pathway.
Acetazolamide: Concurrent use of aspirin and acetazolamide can lead to high serum concentrations of acetazolamide (and toxicity) due to competition at the renal tubule for secretion.
Anticoagulant Therapy (Heparin and Warfarin): Patients on anticoagulation therapy are at increased risk for bleeding because of drug-drug interactions and the effect on platelets. Aspirin can displace warfarin from protein binding sites, leading to prolongation of both the prothrombin time and the bleeding time. Aspirin can increase the anticoagulant activity of heparin, increasing bleeding risk.
Anticonvulsants: Salicylate can displace protein-bound phenytoin and valproic acid, leading to a decrease in the total concentration of phenytoin and an increase in serum valproic acid levels.
Beta Blockers: The hypotensive effects of beta blockers may be diminished by the concomitant administration of aspirin due to inhibition of renal prostaglandins, leading to decreased renal blood flow, and salt and fluid retention.
Diuretics: The effectiveness of diuretics in patients with underlying renal or cardiovascular disease may be diminished by the concomitant administration of aspirin due to inhibition of renal prostaglandins, leading to decreased renal blood flow and salt and fluid retention.

Methotrexate: Salicylate can inhibit renal clearance of methotrexate, leading to bone marrow toxicity, especially in the elderly or renal impaired.
Nonsteroidal Anti-Inflammatory Drugs (NSAID's): The concurrent use of aspirin with other NSAID's should be avoided because this may increase bleeding or lead to decreased renal function.
Oral Hypoglycemics: Moderate doses of aspirin may increase the effectiveness of oral hypoglycemic drugs, leading to hypoglycemia.
Uricosuric Agents (Probenecid and Sulfinpyrazone): Salicylates antagonize the uricosuric action of uricosuric agents.
Carcinogenesis, Mutagenesis, Impairment of Fertility: Administration of aspirin for 68 weeks at 0.5 percent in the feed of rats was not carcinogenic. In the Ames Salmonella assay, aspirin was not mutagenic; however, aspirin did induce chromosome aberrations in cultured human fibroblasts. Aspirin inhibits ovulation in rats. (See Pregnancy.)
Pregnancy: Pregnant women should only take aspirin if clearly needed. Because of the known effects of NSAID's on the fetal cardiovascular system (closure of the ductus arteriosus), use during the third trimester of pregnancy should be avoided. Salicylate products have also been associated with alterations in maternal and neonatal hemostasis mechanisms, decreased birth weight, and with perinatal mortality.
Labor and Delivery: Aspirin should be avoided 1 week prior to and during labor and delivery because it can result in excessive blood loss at delivery. Prolonged gestation and prolonged labor due to prostaglandin inhibition have been reported.
Nursing Mothers: Nursing mothers should avoid using aspirin because salicylate is excreted in breast milk. Use of high doses may lead to rashes, platelet abnormalities, and bleeding in nursing infants.
Pediatric Use: Pediatric dosing recommendations for juvenile rheumatoid arthritis are based on well-controlled clinical studies. An initial dose of 90–130 mg/kg/day in divided doses, with an increase as needed for anti-inflammatory efficacy (target plasma salicylate levels of 150–300 µg/mL) are effective. At high doses (i.e., plasma levels of greater than 200 µg/mL), the incidence of toxicity increases.

Adverse Reactions: Many adverse reactions due to aspirin ingestion are dose-related. The following is a list of adverse reactions that have been reported in the literature. (See Warnings.)
Body as a Whole: Fever, hypothermia, thirst.
Cardiovascular: Dysrhythmias, hypotension, tachycardia.
Central Nervous System: Agitation, cerebral edema, coma, confusion, dizziness, headache, subdural or intracranial hemorrhage, lethargy, seizures.

Fluid and Electrolyte: Dehydration, hyperkalemia, metabolic acidosis, respiratory alkalosis.

Gastrointestinal: Dyspepsia, GI bleeding, ulceration and perforation, nausea, vomiting, transient elevations of hepatic enzymes, hepatitis, Reye's Syndrome, pancreatitis.

Hematologic: Prolongation of the prothrombin time, disseminated intravascular coagulation, coagulopathy, thrombocytopenia.

Hypersensitivity: Acute anaphylaxis, angioedema, asthma, bronchospasm, laryngeal edema, urticaria.

Musculoskeletal: Rhabdomyolysis.

Metabolism: Hypoglycemia (in children), hyperglycemia.

Reproductive: Prolonged pregnancy and labor, stillbirths, lower birth weight infants, antepartum and postpartum bleeding.

Special Senses: Hearing loss, tinnitus. Patients with high frequency hearing loss may have difficulty perceiving tinnitus. In these patients, tinnitus cannot be used as a clinical indicator of salicylism.

Urogenital: Interstitial nephritis, papillary necrosis, proteinuria, renal insufficiency and failure.

Drug Abuse and Dependence: Aspirin is nonnarcotic. There is no known potential for addiction associated with the use of aspirin.

Overdosage: Salicylate toxicity may result from acute ingestion (overdose) or chronic intoxication. The early signs of salicylic overdose (salicylism), including tinnitus (ringing in the ears), occur at plasma concentrations approaching 200 µg/mL. Plasma concentrations of aspirin above 300 µg/mL are clearly toxic. Severe toxic effects are associated with levels above 400 µg/mL (See Clinical Pharmacology.) A single lethal dose of aspirin in adults is not known with certainty but death may be expected at 30 g. For real or suspected overdose, a Poison Control Center should be contacted immediately. Careful medical management is essential.

Signs and Symptoms: In acute overdose, severe acid-base and electrolyte disturbances may occur and are complicated by hyperthermia and dehydration. Respiratory alkalosis occurs early while hyperventilation is present, but is quickly followed by metabolic acidosis.

Treatment: Treatment consists primarily of supporting vital functions, increasing salicylate elimination, and correcting the acid-base disturbance. Gastric emptying and/or lavage is recommended as soon as possible after ingestion, even if the patient has vomited spontaneously. After lavage and/or emesis, administration of activated charcoal, as a slurry, is beneficial, if less than 3 hours have passed since ingestion. Charcoal adsorption should not be employed prior to emesis and lavage. Severity of aspirin intoxication is determined by measuring the blood salicylate level. Acid-base status should be closely followed with serial

blood gas and serum pH measurements. Fluid and electrolyte balance should also be maintained. In severe cases, hyperthermia and hypovolemia are the major immediate threats to life. Children should be sponged with tepid water. Replacement fluids should be administered intravenously and augmented with correction of acidosis. Plasma electrolytes and pH should be monitored to promote alkaline diuresis of salicylate if renal function is normal. Infusion of glucose may be required to control hypoglycemia. Hemodialysis and peritoneal dialysis can be performed to reduce the body drug content. In patients with renal insufficiency or in cases of life-threatening intoxication, dialysis is usually required. Exchange transfusion may be indicated in infants and young children.

Dosage and Administration: Each dose of aspirin should be taken with a full glass of water unless the patient is fluid restricted. Anti-inflammatory and analgesic dosages should be individualized. When aspirin is used in high doses, the development of tinnitus may be used as a clinical sign of elevated plasma salicylate levels except in patients with high frequency hearing loss.

Ischemic Stroke and TIA: 50–325 mg once a day. Continue therapy indefinitely

Suspected Acute MI: The initial dose of 160–162.5 mg is administered as soon as an MI is suspected. The maintenance dose of 160–162.5 mg a day is continued for 30 days post-infarction. After 30 days, consider further therapy based on dosage and administration for prevention of recurrent MI.

Prevention of Recurrent MI: 75–325 mg once a day. Continue therapy indefinitely.

Unstable Angina Pectoris: 75–325 mg once a day. Continue therapy indefinitely.

Chronic Stable Angina Pectoris: 75–325 mg once a day. Continue therapy indefinitely.

CABG: 325 mg daily starting 6 hours post-procedure. Continue therapy for 1 year post-procedure.

PTCA: The initial dose of 325 mg daily should be given 2 hours pre-surgery. Maintenance dose is 160–325 mg daily. Continue therapy indefinitely.

Carotid Endarterectomy: Doses of 80 mg once daily to 650 mg twice daily, started presurgery, are recommended. Continue therapy indefinitely.

Rheumatoid Arthritis: The initial dose is 3 g a day in divided doses. Increase as needed for anti-inflammatory efficacy with target plasma salicylate levels of 150–300 µg/mL. At high doses (i.e., plasma levels of greater than 200 µg/mL), the incidence of toxicity increases.

Juvenile Rheumatoid Arthritis: Initial dose is 90–130 mg/kg/day in divided doses. Increase as needed for anti-inflammatory efficacy with target plasma salicylate levels of 150–300 µg/mL. At high doses (i.e., plasma levels of greater than 200 µg/mL), the incidence of toxicity increases.

Spondyloarthropathies: Up to 4 g per day in divided doses.

Osteoarthritis: Up to 3 g per day in divided doses.

Arthritis and Pleurisy of SLE: The initial dose is 3 g a day in divided doses. Increase as needed for anti-inflammatory efficacy with target plasma salicylate levels of 150–300 µg/mL. At high doses (i.e., plasma levels of greater than 200 µg/mL), the incidence of toxicity increases.

How Supplied: *St. Joseph Adult Low Strength Aspirin Chewable Tablets* are round, concave, orange-flavored, orange-colored tablets that are debossed with the "SJ" logo. Available as follows:
NDC 50580-173-36 Bottle of 36 tablets
NDC Coated Tablets 50580-173-08 Tri-Pack
St Joseph Adult Low Strength Enteric Coated Tablets are round, concave, pink-coated tablets that are printed with the "St J" logo. Available as follows:
NDC 50580-126-36 Bottle of 36 tablets
NDC 50580-126-10 Bottle of 100 tablets
NDC 50580-126-18 Bottle of 180 tablets
NDC 50580-126-03 Bottle of 300 tablets
NDC 50580-126-39 Bottle of 395 tablets
Store in tight container at 25 deg.C (77 deg.F); excursions permitted to 15–30 deg.C (59–86 deg.F).

Shown in Product Identification Guide, page 508

SIMPLY COUGH™ LIQUID

Description: *Simply Cough™ Liquid* is Cherry Berry-flavored and contains no alcohol or aspirin. Each teaspoonful (5 mL) contains dextromethorphan HBr 5 mg.

Actions: *Simply Cough™ Liquid* is a single ingredient product that contains the cough suppressant dextromethorphan hydrobromide to provide fast, effective, temporary relief of your child's cough.

Uses: temporarily relieves cough occurring with a cold

Directions:
• find right dose on chart below. If possible, use weight to dose; otherwise use age.
• only use with enclosed measuring cup
• if needed, repeat dose every 4 hours
• do not use more than 4 times in 24 hours

AccuDose™ Chart

Weight (lb)	Age (yr)	Dose (teaspoon)
under 24	under 2	call a doctor
24–47	2–5	1 tsp
48–95	6–11	2 tsp

Professional Dosage Schedule: 4–11 mos (12–17 lbs): ½ teaspoonful; 12–23

Continued on next page

Simply Cough—Cont.

mos (18–23 lbs): ¾ teaspoonful; 2–3 years (24–35 lbs) 1 teaspoonful; 4–5 yrs (36–47 lbs): 1½ teaspoonsfuls; 6–8 yrs (48–59 lbs): 2 teaspoonsfuls; 9–10 yrs (60–71 lbs): 2½ teaspoonsfuls; 11 yrs (72–95 lbs): 3 teaspoonsfuls.
If needed, repeat dose every 4 hours. Do not use more than 4 times in 24 hours.

Warnings: Do not use in a child who is taking a prescription monoamine oxidase inhibitor (MAOI) (certain drugs for depression, psychiatric or emotional conditions, or Parkinson's disease), or for 2 weeks after stopping the MAOI drug. If you do not know if your child's prescription drug contains an MAOI, ask a doctor or pharmacist before giving this product.
Ask a doctor before use if this child has
• cough that occurs with too much phlegm (mucus)
• chronic cough that lasts or occurs with asthma
Stop use and ask a doctor if
• cough gets worse or lasts for more than 5 days, comes back or occurs with fever, rash or headache that lasts. These could be signs of a serious condition.
Keep out of reach of children. In case of overdose, get medical help or contact a Poison Control Center right away.
Other Information: • **do not use if carton is opened, or if neck wrap or foil inner seal imprinted with "Safety Seal®" is broken or missing**
• store at room temperature
• see top panel for lot and expiration date

Professional Information:
Overdosage Information:
Acute dextromethorphan overdose usually does not result in serious signs and symptoms unless massive amounts have been ingested. Signs and symptoms of a substantial overdose may include nausea and vomiting, visual disturbances, CNS disturbances and urinary retention.

Inactive Ingredients: citric acid, corn syrup, FD&C Red #40, flavor, glycerin, purified water, sodium benzoate, sucralose

How Supplied: Cherry Berry flavored liquid in child resistant tamper-evident bottles of 4 fl. oz.
Shown in Product Identification Guide, page 508

SIMPLY SLEEP™
Nighttime Sleep Aid

Description: SIMPLY SLEEP™ is a non habit-forming nighttime sleep aid. Each SIMPLY SLEEP™ Caplet contains diphenhydramine HCl 25 mg.

Actions: SIMPLY SLEEP™ contains an antihistamine (diphenhydramine HCl) which has sedative properties.

Use: relief of occasional sleeplessness
Directions:

adults and children 12 years and over	take 2 caplets at bedtime if needed or as directed by a doctor
children under 12 years	do not use

Warnings:
Do not use
• with any other product containing diphenhydramine, even one used on skin
• in children under 12 years of age
Ask a doctor before use if you have
• a breathing problem such as emphysema or chronic bronchitis
• trouble urinating due to an enlarged prostate gland
• glaucoma
Ask a doctor or pharmacist before use if you are taking sedatives or tranquilizers
When using this product
• drowsiness may occur
• avoid alcoholic drinks
• do not drive a motor vehicle or operate machinery
Stop use and ask a doctor if
• sleeplessness persists continuously for more than 2 weeks. Insomnia may be a symptom of serious underlying medical illness.
If pregnant or breast-feeding, ask a health professional before use.
Keep out of reach of children. In case of overdose, get medical help or contact a Poison Control Center right away.
Other Information:
• **Do not use if carton is opened or neck wrap or foil inner seal imprinted with "Safety Seal®" is broken.**
• Store at room temperature
• see side panel for lot and expiration

Inactive Ingredients: carnauba wax, cellulose, croscarmellose sodium, dibasic calcium phosphate, FD&C Blue #1, hypromellose, magnesium stearate, polyethylene glycol, polysorbate 80, titanium dioxide.

How Supplied: Light blue mini-caplets embossed with "SL" on one side in blister packs of 24 and 48, 100 & 130 count bottles.
Shown in Product Identification Guide, page 508

SIMPLY STUFFY™ LIQUID

Description: *Simply Stuffy™ Liquid* is Cherry Berry-flavored and contains no alcohol or aspirin. Each teaspoonful (5 mL) contains pseudoephedrine HCL 15 mg.

Actions: *Simply Stuffy™ Liquid* is a single ingredient product that contains the decongestant pseudoephedrine hydrochloride to provide fast, effective, temporary relief of your child's nasal congestion.

Uses: temporarily relieves nasal congestion due to:

• the common cold • hay fever • upper respiratory allergies • sinusitis

Directions:
• find right dose on chart below. If possible, use weight to dose; otherwise use age.
• only use with enclosed measuring cup
• if needed, repeat dose every 4 to 6 hours
• do not use more than 4 times in 24 hours

AccuDose™ Chart

Weight (lb)	Age (yr)	Dose (teaspoon)
under 24	under 2	call a doctor
24–47	2–5	1 tsp
48–95	6–11	2 tsp

Professional Dosage Schedule: 4–11 mos (12–17 lbs): ½ teaspoonful; 12–23 mos (18–23 lbs): ¾ teaspoonful; 2–3 yrs (24–35 lbs) 1 teaspoonful; 4–5 yrs (36–47 lbs): 1½ teaspoonsful; 6–8 yrs (48–59 lbs): 2 teaspoonsful; 9–10 yrs (60–71 lbs): 2½ teaspoonsful; 11 yrs (72–95 lbs): 3 teaspoonsful
If needed, repeat dose every 4 hours. Do not use more than 4 times in 24 hours.

Warnings: Do not use in a child who is taking a prescription monoamine oxidase inhibitor (MAOI) (certain drugs for depression, psychiatric or emotional conditions, or Parkinson's disease), or for 2 weeks after stopping the MAOI drug. If you do not know if your child's prescription drug contains an MAOI, ask a doctor or pharmacist before giving this product.
Ask a doctor before use if this child has
• heart disease • high blood pressure • thyroid disease • diabetes
When using this product
• do not exceed recommended dosage
Stop use and ask a doctor if
• nervousness, dizziness, or sleeplessness occur
• symptoms do not get better within 7 days or occur with a fever
Keep out of reach of children. In case of overdose, get medical help or contact a Poison Control Center right away.
Other Information:
• **do not use if carton is opened, of if neck wrap or foil inner seal imprinted with "Safety Seal®" is broken or missing**
• store at room temperature
• see top panel for lot number and expiration date

Professional Information:
Overdosage Information:
Symptoms from pseudoephedrine overdose consist most often of mild anxiety, tachycardia and/or mild hypertension. Symptoms usually appear within 4 to 8 hours of ingestion and are transient, usually requiring no treatment.

Inactive Ingredients: citric acid, corn syrup, FD&C Red #40, flavor, glycerin, purified water, sodium benzoate, sucralose

How Supplied: Cherry Berry flavored liquid in child resistant tamper-evident bottles of 4 fl. oz.

Shown in Product Identification Guide, page 508

Regular Strength TYLENOL® acetaminophen Tablets

Extra Strength TYLENOL® acetaminophen Gelcaps, Geltabs, Caplets, Cool Caplets, Tablets

Extra Strength TYLENOL® acetaminophen Rapid Release Gels

Extra Strength TYLENOL® acetaminophen Adult Liquid Pain Reliever

TYLENOL® Arthritis Pain Acetaminophen Extended Release Geltabs/Caplets

TYLENOL® 8 Hour Acetaminophen Extended Release Geltabs/Caplets

Product information for all dosage forms of Adult TYLENOL actaminophen have been combined under this heading.

Description: *Each Regular Strength TYLENOL® Tablet contains acetaminophen 325 mg. Each Extra Strength TYLENOL® Gelcap, Geltab, Caplet, Cool Caplets, Tablet or Rapid Release Gel contains acetaminophen 500 mg. Extra Strength TYLENOL® Adult Liquid is alcohol-free and each 15 mL (1/2 fl oz or one tablespoonful) contains 500 mg acetaminophen. Each TYLENOL® Arthritis Pain Extended Relief Caplet and each TYLENOL® 8 Hour Extended Release Geltab/caplet contains acetaminophen 650 mg.*

Actions: Acetaminophen is a clinically proven analgesic/antipyretic. Acetaminophen produces analgesia by elevation of the pain threshold and antipyresis through action on the hypothalamic heat-regulating center. Acetaminophen is equal to aspirin in analgesic and antipyretic effectiveness and it is unlikely to produce many of the side effects associated with aspirin and aspirin-containing products. *Tylenol Arthritis Pain Extended Release* and *TYLENOL 8 Hour Extended Release* use a unique, patented, bilayer geltab/caplet. The first layer dissolves quickly to provide prompt relief while the second layer is time released to provide up to 8 hours of relief.

Uses: *Regular Strength TYLENOL® Tablets, Extra Strength TYLENOL® Gelcaps, Geltabs, Caplets, Cool Caplets, Tablets, or Rapid Release Gels:* temporarily relieves minor aches and pains due to:
- headache • muscular aches • backache • arthritis
- the common cold • toothache • menstrual cramps
- temporarily reduces fever

Extra Strength TYLENOL® Adult Liquid: temporarily relieves minor aches and pains due to:
- headache • muscular aches • backache • arthritis
- the common cold • toothache • menstrual cramps
- reduces fever

TYLENOL® Arthritis Pain Extended Release Geltabs/Caplets: temporarily relieves minor aches and pains due to:
- arthritis • the common cold • headache • toothache
- muscular aches • backache • menstrual cramps

TYLENOL® 8 Hour Extended Release Geltabs/Caplets: temporarily relieves minor aches and pains due to:
- muscular aches • backache • headache • toothache • the common cold
- menstrual cramps • minor pain of arthritis
- temporarily reduces fever

Directions:

Regular Strength TYLENOL® Tablets:
- **do not take more than directed (see overdose warning)**

adults and children 12 years and over	• take 2 tablets every 4 to 6 hours as needed • do not take more than 12 tablets in 24 hours
children 6–11 years	• take 1 tablet every 4 to 6 hours as needed • do not take more than 5 in 24 hours
children under 6 years	do not use this adult Regular Strength product in children under 6 years of age; this will provide more than the recommended dose (overdose) of TYLENOL® and may cause liver damage

Extra Strength TYLENOL® Gelcaps, Geltabs, Caplets, Cool Caplets, Tablets; or Rapid Release Gels:
- **do not take more than directed (see overdose warning)**

adults and children 12 years and over	• take 2 gelcaps, geltabs, caplets, cool caplets or tablets every 4 to 6 hours as needed • do not take more than 8 gelcaps, geltabs, caplets, cool caplets or tablets in 24 hours
children under 12 years	do not use this adult Extra Strength product in children under 12 years of age; this will provide more than the recommended dose (overdose) of TYLENOL® and may cause liver damage

Extra Strength TYLENOL® Adult Liquid:
- **do not take more than directed (see overdose warning)**

adults and children 12 years and over	• take 2 tablespoons (tbsp.) in dose cup provided every 4 to 6 hours as needed • do not take more than 8 tablespoons in 24 hours
children under 12 years	do not use this adult Extra Strength product in children under 12 years of age; this will provide more than the recommended dose (overdose) of TYLENOL® and may cause liver damage

TYLENOL® 8 Hour Extended Release Geltabs/Caplets
- **do not take more than directed (see overdose warning)**

adults and children 12 years and over	• take 2 geltabs/ caplets every 8 hours with water • swallow whole – do not crush, chew or dissolve • do not take more than 6 geltabs/ caplets in 24 hours • do not use for more than 10 days unless directed by a doctor
children under 12 years	• do not use

TYLENOL® Arthritis Pain Extended Release Geltabs/Caplets
- **do not take more than directed (see overdose warning)**

adults	• take 2 geltabs or caplets every 8 hours with water • swallow whole – do not crush, chew or dissolve • do not take more than 6 geltabs or caplets in 24 hours • do not use for more than 10 days unless directed by a doctor
under 18 years of age	• ask a doctor

Continued on next page

Tylenol—Cont.

Warnings: *Regular Strength TYLENOL® Tablets, Extra Strength TYLENOL® Gelcaps, Geltabs, Caplets, Cool Caplets, Tablets or Rapid Release Gels, Extra Strength TYLENOL® Liquid*

Alcohol warning: If you consume 3 or more alcoholic drinks every day, ask your doctor whether you should take acetaminophen or other pain relievers/fever reducers. Acetaminophen may cause liver damage.

Do not use:
- with any other product containing acetaminophen.

Stop using and ask a doctor if:
- new symptoms occur
- redness or swelling is present
- pain gets worse or lasts for more than 10 days
- fever gets worse or lasts for more than 3 days

If pregnant or breast-feeding, ask a health professional before use.

Keep out of reach of children.

Overdose warning: Taking more than the recommended dose (overdose) may cause liver damage. In case of overdose, get medical help or contact a Poison Control Center right away. Quick medical attention is critical for adults as well as for children even if you do not notice any signs or symptoms.

TYLENOL® Arthritis Pain Extended Release Geltabs/Caplets:

Alcohol warning: If you consume 3 or more alcoholic drinks every day, ask your doctor whether you should take acetaminophen or other pain relievers/fever reducers. Acetaminophen may cause liver damage.

Do not use
- with any other product containing acetaminophen.

Stop use and ask a doctor if
- new symptoms occur
- redness or swelling is present
- pain gets worse or lasts for more than 10 days

If pregnant or breast-feeding, ask a health professional before use.

Keep out of reach of children.

Overdose warning: Taking more than the recommended dose (overdose) may cause liver damage. In case of overdose, get medical help or contact a Poison Control Center right away. Quick medical attention is critical for adults as well as for children even if you do not notice any signs or symptoms.

TYLENOL® 8 Hour Extended Release Geltab/Caplets:

Alcohol warning: If you consume 3 or more alcoholic drinks every day, ask your doctor whether you should take acetaminophen or other pain relievers/fever reducers. Acetaminophen may cause liver damage.

Do not use
- with any other product containing acetaminophen.

Stop use and ask a doctor if
- new symptoms occur
- redness or swelling is present

- pain gets worse or lasts for more than 10 days
- fever gets worse or lasts for more than 3 days.

If pregnant or breast-feeding, ask a health professional before use.

Keep out of reach of children.

Overdose warning: Taking more than the recommended dose (overdose) may cause liver damage. In case of overdose, get medical help or contact a Poison Control Center right away. Quick medical attention is critical for adults as well as for children even if you do not notice any signs or symptoms.

Other Information:

Regular Strength TYLENOL® Tablets
- **do not use if carton is opened or red neck wrap or foil inner seal imprinted with "Safety Seal®" is broken**
- store between 20–25°C (68–77°F)

Extra Strength TYLENOL® Gelcaps, Geltabs, Caplets, Cool Caplets, Tablets, or Rapid Release Gels:
- **do not use if carton is opened or red neck wrap or foil inner seal imprinted with "Safety Seal®" is broken**
- store between 20–25°C (68–77°F) (*tablet caplet, and Cool Caplets*)
- store between 20–25°C (68–77°F); avoid high humidity (*Gelcap, Geltab, and Rapid Release Gel*)

Extra Strength TYLENOL® Adult Liquid
- **do not use if carton is opened, or if bottle wrap or foil inner seal imprinted "Safety Seal®" is broken or missing.**
- store between 20–25°C (68–77°F)

TYLENOL® Arthritis Pain Extended Release Geltabs/Caplets and TYLENOL® 8 Hour Extended Release Geltabs/Caplets
- **do not use if carton is opened or neck wrap or foil inner seal with "Safety Seal®" is broken**
- store at 20–25°C (68–77°F)
- avoid excessive heat at 40°C (104°F)

Professional Information:

Overdose Information for all Adult Tylenol products

Acetaminophen: Acetaminophen in massive overdosage may cause hepatic toxicity in some patients. In adults and adolescents ($\geq$ 12 years of age), hepatic toxicity may occur following ingestion of greater than 7.5 to 10 grams over a period of 8 hours or less. Fatalities are infrequent (less than 3–4% of untreated cases) and have rarely been reported with overdoses of less than 15 grams. In children (<12 years of age), an acute overdosage of less than 150 mg/kg has not been associated with hepatic toxicity. Early symptoms following a potentially hepatotoxic overdose may include: nausea, vomiting, diaphoresis and general malaise. Clinical and laboratory evidence of hepatic toxicity may not be apparent until 48 to 72 hours postingestion. In adults and adolescents, any individual presenting with an unknown amount of acetaminophen ingested or with a questionable or unreliable history about the time of ingestion should have a plasma acetaminophen level drawn and be treated with N-acetylcysteine. For full

prescribing information, refer to the N-acetylcysteine package insert. Do not await results of assays for plasma acetaminophen levels before initiating treatment with N-acetylcysteine. The following additional procedures are recommended: Promptly initiate gastric decontamination of the stomach. A plasma acetaminophen assay should be obtained as early as possible, but no sooner than four hours following ingestion. If an acetaminophen *extended release* product is involved, it may be appropriate to obtain an additional plasma acetaminophen level 4–6 hours following the initial acetaminophen level. If either acetaminophen level plots above the treatment line on the acetaminophen overdose nomogram, N-acetylcysteine treatment should be continued for a full course of therapy. Liver function studies should be obtained initially and repeated at 24-hour intervals. Serious toxicity or fatalities have been extremely infrequent following an acute acetaminophen overdose in young children, possibly because of differences in the way they metabolize acetaminophen. In children, the maximum potential amount ingested can be more easily estimated. If more than 150 mg/kg or an unknown amount was ingested, obtain a plasma acetaminophen level as soon as possible, but no sooner than 4 hours following ingestion. If an acetaminophen *extended release* product is involved, it may be appropriate to obtain an additional plasma acetaminophen level 4–6 hours following the initial acetaminophen level. If either acetaminophen level plots above the treatment line on the acetaminophen overdose nomogram, N-acetylcysteine treatment should be initiated and continued for a full course of therapy. If an assay cannot be obtained and the estimated acetaminophen ingestion exceeds 150 mg/kg, dosing with N-acetylcysteine should be initiated and continued for a full course of therapy. For additional emergency information, call your regional poison center or call the Rocky Mountain Poison Center toll-free, (1-800-525-6115).

Our adult Tylenol® combination products contain active ingredients in addition to acetaminophen. The following is basic overdose information regarding those ingredients.

Chlorpheniramine: Chlorpheniramine toxicity should be treated as you would an antihistamine/anticholinergic overdose and is likely to be present within a few hours after acute ingestion.

Dextromethorhphan: Acute dextromethorphan overdose usually does not result in serious signs and symptoms unless massive amounts have been ingested. Signs and symptoms of a substantial overdose may include nausea and vomiting, visual disturbances, CNS disturbances and urinary retention.

Diphenhydramine: Diphenhydramine toxicity should be treated as you would an antihistamine/anticholinergic overdose and is likely to be present within a few hours after acute ingestion.

Doxylamine: Doxylamine toxicity should be treated as you would an antihistamine/anticholinergic overdose and is likely to be present within a few hours after acute ingestion.

Guaifenesin: Guaifenesin should be treated as a nontoxic ingestion.

Pamabrom: Acute overexposure of diuretics is primarily associated with fluid and electrolyte loss. Fluid loss should be treated with the appropriate intravenous and/or oral fluids.

Pseudoephedrine: Symptoms from pseudoephedrine overdose consist most often of mild anxiety, tachycardia and/or mild hypertension. Symptoms usually appear within 4 to 8 hours of ingestion and are transient, usually requiring no treatment.

For additional emergency information, please contact your local poison control center.

Alcohol Information: Chronic heavy alcohol abusers may be at increased risk of liver toxicity from excessive acetaminophen use, although reports of this event are rare. Reports usually involve cases of severe chronic alcoholics and the dosages of acetaminophen most often exceed recommended doses and often involve substantial overdose. Healthcare professionals should alert their patients who regularly consume large amounts of alcohol not to exceed recommended doses of acetaminophen.

Inactive Ingredients:

Regular Strength TYLENOL® Tablets: cellulose, corn starch, magnesium stearate, sodium starch glycolate.

Extra Strength TYLENOL® Tablets: cellulose, corn starch, magnesium stearate, sodium starch glycolate. **Caplets:** cellulose, corn starch, FD&C Red #40, hypromellose, magnesium stearate, polyethylene glycol, sodium starch glycolate, titanium dioxide. **Cool Caplets (LP):** cellulose, corn starch, FD&C Red #40, hypromellose, magnesium stearate, polyethylene glycol, sodium starch glycolate, titanium dioxide or **Cool Caplets (BASF):** carnauba wax, castor oil, cellulose, corn starch, FD&C red #40, hypromellose, magnesium stearate, sodium starch glycolate, titanium dioxide. **Gelcaps:** benzyl alcohol, butylparaben, castor oil, cellulose, corn starch, D&C Yellow #10, edetate calcium disodium, FD&C Blue #1, FD&C Blue #2, FD&C Red #40, gelatin, hypromellose, magnesium stearate, methylparaben, propylparaben, sodium lauryl sulfate, sodium propionate, sodium starch glycolate, titanium dioxide. **Geltabs:** benzyl alcohol, butylparaben, castor oil, cellulose, corn starch, D&C Yellow #10, edetate calcium disodium, FD&C Blue #1, FD&C Blue #2, FD&C Red #40, gelatin, hypromellose, magnesium stearate, methylparaben, propylparaben, sodium lauryl sulfate, sodium

starch glycolate, titanium dioxide. **Rapid Release Gels:** benzyl alcohol, black iron oxide, butylparaben, cellulose, corn starch, D&C yellow #10, edetate calcium disodium, FD&C blue #2, FD&C red #40 gelatin, hypromellose, magnesium stearate, methylparaben, polyethylene glycol, polysorbate 80, propylparaben, red iron oxide, sodium lauryl sulfate, sodium propionate, sodium starch glycolate, titanium dioxide, yellow iron oxide.

Extra Strength TYLENOL® Adult Liquid: citric acid, corn syrup, D&C Red #33, FD&C Red #40, flavor, polyethylene glycol, purified water, saccharin sodium, sodium benzoate, sorbitol

TYLENOL® Arthritis Pain Extended Release **Caplets:** corn starch, hydroxyethyl cellulose, hypromellose, magnesium stearate, microcrystalline cellulose, povidone, powdered cellulose, pregelatinized starch, sodium starch glycolate, titanium dioxide, triacetin. **Geltabs:** benzyl alcohol, butylparaben, castor oil, cellulose, corn starch, edetate calcium disodium, FD&C Blue #1, FD&C Blue #2, gelatin, hydroxyethyl cellulose, hypromellose, magnesium stearate, methylparaben, povidone, propylparaben, sodium lauryl sulfate, sodium propionate, sodium starch glycolate, titanium dioxide.

Tylenol 8 Hour Extended Release **Caplets:** corn starch, D&C Yellow #10, FD&C Red #40, FD&C Yellow #6, hydroxyethyl cellulose, magnesium stearate, microcrystalline cellulose, polyethylene glycol, polyvinyl alcohol, povidone, powdered cellulose, pregelantinized starch, sodium starch glycolate, sucralose, talc, titanium dioxide. Tylenol 8 Hour Extended Release **Caplets (White):** corn starch, hydroxyethyl cellulose, hypromellose, magnesium stearate, microcrystalline cellulose, povidone, powdered cellulose, pregelantinized starch, sodium starch glycolate, titanium dioxide, triacetin. **Geltabs:** benzyl alcohol, butylparaben, castor oil, cellulose, corn starch, edetate calcium disodium, FD & C Blue #1, FD & C Blue #2, FD & C Red #40, gelatin, hydroxyethyl cellulose, hypromellose, magnesium stearate, methylparaben, povidone, propylparaben, sodium lauryl sulfate, sodium propionate, sodium starch glycolate, titanium dioxide

How Supplied:

Regular Strength TYLENOL® Tablets: (colored white, scored, imprinted "TYLENOL" and "325")—tamper-evident bottles of 100.

Extra Strength TYLENOL® Tablets: (colored white, imprinted "TYLENOL" and "500")—tamper-evident bottles of 30, 60, 100, and 200. *Caplets* (colored white, imprinted "TYLENOL 500 mg")— vials of 10, and tamper-evident bottles of 8, 16, 40, 325, 24, 50, 100, 150, and 250. *Cool Caplets* 8, 24, 50, 100, 150, 250. *Gelcaps* (colored yellow and red, imprinted "Tylenol 500") tamper-evident bottles of 40, 24, 50, 100, 150 and 225. *Geltabs* (col-

ored yellow and red, imprinted "Tylenol 500") tamper-evident bottles of 24, 50, 40, 100, and 150. Rapid Release Gels (colored red and light blue with an exposed grey band; gelcaps are imprinted with "TY 500") tamper-evident bottles of 8, 24, 50, 100, 150, and 290.

Extra Strength TYLENOL® Adult Liquid: Cherry-flavored liquid (colored red) 8 fl. oz. tamper-evident bottle with child resistant safety cap and special dosage cup.

TYLENOL® Arthritis Pain Extended Release Caplets: (colored white, engraved "TYLENOL ER") tamper-evident bottles of 24, 50, and 100, 150, 250 and 290

TYLENOL® 8 Hour Extended Release Geltabs/caplet: (colored white and red, imprinted "8 HOUR") tamper-evident bottles of 20, 40 and 80. Caplets: (colored red, imprinted "8 hour") available in 24's, 50's, 100's, 150's and 200's.

Shown in Product Identification Guide, page 510

TYLENOL® Severe Allergy Caplets

TYLENOL® Allergy Complete Night Time Caplets

TYLENOL® Allergy Complete Multi-Symptom Caplets with Cool Burst™, Gelcaps and Geltabs

Product information for all dosage forms of TYLENOL Allergy have been combined under this heading.

Description: Each *TYLENOL® Severe Allergy Caplet* contains acetaminophen 500 mg and diphenhydramine HCl 12.5 mg. Each *TYLENOL® Allergy Complete Night Time Caplet* contains acetaminophen 500 mg, diphenhydramine HCl 25 mg, and pseudoephedrine HCl 30 mg. Each *TYLENOL® Allergy Complete Multi-Symptom Caplet with Cool Burst™ Gelcap and Geltab* contains acetaminophen 500 mg, chlorpheniramine maleate 2 mg, and pseudoephedrine HCl 30 mg.

Actions: *TYLENOL® Severe Allergy Caplets* contain a clinically proven analgesic-antipyretic and antihistamine. Acetaminophen produces analgesia by elevation of the pain threshold and antipyresis through action on the hypothalamic heat regulating center. Acetaminophen is equal to aspirin in analgesic and antipyretic effectiveness, and it is unlikely to produce many of the side effects associated with aspirin and aspirin-containing products.

Diphenhydramine HCl is an antihistamine which helps provide temporary relief of itchy, watery eyes, runny nose, sneezing, itching of the nose or throat due to hay fever or other respiratory allergies.

Continued on next page

Tylenol Severe Allergy—Cont.

TYLENOL® Allergy Complete Night Time Caplets contain, in addition to the above ingredients, a decongestant, pseudoephedrine HCl. Pseudoephedrine is a sympathomimetic amine which provides temporary relief of nasal and sinus congestion.

TYLENOL® Allergy Complete Multi-Symptom Caplets with Cool Burst™, Gelcaps and Geltabs contain acetaminophen, pseudoephedrine HCl and the antihistamine, chlorpheniramine maleate. Chlorpheniramine is an antihistamine which helps provide temporary relief of runny nose, sneezing and watery and itchy eyes.

Uses: *TYLENOL® Severe Allergy:* temporarily relieves these symptoms due to hay fever or other upper respiratory allergies:

• itchy, watery eyes • runny nose
• sneezing • sore throat
• itching of nose or throat

TYLENOL® Allergy Complete Night Time and TYLENOL® Allergy Complete Multi-Symptom: temporarily relieves these symptoms due to hay fever or other upper respiratory allergies:

• nasal congestion • sinus pressure
• sinus pain • headache
• runny nose • sneezing
• itchy, watery eyes • itchy throat

Directions: *TYLENOL® Severe Allergy:*
• **do not take more than directed (see overdose warning)**

adults and children 12 years and over	• take 2 caplets every 4 to 6 hours as needed • do not take more than 8 caplets in 24 hours
children under 12 years	• do not use this adult product in children under 12 years of age; this will provide more than the recommended dose (overdose) and may cause liver damage.

TYLENOL® Allergy Complete Night Time:
• **do not take more than directed (see overdose warning)**

adults and children 12 years and over	• take 2 caplets every 4 to 6 hours as needed • do not take more than 8 caplets in 24 hours
children under 12 years	• do not use this adult product in children under 12 years of age; this will provide more than the recommended dose (overdose) and may cause liver damage.

TYLENOL® Allergy Complete Multi-Symptom geltab with Cool Burst™:
• **do not take more than directed (see overdose warning)**

adults and children 12 years and over	• take two caplets, gelcaps, or geltabs every 4 to 6 hours as needed • swallow whole - do not crush, chew or dissolve • do not take more than 8 caplets, gelcaps, or geltabs in 24 hours
children under 12 years	• do not use this adult product in children under 12 years of age; this will provide more than the recommended dose (overdose) and may cause liver damage.

Warnings:

Alcohol warning: If you consume 3 or more alcoholic drinks every day, ask your doctor whether your should take acetaminophen or other pain relievers/fever reducers. Acetaminophen may cause liver damage.

Sore throat warning: If sore throat is severe, persists for more than 2 days, is accompanied or followed by fever, headache, rash, nausea or vomiting, consult a doctor promptly. *(applies to TYLENOL® Severe Allergy only)*

Do not use
• if you are now taking a prescription monoamine oxidase inhibitor (MAOI) (certain drugs for depression, psychiatric or emotional conditions, or Parkinson's disease) or for 2 weeks after stopping the MAOI drug. If you do not know if your prescription drug contains an MAOI, ask a doctor or pharmacist before taking this product (does not apply to *TYLENOL® Severe Allergy*)
• with any other product containing acetaminophen
• with any other product containing diphenhydramine, even one used on skin. (does not apply to TYLENOL® Allergy Complete Multi-Symptom)

Ask a doctor or pharmacist before use if you are taking sedatives or tranquilizers

Stop use and ask a doctor if
• new symptoms occur
• redness or swelling is present
• pain gets worse or lasts for more than 7 days
• fever gets worse or lasts for more than 3 days
• you get nervous, dizzy or sleepless (does not apply to TYLENOL® Severe Allergy)

If pregnant or breast feeding, ask a health professional before use.

Keep out of reach of children.

Overdose warning: Taking more than the recommended dose (overdose) may cause liver damage. In case of overdose, get medical help or contact a Poison Control Center right away. Quick medical attention is critical for adults as well as for children even if you do not notice any signs or symptoms.

When using this product
• **do not exceed recommended dosage**
• marked drowsiness may occur (does not apply to TYLENOL® Allergy Complete Multi-Symptom)
• drowsiness may occur (applies to TYLENOL® Allergy Complete Multi-Symptom only)
• avoid alcoholic drinks
• alcohol, sedatives and tranquilizers may increase drowsiness
• be careful when driving a motor vehicle or operating machinery
• excitability may occur, especially in children

TYLENOL® Severe Allergy

Ask a doctor before use if you have
• glaucoma
• trouble urinating due to an enlarged prostate gland
• a breathing problem such as emphysema or chronic bronchitis

TYLENOL® Allergy Complete Night Time and TYLENOL® Allergy Complete Multi-Symptom

Ask a doctor before use if you have
• heart disease • glaucoma • diabetes
• thyroid disease • high blood pressure
• trouble urinating due to an enlarged prostate gland
• a breathing problem such as emphysema or chronic bronchitis

Other Information:
• **do not use if carton is opened or if blister unit is broken**

Tylenol Severe Allergy Caplets:
• store between 20–25°C (68–77°F)

TYLENOL® Allergy Complete Multi-Symptom Caplet with Cool Burst™ and TYLENOL® Allergy Complete Night Time Caplet:
• store between 20–25°C (68–77°F)

TYLENOL® Allergy Complete Multi-Symptom Gelcap & Geltabs
• store between 20–25°C (68–77°F). Avoid high humidity
• see side panel for lot number and expiration date (for all products)

Professional Information:
Overdosage Information:
For overdosage information, please refer to pgs. 656–657.

Inactive Ingredients:
TYLENOL® Severe Allergy: **Caplets:** carnauba wax, cellulose, corn starch, D&C Yellow #10, FD&C Yellow #6, hydroxypropyl cellulose, hypromellose, iron

oxide, magnesium stearate, polyethylene glycol, sodium citrate, sodium starch glycolate, titanium dioxide.

TYLENOL® Allergy Complete Night Time: **Caplets:** carnauba wax, cellulose, corn starch, D&C Yellow #10, FD&C Blue #1, hypromellose, iron oxide, magnesium stearate, polyethylene glycol, polysorbate 80, sodium citrate, sodium starch glycolate, titanium dioxide.

TYLENOL® Allergy Complete Multi-Symptom: **Caplets:** carnauba wax, cellulose, corn starch, flavor, hypromellose, magnesium stearate, mannitol, sodium starch glycolate, sucralose. **Gelcaps and Geltabs:** benzyl alcohol, butylparaben, castor oil, cellulose, corn starch, D&C Yellow #10, edetate calcium disodium, FD&C Blue #1, FD&C Blue #2, gelatin, hypromellose, magnesium stearate, methylparaben, propylparaben, sodium lauryl sulfate, sodium propionate, sodium starch glycolate, titanium dioxide.

How Supplied:
TYLENOL® Severe Allergy: **Caplets:** Yellow film-coated, imprinted with "TYLENOL SEVERE ALLERGY" on one side—blister packs of 24.
TYLENOL® Allergy Complete Night Time: **Caplets:** blue film-coated, imprinted with "TYLENOL A/C Night Time" on one side—blister packs of 24.
TYLENOL® Allergy Complete Multi-Symptom: **Caplets with Cool Burst™:** white film-coated, imprinted with "TYLENOL Allergy Complete" on one side—blister packs of 24.
Gelcaps and Geltabs: Green and yellow-colored, imprinted with "TYLENOL A/S"—blister packs of 24 and 48.
These products are also available in a convenience pack containing Tylenol Allergy Complete Multi-Symptom (pack of 12) and Tylenol Allergy Complete Night (pack of 12).

Shown in Product Identification Guide, page 510

TYLENOL® Cold Day Non-Drowsy Caplets with Cool Burst™ and Gelcaps
TYLENOL® Cold Night Caplets with Cool Burst™

Product information for all dosage forms of TYLENOL Cold have been combined under this heading.

Description: Each *TYLENOL® Cold Day Non-Drowsy Caplet with Cool Burst™ and Gelcap* contains acetaminophen 325 mg, dextromethorphan HBr 15 mg, and pseudoephedrine HCl 30 mg. Each *TYLENOL® Cold Night Time with Cool Burst™ Caplet* contains acetaminophen 325 mg, chlorpheniramine maleate 2 mg, dextromethorphan HBr 15 mg, and pseudoephedrine HCl 30 mg.

Actions: *TYLENOL® Cold Day Non-Drowsy* contains a clinically proven analgesic-antipyretic, a decongestant and a cough suppressant. Acetaminophen produces analgesia by elevation of the pain threshold and antipyresis through action on the hypothalamic heat regulating center. Acetaminophen is equal to aspirin in analgesic and antipyretic effectiveness and it is unlikely to produce many of the side effects associated with aspirin and aspirin-containing products. Pseudoephedrine is a sympathomimetic amine which provides temporary relief of nasal congestion. Dextromethorphan is a cough suppressant which provides temporary relief of coughs due to minor throat irritations that may occur with the common cold.

TYLENOL® Cold Night Time contain, in addition to the above ingredients, an antihistamine. Chlorpheniramine is an antihistamine which helps provide temporary relief of runny nose, sneezing and watery and itchy eyes.

Uses: *TYLENOL® Cold Day Non-Drowsy:* temporarily relieves these cold symptoms:
• cough • sore throat • minor aches and pains • headaches • nasal congestion • temporarily reduces fever
TYLENOL® Cold Night Time: temporarily relieves these cold symptoms:
• cough • sore throat • minor aches and pains • headache • nasal congestion • runny nose • sneezing • watery and itchy eyes • temporarily reduces fever

Directions:
TYLENOL® Cold Day Non-Drowsy Gelcaps
• **do not take more than directed (see overdose warning)**

adults and children 12 years and over	• take 2 gelcaps every 6 hours as needed • do not take more than 8 gelcaps in 24 hours.
children under 12 years	• not intended for use in children under 12. Ask your doctor.

TYLENOL® Cold Day Non-Drowsy and Night Caplets with Cool Burst™

adults and children 12 years and over	• take 2 caplets every 6 hours as needed • swallow whole – do not crush, chew or dissolve • do not take more than 8 caplets in 24 hours.
children under 12 years	• not intended for use in children under 12. Ask your doctor.

Warnings:
Alcohol Warning: If you consume 3 or more alcoholic drinks every day, ask your doctor whether you should take acetaminophen or other pain relievers/fever reducers. Acetaminophen may cause liver damage.
Sore throat warning: If sore throat is severe, persists for more than 2 days, is accompanied or followed by fever, headache, rash, nausea or vomiting, consult a doctor promptly.
Do not use
• if you are now taking a prescription monoamine oxidase inhibitor (MAOI) (certain drugs for depression, psychiatric or emotional conditions or Parkinson's disease), or for 2 weeks after stopping the MAOI drug. If you do not know if your prescription drug contains an MAOI, ask a doctor or pharmacist before taking this product.
• with any other product containing acetaminophen
Stop use and ask a doctor if
• new symptoms occur
• redness or swelling is present
• pain or nasal congestion gets worse or lasts for more than 7 days
• fever gets worse or lasts for more than 3 days
• you get nervous, dizzy or sleepless
• cough comes back or occurs with rash or headache that lasts. These could be signs of a serious condition.
If pregnant or breast-feeding, ask a health professional before use.
Keep out of reach of children.
Overdose warning: Taking more than the recommended dose (overdose) may cause liver damage. In case of overdose, get medical help or contact a Poison Control Center right away. Quick medical attention is critical for adults as well as for children even if you do not notice any signs or symptoms.
TYLENOL® Cold Day Non-Drowsy
Ask a doctor before use if you have
• heart disease • diabetes • thyroid disease • cough that occurs with too much phlegm (mucus) • high blood pressure • trouble urinating due to an enlarged prostate gland • chronic cough that lasts as occurs with smoking, asthma, chronic bronchitis or emphysema
When using this product
• do not exceed recommended dosage
TYLENOL® Cold Night Time:
Ask a doctor before use if you have
• heart disease • glaucoma • diabetes • thyroid disease • cough that occurs with too much phlegm (mucus) • high blood pressure • a breathing problem or chronic cough that lasts as occurs with smoking, asthma, chronic bronchitis or emphysema • trouble urinating due to an enlarged prostate gland
Ask a doctor or pharmacist before use if you are taking sedatives or tranquilizers
When using this product
• do not exceed recommended dosage
• drowsiness may occur • avoid alcoholic drinks • alcohol, sedatives and tranquilizers may increase drowsiness • be careful when driving a motor vehicle or operating machinery • excitability may occur, especially in children

Continued on next page

Tylenol Cold—Cont.

OTHER INFORMATION:
- **do not use if carton is opened or if blister unit is broken**
- store between 20–25°C (68–77°F)
- store at room temperature;

Avoid high humidity and excessive heat 40°C (104°F)
Applies to TYLENOL® Cold Non-Drowsy Gelcap only

Professional Information:
Overdosage Information
For overdosage information, please refer to pgs. 656–657.

Inactive Ingredients:
TYLENOL® Cold Day Non Drowsy Formula: **Caplets:** carnauba wax, cellulose, corn starch, FD&C Blue #1 flavor, hypromellose, magnesium stearate, mannitol, sodium starch glycolate, sucralose, titanium dioxide.
Gelcaps: benzyl alcohol, butylparaben, castor oil, cellulose, corn starch, D&C Yellow #10, edetate calcium disodium, FD&C Red #40, gelatin, hypromellose, iron oxide, magnesium stearate, methylparaben, propylparaben, sodium lauryl sulfate, sodium propionate, sodium starch glycolate, titanium dioxide.
TYLENOL® Cold Night Time: **Caplets:** carnauba wax, castor oil, cellulose, corn starch, FD&C Blue #1, flavor hypromellose, magnesium stearate, mannitol, sodium starch glycolate, sucralose, titanium dioxide.

How Supplied:
TYLENOL® Cold Day Non Drowsy Caplets: White-colored, imprinted with "TYLENOL Cold"—blister packs of 12 & 24. **Gelcaps:** Red- and tan-colored, imprinted with "TYLENOL COLD"—blister packs of 24.
TYLENOL® Cold Night Time Caplets: Yellow-colored, imprinted with "TYLENOL Cold"—blister packs of 12 & 24.
These products are also available in a convenience pack containing TYLENOL® Cold Day Non-Drowsy (pack of 12) and TYLENOL® Cold Night Time (pack of 12).

Shown in Product Identification Guide, page 511

TYLENOL® COLD
Severe Congestion Non-Drowsy Caplets with Cool Burst™

Description: Each *TYLENOL® Cold Severe Congestion Non-Drowsy Caplet with Cool Burst*™ contains acetaminophen 325 mg, dextromethorphan HBr 15 mg, guaifenesin 200 mg and pseudoephedrine HCl 30 mg.

Actions: *TYLENOL® Cold Severe Congestion Non-Drowsy Caplets with Cool Burst*™ contain a clinically proven analgesic-antipyretic, decongestant, expectorant and cough suppressant. Acetaminophen produces analgesia by eleva-tion of the pain threshold and antipyresis through action on the hypothalamic heat regulating center. Acetaminophen is equal to aspirin in analgesic and antipyretic effectiveness and is unlikely to produce many of the side effects associated with aspirin and aspirin-containing products. Pseudoephedrine is a sympathomimetic amine which provides temporary relief of nasal congestion. Guaifenesin is an expectorant which helps loosen phlegm (mucus) and thin bronchial secretions to make coughs more productive. Dextromethorphan is a cough suppressant which provides temporary relief of coughs due to minor throat irritations that may occur with the common cold.

Uses: temporarily relieves these cold symptoms:
- cough • sore throat • minor aches and pains • headaches
- nasal congestion
- helps loosen phlegm (mucus) and thin bronchial secretions to make coughs more productive
- temporarily reduces fever

Directions:
- **do not take more than directed (see overdose warning)**

adults and children 12 years and over	• take 2 caplets every 6–8 hours as needed swallow whole – do not crush, chew, dissolve. • do not take more than 8 caplets in 24 hours
children under 12 years	• not intended for use in children under 12. Ask your doctor.

Warnings:
Alcohol warning: If you consume 3 or more alcoholic drinks every day, ask your doctor whether you should take acetaminophen or other pain relievers/fever reducers. Acetaminophen may cause liver damage.
Sore throat warning: If sore throat is severe, persists for more than 2 days, is accompanied or followed by fever, headache, rash, nausea or vomiting, consult a doctor promptly.
Do not use
- if you are now taking a prescription monoamine oxidase inhibitor (MAOI) (certain drugs for depression, psychiatric or emotional conditions, or Parkinson's disease), or for 2 weeks after stopping the MAOI drug. If you do not know if your prescription drug contains an MAOI, ask a doctor or pharmacist before taking this product.
- with any other product containing acetaminophen
Ask a doctor before use if you have
- heart disease • diabetes • thyroid disease • cough that occurs with too much phlegm (mucus) • high blood pressure • trouble urinating due to an enlarged prostate gland • chronic cough that lasts as occurs with smoking, asthma, chronic bronchitis or emphysema
When using this product
- **do not exceed recommended dosage**
Stop use and ask a doctor if
- new symptoms occur
- redness or swelling is present
- pain nasal congestion or cough gets worse or lasts for more than 7 days
- fever gets worse or lasts for more than 3 days
- you get nervous, dizzy or sleepless
- cough comes back or occurs with rash or headache that lasts. These could be signs of a serious condition.
If pregnant or breast-feeding, ask a health professional before use.
Keep out of reach of children.

Overdose Warning: Taking more than the recommended dose (overdose) may cause liver damage. In case of overdose, get medical help or contact a Poison Control Center right away. Quick medical attention is critical for adults as well as for children even if you do not notice any signs or symptoms.
Other Information:
- **do not use if carton is opened or if blister unit is broken**
- Store at 20–25°C (68–77°F)

See side panel for lot # and expiration date.

Professional Information:
Overdosage Information: For overdosage information, please refer to pgs. 656–657.

Inactive Ingredients: carnauba wax, cellulose, corn starch, croscamellose sodium, FD&C Blue #1 flavor, hypromellose, mannitol, povidone, silicon dioxide, stearic acid, sucralose, titanium dioxide

How Supplied:
Caplets: White-colored, imprinted with *"TYLENOL COLD SC"* in blue ink—blister packs of 24 & 48 ct.

Shown in Product Identification Guide, page 511

TYLENOL®
Flu Day Non-Drowsy Gelcaps

TYLENOL® Flu NightTime Gelcaps

TYLENOL® Cold & Flu Severe NightTime Liquid with Cool Burst™

TYLENOL® Cold & Flu Severe Daytime Liquid with Cool Burst™

Product information for all dosage forms of TYLENOL Flu have been combined under this heading.

Description: Each *TYLENOL® Flu Day Non-Drowsy Gelcap* contains acetaminophen 500 mg, dextromethorphan HBr 15 mg and pseudoephedrine HCl 30 mg. Each *TYLENOL® Flu NightTime Gelcap* contains acetaminophen 500 mg, diphenhydramine HCl 25 mg and pseudoephedrine HCl 30 mg. *TYLENOL® Cold & Flu Severe NightTime Liquid with Cool Burst™:* Each 30 mL (2 tablespoonsful) contains acetaminophen 1000 mg, dextromethorphan HBr 30 mg, doxylamine succinate 12.5 mg, and pseudoephedrine HCl

60 mg. *TYLENOL Cold & Flu Severe Daytime Liquid with Cool Burst™:* Each 30mL (2 tablespoonful) contains acetaminophen 1000 mg, dextromethorphan HBr 30 mg, pseudoephedrine HCl 60 mg.

Actions: *TYLENOL® Flu Day Non-Drowsy Gelcaps* contain a clinically proven analgesic-antipyretic, a decongestant and a cough suppressant. Acetaminophen produces analgesia by elevation of the pain threshold and antipyresis through action on the hypothalamic heat regulating center. Acetaminophen is equal to aspirin in analgesic and antipyretic effectiveness and it is unlikely to produce many of the side effects associated with aspirin and aspirin-containing products. Pseudoephedrine hydrochloride is a sympathomimetic amine which provides temporary relief of nasal congestion. Dextromethorphan is a cough suppressant which provides temporary relief of coughs due to minor throat irritations that may occur with the common cold.

TYLENOL® Flu NightTime Gelcaps contains the same clinically proven analgesic-antipyretic and decongestant as *TYLENOL Flu Day Non-Drowsy Gelcaps* along with an antihistamine. Diphenhydramine is an antihistamine which helps provide temporary relief of runny nose and sneezing. *TYLENOL Cold & Flu Severe Daytime Liquid with Cool Burst™* contains the same clinically proven analgesic - antipyretic decongestant and cough suppressant as *TYLENOL Flu Day Non-Drowsy Gelcaps. TYLENOL® Cold & Flu Severe NightTime Liquid with Cool Burst™* contains the same clinically proven analgesic-antipyretic, decongestant and cough suppressant as *TYLENOL Flu Day Non-Drowsy Gelcaps* along with an antihistamine. Doxylamine succinate is an antihistamine which helps provide temporary relief of runny nose and sneezing.

Uses: *TYLENOL® Flu Day Non-Drowsy Gelcaps:*
temporarily relieves these cold and flu symptoms:
• minor aches and pains • headaches
• sore throat • nasal congestion
• coughs
• temporarily reduces fever
TYLENOL® Flu NightTime Gelcaps:
temporarily relieves these cold and flu symptoms:
• minor aches and pains • headaches
• sore throat • nasal congestion • runny nose • sneezing
• temporarily reduces fever
TYLENOL® Cold & Flu Severe Daytime and TYLENOL Cold & Flu Severe NightTime Liquid with Cool Burst™:
temporarily relieves these cold and flu symptoms:
• minor aches and pains • coughs
• nasal congestion • sore throat • runny nose • sneezing (NightTime only)
• temporarily reduces fever • headache

Directions:
• **do not take more than directed (see overdose warning)**

TYLENOL® Flu Day Non-Drowsy Gelcaps:

adults and children 12 years and over	• take 2 gelcaps every 6 hours as needed • do not take more than 8 gelcaps in 24 hours
children under 12 years	• do not use this adult product in children under 12 years of age; this will provide more than the recommended dose (overdose) and may cause liver damage.

TYLENOL® Flu NightTime Gelcaps:
• **do not take more than directed (see overdose warnings)**

adults and children 12 years and over	• take 2 gelcaps at bedtime • may repeat every 6 hours • do not take more than 8 gelcaps in 24 hours
children under 12 years	• do not use this adult product in children under 12 years of age; this will provide more than the recommended dose (overdose) and may cause liver damage.

TYLENOL® Cold & Flu Severe Daytime and TYLENOL Cold & Flu Severe NightTime Liquid with Cool Burst:
• **do not take more than directed (see overdose warnings)**

adults and children 12 years and over	• take 2 tablespoons (tbsp) in dose cup provided every 6 hours as needed • do not take more than 8 tablespoons in 24 hours
children under 12 years	• do not use this adult product in children under 12 years of age; this will provide more than the recommended dose (overdose) and may cause serious liver damage.

Warnings:
Alcohol Warning: If you consume 3 or more alcoholic drinks every day, ask your doctor whether you should take acetaminophen or other pain relievers/fever reducers. Acetaminophen may cause liver damage.
Sore throat warning: If sore throat is severe, persists for more than 2 days, is accompanied or followed by fever, headache, rash, nausea or vomiting, consult a doctor promptly.
Do not use
• if you are now taking a prescription monoamine-oxidase inhibitor (MAOI) (certain drugs for depression, psychiatric or emotional conditions, or Parkinson's disease), or for 2 weeks after stopping the MAOI drug. If you do not know if your prescription drug contains an MAOI, ask a doctor or pharmacist before taking this product.
• with any other product containing acetaminophen
• with any other product containing diphenhydramine, even one used on skin (applies to *TYLENOL Flu NightTime Gelcaps*)
If pregnant or breast-feeding, ask a health professional before use.
Keep out of reach of children.

Overdose Warning: Taking more than the recommended dose (overdose) may cause liver damage. In case of overdose, get medical help or contact a Poison Control Center right away. Quick medical attention is critical for adults as well as for children even if you do not notice any signs or symptoms.
TYLENOL® Flu Day Non-Drowsy Gelcaps
Ask a doctor before use if you have
• heart disease • diabetes • thyroid disease • cough that occurs with too much phlegm (mucus) • high blood pressure • trouble urinating due to an enlarged prostate gland • chronic cough that lasts as occurs with smoking, asthma, chronic bronchitis or emphysema
When using this product
• **do not exceed recommended dosage**
Stop use and ask a doctor if
• new symptoms occur
• redness or swelling is present
• pain gets worse or lasts for more than 7 days
• fever gets worse or lasts for more than 3 days
• you get nervous, dizzy or sleepless
• cough lasts more than 7 days, comes back or occurs with fever, rash or headache that lasts. These could be signs of a serious condition.
TYLENOL® Flu NightTime Gelcaps
Ask a doctor before use if you have
• heart disease • glaucoma • diabetes
• thyroid disease • high blood pressure
• trouble urinating due to an enlarged prostate gland • a breathing problem such as emphysema or chronic bronchitis
Ask a doctor or pharmacist before use if you are taking sedatives or tranquilizers
When using this product
• **do not exceed recommended dosage**
• marked drowsiness may occur

Continued on next page

Tylenol Flu—Cont.

- avoid alcoholic drinks
- alcohol, sedatives and tranquilizers may increase drowsiness
- be careful when driving a motor vehicle or operating machinery
- excitability may occur, especially in children

Stop use and ask a doctor if
- new symptoms occur
- redness or swelling is present
- pain gets worse or lasts for more than 7 days
- fever gets worse or lasts for more than 3 days
- you get nervous, dizzy or sleepless

TYLENOL® Cold & Flu Severe Daytime and TYLENOL Cold & Flu Severe NightTime Liquid with Cool Burst™

Ask a doctor before use if you have
- heart disease • glaucoma • diabetes
- thyroid disease • cough that occurs with too much phlegm (mucus)
- high blood pressure • a breathing problem such as emphysema or chronic bronchitis • trouble urinating due to an enlarged prostate gland

Ask a doctor or pharmacist before use if you are taking sedatives or tranquilizers (applies to *TYLENOL Cold & Flu Severe NightTime* only)

When using this product
- **do not exceed recommended dosage**
- The following apply to *TYLENOL Cold & Flu Severe NightTime* only
  - marked drowsiness may occur
  - avoid alcoholic drinks
  - alcohol, sedatives and tranquilizers may increase drowsiness
  - be careful when driving a motor vehicle or operating machinery
  - excitability may occur, especially in children

Stop use and ask a doctor if
- pain, cough or nasal congestion gets worse or lasts for more than 7 days
- redness or swelling is present
- new symptoms occur
- fever gets worse or lasts for more than 3 days
- you get nervous, dizzy or sleepless (applies to *TYLENOL Cold & Flu Severe NightTime* only)
- cough comes back or occurs with rash or headache that lasts. These could be signs of a serious condition.

Other Information:
TYLENOL® Flu Day Non-Drowsy Gelcaps and TYLENOL® Flu NightTime Gelcaps:
- **do not use if carton is opened or if blister unit is broken**
- Store at room temperature; Avoid high humidity and excessive heat 40°C (104°F)
- **Tylenol Cold & Flu Severe Daytime and NightTime Liquid with Cool Burst™**
- **do not use if dose cup seal, neck band or foil inner seal imprinted "Safety Seal®" is broken or missing**
- Store at room temperature

Professional Information:
Overdosage Information
For overdosage information, please refer to pgs. 656–657.

Inactive Ingredients: *TYLENOL® Flu Day Non-Drowsy Gelcaps:* benzyl alcohol, butylparaben, castor oil, cellulose, corn starch, edetate calcium disodium, FD&C Blue #1, FD&C Red #40, gelatin, hypromellose, iron oxide, magnesium stearate, methylparaben, propylparaben, sodium lauryl sulfate, sodium propionate, sodium starch glycolate, titanium dioxide.
TYLENOL® Flu NightTime Gelcaps: benzyl alcohol, butylparaben, castor oil, cellulose, corn starch, D&C Red #28, edetate calcium disodium, FD&C Blue #1, gelatin, hypromellose, iron oxide, magnesium stearate, methylparaben, propylparaben, sodium citrate, sodium lauryl sulfate, sodium propionate, sodium starch glycolate, titanium dioxide.
Tylenol Cold & Flu Severe Daytime liquid with Cool Burst™: citric acid, FD&C blue #1, flavors, polyethylene glycol, propylene glycol, purified water, sodium benzoate, sodium carboxymethyl cellulose, sorbitol, sucralose, sucrose
Tylenol Cold & Flu Severe NightTime liquid with Cool Burst™: citric acid, FD&C blue #1, flavors, polyethylene glycol, propylene glycol, purified water, sodium benzoate, sodium carboxymethyl cellulose, sorbitol, sucralose, sucrose

How Supplied:
TYLENOL® Flu Day Non-Drowsy Gelcaps: Burgundy- and white-colored gelcap, imprinted with "TYLENOL FLU" in gray ink—blister packs of 12 & 24. Liquid: Blue-colored—bottles of 8 fl oz with child resistant safety cap and tamper evident packaging.
TYLENOL® Flu NightTime: **Gelcaps:** Blue and white-colored gelcap, imprinted with "TYLENOL FLU NT" gray ink—blister packs of 12 and 24.
These products are also available in a convenience pack containing *TYLENOL Flu Day* (pack of 12) and *TYLENOL Flu Night* (pack of 12).
Tylenol Cold & Flu Severe NightTime and Daytime Liquid with Cool Burst™: Blue colored – bottles of 8 fl. oz with child resistant safety cap and tamper evident packaging

---

Extra Strength
TYLENOL® PM
Pain Reliever/Sleep Aid Caplets, Geltabs and Gelcaps

Description: Each *Extra Strength TYLENOL® PM Caplet, Geltab* or *Gelcap* contains acetaminophen 500 mg and diphenhydramine HCl 25 mg.

Actions: *Extra Strength TYLENOL® PM Caplets, Geltabs* and *Gelcaps* contain a clinically proven analgesic-antipyretic and an antihistamine. Maximum allowable non-prescription levels of acetaminophen and diphenhydramine provide temporary relief of occasional headaches and minor aches and pains with accompanying sleeplessness. Acetaminophen is equal to aspirin in analgesic and antipyretic effectiveness and it is unlikely to produce many of the side effects associated with aspirin-containing products. Acetaminophen produces analgesia by elevation of the pain threshold. Diphenhydramine HCl is an antihistamine with sedative properties.

Uses: temporary relief of occasional headaches and minor aches and pains with accompanying sleeplessness.

Directions:
- **do not take more than directed (see overdose warning)**
adults and children 12 years and over: Take 2 caplets, geltabs or gelcaps at bedtime or as directed by a doctor. Children under 12 years: do not use this adult product in children under 12 years of age; this will provide more than the recommended dose (overdose) and may cause liver damage.

Warnings: Alcohol Warning: If you consume 3 or more alcoholic drinks every day, ask your doctor whether you should take acetaminophen or other pain relievers/fever reducers. Acetaminophen may cause liver damage.

Do not use
- with any other product containing acetaminophen
- with any other product containing diphenhydramine, even one used on skin.
- in children under 12 years of age

Ask a doctor before use if you have
- a breathing problem such as emphysema or chronic bronchitis
- trouble urinating due to an enlarged prostate gland
- glaucoma

Ask a doctor or pharmacist before use if you are
- taking sedatives or tranquilizers.

When using this product
- drowsiness will occur
- avoid alcoholic drinks
- do not drive a motor vehicle or operate machinery

Stop use and ask a doctor if
- sleeplessness persists continuously for more than 2 weeks. Insomnia may be a symptom of serious underlying medical illness.
- new symptoms occur
- redness or swelling is present
- pain gets worse or lasts for more than 10 days
- fever gets worse or lasts for more than 3 days

If pregnant or breast-feeding, ask a health professional before use.

Keep out of reach of children.

Overdose warning: Taking more than the recommended dose (overdose) may cause liver damage. In case of overdose, get medical help or contact a Poison Control Center right away. Quick medical attention is critical for adults as well as for children even if you do not notice any signs or symptoms.

Other Information:
- Carton:
- Label: do not use if neck wrap or foil inner seal imprinted with "Safety Seal" is broken or missing
- Pouch: do not use if pouch is opened **do not use if carton is opened or neck wrap or foil inner seal imprinted with "Safety Seal®" is broken**

- Store between 20–25°C (68–77°F). Avoid high humidity. (Applies only to Tylenol® PM Geltabs/Gelcaps)
- see end panel for lot number and expiration date

Professional Information:
Overdosage Information:
For overdosage information, please refer to pgs. 656–657.

Inactive Ingredients:
Caplets: carnauba wax, cellulose, corn starch, FD&C Blue #1, FD&C Blue #2, hypromellose, magnesium stearate, polyethylene glycol, polysorbate 80, sodium citrate, sodium starch glycolate, titanium dioxide.
Geltabs/Gelcaps: benzyl alcohol, butylparaben, castor oil, cellulose, corn starch, D&C Red #28, edetate calcium disodium, FD&C Blue #1, gelatin, hypromellose, iron oxide, magnesium stearate, methylparaben, propylparaben, sodium citrate, sodium lauryl sulfate, sodium propionate, sodium starch glycolate, titanium dioxide,

How Supplied:
Caplets (colored light blue imprinted "Tylenol PM") tamper evident bottles of 24, 50, 100, and 150 and 225.
Gelcaps (colored blue and white imprinted "TYLENOL PM") tamper-evident bottles of 24 and 50.
Geltabs (colored blue and white imprinted "TYLENOL PM") tamper-evident bottles of 24, 50, and 100 and 150.

Shown in Product Identification Guide, page 511

Maximum Strength
TYLENOL® Sinus Day
Non-Drowsy
Geltabs, Gelcaps and Caplets

Maximum Strength
TYLENOL® Sinus
Night Time Caplets

TYLENOL® Sinus Severe
Congestion
Caplets with Cool Burst™

Product information for all dosage forms of TYLENOL Sinus have been combined under this heading.

Description: Each *Maximum Strength TYLENOL® Sinus Day Non-Drowsy Geltab, Gelcap, or Caplet* contains acetaminophen 500 mg and pseudoephedrine HCl 30 mg. Each *Maximum Strength TYLENOL® Sinus Night Time Caplet* contains acetaminophen 500 mg, doxylamine succinate 6.25 mg and pseudoephedrine HCl 30 mg. Each *Tylenol Sinus Severe Congestion Caplet with Cool Burst™* contains acetaminophen 325 mg, guaifenesin 200 mg, and pseudoephedrine HCl 30 mg.

Actions: *Maximum Strength TYLENOL® Sinus Day Non-Drowsy* contains a clinically proven analgesic-antipyretic and a decongestant. Maximum allowable non-prescription levels of acetaminophen and pseudoephedrine provide temporary relief of sinus pain and headache and congestion. Acetaminophen is equal to aspirin in analgesic and antipyretic effectiveness and it is unlikely to produce many of the side effects associated with aspirin and aspirin-containing products. Acetaminophen produces analgesia by elevation of the pain threshold and antipyresis through action on the hypothalamic heat regulating center. Pseudoephedrine hydrochloride is a sympathomimetic amine which promotes sinus cavity drainage by reducing nasopharyngeal mucosal congestion.
Maximum Strength TYLENOL® Sinus Night Time Caplets contain, in addition to the above ingredients, an antihistamine which provides temporary relief of runny nose and itching of the nose or throat.
Tylenol Sinus Severe Congestion contains a clinically proven analgesic-antipyretic, an expectorant, and a decongestant. Maximum allowable non-prescription levels of acetaminophen, guaifenesin, and pseudoephedrine HCl provide temporary relief of sinus pain, headache, and congestion. Acetaminophen is equal to aspirin in analgesic and antipyretic effectiveness and its unlikely to produce many of the side effects associated with aspirin and aspirin-containing products. Acetaminophen produces analgesia by elevation of the pain threshold and antipyresis through action on the hypothalamic heat regulating center. Guaifenesin is an expectorant which helps loosen phlegm (mucus) and thin bronchial secretions to make coughs more productive. Pseudoephedrine hydrochloride is a sympathomimetic amine which promotes sinus cavity drainage by reducing nasopharyngeal mucosal congestion.

Uses:
Maximum Strength TYLENOL® Sinus Day Non-Drowsy: temporarily relieves:
- sinus pain • headache • nasal and sinus congestion
Maximum Strength TYLENOL® Sinus Night Time: temporarily relieves:
- nasal congestion • sinus pressure • sinus pain • headache • runny nose • sneezing • itchy, watery eyes • itching of the nose or throat
Tylenol Sinus Severe Congestion temporarily relieves:
- minor aches and pains
- sinus headache
- temporarily relieves nasal congestion associated with sinusitis
- promotes nasal and/or sinus drainage
- helps loosen phlegm (mucus) and thin bronchial secretions to make coughs more productive

Directions:
Maximum Strength TYLENOL® Sinus Day Non-Drowsy:
- **do not take more than directed (see overdose warning)**

adults and children 12 years and over	• take 2 Geltabs, Gelcaps or Caplets every 4–6 hours as needed • do not take more than 8 Geltabs, Gelcaps or Caplets in 24 hours
children under 12 years	• do not use this adult product in children under 12 years of age; this will provide more than the recommended dose (overdose) and may cause liver damage.

Maximum Strength TYLENOL® Sinus Night Time:
- **do not take more than directed (see overdose warning)**

adults and children 12 years and over	• take 2 caplets every 4–6 hours as needed • do not take more than 8 caplets in 24 hours
children under 12 years	• do not use this adult product in children under 12 years of age; this will provide more than the recommended dose (overdose) and may cause liver damage.

Tylenol Sinus Severe Congestion
- **Do not take more than directed (see overdose warning)**

adults and children 12 years and over	• take 2 caplets every 4–6 hours as needed • swallow whole- do not crush, chew or dissolve • do not take more than 8 caplets in 24 hours
children under 12 years	• not intended for use in children under 12. Ask your doctor.

Warnings: Alcohol warning: If you consume 3 or more alcoholic drinks every day, ask your doctor whether you should take acetaminophen or other pain relievers/fever reducers. Acetaminophen may cause liver damage.

Continued on next page

Tylenol Sinus—Cont.

Do not use
- if you are now taking a prescription monamine oxidase inhibitor (MAOI) (certain drugs for depression, psychiatric or emotional conditions or Parkinson's disease), or for 2 weeks after stopping the MAOI drug. If you do not know if your prescription drug contains an MAOI, ask a doctor or pharmacist before taking this product
- with any other product containing acetaminophen

Maximum Strength TYLENOL® Sinus Day Non-Drowsy Geltabs, Gelcaps and Caplets

Ask a doctor before use if you have
- heart disease • high blood pressure
- thyroid disease • diabetes
- trouble urinating due to an enlarged prostate gland

When using this product
- do not exceed recommend dosage

Maximum Strength TYLENOL® Sinus Night Time Caplets

Ask a doctor before use if you have
- heart disease • glaucoma • diabetes
- thyroid disease • high blood pressure
- trouble urinating due to an enlarged prostate gland • a breathing problem such as emphysema or chronic bronchitis

Ask a doctor or pharmacist before use if
you are taking sedatives or tranquilizers
TYLENOL® Sinus Severe Congestion

Ask doctor before use if you have
- heart disease • diabetes • thyroid disease
- cough that occurs with too much phlegm (mucus)
- high blood pressure
- trouble urinating due to an enlarged prostate gland
- chronic cough that lasts as occurs with smoking, asthma, chronic bronchitis or emphysema

Stop use and ask doctor if
- new symptoms occur
- redness or swelling is present
- pain, nasal congestion, or cough gets worse or lasts for more than 7 days
- you get nervous, dizzy or sleepless
- cough comes back or occurs with rash or headache that lasts. These could be signs of a serious condition.

When using this product
- do not exceed recommended dosage
- marked drowsiness may occur
- avoid alcoholic drinks
- alcohol, sedatives and tranquilizers may increase drowsiness
- be careful when driving a motor vehicle or operating machinery
- excitability may occur, especially in children

Tylenol Sinus Severe Congestion Caplets

Ask a doctor before use if you have
- heart disease • diabetes • thyroid disease • cough that occurs with too much phlegm (mucus) • high blood pressure • trouble urinating due to an enlarged prostate gland • chronic cough that lasts as occurs with smoking, asthma, chronic bronchitis or emphysema

When using this product
- do not exceed recommended dosage

Stop use and ask a doctor if
- new symptoms occur
- redness or swelling is present

- pains gets worse or last for more than 7 days
- fever gets worse or lasts for more than 3 days
- you get nervous, dizzy or sleepless

Tylenol Sinus Severe Congestion

Stop use and ask a doctor if
- new symptoms occur
- redness or swelling is present
- pain, nasal congestion, or cough gets worse or lasts for more than 7 days
- you get nervous, dizzy or sleepless
- cough comes back or occurs with rash or headache that lasts. These could be signs of a serious condition.

If pregnant or breast feeding, ask a health professional before use.
Keep out of reach of children.

Overdose Warning: Taking more than the recommended dose (overdose) may cause liver damage. In case of overdose get medical help or contact a Poison Control Center right away. Quick medical attention is critical for adults as well as for children even if you do not notice any signs or symptoms.

Other Information:
- **do not use if carton is opened or if blister unit is broken**

Maximum Strength TYLENOL® Sinus Geltabs and Gelcaps
- store at room temperature; avoid high humidity and excessive heat 40°C (104°F)

Maximum Strength TYLENOL® Sinus Caplets and Maximum Strength TYLENOL® Sinus Night Time Caplets
- store at room temperature
- do not use if carton is opened or if blister unit is broken

Tylenol Sinus Severe Congestion
- Store at 20–25° C (68–77° F)

Professional Information:
Overdosage Information
For overdosage information, please refer to pgs. 656–657.

Inactive Ingredients:
Maximum Strength TYLENOL® Sinus Day Non-Drowsy Formula: **Caplets:** carnauba wax, cellulose, corn starch, D&C Yellow #10, FD&C Blue #1, FD&C Red #40, hypromellose, iron oxide, magnesium stearate, polyethylene glycol, polysorbate 80, sodium starch glycolate, titanium dioxide.

Gelcaps and Geltabs: benzyl alcohol, butylparaben, castor oil, cellulose, corn starch, D&C Yellow #10, edetate calcium disodium, FD&C Blue #1, gelatin, hypromellose, iron oxide, magnesium stearate, methylparaben, propylparaben, sodium lauryl sulfate, sodium propionate, sodium starch glycolate, titanium dioxide.

Maximum Strength TYLENOL® Sinus Night Time Caplets: black iron oxide, carnauba wax, cellulose, corn starch, FD&C Blue #1, FD&C Blue #2, hypromellose, propylene glycol, silicon dioxide, sodium starch glycolate, stearic acid, titanium dioxide, triacetin, yellow iron oxide.

Tylenol Sinus Severe Congestion: cellulose, corn starch, croscarmellose sodium, D&C Yellow #10, FD&C Blue #1, FD&C Red #40, flavor, iron oxide, mannitol,

polyethylene glycol, polyvinyl alcohol, povidone, silicon dioxide, stearic acid, sucralose, talc, titanium dioxide

How Supplied:
Maximum Strength TYLENOL® Sinus Day Non-Drowsy Formula:
Caplets: Light green-colored, imprinted with "TYLENOL Sinus" in green ink—blister packs of 24 and 48.
Gelcaps: Green- and white-colored, imprinted with "TYLENOL Sinus" in dark green ink—blister packs of 24 and 48.
Geltabs: Green-colored on one side and white-colored on opposite side, imprinted with "TYLENOL Sinus" in gray ink—blister packs of 24 and 48.
Maximum Strength TYLENOL® Sinus Night Time Caplets: Green-colored, imprinted with "Tylenol Sinus NT"—blister packs of 24.
These products are also available in a convenience pack containing Maximum Strength TYLENOL® Sinus Day Non-Drowsy (pack of 12) and Maximum Strength TYLENOL® Sinus Night Time (pack of 12).
Tylenol Sinus Severe Congestion are light green-colored caplets printed with "Tylenol Sinus SC" in black ink and are available in blister packs of 12, 24, and 48.

Shown in Product Identification Guide, page 511

TYLENOL® Cough & Sore Throat Daytime Liquid with Cool Burst™

TYLENOL® Cough & Sore Throat NightTime Liquid with Cool Burst™

Maximum Strength TYLENOL® Sore Throat Adult Liquid

Description: *TYLENOL® Cough & Sore Throat Daytime Liquid with Cool Burst™* contains acetaminophen 1000 mg and dextromethorphan HBr 30 mg in each 30 mL (2 tablespoonsful). *TYLENOL® Cough & Sore Throat NightTime Liquid with Cool Burst™* contains acetaminophen 1000 mg, dextromethorphan HBr 30 mg and doxylamine succinate 12.5 mg in each 30 mL (2 tablespoonsful). *Maximum Strength TYLENOL® Sore Throat Liquid* is available in Honey Lemon Flavor or Wild Cherry Flavor and contains acetaminophen 1000 mg in each 30 mL (2 Tablespoonsful).

Actions: Acetaminophen is a clinically proven analgesic/antipyretic. Acetaminophen produces analgesia by elevation of the pain threshold and antipyresis through action on the hypothalamic heat regulating center. Acetaminophen is equal to aspirin in analgesic and antipyretic effectiveness and it is unlikely to produce many of the side effects associated with aspirin and aspirin-containing products. TYLENOL® Cough & Sore *Throat Daytime Liquid with Cool*

Burst™, in addition to acetaminophen, contains the cough suppressant dextromethorphan hydrobromide.

TYLENOL® Cough & Sore Throat NightTime Liquid with Cool Burst™, in addition to acetaminophen and dextromethorphan hydrobromide, contains the antihistamine doxylamine succinate.

Uses: *Maximum Strength TYLENOL® Sore Throat Liquid* temporarily relieves minor aches and pains due to:
• sore throat • headache • muscular aches • the common cold
• temporarily reduces fever
TYLENOL® Cough & Sore Throat Daytime Liquid temporarily relieves:
• sore throat • headache • minor aches and pains • coughs
TYLENOL® Cough & Sore Throat NightTime Liquid temporarily relieves:
• sore throat • headache • minor aches and pains • coughs • runny nose
• sneezing

Directions:
Maximum Strength TYLENOL® Sore Throat Liquid
• **do not take more than directed (see overdose warning)**

adults and children 12 years and over	• take 2 tablespoons (tbsp) in dose cup provided every 4 to 6 hours as needed • do not take more than 8 tablespoons in 24 hours
children under 12 years	do not use this adult product in children under 12 years of age; this will provide more than the recommended dose (overdose) of TYLENOL® and may cause liver damage.

TYLENOL® Cough & Sore Throat Daytime and NightTime Liquid

adults and children 12 years and over	• take 2 tablespoons (tbsp) in dose cup provided every 6 hours as needed • do not take more than 8 tablespoons in 24 hours
children under 12 years	do not use this adult product in children under 12 years of age; this will provide more than the recommended dose (overdose) of TYLENOL® and may cause liver damage.

Warnings:
Alcohol warning: If you consume 3 or more alcoholic drinks every day, ask your doctor whether you should take acetaminophen or other pain relievers/fever reducers. Acetaminophen may cause liver damage.

Sore throat warning: If sore throat is severe, persists for more than 2 days, is accompanied or followed by fever, headache, rash, nausea or vomiting, consult a doctor promptly.

Do not use
• with any other product containing acetaminophen
• if you are now taking a prescription monoamine oxidase inhibitor (MAOI) (certain drugs for depression, psychiatric or emotional conditions, or Parkinson's disease), or for 2 weeks after stopping the MAOI drug. If you do not know if your prescription drug contains an MAOI, ask a doctor or pharmacist before taking this product. (for *TYLENOL® Cough & Sore Throat Daytime & NightTime Liquid with Cool Burst*™ products)

Ask a doctor before use if you have
(for *TYLENOL® Cough & Sore Throat Daytime*)
• cough that occurs with too much phlegm (mucus)
• chronic cough that lasts or occurs with smoking, asthma, chronic bronchitis, or emphysema
(for *TYLENOL® Cough & Sore Throat NightTime*)
• glaucoma
• cough that occurs with too much phlegm (mucus)
• chronic cough that lasts or occurs with smoking, asthma, chronic bronchitis, or emphysema
• trouble urinating due to an enlarged prostate gland

Ask a doctor or pharmacist before use if you are taking sedatives or tranquilizers (for *TYLENOL® Cough & Sore Throat NightTime Liquid with Cool Burst*™ only)

When using this product
(for *TYLENOL® Cough & Sore Throat Liquid with Cool Burst*™ only)
• marked drowsiness may occur
• avoid alcoholic drinks
• alcohol, sedatives and tranquilizers may increase drowsiness
• be careful when driving a motor vehicle or operating machinery
• excitability may occur, especially in children

Stop use and ask a doctor if
• new symptoms occur
• redness or swelling is present
• pain gets worse or lasts for more than 10 days
• fever gets worse or lasts for more than 3 days
(for *TYLENOL® Cough & Sore Throat Daytime and NightTime Liquid with Cool Burst*™ products)
• pain or cough gets worse or lasts for more than 7 days
• fever gets worse or lasts for more than 3 days
• redness or swelling is present
• new symptoms occur
• cough comes back or occurs with rash or headache that lasts. These could be signs of a serious condition
• you get nervous, dizzy or sleepless (for *TYLENOL® Cough & Sore Throat NightTime Liquid with Cool Burst*™ only)

If pregnant or breast-feeding, ask a health professional before use.
Keep out of the reach of children.
Overdose warning: Taking more than the recommended dose (overdose) may cause liver damage. In case of overdose, get medical help or contact a Poison Control Center right away. Quick medical attention is critical for adults as well as for children even if you do not notice any signs or symptoms.

Other Information:
• **Do not use if carton is opened or if bottle wrap or foil inner seal imprinted "Safety Seal®" is broken or missing**
• store 20–25°C (68–77°F)
• see back label for lot number and expiration date

Professional Information:
Overdosage Information
For overdosage information, please refer to pgs. 656–657.

Inactive Ingredients:
Maximum Strength TYLENOL® Sore Throat Honey-Lemon-Flavored Adult Liquid: caramel color, citric acid, flavor, high fructose corn syrup, polyethylene glycol, propylene glycol, purified water, saccharin sodium, sodium benzoate, sorbitol
Maximum Strength TYLENOL® Sore Throat Wild Cherry-Flavored Adult Liquid: citric acid, D&C Red # 33, FD&C Red # 40, flavor, high fructose corn syrup, polyethylene glycol, propylene glycol, purified water, saccharin sodium, sodium benzoate, sorbitol
TYLENOL® Cough & Sore Throat Daytime Liquid with Cool Burst™: citric acid, FD&C blue # 1, flavors, polyethylene glycol, propylene glycol, purified water, sodium benzoate, sodium carboxymethylcellulose, sorbitol, sucralose, sucrose
TYLENOL® Cough & Sore Throat NightTime Liquid with Cool Burst™: citric acid, FD&C blue # 1, flavors, polyethylene glycol, propylene glycol, purified water, sodium benzoate, sodium carboxymethylcellulose, sorbitol, sucralose, sucrose

How Supplied:
Maximum Strength TYLENOL® Sore Throat Adult Liquid Honey lemon-flavored or wild cherry-flavored liquid in child-resistant tamper-evident bottles of 8 fl. oz.
TYLENOL® Cough & Sore Throat Daytime and NightTime Liquid with Cool Burst™ in child-resistant tamper-evident bottles of 8 fl. oz.
Shown in Product Identification Guide, page 511 & 512

WOMEN'S TYLENOL®
Menstrual Relief Pain Reliever/ Diuretic Caplets

Description: Each *Women's Tylenol® Menstrual Relief Caplet* contains acetaminophen 500 mg and pamabrom 25 mg.

Continued on next page

Tylenol Women's—Cont.

Actions: *Women's TYLENOL® Menstrual Relief Caplets* contain a clinically proven analgesic-antipyretic and a diuretic. Maximum allowable non-prescription levels of acetaminophen and pamabrom provide temporary relief of minor aches and pains due to cramps, headache, and backache and water retention, weight gain, bloating, swelling and full feeling associated with the premenstrual and menstrual periods. Acetaminophen is equal to aspirin in analgesic and antipyretic effectiveness and it is unlikely to produce many of the side effects associated with aspirin containing products. Acetaminophen produces analgesia by elevation of the pain threshold. Pamabrom is a diuretic which relieves water retention.

Uses:
- temporarily relieves minor aches and pains due to:
  - cramps • headache • backache
- temporarily relieves water-weight gain, bloating, swelling and full feeling associated with the premenstrual and menstrual periods

Directions:
- **do not take more than directed (see overdose warning)**

adults and children 12 years and over: take 2 caplets every 4 to 6 hours; do not take more than 8 caplets in 24 hours

children under 12 years: do not use this adult product in children under 12 years of age; this will provide more than the recommended dose (overdose) and may cause liver damage

Warnings: Alcohol warning: If you consume 3 or more alcoholic drinks every day, ask your doctor whether you should take acetaminophen or other pain relievers/fever reducers. Acetaminophen may cause liver damage.

Do not use
- with any other product containing acetaminophen

Stop use and ask a doctor if
- new symptoms occur
- redness or swelling is present
- pain gets worse or lasts for more than 10 days

If pregnant or breast-feeding, ask a health professional before use.

Keep out of reach of children.

Overdose Warning: Taking more than the recommended dose (overdose) may cause liver damage. In case of overdose, get medical help or contact a Poison Control Center right away. Quick medical attention is critical for adults as well as for children even if you do not notice any signs or symptoms.

Other Information:
- **do not use if carton is opened, or if neck wrap or foil inner seal imprinted "Safety Seal®" is broken or missing**
- store at room temperature; avoid excessive heat at 104°F (40°C)
- see end panel for lot number and expiration date

Professional Information: Overdosage Information
For overdosage information, please refer to pgs. 656–657.

Inactive Ingredients:
cellulose, corn starch, hypromellose, magnesium stearate, polydextrose, polyethylene glycol, sodium starch glycolate, titanium dioxide, triacetin.

How Supplied:
White capsule shaped caplets with TYME printed on one side in tamper-evident bottles of 24.

Shown in Product Identification Guide, page 512

Concentrated TYLENOL® acetaminophen Infants' Drops

Children's TYLENOL® acetaminophen Suspension Liquid and Meltaways

Jr. TYLENOL® acetaminophen Meltaways

Product information for all dosages of Children's TYLENOL have been combined under this heading

Description: *Concentrated TYLENOL® Infants' Drops* are stable, alcohol-free, grape-flavored and purple in color or cherry-flavored and red in color. Each 1.6 mL contains 160 mg acetaminophen. *Concentrated TYLENOL® Infants' Drops* features the SAFE-TY-LOCK™ Bottle. The SAFE-TY-LOCK™ Bottle has a unique safety barrier inside the bottle which helps make administration easier. The integrated dropper promotes proper administration. The innovative design eliminates excess product on dropper. The star-shaped barrier inside the bottle minimizes spills and discourages pouring into a spoon. *Children's TYLENOL® Suspension Liquid* is stable, alcohol-free, cherry blast-flavored and red in color, or bubblegum yum-flavored and pink in color, grape splash-flavored and purple in color, or very berry strawberry-flavored and red in color. Each 5 mL (one teaspoonful) contains 160 mg acetaminophen. Each *Children's TYLENOL® Meltaways* contains 80 mg acetaminophen in a grape punch, bubblegum burst or wacky watermelon flavor. *Each Jr. TYLENOL® Meltaways* contains 160 mg acetaminophen in grape punch or bubblegum burst flavor.

Actions: Acetaminophen is a clinically proven analgesic/antipyretic. Acetaminophen produces analgesia by elevation of the pain threshold and antipyresis through action on the hypothalamic heat-regulating center. Acetaminophen is equal to aspirin in analgesic and antipyretic effectiveness and it is unlikely to produce many of the side effects associated with aspirin and aspirin-containing products.

Uses:
Concentrated TYLENOL® Infants' Drops: temporarily:
- reduces fever
- relieves minor aches and pains due to:
  - the common cold • flu • headaches
  - sore throat • immunizations • toothaches

Children's TYLENOL® Suspension Liquid and Children's TYLENOL® Meltaways: temporarily relieves minor aches and pains due to: • the common cold • flu • headaches • sore throat • immunizations • toothache
- temporarily reduces fever

Jr. TYLENOL® Meltaways: temporarily relieves minor aches and pains due to:
- the common cold • flu • headache
- muscle aches • sprains • overexertion
- temporarily reduces fever

Directions: See Table 1: Children's Tylenol Dosing Chart on pgs. 670-672.

Warnings: Sore throat warning: if sore throat is severe, persists for more than 2 days, is accompanied or followed by fever, headache, rash, nausea, or vomiting, consult a doctor promptly (excluding *Jr. TYLENOL® Meltaways*).

Do not use
- with any other product containing acetaminophen

When using this product
- **do not exceed recommended dose (see overdose warning)**

Stop use and ask a doctor if
- new symptoms occur
- redness or swelling is present
- pain gets worse or lasts for more than 5 days
- fever gets worse or lasts for more than 3 days

Keep out of the reach of children.

Overdose Warning: Taking more than the recommended dose (overdose) may cause liver damage. In case of overdose, get medical help or contact a Poison Control Center right away. Quick medical attention is critical even if you do not notice any signs or symptoms.

Other Information:
Concentrated TYLENOL® Infants' Drops:
- **Do not use if plastic carton wrap or bottle wrap imprinted "Safety Seal®" is broken or missing.**
- Store at room temperature
- see bottom panel for expiration date and lot number

Children's TYLENOL® Suspension Liquid:
- **Do not use if bottle wrap, or foil inner seal imprinted "Safety Seal®" is broken or missing**
- Store between 20–25°C (68–77°F)
- see bottom panel for expiration and lot number

Children's TYLENOL® Meltaways:
- **Do not use if carton is opened or if neck wrap or foil inner seal imprinted "Safety Seal®" is broken or missing.** Store between 20–25°C (68–77°F). (Grape Punch: Protect from light). Avoid high humidity.
- see end panel for lot number and expiration date

Jr. TYLENOL® Meltaways:

• **Do not use if carton is opened or if blister unit is broken**

• Store between 20–25°C (68–77°F). (Grape Punch: Protect from light). Avoid high humidity.

• see end panel for lot number and expiration date

Professional Information:
Overdosage Information for all Infants', Children's & Jr. Tylenol® Products

Acetaminophen: Acetaminophen in massive overdosage may cause hepatic toxicity in some patients. In adults and adolescents (≥ 12 years of age), hepatic toxicity may occur following ingestion of greater than 7.5 to 10 grams over a period of 8 hours or less. Fatalities are infrequent (less than 3–4% of untreated cases) and have rarely been reported with overdoses of less than 15 grams. In children (<12 years of age), an acute overdosage of less than 150 mg/kg has not been associated with hepatic toxicity. Early symptoms following a potentially hepatotoxic overdose may include: nausea, vomiting, diaphoresis and general malaise. Clinical and laboratory evidence of hepatic toxicity may not be apparent until 48 to 72 hours postingestion. In adults and adolescents, any individual presenting with an unknown amount of acetaminophen ingested or with a questionable or unreliable history about the time of ingestion should have a plasma acetaminophen level drawn and be treated with *N*-acetylcysteine. For full prescribing information, refer to the *N*-acetylcysteine package insert. Do not await results of assays for plasma acetaminophen levels before initiating treatment with *N*-acetylcysteine. The following additional procedures are recommended: Promptly initiate gastric decontamination of the stomach. A plasma acetaminophen assay should be obtained as early as possible, but no sooner than four hours following ingestion. If an acetaminophen *extended release* product is involved, it may be appropriate to obtain an additional plasma acetaminophen level 4–6 hours following the initial acetaminophen level. If either acetaminophen level plots above the treatment line on the acetaminophen overdose nomogram, *N*-acetylcysteine treatment should be continued for a full course of therapy. Liver function studies should be obtained initially and repeated at 24-hour intervals. Serious toxicity or fatalities have been extremely infrequent following an acute acetaminophen overdose in young children, possibly because of differences in the way they metabolize acetaminophen. In children, the maximum potential amount ingested can be more easily estimated. If more than 150 mg/kg or an unknown amount was ingested, obtain a plasma acetaminophen level as soon as possible, but no sooner than 4 hours following ingestion. If an acetaminophen *extended release* product is involved, it may be appropri-ate to obtain an additional plasma acetaminophen level 4–6 hours following the initial acetaminophen level. If either acetaminophen level plots above the treatment line on the acetaminophen overdose nomogram, *N*-acetylcysteine treatment should be initiated and continued for a full course of therapy. If an assay cannot be obtained and the estimated acetaminophen ingestion exceeds 150 mg/kg, dosing with *N*-acetylcysteine should be initiated and continued for a full course of therapy. For additional emergency information, call your regional poison center or call the Rocky Mountain Poison Center toll-free, (1-800-525-6115).

Our pediatric Tylenol® combination products contain active ingredients in addition to acetaminophen. The following is basic overdose information regarding those ingredients.

Chlorpheniramine: Chlorpheniramine toxicity should be treated as you would an anthihistamine/anticholinergic overdose and is likely to be present within a few hours after acute ingestion.

Dextromethorphan: Acute dextromethorphan overdose usually does not result in serious signs and symptoms unless massive amounts have been ingested. Signs and symptoms of a substantial overdose may include nausea and vomiting, visual disturbances, CNS disturbances and urinary retention.

Diphenhydramine: Diphenhydramine toxicity should be treated as you would an antihistamine/anticholinergic overdose and is likely to be present within a few hours after acute ingestion.

Pseudoephedrine: Symptoms from pseudoephedrine overdose consist most often of mild anxiety, tachycardia and/or mild hypertension. Symptoms usually appear within 4 to 8 hours of ingestion and are transient, usually requiring no treatment.

For additional emergency information, please contact your local poison control center.

Inactive Ingredients:
***Concentrated TYLENOL® Infants' Drops:* Cherry-Flavored:** cellulose, citric acid, corn syrup, FD&C Red #40, flavors, glycerin, purified water, sodium benzoate, sorbitol, xanthan gum. **Grape-Flavored:** cellulose, citric acid, corn syrup, D&C Red #33, FD&C Blue #1, flavors, glycerin, purified water, sodium benzoate, sorbitol, xanthan gum.
Children's TYLENOL® Suspension Liquid: butylparaben, carboxymethylcellulose sodium, cellulose, citric acid, corn syrup, flavors, glycerin, propylene glycol, purified water, sodium benzoate, sorbitol sucralose, xanthan gum. In addition to the above ingredients cherry blast-flavored suspension contains FD&C Red #40, bubblegum-yum suspension contains D&C Red #33 and FD&C Red #40, grape splash-flavored suspension contains D&C Red #33 and FD&C Blue #1 and very berry strawberry-fla-vored suspension contains FD&C Red #40.
Children's TYLENOL® Meltaways: **Wacky Watermelon-Flavored:** cellulose acetate, citric acid, crospovidone, D&C Red #30, dextrose, flavors, magnesium stearate, povidone, sucralose. **Grape-Punch-Flavored:** cellulose acetate, citric acid, crospovidone, dextrose, D&C Red #7, D&C Red #30, FD&C Blue #1, flavors, magnesium stearate, povidone, sucralose. **Bubblegum Burst-Flavored:** cellulose acetate, citric acid, crospovidone, D&C Red #7, dextrose, flavors, magnesium stearate, povidone, sucralose.
***Jr. TYLENOL® Meltaways* Bubblegum Burst Flavored:** cellulose acetate, citric acid, crospovidone, D&C red #7, dextrose, flavors, magnesium stearate, povidone, sucralose. **Grape Punch Flavored:** cellulose acetate, citric acid, crospovidone, D&C Red #7, D&C Red #30, dextrose, FD&C Blue #1, flavors, magnesium stearate, povidone, sucralose.

How Supplied:
Concentrated TYLENOL® Infants' Drops: (purple-colored grape): bottles of ½ oz (15 mL) and 1 oz (30 mL); (red-colored cherry): bottles of ½ oz and 1 oz., each with calibrated plastic dropper.
Children's TYLENOL® Suspension Liquid: (red-colored cherry blast): bottles of 2 and 4 fl oz. (pink-colored bubblegum yum, purple-colored grape splash and red-colored very berry strawberry): bottles of 4 fl. oz.
Children's TYLENOL® Meltaways: (red-colored wacky watermelon, purple-colored grape punch, pink-colored bubblegum burst, scored, imprinted "TY80"). Bottles of 30 and also blister packaged 48's and 64's.
Jr. TYLENOL® Meltaways: (purple-colored grape punch or pink-colored bubblegum burst, imprinted "TY 160"). Blister packaged 24's and 48's. All packages listed above are safety sealed and use child-resistant safety caps or blisters.

Shown in Product Identification Guide, page 509 & 510

CHILDREN'S TYLENOL® Plus Cold & Allergy

Description: *Children's TYLENOL® Plus Cold & Allergy* is Bubble Gum flavored and contains no alcohol or aspirin. Each teaspoon (5 mL) contains acetaminophen 160 mg, diphenhydramine HCl 12.5 mg and pseudoephedrine HCl 15 mg.

Actions: *Children's TYLENOL® Plus Cold & Allergy* combines the analgesic-antipyretic acetaminophen with the antihistamine diphenhydramine hydrochloride and the decongestant pseudoephedrine hydrochloride to pro-

Continued on next page

Tylenol Children—Cont.

vide fast, effective, temporary relief of all your child's symptoms associated with hay fever and other respiratory allergies including sneezing, sore throat, itchy throat, itchy/watery eyes, runny nose, stuffy nose and nasal congestion. Acetaminophen is equal to aspirin in analgesic and antipyretic effectiveness and it is unlikely to produce the side effects often associated with aspirin or aspirin-containing products.

Uses: temporarily relieves these cold and upper respiratory allergy symptoms:
• sore throat • headache
• runny nose • sneezing
• stuffy nose • minor aches and pains
• itchy, watery eyes
• temporarily reduces fever

Directions: See Table 1: Children's Tylenol Dosing Chart on pgs. 670-672.

Warnings: Sore throat warning: If sore throat is severe, persists for more than 2 days, is accompanied or followed by fever, headache, rash, nausea or vomiting, consult a doctor promptly.

Do not use
• in a child who is taking a prescription monoamine oxidase inhibitor (MAOI) (certain drugs for depression, psychiatric, or emotional conditions, or Parkinson's disease) or for 2 weeks after stopping the MAOI drug. If you do not know if your child's prescription drug contains an MAOI, ask a doctor or pharmacist before giving this product.
• with any other product containing acetaminophen.
• with any other product containing diphenhydramine, even one used on skin

Ask a doctor before use if the child has
• heart disease • high blood pressure
• thyroid disease • diabetes
• glaucoma • a breathing problem such as chronic bronchitis

When using this product
• **do not exceed recommended dosage (see overdose warning)**
• marked drowsiness may occur
• excitability may occur, especially in children

Stop use and ask a doctor if
• pain or nasal congestion gets worse or lasts for more than 5 days
• fever gets worse or lasts for more than 3 days
• redness or swelling is present
• new symptoms occur
• nervousness, dizziness or sleeplessness occurs

Keep out of reach of children.

OVERDOSE WARNING

Taking more than the recommended dose (overdose) may cause liver damage. In case of overdose, get medical help or contact a Poison Control Center right away. Quick medical attention is critical even if you do not notice any signs or symptoms

Other Information:
• **do not use if plastic carton wrap or bottle wrap imprinted "Safety Seal®" is broken or missing.**
• store between 20–25° C (68–77° F)
• see bottom panel of carton for lot and expiration date

Professional Information:
Overdosage Information:
For overdosage information, please refer to pg. 667.

Inactive Ingredients:
carboxymethylcellulose sodium, cellulose, citric acid, corn syrup, D&C Red #33, FD&C Red #40, flavors, glycerin, purified water, sodium benzoate, sorbitol, sucralose, xanthan gum

How Supplied:
Pink-colored, Bubble Gum flavored liquid in child resistant tamper-evident bottles of 4 fl. oz.

Shown in Product Identification Guide, page 509

Concentrated TYLENOL® Infants' Drops Plus Cold Nasal Decongestant, Fever Reducer & Pain Reliever

Concentrated TYLENOL® Infants' Drops Plus Cold & Cough Nasal Decongestant, Fever Reducer & Pain Reliever, Cough Suppressant

Children's TYLENOL® Plus Cold Nighttime Suspension Liquid

Children's TYLENOL® Plus Cold Chewable Tablets

Children's TYLENOL® Plus Cold & Cough Suspension Liquid and Chewable Tablets

Children's TYLENOL® Plus Cold Daytime Non-Drowsy

Description: *Concentrated TYLENOL® Infants' Drops Plus Cold* are alcohol-free, aspirin-free, Bubble-Gum-flavored and red in color. Each 1.6 mL contains acetaminophen 160 mg and pseudoephedrine HCl 15 mg. *Concentrated TYLENOL® Infants' Drops Plus Cold & Cough* are alcohol-free, aspirin-free, Cherry-flavored and red in color. Each 1.6 mL contains acetaminophen 160 mg, dextromethorphan HBr 5 mg, and pseudoephedrine HCl 15 mg. *Children's TYLENOL® Plus Cold Nighttime Suspension Liquid* is Grape-flavored and contains no alcohol or aspirin. Each teaspoon (5 mL) contains acetaminophen 160 mg, chlorpheniramine maleate 1 mg and pseudoephedrine HCl 15 mg. *Children's TYLENOL® Plus Cold Chewable Tablets* are Grape-flavored and each tablet contains acetaminophen 80 mg, chlorpheniramine maleate 0.5 mg and pseudoephedrine HCl 7.5 mg. *Children's TYLENOL® Plus Cold & Cough Suspension Liquid* is Cherry-flavored and contains no alcohol or aspirin. Each teaspoonful (5 mL) contains acetaminophen 160 mg, chlorpheniramine maleate 1 mg, dextromethorphan HBr 5 mg and pseudoephedrine HCl 15 mg. *Children's TYLENOL® Plus Cold & Cough Chewable Tablets* are Cherry-flavored and each tablet contains acetamin-

ophen 80 mg, chlorpheniramine maleate 0.5 mg, dextromethorphan HBr 2.5 mg, and pseudoephedrine HCl 7.5 mg.
Children's TYLENOL® Plus Cold Daytime Non-Drowsy Suspension Liquid is Fruit flavored and contains no alcohol or aspirin. Each teaspoon (5 mL) contains acetaminophen 160 mg and pseudoephedrine HCl 15 mg.

Actions: Acetaminophen is a clinically proven analgesic/antipyretic. Acetaminophen produces analgesia by elevation of the pain threshold and antipyresis through action on the hypothalamic heat-regulating center. Acetaminophen is equal to aspirin in analgesic and antipyretic effectiveness and it is unlikely to produce many of the side effects associated with aspirin and aspirin-containing products.
Pseudoephedrine hydrochloride is a sympathomimetic amine which provides temporary relief of nasal congestion.
Chlorpheniramine maleate is an antihistamine that provides temporary relief of runny nose, sneezing and watery and itchy eyes.
Dextromethorphan hydrobromide is a cough suppressant which helps relieve coughs.

Uses: *Concentrated TYLENOL® Infants' Drops Plus Cold,* temporarily relieves these cold symptoms:
• minor aches and pains
• nasal congestion • headaches
• temporarily reduces fever
Concentrated TYLENOL® Infants' Drops Plus Cold & Cough, temporarily relieves these cold symptoms:
• coughs • nasal congestion
• minor aches and pains
• sore throat • headaches
• temporarily reduces fever
Children's TYLENOL® Plus Cold Nighttime Suspension Liquid: temporarily relieves these cold symptoms:
• nasal congestion • sore throat • runny nose • sneezing • headache • minor aches and pains
• temporarily reduces fever
Children's TYLENOL® Plus Cold Chewable Tablets: temporarily relieves these cold symptoms:
• nasal congestion • sore throat • runny nose • sneezing • headache • minor aches and pains
• temporarily reduces fever
Children's TYLENOL® Plus Cold & Cough Suspension Liquid and *Chewable Tablets:* temporarily relieves these cold symptoms:
• nasal congestion • sore throat • runny nose • sneezing • headache • minor aches and pains • coughs
temporarily reduces fever
Children's Tylenol® Plus Cold Daytime Non-Drowsy temporarily relieves: • sinus congestion • stuffy nose • sinus pressure • minor aches, pains and headache • temporarily reduces fever

Directions:
See Table 1: Children's Tylenol Dosing Chart on pgs. 670-672.

Warnings:
Sore throat warning: If sore throat is severe, persists for more than 2 days, is

accompanied by or followed by fever, headache, rash, nausea or vomiting, consult a doctor promptly (does not apply to *Concentrated TYLENOL® Infants' Drops Plus Cold* or *Children's TYLENOL® Plus Cold Daytime Non-Drowsy*)

Do not use
- in a child who is taking a prescription monoamine oxidase inhibitor (MAOI) (certain drugs for depression, psychiatric or emotional conditions, or Parkinson's disease), or for 2 weeks after stopping the MAOI drug. If you do not know if your child's prescription drug contains an MAOI, ask a doctor or pharmacist before giving this product.
- with any other products containing acetaminophen

Keep out of reach of children.

Overdose Warning: Taking more than the recommended dose (overdose) may cause liver damage. In case of overdose, get medical help or contact a Poison Control Center right away. Quick medical attention is critical even if you do not notice any signs or symptoms.

Stop use and ask a doctor if
- new symptoms occur
- redness or swelling is present
- pain gets worse or lasts for more than 5 days *for Children's Tyl. Plus Cold D.T. and N.T. liquid: pain or nasal congestion gets worse or lasts more than 5 days *for Children's TYLENOL® cold plus cough suspension liquid:—pain, cough, or nasal congestion gets worse or lasts more than 5 days.—comes back or occurs with rash or headache that lasts. These could be signs of a serious condition.
- fever gets worse or lasts for more than 3 days
- nervousness, dizziness or sleeplessness occurs
- cough lasts for more than 7 days, comes back or occurs with fever, rash or headache that lasts. These could be signs of a serious condition. (*Concentrated TYLENOL® Infants' Drops Plus Cold & Cough* only)
- cough comes back or occurs with rash or headache that lasts (*Children's Tylenol® Plus Cold & Cough* product only)

Concentrated TYLENOL® Infants' Drops Plus Cold,

Ask a doctor before use if the child has
- heart disease • high blood pressure
- thyroid disease • diabetes

When using this product
- **do not exceed recommended dosage (see overdose warning)**

Concentrated TYLENOL® Infants' Drops Plus Cold & Cough

Ask a doctor before use if the child has
- heart disease • high blood pressure
- cough that occurs with too much phlegm (mucus) • thyroid disease • diabetes • chronic cough that lasts as occurs with asthma

When using this product
- **do not exceed recommended dosage (see Overdose warning)**

Children's TYLENOL® Plus Cold Nighttime Suspension Liquid and Plus Cold Chewable Tablets

Ask a doctor before use if the child has
- heart disease • thyroid disease • glaucoma • high blood pressure • diabetes

- a breathing problem such as chronic bronchitis

When using this product
- **do not exceed recommended dosage (see overdose warning)**
- drowsiness may occur
- excitability may occur, especially in children

Children's TYLENOL® Plus Cold & Cough Nighttime Suspension Liquid and Chewable Tablets

Ask a doctor before use if the child has
- heart disease • thyroid disease • glaucoma • high blood pressure • diabetes
- cough that occurs with too much phlegm (mucus)
- chronic cough that lasts as occurs with asthma

When using this product
- **do not exceed recommended dosage (see overdose warning)**
- drowsiness may occur
- excitability may occur, especially in children

Other Information:
Concentrated TYLENOL® Infants' Drops Plus Cold, Concentrated TYLENOL® Infants' Drops Plus Cold & Cough
- **do not use if plastic carton wrap or bottle wrap imprinted "Safety Seal®" is broken or missing**
- store at room temperature
- see bottom panel for lot number and expiration date

Children's TYLENOL® Plus Cold & Cough Suspension Liquid, Children's TYLENOL® Plus Cold Nighttime Suspension Liquid and Children's TYLENOL® Plus Cold Daytime Non-Drowsy
- **do not use if bottle wrap or foil inner seal imprinted "Safety Seal®" is broken or missing**
- store between 20°–25°C (68°–77°F)
- see bottom panel for lot number and expiration date

Children's TYLENOL® Plus Cold Chewable Tablets
- **phenylketonurics: contains phenylalanine 6 mg per tablet**
- **do not use if carton is opened or if blister unit is broken**
- store at room temperature

Children's TYLENOL® Plus Cold & Cough Chewable Tablets
- **phenylketonurics: contains phenylalanine 4 mg per tablet**
- **do not use if carton is opened or if blister unit is broken**
- store at room temperature
- see side panel for lot number and expiration date

Professional Information:
Overdosage Information: For overdosage information, please refer to pg. 667.

Inactive Ingredients:
Concentrated TYLENOL® Infants' Drops Plus Cold: citric acid, corn syrup, FD&C Red #40, flavors, polyethylene glycol, propylene glycol, sodium benzoate, sodium saccharin.

Concentrated TYLENOL® Infants' Drops Plus Cold & Cough: acesulfame potassium, citric acid, corn syrup, FD&C

Red #40, flavors, polyethylene glycol, propylene glycol, sodium benzoate.

Children's TYLENOL® Plus Cold: Nighttime Suspension Liquid: acesulfame potassium, carboxymethylcellulose sodium, cellulose, citric acid, corn syrup, D&C Red #33, FD&C Blue #1, FD&C Red #40, flavors, glycerin, purified water, sodium benzoate, sorbitol, xanthan gum. **Chewable Tablets:** aspartame, basic polymethacrylate, cellulose, cellulose acetate, citric acid, D&C Red #7, FD&C Blue #1, flavors, hypromellose, magnesium stearate, mannitol.

Children's TYLENOL® Plus Cold & Cough: Suspension Liquid: acesulfame potassium, carboxymethylcellulose sodium, cellulose, citric acid, corn syrup, D&C Red #33, FD&C Red #40, flavors, glycerin, purified water, sodium benzoate, sorbitol, xanthan gum. **Chewable Tablets:** aspartame, basic polymethacrylate, cellulose, cellulose acetate, D&C Red #7, flavors, hypromellose, magnesium stearate, mannitol.

Children's Tylenol® Plus Cold Daytime Non-Drowsy acesulfame potassium, carboxymethylcellulose sodium, cellulose, citric acid, corn syrup, D&C Red #33, FD&C Red #40, flavors, glycerin, purified water, sodium benzoate, sorbitol, xanthan gum.

How Supplied:
Concentrated TYLENOL® Infants' Drops Plus Cold: Red colored, Bubble Gum flavored drops in child resistant tamper-evident bottles of $1/2$ fl. oz.

Concentrated TYLENOL® Infants' Drops Plus Cold & Cough: Red colored, Cherry Flavored drops in Child resistant tamper evident bottles of $1/2$ fl. oz.

Children's TYLENOL® Plus Cold: Nighttime Suspension Liquid: Purple-colored-bottles of 4 fl. oz. Store between 20°–25°C (68°–77°F). **Chewable Tablets:** Purple-colored, imprinted "TYLENOL COLD" on one side and "TC" on opposite side- blisters of 24.

Children's TYLENOL® Plus Cold & Cough: Suspension Liquid: Red colored, Cherry flavored liquid in child resistant tamper-evident bottles of 4 fl. oz.

Chewable Tablets: Red-colored, imprinted TYLENOL C/C" on one side and "TC/C" on the opposite side- blisters of 24.

Cold Daytime 4oz is in white (opaque) bottle

Children's Tylenol® Plus Cold Daytime Non-Drowsy Red-colored, Fruit flavored liquid in child resistant tamper-evident bottles of 4 fl. oz.

Shown in Product Identification Guide, page 509 & 510

Children's TYLENOL® Plus Flu

Description: *Children's TYLENOL® Plus Flu* Suspension Liquid is Bubble

Continued on page 673

TABLE 1
Children's Tylenol® Dosing Chart

AGE GROUP	0–3 mos	4–11 mos	12–23 mos	2–3 yrs	4–5 yrs	6–8 yrs	9–10 yrs	11 yrs	12 yrs	**Maximum doses/24 hrs**
WEIGHT (if possible use weight to dose; otherwise use age)	6–11 lbs	12–17 lbs	18–23 lbs	24–35 lbs	36–47 lbs	48–59 lbs	60–71 lbs	72–95 lbs	96 lbs and over	
PRODUCT FORM / **INGREDIENTS**	Dose to be administered based on weight or age†									
Infants' Drops in each (0.8 mL)										
Concentrated Tylenol Infants' Drops — Acetaminophen 80 mg	(0.4 mL)*	(0.8 mL)*	1.2 mL (0.8 + 0.4 mL)*	1.6 mL (0.8 + 0.8 mL)	—	—	—	—	—	5 times in 24 hrs
Concentrated Tylenol Infants' Drops Plus Cold — Acetaminophen 80 mg, Pseudoephedrine HCl 7.5 mg	(0.4 mL)*	(0.8 mL)*	1.2 mL (0.8 + 0.4 mL)*	1.6 mL (0.8 + 0.8 mL)	—	—	—	—	—	4 times in 24 hrs
Concentrated Tylenol Infants' Drops Plus Cold & Cough — Acetaminophen 80 mg, Dextromethorphan HBr 2.5 mg, Pseudoephedrine HCl 7.5 mg	(0.4 mL)*	(0.8 mL)*	1.2 mL (0.8 + 0.4 mL)*	1.6 mL (0.8 + 0.8 mL)	—	—	—	—	—	4 times in 24 hrs
Children's Liquids Per 5 mL teaspoonful (TSP)										
Children's Tylenol Suspension Liquid — Acetaminophen 160 mg	—	½ TSP*	¾ TSP*	1 TSP	1½ TSP	2 TSP	2½ TSP	3 TSP	—	5 times in 24 hrs
Children's Tylenol Plus Cold Nighttime Suspension Liquid — Acetaminophen 160 mg, Chlorpheniramine Maleate 1 mg, Pseudoephedrine HCl 15 mg	—	½ TSP**	¾ TSP**	1 TSP**	1½ TSP**	2 TSP	2½ TSP	3 TSP	—	4 times in 24 hrs

Product	Ingredients										Max. Dose
Children's Tylenol Plus Cold & Cough Suspension Liquid	Acetaminophen 160 mg Chlorpheniramine Maleate 1 mg Dextromethorphan HBr 5 mg Pseudoephedrine HCl 15 mg	—	½ TSP**	¾ TSP**	1 TSP**	1½ TSP**	2 TSP	2½ TSP	3 TSP	—	4 times in 24 hrs
Children's Tylenol Plus Flu Suspension Liquid†	Acetaminophen 160 mg Chlorpheniramine Maleate 1 mg Dextromethorphan HBr 7.5 mg Pseudoephedrine HCl 15 mg	—	½ TSP**	¾ TSP**	1 TSP**	1½ TSP**	2 TSP	2½ TSP	3 TSP	—	4 times in 24 hrs
Children's Tylenol Plus Cold Daytime Suspension Liquid	Acetaminophen 160 mg Pseudoephedrine HCl 15 mg	—	½ TSP*	¾ TSP*	1 TSP	1½ TSP	2 TSP	2½ TSP	3 TSP	—	4 times in 24 hrs
Children's Tylenol Plus Cold & Allergy Liquid	Acetaminophen 160 mg Diphenhydramine HCl 12.5 mg Pseudoephedrine HCl 15 mg	—	½ TSP**	¾ TSP**	1 TSP**	1½ TSP**	2 TSP	2½ TSP	3 TSP	—	4 times in 24 hrs
Children's Tablets	**Per tablet**										
Children's Tylenol Meltaways	Acetaminophen 80 mg	—	—	—	2 tablets	3 tablets	4 tablets	5 tablets	6 tablets	—	5 times in 24 hrs
Children's Tylenol Plus Cold Chewable Tablets	Acetaminophen 80 mg Chlorpheniramine Maleate 0.5 mg Pseudoephedrine HCl 7.5 mg	—	—	—	2 tablets**	3 tablets**	4 tablets	5 tablets	6 tablets	—	4 times in 24 hrs

(Table continued on next page)

(Continued from previous page)

Product	Ingredients									Frequency
Children's Tylenol Plus Cold & Cough Chewable Tablets	Acetaminophen 80 mg Chlorpheniramine Maleate 0.5 mg Dextromethorphan HBr 2.5 mg Pseudoephedrine HCl 7.5 mg	—	—	2 tablets**	3 tablets**	4 tablets	5 tablets	6 tablets	—	4 times in 24 hrs
JR Tylenol Meltaways	Acetaminophen 160 mg	—	—	—	—	2 tablets	2½ tablets	3 tablets	4 tablets	5 times in 24 hrs
Simply Stuffy Liquid	pseudoephedrine HCl 15 mg	½ tsp.*	¾ tsp.*	1 tsp	1½ tsp	2 tsp	2½ tsp	3 tsp	—	4 times in 24 hours
Simply Cough Liquid	dextromethorphan HBr 5 mg	½ tsp*	¾ tsp*	1 tsp	1½ tsp	2 tsp	2½ tsp	3 tsp	—	4 times in 24 hrs

†All products may be dosed every 4 hours, if needed; except for Children's Tylenol Flu which is dosed every 6–8 hrs, if needed.

*Under 2 years (under 24 lbs), consult a doctor.　　**Under 6 years (under 48 lbs), consult a doctor.

•Infants' Tylenol Drops are more concentrated than Children's Tylenol Liquids. The Infants' Concentrated Drops have been specifically designed for use only with enclosed dropper. Do not use any other dosing device with this product. Shake well before using; fill to prescribed level and dispense liquid slowly into child's mouth, toward inner cheek. Use original bottle cap or dropper to maintain child resistance.

•Children's Tylenol Liquids are less concentrated than Infants' Tylenol Concentrated Drops. The Children's Tylenol Liquids have been specifically designed for use with the enclosed measuring cup. Use only enclosed measuring cup to dose this product. Shake well before using.

•Children's Tylenol Meltaways Tablets are not the same concentration as Junior Tylenol Meltaways Tablets; dissolve in mouth or chew before swallowing.

•Junior Tylenol Meltaways Tablets and Caplets contain twice as much medicine as Children's Tylenol Meltaways Tablets; dissolve in mouth or chew before swallowing.

Gum flavored and contains no alcohol or aspirin. Each teaspoon (5 mL) contains acetaminophen 160 mg, chlorpheniramine maleate 1 mg, dextromethorphan HBr 7.5 mg and pseudoephedrine HCl 15 mg.

Actions: *Children's TYLENOL® Plus Flu* Suspension Liquid combines the analgesic-antipyretic acetaminophen with the decongestant pseudoephedrine hydrochloride, the cough suppressant dextromethorphan hydrobromide and the antihistamine chlorpheniramine maleate to provide fast, effective, temporary relief of all your child's symptoms associated with flu including fever, body aches, headache, stuffy nose, runny nose, sore throat and coughs. Acetaminophen is equal to aspirin in analgesic and antipyretic effectiveness and it is unlikely to produce the side effects often associated with aspirin or aspirin-containing products.

Uses: temporarily relieves these cold and flu symptoms:
• nasal congestion • sore throat
• runny nose • sneezing
• headache • minor aches and pains
• coughs
• temporarily reduces fever

Directions: See Table 1: Children's Tylenol Dosing Chart on pgs. 670-672.

Warnings:
Sore throat warning:
If sore throat is severe, persists for more than 2 days, is accompanied or followed by fever, headache, rash, nausea or vomiting, consult a doctor promptly.
Do not use
• in a child who is taking a prescription monoamine oxidase inhibitor (MAOI) (certain drugs for depression, psychiatric or emotional conditions, or Parkinson's disease), or for 2 weeks after stopping the MAOI drug. If you do not know if your child's prescription drug contains an MAOI, ask a doctor or pharmacist before giving this product.
• with any other product containing acetaminophen.
Ask a doctor before use if the child has
• heart disease • thyroid disease
• glaucoma • high blood pressure
• diabetes • cough that occurs with too much phlegm (mucus)
• chronic cough that lasts as occurs with asthma
When using this product
• do not exceed recommended dosage (see overdose warning)
• drowsiness may occur
• excitability may occur, especially in children
Stop use and ask a doctor if
• new symptoms occur
• fever gets worse or lasts for more than 3 days
• redness or swelling is present
• nervousness, dizziness or sleeplessness occurs
• pain, cough or nasal congestion gets worse or lasts for more than 5 days
• cough comes back or occurs with rash or headache that lasts. These could be signs of a serious condition.
Keep out of reach of children.
Overdose Warning: Taking more than the recommended dose (overdose)

may cause liver damage. In case of overdose, get medical help or contact a Poison Control Center right away. Quick medical attention is critical even if you do not notice any signs or symptoms.

Other Information:
• do not use if bottle wrap or foil inner seal imprinted "Safety Seal®" is broken or missing.
• store between 20–25°C (68–77°F).
• see bottom panel for lot number and expiration date

Professional Information:
Overdosage Information: For overdosage information, please refer to pg. 667.

Inactive Ingredients: acesulfame potassium, carboxymethylcellulose sodium, cellulose, citric acid, corn syrup, D&C Red #33, FD&C Red #40, flavors, glycerin, purified water, sodium benzoate, sorbitol, xanthan gum.

How Supplied: Pink colored, Bubble Gum flavored liquid in child resistant tamper-evident bottle of 4 fl. oz.
Shown in Product Identification Guide, page 509

Children's TYLENOL® Dosing Chart

[See table on pages 670-672]

Mission Pharmacal Company
**10999 IH 10 WEST
SUITE 1000
SAN ANTONIO, TX 78230-1355**

Direct Inquiries to:
PO Box 786099
San Antonio, TX 78278-6099
TOLL FREE: (800) 292-7364
(210) 696-8400
FAX: (210) 696-6010
For Medical Information Contact:
In Emergencies:
Mary Ann Walter

THERA-GESIC®
[thĕr"ə-jē'zik]
TOPICAL ANALGESIC CREME

Active Ingredients:

| | **Purpose:** |
Menthol 1% .... Analgesic
Methyl Salicylate
  15% .... Counterirritant

Use: Temporary relief of minor aches and pains of muscles and joints associated with: Arthritis, simple backaches, strains, bruises, sprains.

Warnings:
For external use only. Use only as directed. Avoid contact with eyes or mucous membranes.

Do not bandage tightly, wrap or cover until after washing the areas where THERA-GESIC has been applied.
Do not use
• immediately after shower or bath
• if skin is sensitive to oil of wintergreen (methyl salicylate)
• on wounds or damaged skin
Ask a doctor before use
• for children under 2 and through 12 years of age
• if prone or sensitive to allergic reactions from aspirin or salicylate
When using this product
• discontinue use if skin irritation develops, or redness is present
• do not swallow
• do not use a heating pad after application of THERA-GESIC
Stop use and ask a doctor if condition worsens, or if symptoms persist for more than 7 days or clear up and occur again within a few days.
If pregnant or breast-feeding, ask a health professional before use.
Keep out of reach of children to avoid accidental poisoning. If swallowed, get medical help or contact a Poison Control Center right away.

Directions: Adults and children 12 or more years of age: Apply thin layers of creme into and around the sore or painful area, not more than 3 to 4 times daily. The number of thin layers controls the intensity of the action of THERA-GESIC. One thin layer provides a mild effect, two thin layers provide a strong effect and three thin layers provide a very strong effect. SEE WARNINGS. Wash hands thoroughly after application.
Other Information: Once THERA-GESIC has penetrated the skin, the area may be washed, leaving it dry, clean and fragrance-free without decreasing the effectiveness of the product. Avoid contact with clothing or other surfaces. Store at 20–25° C (68–77° F).

Inactive Ingredients: Carbomer 934, Dimethicone, Glycerine, Methylparaben, Propylparaben, Sodium Lauryl Sulfate, Trolamine, Water.

How Supplied:
NDC 0178-0320-03   3 oz. tube
NDC 0178-0320-05   5 oz. tube

THERA-GESIC® PLUS
[thĕr" ə-jē'zik]
TOPICAL ANALGESIC CREME

Active Ingredients: **Purpose:**
Methyl Salicylate
  25% .... Topical Analgesic
Menthol 4% .... Topical Analgesic

Warnings:
For external use only. Use only as directed. Avoid contact with eyes or mucous membranes.
Do not bandage tightly, wrap or cover until after washing the areas where THERA-GESIC® PLUS has been applied.

Continued on next page

Thera-Gesic Plus—Cont.

Inactive Ingredients: Aloe Vera, Carbomer 980, Dimethicone, Glycerine, Methylparaben, Propylparaben, Sodium Lauryl Sulfate, Trolamine, Water.

How Supplied:
NDC 0178-0350-03   3 oz. tube
NDC 0178-0350-05   5 oz. tube
For all other information, see listing for THERA-GESIC®.

Novartis Consumer Health, Inc.

200 KIMBALL DRIVE
PARSIPPANY, NJ 07054-0622

Direct Product Inquiries to:
Consumer & Professional Affairs
(800) 452-0051
Fax: (800) 635-2801

Or write to above address.

DESENEX® ANTIFUNGALS
All products are Prescription Strength
Shake Powder
Liquid Spray
Spray Powder
Jock Itch Spray Powder

Drug Facts

Active Ingredient: **Purpose:**
Miconazole nitrate 2% .... Antifungal

Uses: *Shake Powder, Liquid Spray, and Spray Powder*
• cures most athlete's foot (tinea pedis) and ringworm (tinea corporis) • relieves itching, scaling, burning, and discomfort that can accompany athlete's foot
Jock Itch Spray Powder
• cures most jock itch (tinea cruris) • relieves itching, scaling, burning and discomfort that can accompany jock itch
For Spray Powder, Spray Liquid, and Jock Itch Spray Powder
Liquid Spray, Spray Powder and Jock Inch Spray Powder

Warnings:
For external use only
Flammability Warning: Contents under pressure. Do not puncture or incinerate. Flammable mixture; do not use near fire or flame, or expose to heat or temperatures above 49°C (120°F). Use only as directed. Intentional misuse by deliberately concentrating and inhaling the contents can be harmful or fatal.
Do not use • in or near the mouth or the eyes • for nail or scalp infections
When using this product • do not get into the eyes or mouth
Stop use and ask a doctor if • irritation occurs or gets worse • no improvement within 4 weeks for athlete's foot and ringworm, or no improvement within 2 weeks for jock itch.

Keep out of reach of children. If swallowed, get medical help or contact a poison control center right away.

Directions:
• adults and children 2 years and older
• wash the affected area with soap and water and dry completely before applying
Shake Powder
• apply a thin layer over affected area twice a day (morning and night) or as directed by a doctor
• pay special attention to the spaces between the toes. Wear well-fitting, ventilated shoes and change shoes and socks at least once a day.
• use every day for 4 weeks
• supervise children in the use of this product
• children under 2 years of age: ask a doctor
Liquid Spray and Spray Powder
• shake can well, hold 4″ to 6″ from skin
• spray a thin layer over affected area twice a day (morning and night) or as directed by a doctor
• for athlete's foot pay special attention to the spaces between the toes. Wear well-fitting, ventilated shoes and change shoes and socks at least once a day.
• use daily for 4 weeks
• supervise children in the use of this product
• children under 2 years of age: ask a doctor
Jock Itch Spray Powder
• shake can well, hold 4″ to 6″ from skin
• spray a thin layer over affected area twice a day (morning and night) or as directed by a doctor
• use daily for 2 weeks
• supervise children in the use of this product
• children under 2 years of age: ask a doctor

Other Information: • store at controlled room temperature 20-25°C (68-77°F) • see bottom of can for lot number and expiration date
Liquid Spray, Spray Powder and Jock Itch Spray Powder
• if clogging occurs, remove button and clean nozzle with a pin

Inactive Ingredients: *Shake Powder*— corn starch, corn starch/acrylamide/sodium acrylate polymer, fragrance, talc
Liquid Spray—polyethylene glycol 300, polysorbate 20, SD alcohol 40-B (15%w/w) Propellant: dimethyl ether
Spray Powder, Jock Itch Spray Powder— aloe vera gel, aluminum starch octenyl succinate, isopropyl myristate, propylene carbonate, SD alcohol 40-B (10% w/w), sorbitan monooleate, stearalkonium hectorite Propellant: isobutane/ propane

How Supplied: *Shake Powder*-1.5 oz, 3 oz, plastic bottles.
Spray Powder-3 oz cans
Liquid Spray-3.5 oz cans
Jock Itch Spray Powder-3 oz cans
Shown in Product Identification Guide, page 512

EX•LAX® Chocolated Laxative Pieces

Active Ingredient: Sennosides, USP, 15mg
Purpose: Stimulant Laxative

Use: For Relief of
• OCCASIONAL   CONSTIPATION (IRREGULARITY). This product generally produces bowel movement in 6 to 12 hours.

Warnings:
Ask a doctor before use if you have
• abdominal pain • nausea • vomiting
• noticed a sudden change in bowel habits that persists over a period of 2 weeks
Ask a doctor or pharmacist before use if you are • taking any other drug. Take this product 2 or more hours before or after other drugs. Laxatives may affect how other drugs work.
Stop use and ask a doctor if • you need to use more than 1 week
• rectal bleeding or failure to have a bowel movement occur after use of a laxative.
These may be signs of a serious condition.
If pregnant or breast-feeding, ask a health care professional before use.
Keep out of reach of children. In case of overdose, get medical help or contact a Poison Control Center right away.

Directions:

adults and children 12 years of age and older	chew 2 chocolated pieces once or twice daily
children 6 to under 12 years of age	chew 1 chocolated piece once or twice daily
children under 6 years of age	ask a doctor

Other Information: • very low sodium • store at controlled room temperature 20–25°C (68–77°F)

Inactive Ingredients: cocoa, confectioners sugar, hydrogenated palm kernel oil, lecithin, non-fat dry milk, vanillin

How Supplied: Available in boxes of 18 ct. and 48 ct. chewable chocolated pieces.
Shown in Product Identification Guide, page 512

EX•LAX® Laxative Pills
Regular Strength Ex•Lax®
Laxative Pills
Maximum Strength Ex•Lax®
Laxative Pills

Active Ingredients: *Regular Strength Ex·Lax Laxative Pills:* Sennosides, USP, 15 mg. *Maximum Strength Ex·Lax Laxative Pills:* Sennosides, USP, 25 mg.
Purpose: Stimulant Laxative

Use: For Relief of
• OCCASIONAL CONSTIPATION (IRREGULARITY). This product generally produces bowel movement in 6 to 12 hours.

Warnings:

Ask a doctor before use if you have
• abdominal pain • nausea • vomiting
• noticed a sudden change in bowel habits that persists over a period of 2 weeks

Ask a doctor or pharmacist before use if you are • taking any other drug. Take this product 2 or more hours before or after other drugs. Laxatives may affect how other drugs work.

Stop use and ask a doctor if • you need to use more than 1 week
• rectal bleeding or failure to have a bowel movement occur after use of a laxative.
These may be signs of a serious condition.

If pregnant or breast-feeding, ask a health care professional before use.

Keep out of reach of children. In case of overdose, get medical help or contact a Poison Control Center right away.

Directions: • take with a glass of water

adults and children 12 years of age and older	2 pills once or twice daily
children 6 to under 12 years of age	1 pill once or twice daily
children under 6 years of age	ask a doctor

Other Information: • very low sodium
• store at controlled room temperature 20–25°C (68–77°F)

Inactive Ingredients: —acacia, alginic acid, carnauba wax, colloidal silicon dioxide, dibasic calcium phosphate, magnesium stearate, microcrystalline cellulose, sodium benzoate, sodium lauryl sulfate, starch, stearic acid, sucrose, talc, titanium dioxide.
Regular Strength Pills also contain iron oxides.
Maximum Strength Pills also contain FD&C Blue No. 1 aluminum lake

How Supplied: *Regular Strength Ex·Lax Laxative Pills*—Available in boxes of 8 ct. and 30 ct. pills. *Maximum Strength Ex·Lax Laxative Pills*—Available in boxes of 24 ct., 48 ct., and 90 ct. pills.

Shown in Product Identification Guide, page 512

GAS–X® REGULAR STRENGTH
Antigas Chewable Tablets
GAS–X® EXTRA STRENGTH
Antigas Softgels and Chewable Tablets
GAS–X® MAXIMUM STRENGTH
Antigas Softgels
GAS–X® WITH MAALOX®
Antigas/Antacid Softgels and Chewable Tablets

Active Ingredients:
Regular Strength—Each chewable tablet contains simethicone 80 mg.

Extra Strength—Each chewable tablet and swallowable softgel contains simethicone, 125 mg.

Maximum Strength—Each Swallowable softgel contains simethicone, 166 mg.

Gas-X® with Maalox® Tablets—Each extra strength chewable tablet contains simethicone 125 mg and calcium carbonate 500 mg.

Gas-X® with Maalox® Softgels—Each swallowable softgel contains simethicone 62.5 mg and calcium carbonate 250 mg.

Inactive Ingredients:
Regular Strength Peppermint Creme: calcium carbonate, dextrose, flavors, maltodextrin, starch

Regular Strength Cherry Creme: calcium carbonate, D&C Red 30 aluminum lake, dextrose, flavors, maltodextrin, propylene glycol, soy protein isolate

Extra Strength Peppermint Creme: calcium phosphate tribasic, colloidal silicon dioxide, D&C Yellow 10 aluminum lake, D&C Red 30 aluminum lake, dextrose, flavors, maltodextrin, starch

Extra Strength Cherry Creme: calcium phosphate tribasic, colloidal silicon dioxide, D&C Red 30 aluminum lake, dextrose, flavors, maltodextrin, propylene glycol, soy protein isolate, starch

Extra Strength Softgels: D&C Yellow 10, FD&C Blue 1, FD&C Red 40, gelatin, glycerin, peppermint oil, purified water, sorbitol, titanium dioxide

Maximum Strength Softgels: FD&C Blue 1, FD&C Red 40, gelatin, glycerin, peppermint oil, purified water, sorbitol

Gas-X® With Maalox® Wildberry Tablets:
colloidal silicon dioxide, D&C Red 30, dextrose, flavors, maltodextrin, mannitol, pregelatinized starch, talc, tribasic calcium phosphate

Gas-X® With Maalox® Orange Tablets:
colloidal silicon dioxide, dextrose, FD&C yellow 6 aluminum lake, flavors, maltodextrin, mannitol, pregelatinized starch, talc, tribasic calcium phosphate

Gas-X® With Maalox® Softgels:
D&C Red 28, FD&C Blue 1, gelatin, glycerin, polyethylene glycol, polysorbate 80, silicon dioxide, sorbitol, titanium dioxide, purified water

Use:
Gas-X®: For the relief of pressure and bloating commonly referred to as gas.
Gas-X® with Maalox®: Relief of the concurrent symptoms of gas associated with heartburn, sour stomach or acid indigestion.

Warning: Keep out of reach of children.

Gas-X®
Drug Interaction Precautions: No known drug interaction.
Gax-X® with Maalox® Tablets and Softgels

Warnings:
Ask a doctor or pharmacist before use if you are now taking a prescription drug. Antacids may interact with certain prescription drugs.

Gas-X®
Dosage and Administration: For Chewable Tablets: Adults: Chew one or two tablets as needed after meals or at bedtime. Do not exceed six Regular Strength chewable tablets or four Extra Strength chewable tablets in 24 hours except under the advice and supervision of a physician.
For Extra Strength Softgels: Adults: Swallow with water 1 or 2 softgels as needed after meals or at bedtime. Do not exceed 4 softgels in 24 hours except under the advice and supervision of a physician.
For Maximum Strength Softgels: Adults: Swallow with water 1 or 2 softgels as needed after meals or at bedtime. Do not exceed 3 softgels in 24 hours except under the advice and supervision of a physician.
For Gas-X® with Maalox® Tablets: Chew 1 to 2 tablets as symptoms occur or as directed by a physician. Do not take more than 4 tablets in a 24-hour period or use the maximum dosage for more than 2 weeks except under the advice and supervision of a physician.
For Gas-X® with Maalox® Softgels: Adults: Swallow with water 2 to 4 softgels as symptoms occur or as directed by a physician. Do not exceed 8 softgels in a 24 hour period or use the maximum dosage for more than 2 weeks except under the advice and supervision of a physician.

Professional Labeling: Gas-X® may be used in the alleviation of postoperative bloating/pressure, and for use in endoscopic examination.

How Supplied:
Regular Strength Chewable tablets are available in peppermint creme and cherry creme flavored, chewable, scored tablets in boxes of 36 tablets.
Extra Strength Chewable tablets are available in peppermint creme and cherry creme flavored, chewable, scored tablets in boxes of 18 tablets.
Easy-to-swallow, tasteless/Extra Strength Softgels are available in boxes of 10 pills, 30 pills, 50 pills and 60 pills.
Easy-to-swallow, tasteless/Maximum Strength Softgels are available in boxes of 50 pills.
Gas-X® With Maalox® Tablets are available in orange and wild berry flavored, chewable tablets in boxes of 8 tablets and 24 tablets

Continued on next page

Information on Novartis Consumer Health, Inc. products appearing on these pages is effective as of November 2004.

Gas-X—Cont.

Easy-to-swallow, tasteless/Gax-X® with Maalox® Softgels are available in boxes of 24 pills and 48 pills.

Shown in Product Identification Guide, page 512 & 513

LAMISIL ᴬᵀ® CREAM

Active Ingredient: **Purpose:**
Terbinafine
  hydrochloride 1% .... Antifungal

Uses:
- **cures most athlete's foot (tinea pedis)**
- **cures most jock itch (tinea cruris) and ringworm (tinea corporis)**
- **relieves itching, burning, cracking and scaling which accompany these conditions**

Warnings:
For external use only
Do not use • on nails or scalp
• in or near the mouth or the eyes
• for vaginal yeast infections
When using this product do not get into the eyes. If eye contact occurs, rinse thoroughly with water.
Stop use and ask a doctor if too much irritation occurs or gets worse.
Keep out of reach of children. If swallowed, get medical help or contact a poison control center right away.

Directions:
- adults and children 12 years and over
  - use the tip of the cap to break the seal and open the tube
  - wash the affected skin with soap and water and dry completely before applying
  - **for athlete's foot** wear well-fitting, ventilated shoes. Change shoes and socks at least once daily.
    - **between the toes only:** apply twice a day (morning and night) for **1 week** or as directed by a doctor.

1 week between the toes

- **on the bottom or sides of the foot:** apply twice a day (morning and night) for **2 weeks** or as directed by a doctor.

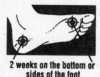
2 weeks on the bottom or sides of the foot

- **for jock itch and ringworm:** apply once a day (morning **or** night) for **1 week** or as directed by a doctor.

- wash hands after each use
- children under 12 years: ask a doctor

Other Information: • do not use if seal on tube is broken or is not visible
• store at controlled room temperature 20–25°C (68–77°F)

Inactive Ingredients: benzyl alcohol, cetyl alcohol, cetyl palmitate, isopropyl myristate, polysorbate 60, purified water, sodium hydroxide, sorbitan monostearate, stearyl alcohol.

How Supplied: Athlete's Foot — Net wt. 12g (.42 oz.) tube and 24g (.85 oz.) tube, Jock Itch — Net wt. 12g (.42 oz.) tube.

Questions? call **1-800-452-0051** 24 hours a day, 7 days a week.

Shown in Product Identification Guide, page 513

MAALOX MAX® MAXIMUM STRENGTH ANTACID/ANTI-GAS Liquid
Oral Suspension Antacid/Anti-Gas

Liquids
☐ **Lemon**
☐ **Cherry**
☐ **Mint**
☐ **Vanilla Crème**
☐ **Wild Berry**

Drug Facts:
[See table below]

Uses: For the relief of
- acid indigestion
- heartburn
- sour stomach
- upset stomach associated with these symptoms
- bloating and pressure commonly referred to as gas

Warnings:
Ask a doctor before use if you have kidney disease.
Ask a doctor or pharmacist before use if you are taking a prescription drug. Antacids may interact with certain prescription drugs.
Stop use and ask a doctor if symptoms last for more than 2 weeks
Keep out of reach of children.

Directions:
- shake well before using
- Adults/children 12 years and older: take 2 to 4 teaspoons four times a day or as directed by a physician

---

- do not take more than 12 teaspoonsful in 24 hours or use the maximum dosage for more than 2 weeks.
- Children under 12 years: consult a physician

To aid in establishing proper dosage schedules, the following information is provided:

MAALOX Max® Maximum Strength Antacid/Anti-Gas

	Per 2 Tsp. (10 mL) (Minimum Recommended Dosage)
Acid neutralizing capacity	38.8 mEq

Inactive Ingredients: butylparaben, carboxymethylcellulose sodium, D&C yellow #10 (lemon flavor only), flavor, hypromellose, microcrystalline cellulose, potassium citrate, propylparaben, purified water, saccharin sodium, sorbitol.

Professional Labeling
Indications: As an antacid for symptomatic relief of hyperacidity associated with the diagnosis of peptic ulcer, gastritis, peptic esophagitis, gastric hyperacidity, or hiatal hernia. As an antiflatulent to alleviate the symptoms of gas, including postoperative gas pain.
Warnings: Prolonged use of aluminum-containing antacids in patients with renal failure may result in or worsen dialysis osteomalacia. Elevated tissue aluminum levels contribute to the development of the dialysis encephalopathy and osteomalacia syndromes. Small amounts of aluminum are absorbed from the gastrointestinal tract and renal excretion of aluminum is impaired in renal failure. Aluminum is not well removed by dialysis because it is bound to albumin and transferrin, which do not cross dialysis membranes. As a result, aluminum is deposited in bone, and dialysis osteomalacia may develop when large amounts of aluminum are ingested orally by patients with impaired renal function.
Aluminum forms insoluble complexes with phosphate in the gastrointestinal tract, thus decreasing phosphate absorp-

Maalox Max® Maximum Strength Antacid/Anti-Gas		
Active Ingredients	**Per Tsp. (5 mL)**	**Purpose**
Aluminum Hydroxide (equivalent to dried gel, USP)	400 mg	antacid
Magnesium Hydroxide	400 mg	antacid
Simethicone	40 mg	antigas

tion. Prolonged use of aluminum-containing antacids by normophosphatemic patients may result in hypophosphatemia if phosphate intake is not adequate. In its more severe forms, hypophosphatemia can lead to anorexia, malaise, muscle weakness, and osteomalacia.

Advantages: In addition to the fast acting antacid ingredients, Aluminum Hydroxide and Magnesium Hydroxide, MAALOX Max® Maximum Strength Antacid/Antigas contains the powerful antigas ingredient, simethicone, to provide concurrent fast relief from discomfort associated with gas.

How Supplied:
MAALOX MAX® MAXIMUM STRENGTH ANTACID/ANTI-GAS Liquid Oral Suspension Antacid/Anti-Gas
Lemon is available in plastic bottles of 12 fl. oz. (355 mL), and 26 fl. oz. (769 mL).
Cherry is available in plastic bottles of 12 fl. oz. (355 mL) and 26 fl. oz. (769 mL).
Mint is available in plastic bottles of 12 fl. oz. (355 mL) and.
Vanilla Crème is available in Plastic Bottles of 12 fl. oz. (355 mL).
Wild Berry is available in Plastic Bottles of 12 fl. oz. (355 mL).
Shown in Product Identification Guide, page 513

MAALOX®
Regular Strength Liquid Antacid/Anti-Gas

Liquids
• Cooling Mint
• Smooth Cherry
[See table above]

Uses: For the relief of
• acid indigestion
• heartburn
• sour stomach
• upset stomach associated with these symptoms
• bloating and pressure commonly referred to as gas

Warnings:
Ask a doctor before use if you have kidney disease
Ask a doctor or pharmacist before use if you are taking a prescription drug. Antacids may interact with certain prescription drugs.
Stop use and ask a doctor if symptoms last for more than 2 weeks
Keep out of reach of children.

Directions:
• shake well before using
• Adults/children 12 years and older: take 2 to 4 teaspoons four times a day or as directed by a physician
• do not take more than 16 teaspoonsful in 24 hours or use the maximum dosage for more than 2 weeks.
• Children under 12 years: consult a physician

Inactive Ingredients: butylparaben, carboxymethylcellulose sodium, flavor, hypromellose, microcrystalline cellulose, propylparaben, purified water, saccharin sodium, sorbitol.

Drug Facts

Active Ingredients	Maalox Suspension 5 mL teaspoon	Purpose
Aluminum Hydroxide (equivalent to dried gel, USP)	200 mg	Antacid
Magnesium Hydroxide	200 mg	Antacid
Simethicone	20 mg	Antigas

Maalox® Suspension Per 2 Tsp. (10 mL) (Minimum Recommended Dosage)	
Acid neutralizing capacity	19.4 mEq

Professional Labeling
Indications: As an antacid for symptomatic relief of hyperacidity associated with the diagnosis of peptic ulcer, gastritis, peptic esophagitis, gastric hyperacidity, or hiatal hernia. As an antiflatulent to alleviate the symptoms of gas, including postoperative gas pain.

Warnings: Prolonged use of aluminum-containing antacids in patients with renal failure may result in or worsen dialysis osteomalacia. Elevated tissue aluminum levels contribute to the development of the dialysis encephalopathy and osteomalacia syndromes. Small amounts of aluminum are absorbed from the gastrointestinal tract and renal excretion of aluminum is impaired in renal failure. Aluminum is not well removed by dialysis because it is bound to albumin and transferrin, which do not cross dialysis membranes. As a result, aluminum is deposited in bone, and dialysis osteomalacia may develop when large amounts of aluminum are ingested orally by patients with impaired renal function. Aluminum forms insoluble complexes with phosphate in the gastrointestinal tract, thus decreasing phosphate absorption. Prolonged use of aluminum-containing antacids by normophosphatemic patients may result in hypophosphatemia if phosphate intake is not adequate. In its more severe forms, hypophosphatemia can lead to anorexia, malaise, muscle weakness, and osteomalacia.

Advantages: In addition to the fast acting antacid ingredients, Aluminum Hydroxide and Magnesium Hydroxide, MAALOX® Regular Strength Antacid/Antigas contains the powerful antigas ingredient, simethicone, to provide concurrent fast relief from discomfort associated with gas.

How Supplied:
Maalox® Cooling Mint Suspension is available in plastic bottles of 5 oz. (148 mL), 12 oz. (355 mL) and 26 oz. (769 mL)

Maalox® Smooth Cherry Suspension is available in plastic bottles of 12 oz. (355 mL)
Shown in Product Identification Guide, page 513

MAXIMUM STRENGTH MAALOX TOTAL STOMACH RELIEF®
Bismuth Subsalicylate/Upset Stomach Reliever Peppermint

Drug Facts

Active Ingredient: (in each 15 mL*)	Purpose:
Bismuth subsalicylate 525 mg	Upset stomach reliever

*15 mL = 1 tablespoon

Uses: • upset stomach • heartburn • nausea • fullness • indigestion

Warnings:
Reye's syndrome: Children and teenagers who have or are recovering from chicken pox or flu-like symptoms should not use this product. When using this product, if changes in behavior with nausea and vomiting occur, consult a doctor because these symptoms could be an early sign of Reye's syndrome, a rare but serious illness.
Allergy alert: Do not take this product if you are: • allergic to salicylates (including aspirin)
Ask a doctor or pharmacist before use if you are • taking a prescription drug for anticoagulation (blood thinning), diabetes, gout, or arthritis • taking other salicylate-containing products (such as aspirin)
When using this product a temporary, but harmless, darkening of the stool and/or tongue may occur
Stop use and ask a doctor if
• symptoms last more than 2 days
• ringing in the ears or a loss of hearing occurs
If pregnant or breast-feeding, ask a health care professional before use.

Continued on next page

***Information* on Novartis Consumer Health, Inc. *products appearing on these pages is effective as of November 2004.*

Maalox Total—Cont.

Keep out of reach of children. In case of overdose, get medical help or contact a poison control center right away.

Directions: • shake well before using
• adults and children 12 years of age and older: 2 tablespoons (30 mL) every 1/2 hour to 1 hour, as required, not to exceed 8 tablespoons (120 mL) in 24 hours.
• children under 12 years of age: ask a doctor

Other Information:
• **each tablespoon contains:** sodium 3.3 mg
• each tablespoon contains: salicylate 232 mg
• store at controlled room temperature 20–25°C (68–77°F)
• keep tightly closed and avoid freezing

Inactive Ingredients: carboxymethylcellulose sodium, ethyl alcohol, flavor, methylparaben, microcrystalline cellulose, propylene glycol, propylparaben, purified water, salicylic acid, sodium salicylate, sorbitol, sucralose, xanthan gum
Questions? call **1-800-452-0051** 24 hours a day, 7 days a week.
U.S. Patent No. 5,904,973
Made in Canada

MAXIMUM STRENGTH MAALOX® TOTAL STOMACH RELIEF®
Bismuth Subsalicylate/Upset Stomach Reliever
Strawberry

Drug Facts

Active Ingredient: (in each 15 mL*)	Purpose:
Bismuth subsalicylate 525 mg	Upset stomach reliever

---
* 15 mL = 1 tablespoon

Uses: • upset stomach • heartburn • nausea • fullness • indigestion

Warnings:
Reye's syndrome: Children and teenagers who have or are recovering from chicken pox or flu-like symptoms should not use this product. When using this product, if changes in behavior with nausea and vomiting occur, consult a doctor because these symptoms could be an early sign of Reye's syndrome, a rare but serious illness.
Allergy alert: Do not take this product if you are allergic to salicylates (including aspirin)
Ask a doctor or pharmacist before use if you are
• taking a prescription drug for anticoagulation (blood thinning), diabetes, gout, or arthritis
• taking other salicylate – containing products (such as aspirin)
When using this product a temporary, but harmless, darkening of the stool and/or tongue may occur

Stop use and ask a doctor if
• symptoms last more than 2 days
• ringing in the ears or a loss of hearing occurs
If pregnant or breast-feeding, ask a health care professional before use.
Keep out of reach of children. In case of overdose, get medical help or contact a poison control center right away.

Directions: • shake well before using
• adults and children 12 years of age and older: 2 tablespoons (30 mL) every ½ hour to 1 hour, as required, not to exceed 8 tablespoons (120 mL) in 24 hours
• children under 12 years of age: ask a doctor

Other Information:
• **each tablespoon contains:** sodium 3.3 mg
• each tablespoon contains: salicylate 232 mg
• store at controlled room temperature 20–25°C (68–77°F)
• keep tightly closed and avoid freezing

Inactive Ingredients: carboxymethylcellulose sodium, flavor, methylparaben, microcrystalline cellulose, propylene glycol, propylparaben, purified water, salicylic acid, sodium salicylate, sorbitol, sucralose, xanthan gum
Questions? call **1-800-452-0051** 24 hours a day, 7 days a week.
U.S. Patent No. 5,904,973
Made in Canada
Shown in Product Identification Guide, page 513

Chewable MAALOX® Regular Strength Antacid
Calcium Carbonate
Chewable Tablets
Lemon and Wild Berry
flavors Chewable Tablets

MAALOX® Regular Strength

Drug Facts

Active Ingredient: (in each tablet)	Purpose:
Calcium carbonate 600 mg	Antacid

Uses: For the relief of
• acid indigestion
• heartburn
• sour stomach
• upset stomach associated with these symptoms

Warnings:
Ask a doctor or pharmacist before use if you are: presently taking a prescription drug. Antacids may interact with certain prescription drugs
Stop use and ask a doctor if symptoms last for more than 2 weeks.
Keep out of reach of children.

Directions:
• Chew 1 to 2 tablets as symptoms occur or as directed by a physician
• do not take more than 12 tablets in a 24-hour period or use the maximum

dosage for more than 2 weeks except under the advice and supervision of a physician

Other Information:
• Phenylketonurics: Contains Phenylalanine, .5 mg per tablet
• store at controlled room temperature 20–25°C (68–77°F)
• keep tightly closed and dry
• Acid neutralizing capacity (per 2 tablets) is 21.6 mEq.

Inactive Ingredients: aspartame, colloidal silicon dioxide, croscarmellose sodium, D&C Red #30 aluminum lake, D&C Yellow #10 aluminum lake, dextrose, FD&C Blue #1 aluminum lake, flavors, magnesium stearate, maltodextrin, mannitol, pregelatinized starch.

How Supplied:
Lemon — Plastic Bottles of 85 ct. Tablets.
Wild Berry — Plastic Bottles of 45 ct. Tablets.
Questions? call **1-800-452-0051** 24 hours a day, 7 days a week.
Shown in Product Identification Guide, page 513

Chewable MAALOX Max® Maximum Strength
Antacid/Antigas.
Calcium Carbonate and Simethicone
Chewable Tablets
Assorted, Lemon and Wild Berry
Flavors. Quick Dissolving Tablets

MAALOX Max® Maximum Strength

Drug Facts:

Active Ingredients: (in each tablet)	Purpose:
Calcium carbonate 1000 mg	Antacid
Simethicone 60 mg	Antigas

Uses: For the relief of
• acid indigestion
• heartburn
• sour stomach
• upset stomach associated with these symptoms
• bloating and pressure commonly referred to as gas

Warnings:
Ask a doctor or pharmacist before use if you are: presently taking a prescription drug. Antacids may interact with certain prescription drugs.
Stop use and ask a doctor if: symptoms last for more than 2 weeks.
Keep out of reach of children.

Directions:
• Chew 1 to 2 tablets as symptoms occur or as directed by a physician
• do not take more than 8 tablets in a 24-hour period or use the maximum dosage for more than 2 weeks except under the advice and supervision of a physician

Other Information:
• store at controlled room temperature 20–25°C (68–77°F)
• keep tightly closed and dry

- Acid neutralizing capacity (per 2 tablets) is 34mEq.

Inactive Ingredients: acesulfame K, colloidal silicon dioxide, croscarmellose sodium, D&C Red #30 aluminum lake, D&C Yellow #10 aluminum lake, dextrose, flavors, magnesium stearate, maltodextrin, mannitol, pregelatinized starch.

How Supplied:
Lemon — Plastic Bottles of 35 and 65 Tablets.
Wild Berry — Plastic Bottles of 35 and 65 Tablets.
Assorted — Plastic Bottles of 35, 65 and 90 Tablets.
Questions? call 1-800-452-0051 24 hours a day, 7 days a week.

Shown in Product Identification Guide, page 513

THERAFLU® Severe Cold Caplets
Pain Reliever-Fever Reducer (Acetaminophen)/Antihistamine (Chlorpheniramine) Cough Suppressant (Dextromethorphan)/ Nasal Decongestant (Pseudoephedrine)

Drug Facts
Active Ingredients:
(in each caplet) **Purpose:**
Acetaminophen
  500 mg .... Pain reliever/
              Fever reducer
Chlorpheniramine maleate
  2 mg .... Antihistamine
Dextromethorphan HBr
  15 mg .... Cough suppressant
Pseudoephedrine HCl
  30 mg .... Nasal decongestant

Uses: temporarily relieves:
- headache • minor aches and pains • runny nose • sneezing • itchy nose or throat • itchy, watery eyes due to hay fever • minor sore throat pain • nasal and sinus congestion • cough due to minor throat and bronchial irritation
- temporarily reduces fever

Warnings:
Alcohol Warning: If you consume 3 or more alcoholic drinks every day, ask your doctor whether you should take acetaminophen or any other pain relievers/fever reducers. Acetaminophen may cause liver damage.
Do not use • if you are now taking a prescription monamine oxidase inhibitor (MAOI) (certain drugs for depression), psychiatric, or emotional conditions, or Parkinson's disease), or for 2 weeks after stopping the MAOI drug. If you do not know if your prescription drug contains an MAOI, ask a doctor or pharmacist before taking this product.
- with any other product containing acetaminophen (**see Overdose Warning**)

Ask a doctor before use if you have
- heart disease • high blood pressure
- thyroid disease • diabetes • glaucoma
- a breathing problem such as emphysema, asthma, or chronic bronchitis
- trouble urinating due to an enlarged prostate gland
- cough that occurs with smoking, too much phlegm (mucus) or chronic cough that lasts

Ask a doctor or pharmacist before use if you are taking sedatives or tranquilizers.

When using this product • do not take more than directed • avoid alcoholic drinks
- may cause marked drowsiness
- alcohol, sedatives, and tranquilizers may increase drowsiness
- be careful when driving a motor vehicle or operating machinery
- excitability may occur, especially in children

Stop use and ask a doctor if • nervousness, dizziness, or sleeplessness occurs
- pain, cough or nasal congestion gets worse or lasts more than 7 days
- fever gets worse or lasts more than 3 days
- redness or swelling is present
- new symptoms occur
- sore throat is severe, persists for more than 2 days, is accompanied or followed by fever, headache, rash, nausea, or vomiting
- cough comes back or occurs with rash or headache that lasts. These could be signs of a serious condition.

If pregnant or breast-feeding, ask a health care professional before use.
Keep out of reach of children.
Overdose Warning: Taking more than the recommended dose can cause serious health problems, including serious liver damage. In case of overdose, get medical help or contact a poison control center right away. Prompt medical attention is critical for adults as well as for children even if you do not notice any signs or symptoms.

Directions:
- do not use more than directed (**see Overdose Warning)**
- take every 6 hours; not more than 8 caplets in 24 hours
- adults and children 12 years of age and over: 2 caplets every 6 hours
- children under 12 years of age: consult a doctor

Other Information: • each caplet contains: **sodium 6 mg** • store at controlled room temperature 20–25°C (68–77°F)

Inactive Ingredients: colloidal silicon dioxide, croscarmellose sodium, D&C Yellow 10 aluminum lake, FD&C Blue 1 aluminum lake, FD&C Yellow 6 aluminum lake, gelatin, hydroxypropyl cellulose, hypromellose, lactose, magnesium stearate, methylparaben, polydextrose, polyethylene glycol, pregelatinized starch, titanium dioxide, triacetin

How Supplied: 24 coated caplets
Shown in Product Identification Guide, page 514

THERAFLU® Severe Cold Non-Drowsy Caplets
Pain Reliever-Fever Reducer (Acetaminophen)/Cough Suppressant (Dextromethorphan) Nasal Decongestant (Pseudoephedrine)

Drug Facts
Active Ingredients:
(in each caplet) **Purpose:**
Acetaminophen 500 mg ... Pain reliever/
              Fever reducer
Dextromethorphan
  HBr 15 mg .... Cough suppressant
Pseudoephedrine
  HCl 30 mg .... Nasal decongestant

Uses: temporarily relieves:
- minor aches and pains • minor sore throat pain • nasal and sinus congestion
- cough due to minor throat and bronchial irritation

Warnings:
Alcohol Warning: If you consume 3 or more alcoholic drinks every day, ask your doctor whether you should take acetaminophen or any other pain relievers/fever reducers. Acetaminophen may cause liver damage.
Do not use • if you are now taking a prescription monoamine oxidase inhibitor (MAOI) (certain drugs for depression, psychiatric, or emotional conditions, or Parkinson's disease), or for 2 weeks after stopping the MAOI drug. If you do not know if your prescription drug contains an MAOI, ask a doctor or pharmacist before taking this product.
- with any other product containing acetaminophen (**see Overdose Warning**)

Ask a doctor before use if you have
- heart disease • high blood pressure
- thyroid disease • diabetes • glaucoma
- a breathing problem such as emphysema, asthma, or chronic bronchitis
- trouble urinating due to an enlarged prostate gland
- cough that occurs with smoking, too much phlegm (mucus) or chronic cough that lasts

When using this product • do not take more than directed

Stop use and ask a doctor if • nervousness, dizziness, or sleeplessness occurs
- pain, cough or nasal congestion gets worse or lasts more than 7 days
- fever gets worse or lasts more than 3 days
- redness or swelling is present
- new symptoms occur
- sore throat is severe, persists for more than 2 days, is accompanied or followed by fever, headache, rash, nausea, or vomiting
- cough comes back or occurs with rash or headache that lasts. These could be signs of a serious condition.

Continued on next page

Information on Novartis Consumer Health, Inc. products appearing on these pages is effective as of November 2003.

Theraflu Severe Cold—Cont.

If pregnant or breast-feeding, ask a health care professional before use.
Keep out of reach of children.
Overdose Warning: Taking more than the recommended dose can cause serious health problems, including serious liver damage. In case of overdose, get medical help or contact a poison control center right away. Prompt medical attention is critical for adults as well as for children even if you do not notice any signs or symptoms.

Directions:
• do not use more than directed **(see Overdose Warning)**
• take every 6 hours; not more than 8 caplets in 24 hours
• adults and children 12 years of age and over: 2 caplets every 6 hours
• children under 12 years of age: consult a doctor
Other Information: • each caplet contains: **sodium 6 mg**
• store at controlled room temperature 20–25°C (68–77°F)

Inactive Ingredients: colloidal silicon dioxide, croscarmellose sodium, D&C Yellow 10 aluminum lake, FD&C Red 40 aluminum lake, FD&C Yellow 6 aluminum lake, gelatin, hydroxypropyl cellulose, hypromellose, lactose, magnesium stearate, methylparaben, polydextrose, polyethylene glycol, pregelatinized starch, titanium dioxide, triacetin

How Supplied: 12 coated caplets
Shown in Product Identification Guide, page 514

THERAFLU® Cold & Cough
Pain Reliever-Fever Reducer (Acetaminophen)
Antihistamine (Chlorpheniramine)
Cough Suppressant (Dextromethorphan)
Nasal Decongestant (Pseudoephedrine)

Drug Facts

Active Ingredients
(in each packet):   **Purpose:**
Acetaminophen
650 mg ..... Pain reliever/Fever reducer
Chlorpheniramine maleate
4 mg .... Antihistamine
Dextromethorphan HBr
20 mg .... Cough suppressant
Pseudoephedrine HCl
60 mg .... Nasal decongestant

Uses: temporarily relieves: • headache • sneezing • runny nose • minor aches and pains • itchy nose or throat • itchy, watery eyes due to hay fever • minor sore throat pain • nasal and sinus congestion • cough due to minor throat and bronchial irritation

Warnings:
Alcohol Warning: If you consume 3 or more alcoholic drinks every day, ask your doctor whether you should take acetamin-

ophen or other pain relievers/fever reducers. Acetaminophen may cause liver damage.
Do not use • if you are now taking a prescription monoamine oxidase inhibitor (MAOI) (certain drugs for depression, psychiatric, or emotional conditions, or Parkinson's disease), or for 2 weeks after stopping the MAOI drug. If you do not know if your prescription drug contains an MAOI, ask a doctor or pharmacist before taking this product.
• with any other product containing acetaminophen **(see Overdose Warning)**
Ask a doctor before use if you have heart disease • high blood pressure • thyroid disease • diabetes • glaucoma • a breathing problem such as emphysema, asthma, or chronic bronchitis • trouble urinating due to an enlarged prostate gland • cough that occurs with smoking, too much phlegm (mucus) or chronic cough that lasts
Ask a doctor or pharmacist before use if you are taking sedatives or tranquilizers.
When using this product • do not take more than directed • avoid alcoholic drinks • may cause marked drowsiness • alcohol, sedatives, and tranquilizers may increase drowsiness • be careful when driving a motor vehicle or operating machinery • excitability may occur, especially in children
Stop use and ask a doctor if • nervousness, dizziness, or sleeplessness occurs
• pain, cough or nasal congestion gets worse or lasts more than 7 days
• fever gets worse or lasts more than 3 days
• redness or swelling is present
• new symptoms occur
• sore throat is severe, persists for more than 2 days, is accompanied or followed by fever, headache, rash, nausea, or vomiting
• cough comes back or occurs with rash or headache that lasts. These could be signs of a serious condition.
If pregnant or breast-feeding, ask a health care professional before use.
Keep out of reach of children.
Overdose Warning: Taking more than the recommended dose can cause serious health problems, including serious liver damage. In case of overdose, get medical help or contact a poison control center right away. Prompt medical attention is critical for adults as well as for children even if you do not notice any signs or symptoms.

Directions:
• do not use more than directed **(see Overdose Warning)**
• take every 4–6 hours; not to exceed 4 packets in 24 hours or as directed by a doctor
• adults and children 12 years of age and over: dissolve contents of one packet into 6 oz. hot water. Sip while hot. Consume entire drink within 10–15 minutes.
• children under 12 years of age: consult a doctor
Sweeten to taste if desired.
If using a microwave, add contents of one packet to 6 oz. of cool water; stir briskly before and after heating. Do not overheat.

Other Information:
• each packet contains: **sodium 19 mg**
• Phenylketonurics: Contains Phenylalanine 13 mg per adult dose
• store at controlled room temperature 20-25°C (68-77°F)

How Supplied: 6 packets

Inactive Ingredients: acesulfame K, aspartame, citric acid, D&C yellow 10, flavors, maltodextrin, silicon dioxide, sodium citrate, sucrose, tribasic calcium phosphate
Questions? call **1-800-452-0051** 24 hours a day, 7 days a week.

THERAFLU® Cold & Sore Throat
Pain Reliever-Fever Reducer (Acetaminophen)
Antihistamine (Chlorpheniramine)
Nasal Decongestant (Pseudoephedrine)

Drug Facts

Active Ingredients
(in each packet):   **Purpose:**
Acetaminophen
650 mg .... Pain reliever/ Fever reducer
Chlorpheniramine maleate
4 mg .... Antihistamine
Pseudoephedrine HCl
60 mg .... Nasal decongestant

Uses: temporarily relieves • headache • minor aches and pains • runny nose • itchy nose or throat • fever • minor sore throat pain • sneezing • nasal and sinus congestion • itchy, watery eyes due to hay fever

Warnings:
Alcohol Warning: If you consume 3 or more alcoholic drinks every day, ask your doctor whether you should take acetaminophen or other pain relievers/ fever reducers. Acetaminophen may cause liver damage.
Do not use • if you are now taking a prescription monoamine oxidase inhibitor (MAOI) (certain drugs for depression, psychiatric, or emotional conditions, or Parkinson's disease), or for 2 weeks after stopping the MAOI drug. If you do not know if your prescription drug contains an MAOI, ask a doctor or pharmacist before taking this product.
• with any other product containing acetaminophen **(see Overdose Warning)**
Ask a doctor before use if you have
• heart disease • high blood pressure
• thyroid disease • diabetes • glaucoma
• a breathing problem such as emphysema or chronic bronchitis
• trouble urinating due to an enlarged prostate gland
Ask a doctor or pharmacist before use if you are taking sedatives or tranquilizers.
When using this product • do not take more than directed • avoid alcoholic drinks • may cause marked drowsiness • alcohol, sedatives, and tranquilizers may increase drowsiness • be careful when driving a motor vehicle or operat-

ing machinery • excitability may occur, especially in children

Stop use and ask a doctor if • nervousness, dizziness, or sleeplessness occurs
• pain, cough or nasal congestion gets worse or lasts more than 7 days
• fever gets worse or lasts more than 3 days
• redness or swelling is present
• sore throat is severe, persists for more than 2 days, is accompanied or followed by fever, headache, rash, nausea, or vomiting
• new symptoms occur. These could be signs of a serious condition.

If pregnant or breast-feeding, ask a health care professional before use.

Keep out of reach of children.

Overdose Warning: Taking more than the recommended dose can cause serious health problems, including serious liver damage. In case of overdose, get medical help or contact a poison control center right away. Prompt medical attention is critical for adults as well as for children even if you do not notice any signs or symptoms.

Directions:
• do not use more than directed **(see Overdose Warning)**
• take every 4 to 6 hours; not to exceed 4 packets in 24 hours or as directed by a doctor
• adults and children 12 years of age and over: dissolve contents of one packet into 6 oz. hot water. Sip while hot. Consume entire drink within 10–15 minutes.
• children under 12 years of age: consult a doctor

Sweeten to taste if desired.

If using a microwave, add contents of one packet to 6 oz. of cool water; stir briskly before and after heating. Do not overheat.

Other Information:
• each packet contains: **sodium 19 mg**
• Phenylketonurics: Contains Phenylalanine 11 mg per adult dose
• store at controlled room temperature 20-25°C (68-77°F)

How Supplied: 6 Packets

Inactive Ingredients: acesulfame K, aspartame, citric acid, D&C Yellow 10, flavors, maltodextrin, silicon dioxide, sodium citrate, sucrose, tribasic calcium phosphate

Questions? call **1-800-452-0051** 24 hours a day, 7 days a week.

THERAFLU®
Flu & Chest Congestion
Pain Reliever-Fever Reducer
(Acetaminophen)
Cough Suppressant
(Dextromethorphan)
Expectorant (Guaifenesin)
Nasal Decongestant
(Pseudoephedrine)

Drug Facts

Active Ingredients (in each packet): **Purpose:**
Acetaminophen
1000 mg .... Pain reliever/ Fever reducer
Dextromethorphan HBr
30 mg .... Cough suppressant
Guaifenesin
400 mg .... Expectorant
Pseudoephedrine HCl
60 mg .... Nasal decongestant

Uses: temporarily relieves:
• minor aches and pains • headache
• minor sore throat pain • nasal congestion • chest congestion by loosening phlegm to help clear bronchial passageways
• temporarily reduces fever

Warnings: Alcohol Warning: If you consume 3 or more alcoholic drinks every day, ask your doctor whether you should take acetaminophen or other pain relievers/fever reducers. Acetaminophen may cause liver damage.

Do not use • if you are now taking a prescription monoamine oxidase inhibitor (MAOI) (certain drugs for depression, psychiatric, or emotional conditions, or Parkinson's disease), or for 2 weeks after stopping the MAOI drug. If you do not know if your prescription drug contains an MAOI, ask a doctor or pharmacist before taking this product.

• with any other product containing acetaminophen **(see Overdose Warning)**

Ask a doctor before use if you have
• heart disease • high blood pressure
• thyroid disease • diabetes • a breathing problem such as emphysema or chronic bronchitis
• trouble urinating due to an enlarged prostate gland
• cough that occurs with smoking, too much phlegm (mucus) or chronic cough that lasts

When using this product • do not use more than directed

Stop use and ask a doctor if • nervousness, dizziness, or sleeplessness occurs
• pain, cough or nasal congestion gets worse or lasts more than 7 days
• fever gets worse or lasts more than 3 days
• redness or swelling is present
• new symptoms occur
• sore throat is severe, persists for more than 2 days, is accompanied or followed by fever, headache, rash, nausea, or vomiting
• cough comes back or occurs with rash or headache that lasts. These could be signs of a serious condition.

If pregnant or breast-feeding, ask a health care professional before use.

Keep out of reach of children.

Overdose Warning: Taking more than the recommended dose can cause serious health problems, including serious liver damage. In case of overdose, get medical help or contact a poison control center right away. Prompt medical attention is critical for adults as well as for children even if you do not notice any signs or symptoms.

Directions:
• do not use more than directed **(see Overdose Warning)**

• take every 6 hours; not to exceed 4 packets in 24 hours or as directed by a doctor.
• adults and children 12 years of age and over: dissolve contents of one packet into 6 oz. hot water. Sip while hot. Consume entire drink within 10–15 minutes.
• children under 12 years of age: consult a doctor

Sweeten to taste if desired.

If using a microwave, add contents of one packet to 6 oz. of cool water; stir briskly before and after heating. Do not overheat.

Other Information:
• each packet contains: **sodium 15 mg**
• Phenylketonurics: Contains Phenylalanine 24 mg per adult dose
• store at controlled room temperature 20-25°C (68-77°F)

How Supplied: 6 Packets

Inactive Ingredients: acesulfame K, aspartame, calcium phosphate, citric acid, D&C Yellow 10, FD&C Red 40, flavors, maltodextrin, silicon dioxide, sodium citrate, sucrose

Questions? call **1-800-452-0051** 24 hours a day, 7 days a week.

THERAFLU® Flu & Sore Throat
Pain Reliever-Fever Reducer
(Acetaminophen)
Antihistamine (Chlorpheniramine)
Nasal Decongestant
(Pseudoephedrine)

Drug Facts

Active Ingredients (in each packet): **Purpose:**
Acetaminophen
1000 mg .... Pain reliever/ Fever reducer
Chlorpheniramine maleate
4 mg .... Antihistamine
Pseudoephedrine
HCl 60 mg .... Nasal decongestant

Uses: temporarily relieves:
• headache • minor aches and pains
• runny nose • itchy nose or throat
• minor sore throat pain • sneezing
• nasal and sinus congestion • itchy, watery eyes due to hay fever
• temporarily reduces fever

Warnings:

Alcohol Warning: If you consume 3 or more alcoholic drinks every day, ask your doctor whether you should take acetaminophen or other pain relievers/fever reducers. Acetaminophen may cause liver damage.

Do not use • if you are now taking a prescription monoamine oxidase inhibitor

Continued on next page

Information on Novartis Consumer Health, Inc. products appearing on these pages is effective as of November 2003.

Theraflu Flu & Sore Th.—Cont.

(MAOI) (certain drugs for depression, psychiatric, or emotional conditions, or Parkinson's disease), or for 2 weeks after stopping the MAOI drug. If you do not know if your prescription drug contains an MAOI, ask a doctor or pharmacist before taking this product.
• with any other product containing acetaminophen (see **Overdose Warning**)

Ask a doctor before use if you have
• heart disease • high blood pressure
• thyroid disease • diabetes • glaucoma
• a breathing problem such as emphysema or chronic bronchitis
• trouble urinating due to an enlarged prostate gland

Ask a doctor or pharmacist before use if you are taking sedatives or tranquilizers.

When using this product • do not take more than directed • avoid alcoholic drinks • may cause marked drowsiness • alcohol, sedatives, and tranquilizers may increase drowsiness • be careful when driving a motor vehicle or operating machinery • excitability may occur, especially in children

Stop use and ask a doctor if • nervousness, dizziness, or sleeplessness occurs
• pain, cough or nasal congestion gets worse or lasts more than 7 days
• fever gets worse or lasts more than 3 days
• redness or swelling is present
• sore throat is severe, persists for more than 2 days, is accompanied or followed by fever, headache, rash, nausea, or vomiting
• new symptoms occur. These could be signs of a serious condition.

If pregnant or breast-feeding, ask a health care professional before use.

Keep out of reach of children.

Overdose Warning: Taking more than the recommended dose can cause serious health problems, including serious liver damage. In case of overdose, get medical help or contact a poison control center right away. Prompt medical attention is critical for adults as well as for children even if you do not notice any signs or symptoms.

Directions:
• do not use more than directed (see **Overdose Warning**)
• take every 6 hours; not to exceed 4 packets in 24 hours or as directed by a doctor
• adults and children 12 years of age and over: dissolve contents of one packet into 6 oz. hot water. Sip while hot. Consume entire drink within 10–15 minutes.
• children under 12 years of age: consult a doctor
Sweeten to taste if desired.
• If using a microwave, add contents of one packet to 6 oz. of cool water; stir briskly before and after heating. Do not overheat.

Other Information:
• each packet contains: **sodium 12 mg**
• Phenylketonurics: Contains Phenylalanine 22 mg per adult dose

• store at controlled room temperature 20-25°C (68-77°F)

How Supplied: 6 Packets

Inactive Ingredients: acesulfame K, aspartame, citric acid, D&C Yellow 10, FD&C Blue 1, FD&C Red 40, flavors, maltodextrin, silicon dioxide, sodium citrate, sucrose, tribasic calcium phosphate
Questions? call **1-800-452-0051**
24 hours a day, 7 days a week.

THERAFLU ® Severe Cold
Pain Reliever-Fever Reducer (Acetaminophen)
Antihistamine (Chlorpheniramine)
Cough Suppressant (Dextromethorphan)
Nasal Decongestant (Pseudoephedrine)

Drug Facts

Active Ingredients
(in each packet):   **Purpose:**
Acetaminophen
    1000 mg .... Pain reliever/
                                Fever reducer
Chlorpheniramine maleate
    4 mg .... Antihistamine
Dextromethorphan HBr
    30 mg .... Cough suppressant
Pseudoephedrine HCl
    60 mg .... Nasal decongestant

Uses: temporarily relieves: • headache • minor aches and pains • runny nose • sneezing • itchy nose or throat • itchy, watery eyes due to hay fever • minor sore throat pain • nasal and sinus congestion • cough due to minor throat and bronchial irritation • temporarily reduces fever

Warnings:

Alcohol Warning: If you consume 3 or more alcoholic drinks every day, ask your doctor whether you should take acetaminophen or other pain relievers/fever reducers. Acetaminophen may cause liver damage.

Do not use • if you are now taking a prescription monoamine oxidase inhibitor (MAOI) (certain drugs for depression, psychiatric, or emotional conditions, or Parkinson's disease), or for 2 weeks after stopping the MAOI drug. If you do not know if your prescription drug contains an MAOI, ask a doctor or pharmacist before taking this product.
• with any other product containing acetaminophen (see **Overdose Warning**)

Ask a doctor before use if you have
• heart disease • high blood pressure
• thyroid disease • diabetes • glaucoma
• a breathing problem such as emphysema, asthma, or chronic bronchitis
• trouble urinating due to an enlarged prostate gland
• cough that occurs with smoking, too much phlegm (mucus) or chronic cough that lasts

Ask a doctor or pharmacist before use if you are taking sedatives or tranquilizers.

When using this product • do not use more than directed • avoid alcoholic drinks
• may cause marked drowsiness • alcohol, sedatives, and tranquilizers may increase drowsiness
• be careful when driving a motor vehicle or operating machinery
• excitability may occur, especially in children

Stop use and ask a doctor if • nervousness, dizziness, or sleeplessness occurs
• pain, cough or nasal congestion gets worse or lasts more than 7 days
• fever gets worse or lasts more than 3 days
• redness or swelling is present
• new symptoms occur
• sore throat is severe, persists for more than 2 days, is accompanied or followed by fever, headache, rash, nausea, or vomiting
• cough comes back or occurs with rash or headache that lasts. These could be signs of a serious condition.

If pregnant or breast-feeding, ask a health care professional before use.

Keep out of reach of children.

Overdose Warning: Taking more than the recommended dose can cause serious health problems, including serious liver damage. In case of overdose, get medical help or contact a poison control center right away. Prompt medical attention is critical for adults as well as for children even if you do not notice any signs or symptoms.

Directions:
• do not use more than directed (see **Overdose Warning**)
• take every 6 hours; not to exceed 4 packets in 24 hours or as directed by a doctor
• adults and children 12 years of age and over: dissolve contents of one packet into 6 oz. hot water. Sip while hot. Consume entire drink within 10–15 minutes.
• children under 12 years of age: consult a doctor
Sweeten to taste if desired.
If using a microwave, add contents of one packet to 6 oz. of cool water; stir briskly before and after heating. Do not overheat.

Other Information:
• each packet contains: **sodium 19 mg**
• Phenylketonurics: Contains Phenylalanine 17 mg per adult dose
• store at controlled room temperature 20-25°C (68-77°F)

How Supplied: 6 Packets

Inactive Ingredients: acesulfame K, aspartame, citric acid, D&C yellow 10, flavors, maltodextrin, silicon dioxide, sodium citrate, sucrose, tribasic calcium phosphate

Questions? call **1-800-452-0051**
24 hours a day, 7 days a week.

Shown in Product Identification Guide, page 513

THERAFLU® Severe Cold
Non-Drowsy
**Pain Reliever-Fever Reducer
(Acetaminophen)
Cough Suppressant
(Dextromethorphan)
Nasal Decongestant
(Pseudoephedrine)**

Drug Facts

**Active Ingredients
(in each packet):**   **Purpose:**

Acetaminophen
   1000 mg .... Pain reliever/
                       Fever reducer
Dextromethorphan HBr
   30 mg .... Cough suppressant
Pseudoephedrine HCl
   60 mg .... Nasal decongestant

Uses: temporarily relieves: • minor
aches and pains
• minor sore throat pain • nasal and sinus congestion • headache
• cough due to minor throat and bronchial irritation
• temporarily reduces fever

Warnings:
Alcohol Warning: If you consume 3 or
more alcoholic drinks every day, ask your
doctor whether you should take acetaminophen or any other pain relievers/fever
reducers. Acetaminophen may cause
liver damage.
Do not use • if you are now taking a prescription monoamine oxidase inhibitor
(MAOI) (certain drugs for depression,
psychiatric, or emotional conditions, or
Parkinson's disease), or for 2 weeks after
stopping the MAOI drug. If you do not
know if your prescription drug contains
an MAOI, ask a doctor or pharmacist before taking this product.
• with any other product containing acetaminophen   **(see**   **Overdose
Warning)**
Ask a doctor before use if you have
• heart disease • high blood pressure
• thyroid disease • diabetes • glaucoma
• a breathing problem such as emphysema, asthma or chronic bronchitis
• trouble urinating due to an enlarged
prostate gland
• cough that occurs with smoking, too
much phlegm (mucus) or chronic
cough that lasts
When using this product • do not use
more than directed
Stop use and ask a doctor if • nervousness, dizziness, or sleeplessness occurs
• pain, cough or nasal congestion gets
worse or lasts more than 7 days
• fever gets worse or lasts more than 3
days
• redness or swelling is present
• new symptoms occur
• sore throat is severe, persists for more
than 2 days, is accompanied or followed by fever, headache, rash, nausea, or vomiting.
• cough comes back or occurs with rash
or headache that lasts. These could be
signs of a serious condition.
If pregnant or breast-feeding, ask a
health care professional before use.
Keep out of reach of children.
Overdose Warning: Taking more
than the recommended dose can cause

serious health problems, including serious liver damage. In case of overdose, get
medical help or contact a poison control
center right away. Prompt medical attention is critical for adults as well as for
children even if you do not notice any
signs or symptoms.

Directions:
• do not use more than directed (**see
Overdose Warning**)
• take every 6 hours; not to exceed 4
packets in 24 hours or as directed by a
doctor
• adults and children 12 years of age
and over: dissolve contents of one
packet into 6 oz. hot water. Sip while
hot. Consume entire drink within
10–15 minutes.
• children under 12 years of age: consult
a doctor
Sweeten to taste if desired.
If using a microwave, add contents of
one packet to 6 oz. of cool water; stir
briskly before and after heating. Do not
overheat.

Other Information:
• each packet contains: **sodium 19 mg**
• Phenylketonurics: Contains Phenylalanine 17 mg per adult dose
• store at controlled room temperature
20-25°C (68-77°F)

How Supplied: 6 Packets

Inactive Ingredients: acesulfame K,
aspartame, citric acid, D&C yellow 10,
flavors, maltodextrin, silicon dioxide, sodium citrate, sucrose, tribasic calcium
phosphate
Questions? call **1-800-452-0051**
24 hours a day, 7 days a week.

THERAFLU® Severe Cold & Cough
**Pain Reliever/Fever Reducer
(Acetaminophen)
Antihistamine (Chlorpheniramine)
Cough Suppressant
(Dextromethorphan)
Nasal Decongestant
(Pseudoephedrine)**

Drug Facts

**Active Ingredients
(in each packet):**   **Purpose:**
Acetaminophen
   1000 mg .... Pain reliever/
                       Fever reducer
Chlorpheniramine maleate
   4 mg .... Antihistamine
Dextromethorphan HBr
   30 mg .... Cough suppressant
Pseudoephedrine HCl
   60 mg .... Nasal decongestant

Uses: temporarily relieves
• headache • minor aches and pains
• runny nose • sneezing • itchy nose or
throat
• itchy, watery eyes due to hay fever
   • minor sore throat pain
• nasal and sinus congestion • cough
due to minor throat and bronchial
irritation
• temporarily reduces fever

Warnings:
Alcohol Warning: If you consume 3 or
more alcoholic drinks every day, ask

your doctor whether you should take
acetaminophen or other pain relievers/
fever reducers. Acetaminophen may
cause liver damage.
Do not use • if you are now taking a prescription monoamine oxidase inhibitor
(MAOI) (certain drugs for depression,
psychiatric, or emotional conditions, or
Parkinson's disease), or for 2 weeks after
stopping the MAOI drug. If you do not
know if your prescription drug contains
an MAOI, ask a doctor or pharmacist before taking this product.
• with any other product containing acetaminophen   **(see**   **Overdose
Warning)**
Ask a doctor before use if you have
• heart disease • high blood pressure
• thyroid disease • diabetes • glaucoma
• a breathing problem such as emphysema, asthma, or chronic bronchitis
• trouble urinating due to an enlarged
prostate gland
• cough that occurs with smoking, too
much phlegm (mucus) or chronic
cough that lasts
**Ask a doctor or pharmacist before use if
you are** taking sedatives or tranquilizers.
When using this product • do not use
more than directed • avoid alcoholic
drinks
• may cause marked drowsiness • alcohol, sedatives, and tranquilizers may
increase drowsiness
• be careful when driving a motor vehicle or operating machinery
• excitability may occur, especially in
children
Stop use and ask a doctor if • nervousness, dizziness, or sleeplessness occurs
• pain, cough or nasal congestion gets
worse or lasts more than 7 days
• fever gets worse or lasts more than 3
days
• redness or swelling is present
• new symptoms occur
• sore throat is severe, persists for more
than 2 days, is accompanied or followed by fever, headache, rash, nausea, or vomiting
• cough comes back or occurs with rash
or headache that lasts. These could be
signs of a serious condition.
If pregnant or breast-feeding, ask a
health care professional before use.
Keep out of reach of children.
Overdose Warning: Taking more
than the recommended dose can cause
serious health problems, including serious liver damage. In case of overdose, get
medical help or contact a poison control
center right away. Prompt medical attention is critical for adults as well as for
children even if you do not notice any
signs or symptoms.

Directions:
• do not use more than directed (**see
Overdose Warning**)

Continued on next page

Information on Novartis Consumer
Health, Inc. *products appearing on
these pages is effective as of
November 2003.*

Theraflu Cold & Cough—Cont.

- take every 6 hours; not to exceed 4 packets in 24 hours or as directed by a doctor
- adults and children 12 years of age and over: dissolve contents of one packet into 6 oz. hot water. Sip while hot. Consume entire drink within 10–15 minutes.
- children under 12 years of age: consult a doctor
Sweeten to taste if desired.
If using a microwave, add contents of packet to 6 oz of cool water; stir briskly before and after heating. Do not overheat.

Other Information:
- each packet contains: **sodium 14 mg**
- Phenylketonurics: Contains Phenylalanine 27 mg per adult dose
- store at controlled room temperature 20-25°C (68-77°F)

How Supplied: 6 packets

Inactive Ingredients: acesulfame K, aspartame, citric acid, FD&C Blue 1, FD& C Red 40, flavors, maltodextrin, silicon dioxide, sodium citrate, sucrose, tribasic calcium phosphate
Questions? call **1-800-452-0051** 24 hours a day, 7 days a week.
Shown in Product Identification Guide, page 513

THERAFLU® THIN STRIPS™ LONG ACTING COUGH
Cough Suppressant

Drug Facts

Active Ingredient: **Purpose:**
(in each strip):
Dextromethorphan 11 mg (equivalent to 15 mg dextromethorphan HBr) .. Cough suppressant

Uses: • temporarily relieves cough due to minor throat and bronchial irritation as may occur with a cold

Warnings:
Do not use if you are now taking a prescription monoamine oxidase inhibitor (MAOI) (certain drugs for depression, psychiatric, or emotional conditions, or Parkinson's disease), or for 2 weeks after stopping the MAOI drug. If you do not know if your prescription drug contains an MAOI, ask a doctor or pharmacist before taking this product.
Ask a doctor before use if you have
- a cough that occurs with too much phlegm (mucus)
- a cough that lasts or is chronic such as occurs with smoking, asthma, or emphysema
When using this product • do not use more than directed
Stop use and ask a doctor if
- cough lasts more than 7 days, comes back, or is accompanied by fever, rash, or persistent headache. These could be signs of a serious condition.
If pregnant or breast-feeding, ask a health care professional before use.
Keep out of reach of children. In case of overdose, get medical help or contact a Poison Control Center right away.

Directions:
- adults and children 12 years of age and over: allow 2 strips to dissolve on your tongue every 6 to 8 hours as needed, not to exceed 8 strips in 24 hours or as directed by a doctor
- children under 12 years of age: ask a doctor
Other Information:
- store at controlled room temperature 20–25° (68–77° F)

Inactive Ingredients: acetone, alcohol, dibasic sodium phosphate, FD&C Red 40, flavors, hydroxypropyl cellulose, hypromellose, maltodextrin, microcrystalline cellulose, polacrilin, polyethylene glycol, pregelatinized starch, propylene glycol, purified water, sorbitol, sucralose, titanium dioxide
Cherry Flavor. Alcohol: less than 5%

How Supplied: Available in 12 ct. cartons
Questions? call **1-800-452-0051** 24 hours a day, 7 days a week.
Shown in Product Identification Guide, page 513

THERAFLU® THIN STRIPS™-MULTISYMPTOM
Antihistamine/Cough Suppressant

Drug Facts
Active Ingredient   **Purpose:**
(in each strip):
Diphenhydramine HCl 25 mg .. Antihistamine/Cough Suppressant

Uses: • temporarily relieves
• cough due to minor throat and bronchial irritation occurring with a cold
• runny nose • sneezing • itchy nose or throat • itchy, watery eyes due to hay fever

Warnings:
Do not use • with any other product containing diphenhydramine, even one used on skin
Ask a doctor before use if you have
- glaucoma
- a breathing problem such as emphysema, asthma or chronic bronchitis
- a cough that occurs with smoking, too much phlegm (mucus) or chronic cough that lasts
- trouble urinating due to an enlarged prostate gland
Ask a doctor or pharmacist before use if you are • taking sedatives or tranquilizers
When using this product • do not take more than directed • avoid alcoholic drinks
• marked drowsiness may occur • alcohol, sedatives, and tranquilizers may increase drowsiness
• be careful when driving a motor vehicle or operating machinery
• excitability may occur, especially in children
Stop use and ask a doctor if
- cough lasts more than more than 7 days, comes back, or is accompanied by fever, rash, or persistent headache. These could be signs of a serious condition.
If pregnant or breast-feeding, ask a health care professional before use.

Keep out of reach of children. In case of overdose, get medical help or contact a Poison Control Center right away.

Directions:
- adults and children 12 years of age and over: allow 1 strip to dissolve on tongue every 4 hours, not to exceed 6 strips in 24 hours, or as directed by a doctor
- children under 12 years of age: consult a doctor
Other Information:
- store at controlled room temperature 20–25° (68–77° F)

Inactive Ingredients: acetone, alcohol, FD&C Red 40, flavors, hydroxypropyl cellulose, hypromellose, maltodextrin, microcrystalline cellulose, polyethylene glycol, pregelatinized starch, propylene glycol, purified water, sodium polystyrene sulfonate, sorbitol, sucralose, titanium dioxide
Questions?
call **1-800-452-0051** 24 hours a day, 7 days a week.
Cherry Flavor. Alcohol: less than 5%

How Supplied: Available in 12 ct. cartons
Shown in Product Identification Guide, page 513

TRIAMINIC® ALLERCHEWS®
Loratadine Orally Disintegrating Tablets
24 Hour Non-Drowsy†
Allergy

Drug Facts

Active Ingredient   **Purpose:**
(in each tablet):
Loratadine 10 mg .... Antihistamine

Uses: temporarily relieves these symptoms due to hay fever or other upper respiratory allergies: • runny nose • sneezing • itchy, watery eyes • itching of the nose or throat

Warnings:
Do not use if you have ever had an allergic reaction to this product or any of its ingredients.
Ask a doctor before use if you have liver or kidney disease.
Your doctor should determine if you need a different dose.
When using this product do not take more than directed.
Taking more than directed may cause drowsiness.
Stop use and ask a doctor if an allergic reaction to this product occurs. Seek medical help right away.
If pregnant or breast-feeding, ask a health professional before use.
Keep out of reach of children. In case of overdose, get medical help or contact a Poison Control Center right away.

Directions: Place one tablet on tongue; tablet disintegrates, with or without water.

adults and children 6 years of age and over	1 tablet daily; not more than 1 tablet in 24 hours
children under 6 years of age	ask a doctor
consumers with liver or kidney disease	ask a doctor

Other Information:
- store between 20 and 25°C (68 and 77°F)
- keep in a dry place
- use tablet immediately after opening individual blister

Inactive Ingredients: croscarmellose sodium, crospovidone, hypromellose, magnesium stearate, mannitol, microcrystalline cellulose
Questions? call **1-800-452-0051** 24 hours a day, 7 days a week.

---

†When used as directed

How Supplied: 8 Orally Disintegrating Tablets
Shown in Product Identification Guide, page 514

TRIAMINIC® Chest & Nasal Congestion (Expectorant, Nasal Decongestant)
Tropical Flavor

Drug Facts

Active Ingredients:
(in each 5 mL, 1 teaspoon):   Purpose:
Guaifenesin,
USP, 50 mg .... Expectorant
Pseudoephedrine HCl,
USP, 15 mg .... Nasal decongestant

Uses: •temporarily relieves
- chest congestion by loosening phlegm (mucus) to help clear bronchial passageways
- nasal and sinus congestion

Warnings:
Do not use •in a child who is taking a prescription monoamine oxidase inhibitor (MAOI) (certain drugs for depression, psychiatric or emotional conditions, or Parkinson's disease), or for 2 weeks after stopping the MAOI drug. If you do not know if the child's prescription drug contains an MAOI, ask a doctor or pharmacist before giving this product.
Ask a doctor before use if the child has
- heart disease • high blood pressure
- thyroid disease • diabetes • glaucoma
- a breathing problem such as asthma or chronic bronchitis
- cough that occurs with too much phlegm (mucus) or chronic cough that lasts
When using this product
- do not exceed recommended dosage
Stop use and ask a doctor if
- nervousness, dizziness, or sleeplessness occur
- symptoms do not improve within 7 days or occur with a fever
- cough persists for more than 7 days, comes back, or occurs with a fever,

rash, or persistent headache. These could be signs of a serious condition.
Keep out of reach of children. In case of overdose, get medical help or contact a poison control center right away.

Directions:
- take every 4 to 6 hours; not to exceed 4 doses in 24 hours or as directed by a doctor

children 6 to under 12 years of age	2 teaspoons
children 2 to under 6 years of age	1 teaspoon
children under 2 years of age	ask a doctor

Other Information:
- contains no aspirin
- store at controlled room temperature 20–25°C (68–77°F)

Inactive Ingredients: benzoic acid, D&C Yellow 10, disodium edetate, FD&C Yellow 6, flavors, glycerin, polyethylene glycol, purified water, sorbitol, sucrose
Questions? call **1-800-452-0051** 24 hours a day, 7 days a week.

How Supplied: 4 fl oz bottle
Shown in Product Identification Guide, page 514

TRIAMINIC® COLD & ALLERGY
Antihistamine, Nasal Decongestant
Orange Flavor

Drug Facts

Active Ingredients
(in each 5 mL, 1 teaspoon):   Purpose:
Chlorpheniramine maleate,
USP, 1 mg .... Antihistamine
Pseudoephedrine HCl,
USP, 15 mg .... Nasal decongestant

Uses: • temporarily relieves
- sneezing • itchy nose or throat
- runny nose
- itchy, watery eyes due to hay fever
- nasal and sinus congestion

Warnings:
Do not use • in a child who is taking a prescription monoamine oxidase inhibitor (MAOI) (certain drugs for depression, psychiatric or emotional conditions, or Parkinson's disease), or for 2 weeks after stopping the MAOI drug. If you do not know if the child's prescription drug contains an MAOI, ask a doctor or pharmacist before giving this product.
Ask a doctor before use if the child has
- heart disease • high blood pressure
- thyroid disease • diabetes • glaucoma
- a breathing problem such as chronic bronchitis
Ask a doctor or pharmacist before use if the child is taking sedatives or tranquilizers.
When using this product
- do not exceed recommended dosage
- may cause drowsiness
- sedatives and tranquilizers may increase drowsiness
- excitability may occur, especially in children

Stop use and ask a doctor if
- nervousness, dizziness, or sleeplessness occurs
- symptoms do not improve within 7 days or occur with a fever. These could be signs of a serious condition.
Keep out of reach of children. In case of overdose, get medical help or contact a poison control center right away.

Directions: • take every 4 to 6 hours; not to exceed 4 doses in 24 hours or as directed by a doctor

children 6 to under 12 years of age	2 teaspoons
children under 6 years of age	ask a doctor

Other Information:
- contains no aspirin
- store at controlled room temperature 20–25°C (68–77°F)

Inactive Ingredients benzoic acid, edetate disodium, FD&C Yellow 6, flavors, purified water, sorbitol, sucrose
Questions? call 1-800-452-0051 24 hours a day, 7 days a week.

How Supplied: 4 fl oz bottle

TRIAMINIC® COLD & COUGH
Antihistamine, Cough Suppressant, Nasal Decongestant
Cherry Flavor
Drug Facts
Active Ingredients
(in each 5 mL, 1 teaspoon):   Purpose:
Chlorpheniramine maleate,
USP, 1 mg .... Antihistamine
Dextromethorphan HBr,
USP, 5 mg .... Cough suppressant
Pseudoephedrine HCl,
USP, 15 mg .... Nasal decongestant

Uses: • temporarily relieves
- sneezing • itchy nose or throat
- runny nose • itchy, watery eyes due to hay fever
- nasal and sinus congestion
- cough due to minor throat and bronchial irritation

Warnings:
Do not use • in a child who is taking a prescription monoamine oxidase inhibitor (MAOI) (certain drugs for depression, psychiatric or emotional conditions, or Parkinson's disease), or for 2 weeks after stopping the MAOI drug. If you do not know if the child's prescription drug contains an MAOI, ask a doctor or pharmacist before giving this product.
Ask a doctor before use if the child has
- heart disease • high blood pressure
- thyroid disease • diabetes • glaucoma
- a breathing problem such as asthma or chronic bronchitis
- cough that occurs with too much phlegm (mucus) or chronic cough that lasts

Continued on next page

Information on **Novartis** *Consumer Health, Inc.* *products appearing on these pages is effective as of November 2003.*

Triaminic—Cont.

Ask a doctor or pharmacist before use if the child is taking sedatives or tranquilizers

When using this product
- do not exceed recommended dosage
- may cause marked drowsiness
- sedatives and tranquilizers may increase drowsiness
- excitability may occur, especially in children

Stop use and ask a doctor if
- nervousness, dizziness, or sleeplessness occurs
- symptoms do not improve within 7 days or occur with a fever
- cough persists for more than 7 days, comes back or occurs with a fever, rash or persistent headache. These could be signs of a serious condition.

Keep out of reach of children. In case of overdose, get medical help or contact a poison control center right away.

Directions: • take every 4 to 6 hours; not to exceed 4 doses in 24 hours or as directed by a doctor

children 6 to under 12 years of age	2 teaspoons
children under 6 years of age	ask a doctor

Other Information:
- each teaspoon contains: sodium 6 mg
- contains no aspirin
- store at controlled room temperature 20–25°C (68–77°F)

Inactive Ingredients: benzoic acid, citric acid, dibasic sodium phosphate, disodium edetate, FD&C Red 40, flavors, propylene glycol, purified water, sorbitol, sucrose

Questions? call 1-800-452-0051 24 hours a day, 7 days a week.

How Supplied: 4 fl oz bottle

TRIAMINIC® FLU COUGH & FEVER
Pain Reliever/Fever Reducer, Antihistamine, Cough Suppressant, Nasal Decongestant
Bubble Gum Flavor
Drug Facts
Active Ingredients
(in each 5 mL, 1 teaspoon):   **Purpose:**
Acetaminophen,
USP, 160 mg .... Pain reliever/fever reducer
Chlorpheniramine maleate,
USP, 1 mg .... Antihistamine
Dextromethorphan HBr,
USP, 7.5 mg .... Cough suppressant
Pseudoephedrine HCl,
USP, 15 mg .... Nasal decongestant

Uses: • temporarily relieves
- minor aches and pains • headache
- minor sore throat pain • sneezing
- itchy nose or throat
- itchy, watery eyes due to hay fever
- nasal and sinus congestion
- cough due to minor throat and bronchial irritation
- temporarily reduces fever

Warnings:
Do not use • in a child who is taking a prescription monoamine oxidase inhibitor (MAOI) (certain drugs for depression, psychiatric or emotional conditions, or Parkinson's disease), or for 2 weeks after stopping the MAOI drug. If you do not know if the child's prescription drug contains an MAOI, ask a doctor or pharmacist before giving this product.
- with any other product containing acetaminophen **(see Overdose Warning)**

Ask a doctor before use if the child has
- heart disease • high blood pressure
- thyroid disease • diabetes • glaucoma
- a breathing problem such as asthma or chronic bronchitis
- cough that occurs with too much phlegm (mucus) or chronic cough that lasts

Ask a doctor or pharmacist before use if the child is taking sedatives or tranquilizers.

When using this product
- do not exceed recommended dosage
- may cause marked drowsiness
- sedatives and tranquilizers may increase drowsiness
- excitability may occur, especially in children

Stop use and ask a doctor if
- nervousness, dizziness, or sleeplessness occurs
- pain, cough or nasal congestion gets worse or lasts more than 5 days
- fever gets worse or lasts more than 3 days
- redness or swelling is present
- new symptoms occur
- sore throat is severe, persists for more than 2 days or occurs with fever, headache, rash, nausea or vomiting
- cough comes back or occurs with a rash or headache that lasts. These could be signs of a serious condition.

Keep out of reach of children.

Overdose Warning: Taking more than the recommended dose can cause serious health problems, including serious liver damage. In case of overdose, get medical help or contact a poison control center right away. Prompt medical attention is critical for adults as well as for children even if you do not notice any signs or symptoms.

Directions: • do not use more than directed **(see Overdose Warning)**
- take every 6 hours; not to exceed 4 doses in 24 hours or as directed by a doctor

children 6 to under 12 years of age	2 teaspoons
children under 6 years of age	ask a doctor

Other Information:
- each teaspoon contains: sodium 6 mg
- contains no aspirin
- store at controlled room temperature 20–25°C (68–77°F)

Inactive Ingredients: benzoic acid, citric acid, dibasic sodium phosphate, edetate disodium, FD&C Red 40, flavors, glycerin, polyethylene glycol, purified water, sorbitol, sucrose

Questions? call 1-800-452-0051 24 hours a day, 7 days a week.

How Supplied: 4 fl oz bottle

TRIAMINIC® NIGHT TIME COLD & COUGH
Antihistamine, Cough Suppressant, Nasal Decongestant
Grape Flavor
Drug Facts
Active Ingredients
(in each 5 mL, 1 teaspoon):   **Purpose:**
Chlorpheniramine maleate,
USP, 1 mg .... Antihistamine
Dextromethorphan HBr,
USP, 7.5 mg .... Cough suppressant
Pseudoephedrine HCl,
USP, 15 mg .... Nasal decongestant

Uses: • temporarily relieves
- sneezing • itchy nose or throat
- runny nose
- itchy, watery eyes due to hay fever
- nasal and sinus congestion
- cough due to minor throat and bronchial irritation

Warnings:
Do not use • in a child who is taking a prescription monoamine oxidase inhibitor (MAOI) (certain drugs for depression, psychiatric or emotional conditions, or Parkinson's disease), or for 2 weeks after stopping the MAOI drug. If you do not know if the child's prescription drug contains an MAOI, ask a doctor or pharmacist before giving this product.

Ask a doctor before use if the child has
- heart disease • high blood pressure
- thyroid disease • diabetes • glaucoma
- a breathing problem such as asthma or chronic bronchitis
- cough that occurs with too much phlegm (mucus) or chronic cough that lasts

Ask a doctor or pharmacist before use if the child is taking sedatives or tranquilizers.

When using this product
- do not exceed recommended dosage
- may cause marked drowsiness
- sedatives and tranquilizers may increase drowsiness
- excitability may occur, especially in children

Stop use and ask a doctor if
- nervousness, dizziness, or sleeplessness occurs
- symptoms do not improve within 7 days or occur with a fever
- cough persists for more than 7 days, comes back, or occurs with a fever, rash, or persistent headache. These could be signs of a serious condition.

Keep out of reach of children. In case of overdose, get medical help or contact a poison control center right away.

Directions: • take every 6 hours; not to exceed 4 doses in 24 hours or as directed by a doctor

children 6 to under 12 years of age	2 teaspoons
children under 6 years of age	ask a doctor

Other Information:
- each teaspoon contains: sodium 8 mg
- contains no aspirin • protect from light

- store at controlled room temperature 20–25°C (68–77°F)

Inactive Ingredients: benzoic acid, citric acid, dibasic sodium phosphate, edetate disodium, FD&C Blue 1, FD&C Red 40, flavors, propylene glycol, purified water, sorbitol, sucrose

Questions? call 1-800-452-0051 24 hours a day, 7 days a week.

How Supplied: 4 fl oz bottle
Shown in Product Identification Guide, page 514

TRIAMINIC® Cough
Cough Suppressant, Nasal Decongestant-Berry Flavor

TRIAMINIC® Cough & Nasal Congestion
Cough Suppressant, Nasal Decongestant-Orange Strawberry Flavor

TRIAMINIC® Cough & Sore Throat
Cough Suppressant, Nasal Decongestant, Pain Reliever/Fever Reducer-Grape Flavor

Triaminic® Cough
Berry Flavor
Drug Facts
Active Ingredients
(in each 5 mL;
1 teaspoon):   Purpose:
Dextromethorphan HBr,
USP, 5 mg .... Cough suppressant
Pseudoephedrine, HCl,
USP, 15 mg .... Nasal decongestant

Uses: • temporarily relieves
- cough due to minor throat and bronchial irritation
- nasal and sinus congestion

Warnings:
Do not use • in a child who is taking a prescription monoamine oxidase inhibitor (MAOI) (certain drugs for depression, psychiatric or emotional conditions, or Parkinson's disease), or for 2 weeks after stopping the MAOI drug. If you do not know if the child's prescription drug contains an MAOI, ask a doctor or pharmacist before giving this product.
- if the child is on a sodium-restricted diet unless directed by a doctor.
Ask a doctor before use if the child has
- heart disease • high blood pressure
- thyroid disease • diabetes • glaucoma
- a breathing problem such as asthma or chronic bronchitis
- cough that occurs with too much phlegm (mucus) or chronic cough that lasts
When using this product
- **do not exceed recommended dosage**
Stop use and ask a doctor if
- nervousness, dizziness, or sleeplessness occurs
- symptoms do not improve within 7 days or occur with a fever
- cough persists for more than 7 days, comes back, or occurs with a fever, rash, or persistent headache. These could be signs of a serious condition.
Keep out of reach of children. In case of overdose, get medical help or contact a poison control center right away.

Directions: • take every 4 to 6 hours; not to exceed 4 doses in 24 hours or as directed by a doctor

children 6 to under 12 years of age	2 teaspoons
children 2 to under 6 years of age	1 teaspoon
children under 2 years of age	ask a doctor

Other Information:
- each teaspoon contains: **sodium 20 mg**
- contains no aspirin
- store at controlled room temperature 20–25°C (68–77°F)

Inactive Ingredients: benzoic acid, FD&C Blue 1, FD&C Red 40, flavors, propylene glycol, purified water, sodium chloride, sorbitol, sucrose

Questions? call **1-800-452-0051** 24 hours a day, 7 days a week.

How Supplied: 4 fl oz Bottle

Triaminic® Cough & Nasal Congestion Cough Suppressant, Nasal Decongestant Orange-Strawberry Flavor
Drug Facts
Active Ingredients
(in each 5 mL,
1 teaspoon):   Purpose:
Dextromethorphan HBr,
USP, 7.5 mg .... Cough suppressant
Pseudoephedrine, HCl,
USP, 15 mg .... Nasal decongestant

Uses: • temporarily relieves
- cough due to minor throat and bronchial irritation
- nasal and sinus congestion

Warnings:
Do not use • in a child who is taking a prescription monoamine oxidase inhibitor (MAOI) (certain drugs for depression, psychiatric or emotional conditions, or Parkinson's disease), or for 2 weeks after stopping the MAOI drug. If you do not know if the child's prescription drug contains an MAOI, ask a doctor or pharmacist before giving this product.
Ask a doctor before use if the child has
- heart disease • high blood pressure
- thyroid disease • diabetes • glaucoma
- a breathing problem such as asthma or chronic bronchitis
- cough that occurs with too much phlegm (mucus) or chronic cough that lasts
When using this product
- **do not exceed recommended dosage**
Stop use and ask a doctor if
- nervousness, dizziness, or sleeplessness occurs
- symptoms do not improve within 7 days or occur with a fever
- cough persists for more than 7 days, comes back, or occurs with a fever, rash, or persistent headache. These could be signs of a serious condition.
Keep out of reach of children. In case of overdose, get medical help or contact a poison control center right away.

Directions: • take every 6 hours; not to exceed 4 doses in 24 hours or as directed by a doctor

children 6 to under 12 years of age	2 teaspoons
children 2 to under 6 years of age	1 teaspoon
children under 2 years of age	ask a doctor

Other Information:
- each teaspoon contains: **sodium 7 mg**
- contains no aspirin
- protect from light
- store at controlled room temperature 20–25°C (68–77°F)

Inactive Ingredients: benzoic acid, citric acid, dibasic sodium phosphate, edetate disodium, flavors, propylene glycol, purified water, sorbitol, sucrose

Questions? call **1-800-452-0051** 24 hours a day, 7 days a week.

How Supplied: 4 fl oz Bottle

Triaminic® Cough & Sore Throat
Cough Suppressant, Nasal Decongestant, Pain Reliever/Fever Reducer
Grape Flavor
Drug Facts
Active Ingredients:
(in each 5 mL,
1 teaspoon):   Purpose:
Acetaminophen,
USP, 160 mg .... Pain reliever/Fever reducer
Dextromethorphan HBr,
USP, 7.5 mg .... Cough suppressant
Pseudoephedrine HCl,
USP, 15 mg .... Nasal decongestant

Uses: • temporarily relieves
- minor aches and pains • headache
- minor sore throat pain
- nasal and sinus congestion
- cough due to minor throat and bronchial irritation
- temporarily reduces fever

Warnings:
Do not use • in a child who is taking a prescription monoamine oxidase inhibitor (MAOI) (certain drugs for depression, psychiatric or emotional conditions, or Parkinson's disease), or for 2 weeks after stopping the MAOI drug. If you do not know if the child's prescription drug contains an MAOI, ask a doctor or pharmacist before giving this product.
- with any other product containing acetaminophen **(see Overdose Warning)**
Ask a doctor before use if the child has
- heart disease • high blood pressure
- thyroid disease • diabetes • glaucoma
- a breathing problem such as asthma or chronic bronchitis
- cough that occurs with too much phlegm (mucus) or chronic cough that lasts

Continued on next page

Information **on Novartis Consumer Health, Inc.** *products appearing on these pages is effective as of November 2004.*

Triaminic Cough—Cont.

When using this product
• do not exceed recommended dosage
Stop use and ask a doctor if
• nervousness, dizziness, or sleeplessness occurs
• pain, cough or nasal congestion gets worse or lasts more than 5 days
• fever gets worse or lasts more than 3 days
• redness or swelling is present
• new symptoms occur
• sore throat is severe, persists for more than 2 days or occurs with fever, headache, rash, nausea or vomiting
• cough comes back or occurs with a rash or headache that lasts. These could be signs of a serious condition.
Keep out of reach of children.
Overdose Warning: Taking more than the recommended dose can cause serious health problems, including serious liver damage. In case of overdose, get medical help or contact a poison control center right away. Prompt medical attention is critical for adults as well as for children even if you do not notice any signs or symptoms.

Directions:
• do not use more than directed **(see Overdose Warning)**
• take every 6 hours; not to exceed 4 doses in 24 hours or as directed by a doctor

children 6 to under 12 years of age	2 teaspoons
children 2 to under 6 years of age	1 teaspoon
children under 2 years of age	ask a doctor

Other Information:
• each teaspoon contains: **sodium 5 mg**
• contains no aspirin
• store at controlled room temperature 20–25°C (68–77°F)

Inactive Ingredients: citric acid, edetate disodium, FD&C Blue 1, FD&C Red 40, flavors, glycerin, polyethylene glycol, purified water, sodium benzoate, sodium citrate, sorbitol, sucrose
Questions? call **1-800-452-0051** 24 hours a day, 7 days a week.

How Supplied: 4 fl oz Bottle
Shown in Product Identification Guide, page 514

TRIAMINIC® Softchews® Allergy
Runny Nose & Congestion
Antihistamine, Nasal Decongestant
Orange Flavor

Drug Facts

Active Ingredients
(in each tablet): **Purpose:**
Chlorpheniramine maleate, USP,
1 mg .... Antihistamine
Pseudoephedrine HCl, USP,
15 mg .... Nasal decongestant

Uses: temporarily relieves •sneezing •itchy nose or throat •runny nose •itchy, watery eyes due to hay fever •nasal and sinus congestion

Warnings:
Do not use • in a child who is taking a prescription monoamine oxidase inhibitor (MAOI) (certain drugs for depression, psychiatric or emotional conditions, or Parkinson's disease), or for 2 weeks after stopping the MAOI drug. If you do not know if the child's prescription drug contains an MAOI, ask a doctor or pharmacist before giving this product.
Ask a doctor before use if the child has
• heart disease • high blood pressure
• thyroid disease • diabetes • glaucoma
• a breathing problem such as chronic bronchitis
Ask a doctor or pharmacist before use if the child is taking sedatives or tranquilizers.
When using this product • do not exceed recommended dosage • may cause drowsiness • sedatives and tranquilizers may increase drowsiness • excitability may occur, especially in children
Stop use and ask a doctor if • nervousness, dizziness, or sleeplessness occurs
• symptoms do not improve within 7 days, or occur with fever.
These could be signs of a serious condition.
Keep out of reach of children. In case of overdose, get medical help or contact a poison control center right away.

Directions: • Let Softchews® tablet dissolve in mouth or chew Softchews® tablet before swallowing, whichever is preferred
• take every 4 to 6 hours; not to exceed 4 doses in 24 hours or as directed by a doctor

children 6 to under 12 years of age	2 tablets
children under 6 years of age	ask a doctor

Other Information:
• each Softchews® tablet contains: **sodium 5 mg**
• Phenylketonurics: Contains **Phenylalanine, 17.6 mg** per Softchews® tablet
• contains no aspirin • store at controlled room temperature 20–25°C (68–77°F).

Inactive Ingredients: aspartame, carnauba wax, citric acid, crospovidone, ethylcellulose, FD&C Yellow 6 aluminum lake, flavors, fractionated coconut oil, hypromellose, magnesium stearate, mannitol, microcrystalline cellulose, mono- and diglycerides, oleic acid, polyethylene glycol, silicon dioxide, sodium bicarbonate, sodium chloride, sorbitol, starch, sucrose, triethyl citrate
Questions? call **1-800-452-0051** 24 hours a day, 7 days a week.

How Supplied: 18 Softchews® tablets
U.S. Pat. No. 5,178,878
Shown in Product Identification Guide, page 514

TRIAMINIC® Softchews®
Cold & Cough
Antihistamine, Cough Suppressant,
Nasal Decongestant
Cherry Flavor

Drug Facts

Active Ingredients
(in each tablet): **Purpose:**
Chlorpheniramine maleate, USP,
1 mg .... Antihistamine
Dextromethorphan HBr, USP,
5 mg .... Cough suppressant
Pseudoephedrine HCl, USP,
15 mg .... Nasal decongestant

Uses: temporarily relieves • sneezing
• itchy nose or throat • runny nose
• itchy, watery eyes due to hay fever
• nasal and sinus congestion
• cough due to minor throat and bronchial irritation

Warnings:
Do not use • in a child who is taking a prescription monoamine oxidase inhibitor (MAOI) (certain drugs for depression, psychiatric, or emotional conditions, or Parkinson's disease), or for 2 weeks after stopping the MAOI drug. If you do not know if the child's prescription drug contains an MAOI, ask a doctor or pharmacist before giving this product.
Ask a doctor before use if the child has
• heart disease • high blood pressure
• thyroid disease • diabetes • glaucoma
• a breathing problem such as asthma or chronic bronchitis
• cough that occurs with too much phlegm (mucus) or chronic cough that lasts
Ask a doctor or pharmacist before use if the child is taking sedatives or tranquilizers.
When using this product • do not exceed recommended dosage • may cause marked drowsiness • sedatives and tranquilizers may increase drowsiness
• excitability may occur, especially in children
Stop use and ask a doctor if • nervousness, dizziness, or sleeplessness occurs
• symptoms do not improve within 7 days or occurs with a fever • cough persists for more than 7 days, comes back or occurs with a fever, rash, or persistent headache. These could be signs of a serious condition.
Keep out of reach of children. In case of overdose, get medical help or contact a poison control center right away.

Directions: • Let Softchews® tablet dissolve in mouth or chew Softchews® tablet before swallowing, whichever is preferred
• take every 4 to 6 hours; not to exceed 4 doses in 24 hours or as directed by a doctor

children 6 to under 12 years of age	2 tablets
children under 6 years of age	ask a doctor

Other Information:
• each Softchews® tablet contains: **sodium 5 mg**
• Phenylketonurics: Contains **Phenylalanine, 17.6 mg** per Softchews® tablet
• contains no aspirin • store at controlled room temperature 20–25°C (68–77°F)

Inactive Ingredients: aspartame, carnauba wax, citric acid, crospovidone, D&C Red 27 aluminum lake, D&C Red 30 aluminum lake, ethylcellulose, FD&C Blue 2 aluminum lake, flavors, fractionated coconut oil, gum arabic, hypromellose, magnesium stearate, maltodextrin, mannitol, microcrystalline cellulose, mono- and di-glycerides, oleic acid, polyethylene glycol, povidone, silicon dioxide, sodium bicarbonate, sodium chloride, sorbitol, starch, sucrose, triethyl citrate
Questions? call **1-800-452-0051** 24 hours a day, 7 days a week.

How Supplied: 18 Softchews® Tablets
U.S. Pat. No. 5,178,878
Shown in Product Identification Guide, page 514

TRIAMINIC® Softchews®
Cough & Sore Throat
Pain Reliever/Fever Reducer,
Cough Suppressant, Nasal Decongestant,
Grape Flavor

Drug Facts:

Active Ingredients
(in each tablet):   **Purpose:**
Acetaminophen, USP,
160 mg ...... Pain reliever/Fever reducer
Dextromethorphan HBr, USP,
5 mg .... Cough suppressant
Pseudoephedrine HCl, USP,
15 mg .... Nasal decongestant

Uses: • temporarily relieves • minor aches and pains • headache • minor sore throat pain • nasal and sinus congestion • cough due to minor throat and bronchial irritation • temporarily reduces fever

Warnings:
Do not use • in a child who is taking a prescription monoamine oxidase inhibitor (MAOI) (certain drugs for depression, psychiatric or emotional conditions, or Parkinson's disease), or for 2 weeks after stopping the MAOI drug. If you do not know if the child's prescription drug contains an MAOI, ask a doctor or pharmacist before giving this product. • with any other product containing acetaminophen (**see Overdose Warning**)
Ask a doctor before use if the child has
• heart disease • high blood pressure
• thyroid disease • diabetes • glaucoma
• a breathing problem such as asthma or chronic bronchitis
• cough that occurs with too much phlegm (mucus) or chronic cough that lasts
When using this product • do not exceed recommended dosage
Stop use and ask a doctor if • nervousness, dizziness, or sleeplessness occurs

• pain, cough or nasal congestion gets worse or lasts more than 5 days
• fever gets worse or lasts more than 3 days
• redness or swelling is present
• new symptoms occur
• sore throat is severe, persists for more than 2 days or occurs with fever, headache, rash, nausea or vomiting
• cough comes back or occurs with a rash or headache that lasts. These could be signs of a serious condition.
Keep out of reach of children.
Overdose Warning: Taking more than the recommended dose can cause serious health problems, including serious liver damage. In case of overdose, get medical help or contact a poison control center right away. Prompt medical attention is critical for adults as well as for children even if you do not notice any signs or symptoms.

Directions: • do not use more than directed (**see Overdose Warning**)
• Let Softchews® tablet dissolve in mouth or chew Softchews® tablet before swallowing, whichever is preferred
• take every 4 to 6 hours; not to exceed 4 doses in 24 hours or as directed by a doctor

children 6 to under 12 years of age	2 tablets
children 2 to under 6 years of age	1 tablet
children under 2 years of age	ask a doctor

Other Information:
• each Softchews® tablet contains: **sodium 8 mg**
• Phenylketonurics: Contains **Phenylalanine, 28.1 mg** per Softchews® tablet
• contains no aspirin
• store at controlled room temperature 20–25°C (68–77°F)

Inactive Ingredients: aspartame, citric acid, crospovidone, D&C Red 27 aluminum lake, dextrin, ethylcellulose, FD&C Blue 1 aluminum lake, flavors, fractionated coconut oil, hypromellose, magnesium stearate, maltodextrin, mannitol, microcrystalline cellulose, oleic acid, polyethylene glycol, povidone, sodium bicarbonate, sodium chloride, sorbitol, starch, sucrose, triethyl citrate
Questions? call **1-800-452-0051** 24 hours a day, 7 days a week.
U.S. Pat. No. 5,178,878
How Supplied: 18 Softchews® Tablets
Shown in Product Identification Guide, page 514

TRIAMINIC® SPRAY Sore Throat
Phenol
Oral Anesthetic/Analgesic
Grape Flavor

Drug Facts
Active Ingredient: **Purpose:**
Phenol, 0.5% .... Anesthetic/Analgesic
Uses: temporarily relieves:
• sore mouth
• minor irritation or injury of the mouth and gums

• pain due to minor dental procedures, or orthodontic appliances
• pain associated with canker sores
• sore throat pain

Warnings:
When using this product
• do not use more than directed
Stop use and ask a doctor if
• sore throat is severe, persists for more than 2 days or is accompanied by difficulty in breathing.
• sore throat is accompanied or followed by fever, headache, rash, swelling, nausea or vomiting.
• sore mouth symptoms do not improve within 7 days or irritation, pain or redness persists or worsens. These could be signs of a serious condition.
Keep out of reach of children. In case of overdose, get medical help or contact a poison control center right away.

Directions: Triaminic Sore Throat Spray may be used every 2 hours or as directed by a dentist or physician.

Children 2 to under 12 years of age (with adult supervision):	For each application, spray up to 5 times into the throat or affected area.
Children under 2 years of age:	ask a physician or dentist.

Other Information:
• contains no aspirin, no alcohol or sugar
• store at controlled room temperature 20–25°C (68–77°F)

Inactive Ingredients: FD&C Blue 1, FD&C Red 40, flavors, glycerin, purified water, sodium saccharin, sorbitol
Questions? call **1-800-452-0051** 24 hours a day, 7 days a week.

How Supplied: 4 fl oz Bottle
Shown in Product Identification Guide, page 514

TRIAMINIC® THIN STRIPS™
LONG ACTING COUGH

Drug Facts

Active Ingredient
(in each strip):   **Purpose:**
Dextromethorphan 5.5 mg
(equivalent to 7.5 mg dextromethorphan HBr) .... Cough suppressant

Uses:
• temporarily relieves cough due to minor throat and bronchial irritation as may occur with a cold

Warnings: Do not use in a child who is taking a prescription monoamine oxi-

Continued on next page

Continued on next page

Information on Novartis Consumer Health, Inc. products appearing on these pages is effective as of November 2003.

Triaminic Thin Strips—Cont.

dase inhibitor (MAOI) (certain drugs for depression, psychiatric, or emotional conditions, or Parkinson's disease), or for 2 weeks after stopping the MAOI drug. If you do not know if your child's prescription drug contains an MAOI, ask a doctor or pharmacist before giving this product.

Ask a doctor before use if the child has
• cough that occurs with too much phlegm (mucus)
• cough that lasts or is chronic such as occurs with asthma

When using this product
• do not use more than directed

Stop use and ask a doctor if • cough lasts more than 7 days, comes back, or is accompanied by fever, rash, or persistent headache.
These could be signs of a serious condition.

Keep out of reach of children. In case of overdose, get medical help or contact a Poison Control Center right away.

Directions:
• children 6 to under 12 years of age: allow 2 strips to dissolve on tongue. May be taken every 6 to 8 hours.
• do not exceed 8 strips in 24 hours or as directed by a doctor
• children under 6 years of age: ask a doctor

Other Information:
• store at controlled room temperature 20–25°C (68–77°F)

Inactive Ingredients: acetone, alcohol, dibasic sodium phosphate, FD&C Red 40, flavors, hydroxypropyl cellulose, hypromellose, maltodextrin, microcrystalline cellulose, polacrilin, polyethylene glycol, pregelatinized starch, propylene glycol, purified water, sorbitol, sucralose, titanium dioxide

Questions? call **1-800-452-0051** 24 hours a day, 7 days a week.

Alcohol: Cherry Flavor, less than 5%

How Supplied: Available in 16 ct cartons.

Shown in Product Identification Guide, page 514

TRIAMINIC® THIN STRIPS™ COUGH & RUNNY NOSE

Drug Facts

Active Ingredient
(in each strip):   **Purpose:**
Diphenhydramine HCl 12.5 mg .. Cough suppressant/ Antihistamine

Uses: • temporarily relieves
• runny nose • sneezing
• itchy nose or throat
• itchy, watery eyes due to hay fever
• cough due to minor throat and bronchial irritation occurring with a cold

Warnings:
• do not use more than directed
• marked drowsiness may occur. Sedatives and tranquilizers may increase the drowsiness effect.
• excitability may occur, especially in children

Stop use and ask a doctor if
• cough lasts more than 7 days, comes back, or is accompanied by fever, rash, or persistent headache. These could be signs of a serious condition.

Keep out of reach of children. In case of overdose, get medical help or contact a Poison Control Center right away.

Do not use • with any other product containing diphenhydramine, even one used on skin

Ask a doctor before use if the child has
• glaucoma
• cough that occurs with too much phlegm (mucus)
• cough that lasts or is chronic such as occurs with asthma or chronic bronchitis

Ask a doctor or pharmacist before use if the child is
• taking sedatives or tranquilizers

When using this product

Directions:
• children 6 to under 12 years of age: allow 1 strip to dissolve on tongue.
May be taken every 4 hours.
• do not exceed 6 strips in 24 hours, or as directed by a doctor
• children under 6 years of age: ask a doctor

Other Information:
• store at controlled room temperature 20–25°C (68–77°F)

Inactive Ingredients: acetone, alcohol, FD&C Blue 1, FD&C Red 40, flavors hydroxypropyl cellulose, hypromellose, maltodextrin, microcrystalline cellulose, polyethylene glycol, pregelatinized starch, propylene glycol, purified water, sodium polystyrene sulfonate, sorbitol, sucralose, titanium dioxide

Questions?
call **1-800-452-0051** 24 hours a day, 7 days a week.

Alcohol: Grape Flavor, less than 5%

How Supplied: Available in 16 ct cartons

Shown in Product Identification Guide, page 514

TRIAMINIC® Vapor Patch® -Mentholated Cherry Scent Cough Suppressant
TRIAMINIC® Vapor Patch® -Menthol Scent Cough Suppressant

Drug Facts Cherry Scent
Active Ingredients
(in each patch):   **Purpose:**
Camphor 4.7% .... Cough suppressant
Menthol 2.6% .... Cough suppressant

Use: temporarily relieves cough due to:
• a cold • minor throat and bronchial irritation to help you sleep

Warnings:
For external use only
Flammable: Keep away from fire or flame
Ask a doctor before use if the child has
• cough that occurs with too much phlegm (mucus)
• a persistent or chronic cough such as occurs with asthma

When using this product do not • use more than directed
• heat • microwave • use near an open flame
• add to hot water or any container where heating water. May cause splattering and result in burns
Additionally, do not
• apply to eyes, wounds, sensitive, irritated or damaged skin
• take by mouth or place in nostrils

Stop use and ask a doctor if • cough persists for more than 7 days, comes back, or occurs with fever, rash, or persistent headache. These could be signs of a serious condition. • too much skin irritation occurs or gets worse

Keep out of reach of children. If swallowed, get medical help or contact a poison control center right away.

Directions:
• see important warnings under 'When using this product'
• Children 2 to under 12 years of age:
  • Remove plastic backing
  • Apply patch to the throat or chest
  • If the child has sensitive skin, the patch may be applied to the same area on clothing*
  • Clothing should be loose about the throat and chest to help the vapors reach the nose and mouth
  • Apply a new patch up to three times daily or as directed by a doctor
  • May use with other cough suppressant products
• Children under 2 years of age: Ask a doctor
* The patch may not adhere to some types of polyester clothing

Other Information:
• store at controlled room temperature 20–25°C (68–77°F) • protect from excessive heat

Inactive Ingredients: acrylic ester copolymer, aloe vera gel, eucalyptus oil, glycerin, karaya, propylene glycol, purified water, wild cherry fragrance
Questions? call **1-800-452-0051** 24 hours a day, 7 days a week.

Drug Facts Menthol Scent
Active Ingredients
(in each patch):   **Purpose:**
Camphor 4.7% .... Cough suppressant
Menthol 2.6% .... Cough suppressant

Use: temporarily relieves cough due to:
• a cold • minor throat and bronchial irritation to help you sleep

Warnings:
For external use only
Flammable: Keep away from fire or flame
Ask a doctor before use if the child has
• cough that occurs with too much phlegm (mucus)
• a persistent or chronic cough such as occurs with asthma

When using this product do not • use more than directed
• heat • microwave • use near an open flame
• add to hot water or any container where heating water. May cause splattering and result in burns
Additionally, do not
• apply to eyes, wounds, sensitive, irritated or damaged skin

• **take by mouth or place in nostrils**
Stop use and ask a doctor if • cough persists for more than 7 days, comes back, or occurs with fever, rash, or persistent headache. These could be signs of a serious condition. • too much skin irritation occurs or gets worse
Keep out of reach of children. If swallowed, get medical help or contact a poison control center right away.

Directions:
• see important warnings under 'When using this product'
• Children 2 to under 12 years of age:
  • Remove plastic backing
  • Apply patch to the throat or chest
  • If the child has sensitive skin, the patch may be applied to the same area on clothing*
  • Clothing should be loose about the throat and chest to help the vapors reach the nose and mouth
  • Apply a new patch up to three times daily or as directed by a doctor
  • May use with other cough suppressant products
• Children under 2 years of age: Ask a doctor
* The patch may not adhere to some types of polyester clothing

Other Information:
• store at controlled room temperature 20–25°C (68–77°F) • protect from excessive heat

Inactive Ingredients: acrylic ester copolymer, aloe vera gel, eucalyptus oil, glycerin, karaya, purified water, spirits or turpentine
Questions? call **1-800-452-0051** 24 hours a day, 7 days a week.

How Supplied: Ointment on a breathable patch
Shown in Product Identification Guide, page 514

Performance Health, Inc.

1017 BOYD ROAD
EXPORT, PA 15632-8997

Direct Inquiries to:
Phone - 724-733-9500
Fax - 724-733-4266
Email - PDR@Biofreeze.com

BIOFREEZE® PAIN RELIEVING GEL

Active Ingredient: Menthol 3.5%

Inactive Ingredients: Camphor (for scent), carbomer, FD&C blue #1, FD&C yellow #5, Glycerine, Herbal Extract (ILEX Paraguariensis), Isopropyl Alcohol, Methylparaben, Propylene Glycol, Silicon Dioxide, Triethanolamine, Water

Indications: Temporary relief from minor aches and pains of sore muscles and joints associated with arthritis, backache, strains and sprains.

Warnings: Ask a doctor before use if you have sensitive skin. Keep away from excessive heat or open flame. Avoid contact with the eyes or mucous membranes. Do not apply to wounds or damaged skin. Do not use with other ointments, creams, sprays or liniments. Do not apply to irritated skin or if excessive irritation develops. Do not bandage. Wash hands after use. If pregnant or breast-feeding, ask a health professional before use. Keep out of reach of children. If accidentally ingested, get medical help or contact a Poison Control Center.

Directions: Adults and children 2 years of age and older: Rub a thin film over affected areas not more than 4 times daily; massage not necessary. Children under 2 years of age: consult physician.

How Supplied: 4 oz. tube, 3 oz. Roll-on and 5 gram packets for home use. 16 oz., 32 oz. and Gallon for professional use.

Pfizer Consumer Healthcare, Pfizer Inc.

201 TABOR ROAD
MORRIS PLAINS, NJ 07950

Address Questions & Comments to:
Consumer Affairs, Pfizer Consumer Healthcare
182 Tabor Road
Morris Plains, NJ 07950
For Medical Emergencies/Information Contact:
1-(800)-223-0182
1-(800)-524-2624 (Spanish)
1-(800)-378-1783 (e.p.t.)
1-(800)-337-7266 (e.p.t.-Spanish)

BENADRYL® Allergy Kapseals® Capsules (also available in Ultratab™ Tablets)
[bĕ 'nă-drĭl]

Drug Facts:

Active Ingredient: **Purpose:**
(in each capsule)
Diphenhydramine HCl
    25 mg .... Antihistamine

Uses:
• temporarily relieves these symptoms due to hay fever or other upper respiratory allergies:
  • runny nose
  • sneezing
  • itchy, watery eyes
  • itching of the nose or throat
• temporarily relieves these symptoms due to the common cold:
  • runny nose
  • sneezing

Warnings:
Do not use with any other product containing diphenhydramine, even one used on skin.
Ask a doctor before use if you have
• glaucoma
• trouble urinating due to an enlarged prostate gland

• a breathing problem such as emphysema or chronic bronchitis
Ask a doctor or pharmacist before use if you are taking sedatives or tranquilizers
When using this product
• marked drowsiness may occur
• avoid alcoholic drinks
• alcohol, sedatives, and tranquilizers may increase drowsiness
• be careful when driving a motor vehicle or operating machinery
• excitability may occur, especially in children
If pregnant or breast-feeding, ask a health professional before use.
Keep out of reach of children. In case of overdose, get medical help or contact a Poison Control Center right away.

Directions:
• take every 4 to 6 hours
• do not take more than 6 doses in 24 hours

adults and children 12 years of age and over	25 mg to 50 mg (1 to 2 capsules)
children 6 to under 12 years of age	12.5 mg** to 25 mg (1 capsule)
children under 6 years of age	ask a doctor

**12.5 mg dosage strength is not available in this package. Do not attempt to break capsules.

Other Information:
• store at 59° to 77°F in a dry place
• protect from light

Inactive Ingredients: Capsules: D&C red no. 28, FD&C blue no. 1, FD&C red no. 3, FD&C red no. 40, gelatin, glyceryl monooleate, lactose, magnesium stearate, talc, and titanium dioxide. Printed with black edible ink.

Tablets: candelilla wax, crospovidone, dibasic calcium phosphate dihydrate, D&C red no. 27 aluminum lake, hypromellose, magnesium stearate, microcrystalline cellulose, polyethylene glycol, polysorbate 80, pregelatinized starch, stearic acid, and titanium dioxide.

Questions? call **1-800-524-2624** (English/Spanish), weekdays, 9 AM–5 PM EST

How Supplied: Benadryl tablets are supplied in boxes of 24 and 48, bottles of

Continued on next page

This product information was prepared in November 2004. On these and other Pfizer Consumer Healthcare Products, detailed information may be obtained by addressing Pfizer Consumer Healthcare, Pfizer, Inc., Morris Plains, NJ 07950

Benadryl Allergy—Cont.

100 and 124; capsules are supplied in boxes of 24 and 48.

**BENADRYL®
Dye-Free
Allergy Liqui-Gels®
Softgels**
[bĕ 'nă-drĭl]

Drug Facts:

Active Ingredient:

(in each softgel):	Purpose:
Diphenhydramine HCl 25 mg	Antihistamine

Uses:
- temporarily relieves these symptoms due to hay fever or other upper respiratory allergies:
  - runny nose
  - sneezing
  - itchy, watery eyes
  - itching of the nose or throat
- temporarily relieves these symptoms due to the common cold:
  - runny nose
  - sneezing

Warnings:
Do not use with any other product containing diphenhydramine, even one used on skin.
Ask a doctor before use if you have:
- glaucoma
- trouble urinating due to an enlarged prostate gland
- a breathing problem such as emphysema or chronic bronchitis
Ask a doctor or pharmacist before use if you are taking sedatives or tranquilizers
When using this product
- marked drowsiness may occur
- avoid alcoholic drinks
- alcohol, sedatives, and tranquilizers may increase drowsiness
- be careful when driving a motor vehicle or operating machinery
- excitability may occur, especially in children
If pregnant or breast-feeding, ask a health professional before use.
Keep out of reach of children. In case of overdose, get medical help or contact a Poison Control Center right away.

Directions:
- take every 4 to 6 hours
- do not take more than 6 doses in 24 hours

adults and children 12 years of age and over	25 mg to 50 mg (1 to 2 softgels)
children 6 to under 12 years of age	12.5 mg** to 25 mg (1 softgel)
children under 6 years of age	ask a doctor

**12.5 mg dosage strength is not available in this package. Do not attempt to break softgels.

Other Information:
- store at 59° to 77°F in a dry place
- protect from heat, humidity, and light

Inactive Ingredients: Gelatin, glycerin, polyethylene glycol 400, and sorbitol. Softgels are imprinted with edible dye-free ink.

Questions? call **1-800-524-2624** (English/Spanish), weekdays, 9 AM–5 PM EST

How Supplied: Benadryl® Dye-Free Allergy Liqui-Gels® Softgels are supplied in boxes of 24.

Liqui-Gels is a registered trademark of R.P. Scherer Corporation.

BENADRYL® ALLERGY & COLD
[bĕ nă-drĭl]

Acetaminophen, Diphenhydramine HCl, Pseudoephedrine HCl

Pain Reliever/Fever Reducer, Antihistamine, Nasal Decongestant

Active Ingredients

(in each caplet):	Purposes:
Acetaminophen 500 mg	Pain reliever/fever reducer
Diphenhydramine HCl 12.5 mg	Antihistamine
Pseudoephedrine HCl 30 mg	Nasal decongestant

Uses:
- temporarily relieves these symptoms of hay fever and the common cold:
  - sneezing
  - runny nose
  - headache
  - minor aches and pains
  - sore throat
  - nasal congestion
- temporarily relieves these additional symptoms of hay fever:
  - itching of the nose or throat
  - itchy, watery eyes
- temporarily reduces fever

Warnings:

Alcohol warning: If you consume 3 or more alcoholic drinks every day, ask your doctor whether you should take acetaminophen or other pain relievers/fever reducers. Acetaminophen may cause liver damage.

Do not use:
- with another product containing any of these active ingredients
- if you are now taking a prescription monoamine oxidase inhibitor (MAOI) (certain drugs for depression, psychiatric, or emotional conditions, or Parkinson's disease), or for 2 weeks after stopping the MAOI drug. If you do not know if your prescription drug contains an MAOI, ask a doctor or pharmacist before taking this product.
- with any other product containing diphenhydramine, even one used on skin.

Ask a doctor before use if you have:
- heart disease
- high blood pressure
- thyroid disease
- trouble urinating due to an enlarged prostate gland
- glaucoma
- diabetes
- a breathing problem such as emphysema or chronic bronchitis
Ask a doctor or pharmacist before use if you are taking sedatives or tranquilizers

When using this product:
- **do not use more than directed**
- marked drowsiness may occur
- avoid alcoholic drinks
- alcohol, sedatives, and tranquilizers may increase drowsiness
- be careful when driving a motor vehicle or operating machinery
- excitability may occur, especially in children

Stop use and ask a doctor if:
- you get nervous, dizzy or sleepless
- new symptoms occur
- pain or nasal congestion gets worse or lasts more than 7 days
- fever gets worse or lasts more than 3 days
- sore throat is severe
- redness or swelling is present
- sore throat lasts for more than 2 days, is accompanied or followed by fever, headache, rash, swelling, nausea, or vomiting

If pregnant or breast-feeding, ask a health professional before use.

Keep out of reach of children.

Overdose warning: Taking more than the recommended dose may cause liver damage. In case of overdose, get medical help or contact a Poison Control Center right away. Quick medical attention is critical for adults as well as for children even if you do not notice any signs or symptoms.

Directions:
- do not use more than directed (see overdose warning)
- take every 6 hours while symptoms persist
- adults and children 12 years of age and over: 2 caplets
- children under 12 years of age: ask a doctor
- do not take more than 8 caplets in 24 hours or as directed by a doctor

Other Information:
- store at 59° to 77°F in a dry place

Inactive Ingredients: candelilla wax, corn starch, croscarmellose sodium, hydroxypropyl cellulose, hypromellose, microcrystalline cellulose, polyethylene glycol, pregelatinized starch, sodium starch glycolate, stearic acid, titanium dioxide, and zinc stearate

Questions:

Call 1-800-524-2624 (English/Spanish), weekdays, 9 AM - 5 PM EST

How Supplied: Available in boxes of 24 tablets

BENADRYL® Allergy & Sinus Headache Caplets*
(also available in Gelcaps)
[bě 'nă-drĭl]
*Capsule Shaped Tablets

Drug Facts:

Active Ingredients:
(in each caplet)   **Purpose:**
Acetaminophen 500 mg .... Pain reliever
Diphenhydramine HCl
  12.5 mg .... Antihistamine
Pseudoephedrine HCl
  30 mg .... Nasal decongestant

Uses:
- temporarily relieves these symptoms of hay fever and the common cold:
  - runny nose
  - sneezing
  - headache
  - minor aches and pains
  - nasal congestion
- temporarily relieves these additional symptoms of hay fever:
  - itching of the nose or throat
  - itchy, watery eyes

Warnings:
Alcohol warning: If you consume 3 or more alcoholic drinks every day, ask your doctor whether you should take acetaminophen or other pain relievers/fever reducers. Acetaminophen may cause liver damage.

Do not use:
- with another product containing any of these active ingredients.
- if you are now taking a prescription monoamine oxidase inhibitor (MAOI) (certain drugs for depression, psychiatric, or emotional conditions, or Parkinson's disease), or for 2 weeks after stopping the MAOI drug. If you do not know if your prescription drug contains an MAOI, ask a doctor or pharmacist before taking this product.
- with any other product containing diphenhydramine, even one used on skin.

Ask a doctor before use if you have:
- heart disease
- glaucoma
- thyroid disease
- diabetes
- high blood pressure
- trouble urinating due to an enlarged prostate gland
- a breathing problem such as emphysema or chronic bronchitis

Ask a doctor or pharmacist before use if you are taking sedatives or tranquilizers
When using this product:
- do not use more than directed
- marked drowsiness may occur
- excitability may occur, especially in children
- avoid alcoholic drinks
- alcohol, sedatives, and tranquilizers may increase drowsiness
- be careful when driving a motor vehicle or operating machinery

Stop use and ask a doctor if:
- you get nervous, dizzy, or sleepless
- new symptoms occur
- pain or nasal congestion gets worse or lasts more than 7 days
- redness or swelling is present
- fever gets worse or lasts more than 3 days

If pregnant or breast-feeding, ask a health professional before use.

Keep out of reach of children.
Overdose warning: Taking more than the recommended dose may cause liver damage. In case of overdose, get medical help or contact a Poison Control Center right away. Quick medical attention is critical for adults as well as for children even if you do not notice any signs or symptoms.

Directions:
- do not use more than directed (see overdose warning)
- take every 6 hours while symptoms persist
- do not take more than 8 caplets in 24 hours or as directed by a doctor
- adults and children 12 years of age and over: 2 caplets
- children under 12 years of age: ask a doctor

Other Information:
- store at 59° to 77°F in a dry place

Inactive Ingredients: (Caplets): Candelilla wax, corn starch, croscarmellose sodium, D&C yellow no. 10 aluminum lake, FD&C blue no. 1 aluminum lake, FD&C yellow no. 6 aluminum lake, hydroxypropyl cellulose, hypromellose, microcrystalline cellulose, polyethylene glycol, polysorbate 80, pregelatinized starch, sodium starch glycolate, stearic acid, titanium dioxide, and zinc stearate (Gelcaps): Colloidal silicon dioxide, croscarmellose sodium, D&C yellow no. 10 Al lake, FD&C green no. 3 Al lake, gelatin, hypromellose, polysorbate 80, stearic acid and titanium dioxide.

Questions? call **1-800-524-2624** (English/Spanish), weekdays, 9 AM - 5 PM EST

How Supplied: Benadryl Allergy & Sinus Headache is available in boxes of 24 and 48 caplets, and boxes of 24, 48 and 72 gelcaps.

Children's BENADRYL D® Liquid Medication
[bě'nă-drĭl]
Diphenhydramine HCl and pseudoephedrine HCl liquid
Antihistamine, Nasal decongestant

Drug Facts

Active Ingredients
  (in each 5 mL)*:   **Purpose:**
Diphenhydramine HCl 12.5 mg .... Antihistamine
Pseudoephedrine HCl 30 mg . Nasal decongestant

*5 mL = one teaspoonful

Uses:
- temporarily relieves these symptoms due to hay fever or other upper respiratory allergies:
  - runny nose • sneezing • itchy, watery eyes • nasal congestion
  - itching of the nose or throat
- temporarily relieves these symptoms due to the common cold:
  - runny nose • sneezing • nasal congestion

Warnings:
Do not use
- if you are now taking a prescription monoamine oxidase inhibitor (MAOI) (certain drugs for depression, psychiatric, or emotional conditions, or Parkinson's disease), or for 2 weeks after stopping the MAOI drug. If you do not know if your prescription drug contains an MAOI, ask a doctor or pharmacist before taking this product
- with any other product containing diphenhydramine, even one used on skin

Ask a doctor before use if you have
- heart disease • glaucoma • thyroid disease • diabetes
- high blood pressure • trouble urinating due to an enlarged prostate gland
- a breathing problem such as emphysema or chronic bronchitis

Ask a doctor or pharmacist before use if you are taking sedatives or tranquilizers
When using this product
- do not use more than directed
- marked drowsiness may occur • avoid alcoholic drinks
- alcohol, sedatives, and tranquilizers may increase drowsiness
- be careful when driving a motor vehicle or operating machinery
- excitability may occur, especially in children

Stop use and ask a doctor if
- you get nervous, dizzy, or sleepless
- symptoms do not improve within 7 days or are accompanied by fever

If pregnant or breast-feeding, ask a health professional before use.
Keep out of reach of children. In case of overdose, get medical help or contact a Poison Control Center right away.

Directions:
- take every 4 to 6 hours • do not take more than 4 doses in 24 hours

children under 6 years of age	ask a doctor
children 6 to under 12 years of age	1 teaspoonful
adults and children 12 years of age and over	2 teaspoonfuls

Other Information:
- store at 59° to 77°F

Inactive Ingredients: citric acid, FD&C blue no. 1, FD&C red no. 40, flavors, glycerin, mono ammonium glycyrrhizinate, poloxamer 407, polysorbate 20,

Continued on next page

This product information was prepared in November 2003. On these and other Pfizer Consumer Healthcare Products, detailed information may be obtained by addressing Pfizer Consumer Healthcare, Pfizer, Inc., Morris Plains, NJ 07950

Children's Benadryl D—Cont.

purified water, saccharin sodium, sodium benzoate, sodium chloride, sodium citrate, and sorbitol solution

Questions? call **1-800-524-2624** (English/Spanish), weekdays, 9 AM – 5 PM EST

How Supplied: Benadryl D® Liquid Medication is available in a 4 fl oz bottle.

BENADRYL-D Tablets
(Formerly Benadryl Allergy & Sinus)
[bĕ'nă-drĭl]

Drug Facts:

Active Ingredients
(in each tablet):   **Purpose:**
Diphenhydramine HCl
  25 mg .... Antihistamine
Pseudoephedrine HCl
  60 mg .... Nasal decongestant

Uses:
- temporarily relieves these symptoms due to hay fever or other upper respiratory allergies:
  - runny nose
  - sneezing
  - itchy, watery eyes
  - nasal congestion
  - itching of the nose or throat
- temporarily relieves these symptoms due to the common cold:
  - runny nose
  - sneezing
  - nasal congestion

Warnings:
Do not use
- if you are now taking a prescription monoamine oxidase inhibitor (MAOI) (certain drugs for depression, psychiatric, or emotional conditions, or Parkinson's disease), or for 2 weeks after stopping the MAOI drug. If you do not know if your prescription drug contains an MAOI, ask a doctor or pharmacist before taking this product.
- with any other product containing diphenhydramine, even one used on skin.

Ask a doctor before use if you have:
- heart disease
- glaucoma
- thyroid disease
- diabetes
- high blood pressure
- trouble urinating due to an enlarged prostate gland
- a breathing problem such as emphysema or chronic bronchitis

Ask a doctor or pharmacist before use if you are taking sedatives or tranquilizers
When using this product
- do not use more than directed
- marked drowsiness may occur
- avoid alcoholic drinks
- alcohol, sedatives, and tranquilizers may increase drowsiness
- be careful when driving a motor vehicle or operating machinery
- excitability may occur, especially in children

Stop use and ask a doctor if
- you get nervous, dizzy, or sleepless
- symptoms do not improve within 7 days or are accompanied by fever

If pregnant or breast-feeding, ask a health professional before use.
Keep out of reach of children. In case of overdose, get medical help or contact a Poison Control Center right away.

Directions:
- adults and children 12 years of age and over: one (1) tablet
- take every 4 to 6 hours
- do not take more than 4 tablets in 24 hours
- children under 12 years of age: ask a doctor

Other Information:
- protect from light
- store at 59° to 77°F in a dry place

Inactive Ingredients: croscarmellose sodium, dibasic calcium phosphate dihydrate, FD&C blue no. 1 aluminum lake, hypromellose, microcrystalline cellulose, polyethylene glycol, polysorbate 80, pregelatinized starch, stearic acid, titanium dioxide, and zinc stearate. Printed with edible black ink.

Questions? call **1-800-524-2624** (English/Spanish), weekdays, 9 AM – 5 PM EST

How Supplied: Benadryl-D Tablets are supplied in boxes of 24.

Children's BENADRYL-D® Allergy & Sinus Fastmelt® Tablets
[bĕ'nă-drĭl]
Diphenhydramine citrate and pseudoephedrine HCl tablets
Antihistamine, Nasal decongestant

Drug Facts

Active Ingredients
(In each tablet):   **Purpose:**
Diphenhydramine citrate
  19 mg* .... Antihistamine
Pseudoephedrine HCl
  30 mg .... Nasal decongestant

*equivalent to 12.5 mg of diphenhydramine HCl

Uses:
- temporarily relieves these symptoms of hay fever or the common cold:
  - runny nose • sneezing • nasal congestion
- temporarily relieves these additional symptoms of hay fever:
  - itching of the nose or throat
  - itchy, watery eyes

Warnings:
Do not use
- if you are now taking a prescription monoamine oxidase inhibitor (MAOI) (certain drugs for depression, psychiatric, or emotional conditions, or Parkinson's disease), or for 2 weeks after stopping the MAOI drug. If you do not know if your prescription drug contains an MAOI, ask a doctor or pharmacist before taking this product.
- with any other product containing diphenhydramine, even one used on skin.

Ask a doctor before use in you have
- heart disease • high blood pressure
- thyroid disease • trouble urinating due to an enlarged prostate gland
- diabetes • glaucoma • a breathing problem such as emphysema or chronic bronchitis

Ask a doctor or pharmacist before use if you are taking sedatives or tranquilizers
When using this product • do not use more than directed • marked drowsiness may occur • alcohol, sedatives, and tranquilizers may increase drowsiness • avoid alcoholic drinks • be careful when driving a motor vehicle or operating machinery • excitability may occur, especially in children

Stop use and ask a doctor if
- you get nervous, dizzy, or sleepless
- symptoms do not improve within 7 days or are accompanied by fever

If pregnant or breast-feeding, ask a health professional before use.
Keep out of reach of children. In case of overdose, get medical help or contact a Poison Control Center right away.

Directions:
- adults and children 12 years of age and over: 2 tablets
- do not take more than 8 tablets in 24 hours, or as directed by a doctor
- children under 12 years of age: ask a doctor
- place in mouth and allow to dissolve
- take every 4 to 6 hours

Other Information: • phenylketonurics: contains phenylalanine 4.6 mg per tablet • store at 59° to 77°F in a dry place

Inactive Ingredients: aspartame, citric acid, D&C red no. 7 calcium lake, ethylcellulose, flavor, lactitol, magnesium stearate, mannitol, polyethylene, soy protein isolate, and stearic acid

Questions? call **1-800-524-2624** (English/Spanish), weekdays, 9 AM - 5 PM EST

How Supplied: 20 Dissolving tablets

BENADRYL® Maximum Strength Severe Allergy† & Sinus Headache Caplets*
[bĕ'nă-drĭl]
* Capsule Shaped Tablets
† Upper Respiratory Allergies Only

Drug Facts:

Active Ingredients:
(in each caplet)   **Purposes:**
Acetaminophen
  500 mg .... Pain reliever
Diphenhydramine
  HCl 25 mg .... Antihistamine
Pseudoephedrine
  HCl 30 mg .... Nasal decongestant

Uses:
- temporarily relieves these symptoms of hay fever and the common cold:
  - runny nose
  - headache
  - sneezing
  - minor aches and pains
  - nasal congestion

- temporarily relieves these additional symptoms of hay fever:
  - itching of the nose or throat
  - itchy, watery eyes

Warnings:

Alcohol warning: If you consume 3 or more alcoholic drinks every day, ask your doctor whether you should take acetaminophen or other pain relievers/fever reducers. Acetaminophen may cause liver damage.

Do not use

- with another product containing any of these active ingredients
- if you are now taking a prescription monoamine oxidase inhibitor (MAOI) (certain drugs for depression, psychiatric, or emotional conditions, or Parkinson's disease), or for 2 weeks after stopping the MAOI drug. If you do not know if your prescription drug contains an MAOI, ask a doctor or pharmacist before taking this product.
- with any other product containing diphenhydramine, even one used on skin.

Ask a doctor before use if you have

- heart disease
- glaucoma
- thyroid disease
- diabetes
- high blood pressure
- trouble urinating due to an enlarged prostate gland
- a breathing problem such as emphysema or chronic bronchitis

Ask a doctor or pharmacist before use if you are taking sedatives or tranquilizers

When using this product

- **do not use more than directed**
- marked drowsiness may occur
- excitability may occur, especially in children
- avoid alcoholic drinks
- alcohol, sedatives, and tranquilizers may increase drowsiness
- be careful when driving a motor vehicle or operating machinery

Stop use and ask a doctor if

- you get nervous, dizzy, or sleepless
- new symptoms occur
- redness or swelling is present
- pain or nasal congestion gets worse or lasts more than 3 days
- fever gets worse or lasts more than 3 days

If pregnant or breast-feeding, ask a health professional before use.

Keep out of reach of children.

Overdose warning: Taking more than the recommended dose may cause liver damage. In case of overdose, get medical help or contact a Poison Control Center right away. Quick medical attention is critical for adults as well as for children even if you do not notice any signs or symptoms.

Directions:

- do not use more than directed (see overdose warning)
- take every 6 hours while symptoms persist
- do not take more than 8 caplets in 24 hours or as directed by a doctor
- adults and children 12 years of age and over: 2 caplets
- children under 12 years of age: ask a doctor

Other Information:

- store at 59° to 77°F in a dry place

Inactive Ingredients: Carnauba wax, crospovidone, FD&C blue no. 1 aluminum lake, hypromellose, magnesium stearate, microcrystalline cellulose, polyethylene glycol, polysorbate 80, povidone, pregelatinized starch, sodium starch glycolate, stearic acid, and titanium dioxide

Questions? call **1-800-524-2624** (English/Spanish), weekdays, 9 AM – 5 PM EST

How Supplied: Available in 20 Caplets (capsule-shaped tablets).

Children's BENADRYL Allergy Liquid (Cherry flavor) and Children's BENADRYL Dye-Free Allergy Liquid (Bubble gum flavor)
[bě 'nă-drĭl]

Drug Facts:

Active Ingredient: **Purpose:**
(in each 5 mL)
Diphenhydramine
  HCl 12.5 mg .... Antihistamine
5 mL = one teaspoonful

Uses:

- temporarily relieves these symptoms due to hay fever or other upper respiratory allergies:
  - runny nose
  - sneezing
  - itchy, watery eyes
  - itching of the nose or throat
- temporarily relieves these symptoms due to the common cold:
  - runny nose
  - sneezing

Warnings:

Do not use with any other product containing diphenhydramine, even one used on skin.

Ask a doctor before use if you have:

- glaucoma
- trouble urinating due to an enlarged prostate gland
- a breathing problem such as emphysema or chronic bronchitis

Ask a doctor or pharmacist before use if you are taking sedatives or tranquilizers

When using this product:

- marked drowsiness may occur
- avoid alcoholic drinks
- alcohol, sedatives, and tranquilizers may increase drowsiness
- be careful when driving a motor vehicle or operating machinery
- excitability may occur, especially in children

If pregnant or breast-feeding, ask a health professional before use.

Keep out of reach of children. In case of overdose, get medical help or contact a Poison Control Center right away.

Directions:

- take every 4 to 6 hours
- do not take more than 6 doses in 24 hours

children under 6 years of age	ask a doctor
children 6 to under 12 years of age	1 to 2 teaspoonfuls (12.5 mg to 25 mg)
adults and children 12 years of age and over	2 to 4 teaspoonfuls (25 mg to 50 mg)

Other Information:

- store at 59° to 77°F

Inactive Ingredients: Children's Benadryl Allergy Liquid: Citric acid, D&C red no. 33, FD&C red no. 40, flavors, glycerin, mono ammonium glycyrrhizinate, poloxamer 407, purified water, sodium benzoate, sodium chloride, sodium citrate, and sugar. Children's Benadryl Dye-Free Allergy Liquid: carboxymethylcellulose sodium, citric acid, flavors, glycerin, purified water, saccharin sodium, sodium benzoate, sodium citrate, and sorbitol solution.

Questions? call **1-800-524-2624** (English/Spanish), weekdays, 9 AM–5 PM EST

How Supplied: Children's Benadryl Allergy Liquid is supplied in 4 and 8 fluid ounce bottles. Children's Benadryl Dye-Free Allergy Liquid is supplied in 4 fl oz bottles. Also available: Children's Benadryl Allergy Chewable Tablets. (Phenylketonurics: contains phenylalanine 4.2 mg per tablet)

Children's BENADRYL® Allergy & Cold
FASTMELT™
Dissolving Tablets
[bě 'nă-drĭl]
Cherry Flavored

Drug Facts:

Active Ingredients: **Purposes:**
(in each tablet)
Diphenhydramine citrate
  19 mg* .... Antihistamine/cough
                                    suppressant
Pseudoephedrine HCl
  30 mg .... Nasal decongestant

*equivalent to 12.5 mg of diphenhydramine HCl

Continued on next page

This product information was prepared in November 2003. On these and other Pfizer Consumer Healthcare Products, detailed information may be obtained by addressing Pfizer Consumer Healthcare, Pfizer, Inc., Morris Plains, NJ 07950

Children's Benadryl—Cont.

Uses:
- temporarily relieves these symptoms of hay fever or the common cold:
  - runny nose
  - sneezing
  - nasal congestion
  - cough
- temporarily relieves these additional symptoms of hay fever:
  - itching of the nose or throat
  - itchy, watery eyes

Warnings:
Do not use
- if you are now taking a prescription monoamine oxidase inhibitor (MAOI) (certain drugs for depression, psychiatric, or emotional conditions, or Parkinson's disease), or for 2 weeks after stopping the MAOI drug. If you do not know if your prescription drug contains an MAOI, ask a doctor or pharmacist before taking this product.
- with any other product containing diphenhydramine, even one used on skin.

Ask a doctor before use if you have
- heart disease
- high blood pressure
- thyroid disease
- trouble urinating due to an enlarged prostate gland
- diabetes
- cough accompanied by excessive phlegm (mucus)
- glaucoma
- a breathing problem such as emphysema or chronic bronchitis
- persistent or chronic cough such as occurs with smoking, asthma, or emphysema

Ask a doctor or pharmacist before use if you are taking sedatives or tranquilizers

When using this product
- do not use more than directed
- marked drowsiness may occur
- excitability may occur, especially in children
- avoid alcoholic drinks
- alcohol, sedatives, and tranquilizers may increase drowsiness
- be careful when driving a motor vehicle or operating machinery

Stop use and ask a doctor if
- you get nervous, dizzy, or sleepless
- symptoms do not improve within 7 days or are accompanied by fever
- cough persists for more than 1 week, tends to recur, or is accompanied by fever, rash, or persistent headache. These could be signs of a serious condition.

If pregnant or breast-feeding, ask a health professional before use.

Keep out of reach of children. In case of overdose, get medical help or contact a Poison Control Center right away.

Directions:
- place in mouth and allow to dissolve
- take every 4 hours

adults and children 12 years of age and over	2 tablets; do not take more than 8 tablets in 24 hours or as directed by a doctor
children 6 to under 12 years of age	1 tablet; do not take more than 4 tablets in 24 hours or as directed by a doctor
children under 6 years of age	ask a doctor

Other Information:
- **phenylketonurics:** contains phenylalanine 4.6 mg per tablet
- store at 59° to 77°F in a dry place

Inactive Ingredients: Aspartame, citric acid, D&C red no. 7 calcium lake, ethylcellulose, flavor, lactitol, magnesium stearate, mannitol, polyethylene, soy protein isolate, and stearic acid

Questions? call **1-800-524-2624** (English/Spanish), weekdays, 9 AM - 5 PM EST

How Supplied: Available in boxes of 20 dissolving tablets.

Children's BENADRYL® Allergy Fastmelt Tablets
[bĕ′nă-drĭl]

Drug Facts

Active Ingredient (in each tablet):   **Purpose:**
Diphenhydramine citrate 19 mg* .... Antihistamine

*equivalent to 12.5 mg of diphenhydramine HCl

Uses:
- temporarily relieves these symptoms due to hay fever or other upper respiratory allergies:
  - runny nose • sneezing • itchy, watery eyes • itching of the nose or throat
- temporarily relieves these symptoms due to the common cold:
  - runny nose • sneezing

Warnings: Do not use with any other product containing diphenhydramine, even one used on skin

Ask a doctor before use if you have
- glaucoma • trouble urinating due to an enlarged prostate gland • a breathing problem such as emphysema or chronic bronchitis

Ask a doctor or pharmacist before use if you are taking sedatives or tranquilizers

When using this product
- marked drowsiness may occur • avoid alcoholic drinks • alcohol, sedatives, and tranquilizers may increase drowsiness • be careful when driving a motor vehicle or operating machinery • excitability may occur, especially in children

If pregnant or breast-feeding, ask a health professional before use.

Keep out of reach of children. In case of overdose, get medical help or contact a Poison Control Center right away.

Directions:
- take every 4 to 6 hours • do not take more than 6 doses in 24 hours

adults and children 12 years of age and over	2 to 4 tablets (38 mg to 76 mg)
children 6 to under 12 years of age	1 to 2 tablets (19 mg to 38 mg)
children under 6 years of age	ask a doctor

Other Information:
- **phenylketonurics:** contains phenylalanine 4.5 mg per tablet • store at 59° to 77°F in a dry place • protect from heat, humidity, and light

Inactive Ingredients: aspartame, citric acid, D&C red no. 7 calcium lake, ethylcellulose, flavors, lactitol monohydrate, magnesium stearate, mannitol, polyethylene, soy protein isolate, stearic acid

Questions? call **1-800-524-2624** (English/Spanish), weekdays, 9 AM – 5 PM EST

How Supplied: Available in boxes of 10 and 20 dissolving tablets.

BENADRYL® Itch Relief Stick Extra Strength
Topical Analgesic/Skin Protectant
[bĕ′nă-drĭl]

Drug Facts

Active Ingredients: **Purpose:**
Diphenhydramine hydrochloride 2% .... Topical analgesic
Zinc acetate 0.1% .... Skin protectant

Uses:
- temporarily relieves pain and itching associated with:
  - insect bites • minor burns
  - sunburn
  - minor skin irritations • minor cuts
  - scrapes
  - rashes due to poison ivy, poison oak, and poison sumac
- dries the oozing and weeping of poison ivy, poison oak and poison sumac

Warnings:
For external use only.
Flammable. Keep away from fire or flame.
Do not use
- on large areas of the body
- with any other product containing diphenhydramine, even one taken by mouth

Ask a doctor before use
- on chicken pox • on measles

When using this product
- avoid contact with eyes

Stop use and ask a doctor if
- condition worsens or does not improve within 7 days
- symptoms persist for more than 7 days or clear up and occur again within a few days

Keep out of reach of children. If swallowed, get medical help or contact a Poison Control Center right away.

Directions:
- do not use more than directed
- hold stick straight down over affected skin area
- press tip of stick repeatedly on affected skin area until liquid flows, then dab sparingly
- adults and children 2 years of age and older: apply to affected area not more than 3 to 4 times daily
- children under 2 years of age: ask a doctor

Other Information: • store at 20° to 25° C (68° to 77° F)

Inactive Ingredients: alcohol, glycerin, povidone, purified water, and tromethamine

Questions? call **1-800-524-2624** (English/Spanish), weekdays, 9 AM - 5 PM EST

How Supplied: Benadryl® Itch Relief Stick is available in a .47 fl. oz (14 mL) dauber.

BENADRYL® Itch Stopping Cream Extra Strength
[bĕ 'nă-drĭl]

Drug Facts
Active Ingredients: **Purpose:**
Diphenhydramine
hydrochloride 2% .... Topical analgesic
Zinc acetate 0.1% .... Skin protectant

Uses:
- temporarily relieves pain and itching associated with:
  - insect bites
  - minor burns
  - sunburn
  - minor skin irritations
  - minor cuts
  - scrapes
  - rashes due to poison ivy, poison oak, and poison sumac
- dries the oozing and weeping of poison ivy, poison oak, and poison sumac

Warnings:
For external use only
Do not use
- on large areas of the body
- with any other product containing diphenhydramine, even one taken by mouth

Ask a doctor before use
- on chicken pox • on measles

When using this product
- avoid contact with eyes

Stop use and ask a doctor if
- condition worsens or does not improve within 7 days
- symptoms persist for more than 7 days or clear up and occur again within a few days

Keep out of reach of children. If swallowed, get medical help or contact a Poison Control Center right away.

Directions:
- do not use more than directed
- adults and children 2 years of age and older: apply to affected area not more than 3 to 4 times daily
- children under 2 years of age: ask a doctor

Other Information: • store at 20° to 25° C (68° to 77° F)

Inactive Ingredients: cetyl alcohol, diazolidinyl urea, methylparaben, polyethylene glycol monostearate 1000, propylene glycol, propylparaben, and purified water

Questions? call **1-800-524-2624** (English/Spanish), Monday to Friday, 9 AM - 5 PM EST

How Supplied: Benadryl Itch Stopping Cream Extra Strength is available in 1 oz (28.3 g) tubes.
Also available in original strength.

BENADRYL® Itch Stopping Gel Extra Strength
[bĕ 'nă-drĭl]

Drug Facts
Active Ingredient: **Purpose:**
Diphenhydramine
hydrochloride 2% .... Topical analgesic

Uses:
- temporarily relieves pain and itching associated with:
  - insect bites
  - minor burns
  - sunburn
  - minor skin irritations
  - minor cuts
  - scrapes
  - rashes due to poison ivy, poison oak, and poison sumac

Warnings:
For external use only
Do not use
- on large areas of the body
- with any other product containing diphenhydramine, even one taken by mouth

Ask a doctor before use
- on chicken pox
- on measles

When using this product
- avoid contact with eyes

Stop use and ask a doctor if
- condition worsens
- symptoms persist for more than 7 days or clear up and occur again within a few days

Keep out of reach of children. If swallowed, get medical help or contact a Poison Control Center right away.

Directions:
- do not use more than directed
- adults and children 12 years of age and older: apply to affected area not more than 3 to 4 times daily
- children under 2 years of age: ask a doctor

Other Information:
- store at 20° to 25° C (68° to 77°F)

Inactive Ingredients: SD alcohol 38-B, camphor, citric acid, diazolidinyl urea, glycerin, hypromellose, methylparaben, propylene glycol, propylparaben, purified water, and sodium citrate

Questions? call **1-800-524-2624** (English/Spanish), Monday to Friday, 9 AM - 5 PM EST

How Supplied: Benadryl Itch Stopping Gel Extra Strength is supplied in 4 fl. oz. (118mL) bottles

---

BENADRYL® Itch Stopping Spray Extra Strength
[bĕ 'nă-drĭl]

Drug Facts
Active Ingredients: **Purpose:**
Diphenhydramine hydrochloride
2% .... Topical analgesic
Zinc acetate 0.1% .... Skin protectant

Uses:
- temporarily relieves pain and itching associated with:
  - insect bites • minor burns
  - sunburn • minor skin irritations
  - minor cuts • scrapes • rashes due to poison ivy, poison oak, and poison sumac
- dries the oozing and weeping of poison ivy, poison oak and poison sumac

Warnings:
For external use only.
Flammable. Keep away from fire or flame.
Do not use
- on large areas of the body
- with any other product containing diphenhydramine, even one taken by mouth

Ask a doctor before use
- on chicken pox • on measles

When using this product
- avoid contact with eyes

Stop use and ask a doctor if
- condition worsens or does not improve within 7 days
- symptoms persist for more than 7 days or clear up and occur again within a few days

Keep out of reach of children. If swallowed, get medical help or contact a Poison Control Center right away.

Directions:
- do not use more than directed
- adults and children 2 years of age and older: apply to affected area not more than 3 to 4 times daily
- children under 2 years of age: ask a doctor

Other Information: • store at 20° to 25° C (68° to 77° F)

Inactive Ingredients: alcohol, glycerin, povidone, purified water, and tris (hydroxymethyl) aminomethane

Questions? call **1-800-524-2624** (English/Spanish), weekdays, 9 AM - 5 PM EST

How Supplied: Benadryl Itch Stopping Spray Extra Strength Spray is available in a 2 fl. oz. (59mL) pump spray bottle.

Continued on next page

This product information was prepared in November 2003. On these and other Pfizer Consumer Healthcare Products, detailed information may be obtained by addressing Pfizer Consumer Healthcare, Pfizer, Inc., Morris Plains, NJ 07950

BENGAY® External Analgesic Products

Description: BENGAY products contain menthol in an alcohol base gel, combinations of methyl salicylate and menthol in cream and ointment bases, as well as a combination of methyl salicylate, menthol and camphor in a non-greasy cream base; all suitable for topical application.

In addition to the Original Formula Pain Relieving Ointment (methyl salicylate, 18.3%; menthol, 16%), BENGAY is offered as BENGAY Greaseless Pain Relieving Cream (methyl salicylate, 15%; menthol, 10%), an Arthritis Formula NonGreasy Pain Relieving Cream (methyl salicylate, 30%; menthol, 8%), an Ultra Strength NonGreasy Pain Relieving Cream (methyl salicylate 30%; menthol 10%; camphor 4%), and Vanishing Scent NonGreasy Pain Relieving Gel (2.5% menthol).

Action and Uses: Methyl salicylate, menthol and camphor are external analgesics which stimulate sensory receptors of warmth and/or cold. This produces a counter-irritant response which provides temporary relief of minor aches and pains of muscles and joints associated with simple backache, arthritis, strains and sprains.

Several double-blind clinical studies of BENGAY products containing menthol-methyl salicylate have shown the effectiveness of this combination in counteracting minor pain of skeletal muscle stress and arthritis.

Three studies involving a total of 102 normal subjects in which muscle soreness was experimentally induced showed statistically significant beneficial results from use of the active product vs. placebo for lowered Muscle Action Potential (spasms), greater rise in threshold of muscular pain and greater reduction in perceived muscular pain.

Six clinical studies of a total of 207 subjects suffering from minor pain due to osteoarthritis and rheumatoid arthritis showed the active product to give statistically significant beneficial results vs. placebo for greater relief of perceived pain, increased range of motion of the affected joints and increased digital dexterity. In two studies designed to measure the effect of topically applied BENGAY vs. placebo on muscular endurance, discomfort, onset of exercise pain and fatigue, 30 subjects performed a submaximal three-hour run and another 30 subjects performed a maximal treadmill run. BENGAY was found to significantly decrease the discomfort during the submaximal and maximal runs, and increase the time before onset of fatigue during the maximal run.

Applied before workouts, BENGAY relaxes tight muscles and increases circulation to make exercising more comfortable, longer.

To help reduce muscle ache and soreness after exercise, BENGAY can be applied and allowed to work before taking a shower.

Directions: Apply to affected area not more than 3 to 4 times daily.

Warnings: For external use only. Use only as directed. Do not use with a heating pad. Keep away from children to avoid accidental ingestion. Do not swallow. If swallowed, get medical help or contact a Poison Control Center immediately. Do not bandage tightly. Keep away from eyes, mucous membranes, broken or irritated skin. If skin redness or excessive irritation develops, pain lasts for more than 10 days, or with arthritis—like conditions in children under 12, do not use and call a physician.

BENGAY® Pain Relieving Patch
[bĕn-gā]

Drug Facts

Active Ingredient: **Purpose:**
Menthol 1.4% .... Topical analgesic (present as crystalline and natural forms)

Uses:
- temporarily relieves minor aches and pains of muscles and joints associated with:
  - simple backache • arthritis • strains
  - bruises • sprains

Warnings:
For external use only.
Do not use
- on wounds or damaged skin
- with a heating pad
- on a child under 12 years of age with arthritis-like conditions

Ask a doctor before use if you have
- redness over the affected area

When using this product
- avoid contact with eyes or mucous membranes
- do not bandage tightly

Stop use and ask a doctor if
- condition worsens or symptoms persist for more than 7 days
- symptoms clear up and occur again within a few days • excessive skin irritation occurs

Keep out of reach of children. If swallowed, get medical help or contact a Poison Control Center immediately.

Directions:
- open pouch and remove patch
- if desired, cut patch to size
- peel off protective backing and apply sticky side to affected area
- adults and children 12 years of age and older: apply to affected area not more than 3 to 4 times daily
- children under 12 years of age: consult a doctor

Other Information: • store at 20° to 25°C (68° to 77°F)

Inactive Ingredients: camphor, carboxymethylcellulose sodium, glycerin, kaolin, methyl acrylate/2-ethylhexyl acrylate copolymer, methyl salicylate, poly-

acrylic acid, polysorbate 80, sodium polyacrylate, tartaric acid, titanium dioxide, and water

Questions? call **1-800-223-0182,** weekdays, 9 AM – 5 PM EST

How Supplied: Bengay Pain Relieving Patch is available in cartons containing 5 individually sealed regular size patches and 4 individually sealed large size patches.

BENGAY® ULTRA STRENGTH Pain Relieving Patch
[bĕn-gā]
Menthol Topical Analgesic Patch
[Menthol 5%]

Drug Facts:

Active Ingredient: **Purpose:**
Menthol 5% .... Topical analgesic

Uses:
- temporarily relieves minor aches and pains of muscles and joints associated with:
  - simple backache • arthritis • strains
  - bruises • sprains

Warnings:
For external use only.
Do not use
- on wounds or damaged skin
- with a heating pad
- on a child under 12 years of age with arthritis-like conditions

Ask a doctor before use if you have
- redness over the affected area

When using this product
- avoid contact with eyes or mucous membranes
- do not bandage tightly

Stop use and ask a doctor if
- condition worsens or symptoms persist for more than 7 days
- symptoms clear up and occur again within a few days
- excessive skin irritation occurs

Keep out of reach of children. If swallowed, get medical help or contact a Poison Control Center immediately.

Directions:
- open pouch and remove patch
- if desired, cut patch to size
- peel off protective backing and apply sticky side to affected area
- adults and children 12 years of age and older: apply to affected area not more than 3 to 4 times daily
- children under 12 years of age: consult a doctor

Other Information:
- store at 20° to 25°C (68° to 77°F)

Inactive Ingredients: carboxymethylcellulose sodium, glycerin, kaolin, methyl acrylate/2-ethylhexyl acrylate copolymer, polyacrylic acid, polysorbate 80, sodium polyacrylate, tartaric acid, titanium dioxide, and water

Questions? call **1-800-223-0182,** weekdays 9AM – 5 PM EST

How Supplied: Available in cartons containing 5 individually sealed regular size patches and 4 individually sealed large size patches.

CORTIZONE•5®
Ointment

Drug Facts

Active Ingredient: **Purpose:**
Hydrocortisone 0.5% .... Anti-itch

Uses:
- temporarily relieves itching of minor skin irritations, inflammation, and rashes due to:
  - eczema
  - insect bites
  - cosmetics
  - psoriasis
  - detergents
  - soaps
  - poison ivy, oak, sumac
  - jewelry
  - seborrheic dermatitis
  - and for external anal and genital itching
- other uses of this product should be only under the advice and supervision of a doctor

Warnings:
For external use only
Do not use
- for the treatment of diaper rash. Consult a doctor.
- in the genital area if you have a vaginal discharge. Consult a doctor.

When using this product
- avoid contact with the eyes
- do not exceed the recommended daily dosage unless directed by a doctor
- do not put directly in rectum by using fingers or any mechanical device

Stop use and ask a doctor if
- rectal bleeding occurs
- condition worsens, or if symptoms persist for more than 7 days or clear up and occur again within a few days, and do not begin use of any other hydrocortisone product unless you have asked a doctor

Keep out of reach of children. If swallowed, get medical help or contact a Poison Control Center right away.

Directions:
- adults and children 2 years of age and older:
  - apply to affected area not more than 3 to 4 times daily
  - children under 2 years of age: do not use, ask a doctor
- for external anal and genital itching, adults:
  - when practical, clean the affected area with mild soap and warm water and rinse thoroughly
  - gently dry by patting or blotting with toilet tissue or a soft cloth before applying
  - apply to affected area not more than 3 to 4 times daily
  - children under 12 years of age: ask a doctor

Other Information:
- store at 15° to 30°C (59° to 86°F)

Inactive Ingredients: aloe barbadensis extract and white petrolatum

Questions? call **1-800-223-0182**, Monday to Friday, 9 AM - 5 PM EST

How Supplied: CORTIZONE•5® ointment: 1 oz. tube.

CORTIZONE•10®
Creme

Drug Facts

Active Ingredient: **Purpose:**
Hydrocortisone 1% .... Anti-itch

Uses:
- temporarily relieves itching associated with minor skin irritations, inflammation, and rashes due to:
  - eczema • psoriasis • poison ivy, oak, sumac • insect bites • detergents
  - jewelry • cosmetics • soaps
  - seborrheic dermatitis
- temporarily relieves external anal and genital itching
- other uses of this product should only be under the advice and supervision of a doctor

Warnings:
For external use only.
Do no use
- in the genital area if you have a vaginal discharge. Consult a doctor.
- for the treatment of diaper rash. Consult a doctor.

When using this product
- avoid contact with the eyes
- do not use more than directed unless told to do so by a doctor
- do not put directly into the rectum by using fingers or any mechanical device or applicator

Stop use and ask a doctor if
- condition worsens, symptoms persist for more than 7 days or clear up and occur again within a few days, and do not begin use of any other hydrocortisone product unless you have asked a doctor
- rectal bleeding occurs

Keep out of reach of children. If swallowed, get medical help or contact a Poison Control Center right away.

Directions:
- **for itching of skin irritation, inflammation, and rashes:**
- adults and children 2 years of age and older: apply to affected area not more than 3 to 4 times daily
- children under 2 years of age: ask a doctor
- **for external anal and genital itching, adults:**
- when practical, clean the affected area with mild soap and warm water and rinse thoroughly
- gently dry by patting or blotting with toilet tissue or a soft cloth before applying
- apply to affected area not more than 3 to 4 times daily
- children under 12 years of age: ask a doctor

Other Information:
- store at 20° to 25°C (68° to 77°F)
- contents filled by weight, not volume

Inactive Ingredients: aloe barbadensis gel, aluminum sulfate, calcium acetate, cetearyl alcohol, glycerin, light mineral oil, maltodextrin, methylparaben, potato dextrin, propylparaben, purified water, sodium cetearyl sulfate, sodium lauryl sulfate, white petrolatum, and white wax

Questions? call **1-800-223-0182**, weekdays, 9 AM - 5 PM EST

How Supplied: CORTIZONE•10® creme: .5 oz., 1 oz. and 2 oz. tubes.

CORTIZONE•10®
Ointment

Drug Facts
Active Ingredient: **Purpose:**
Hydrocortisone 1% .... Anti-itch

Uses:
- temporarily relieves itching of minor skin irritations, inflammation, and rashes due to:
  - eczema
  - insect bites
  - cosmetics
  - psoriasis
  - detergents
  - soaps
  - poison ivy, oak, sumac
  - jewelry
  - seborrheic dermatitis
- temporarily relieves external anal and genital itching
- other uses of this product should be only under the advice and supervision of a doctor

Warnings:
For external use only.
Do not use
- in the genital area if you have a vaginal discharge. Consult a doctor.
- for the treatment of diaper rash. Consult a doctor.

When using this product
- avoid contact with eyes
- do not use more than directed unless told to do so by a doctor
- do not put directly in rectum by using fingers or any mechanical device or applicator

Stop use and ask a doctor if
- condition worsens, or if symptoms persist for more than 7 days or clear up and occur again within a few days, and do not begin use of any other hydrocortisone product unless you have asked a doctor
- rectal bleeding occurs

Keep out of reach of children. If swallowed, get medical help or contact a Poison Control Center right away.

Directions:
- **for itching of skin irritation, inflammation, and rashes:**
  - adults and children 2 years of age and older: apply to affected area not more than 3 to 4 times daily
  - children under 2 years of age: ask a doctor
- **for external anal and genital itching, adults:**
  - when practical, clean the affected area with mild soap and warm water and rinse thoroughly
  - gently dry by patting or blotting with toilet tissue or a soft cloth before applying
  - apply to affected area not more than 3 to 4 times daily

Continued on next page

This product information was prepared in November 2003. On these and other Pfizer Consumer Healthcare Products, detailed information may be obtained by addressing Pfizer Consumer Healthcare, Pfizer, Inc., Morris Plains, NJ 07950

Cortizone•10 Ointment—Cont.

- children under 12 years of age: ask a doctor

Other Information:
- store at 20° to 25°C (68° to 77°F)

Inactive Ingredients: white petrolatum

Questions? call **1-800-223-0182**, weekdays, 9 AM - 5 PM EST

How Supplied: CORTIZONE•10® ointment: 1 oz. and 2 oz. tubes.

CORTIZONE•10® Plus
Creme
Hydrocortisone Anti-Itch Cream

Drug Facts:

Active Ingredient: **Purpose:**
Hydrocortisone 1% .... Anti-itch

Uses:
- temporarily relieves itching of minor skin irritations, inflammation, and rashes due to:
  - eczema
  - insect bites
  - cosmetics
  - psoriasis
  - detergents
  - soaps
  - poison ivy, oak, sumac
  - jewelry
  - seborrheic dermatitis
- temporarily relieves external anal and genital itching
- other uses of this product should only be under the advice and supervision of a doctor

Warnings:
For external use only.
Do not use
- in the genital area if you have a vaginal discharge. Consult a doctor.
- for the treatment of diaper rash. Consult a doctor.
When using this product
- avoid contact with eyes
- do not use more than directed unless told to do so by a doctor
- do not put directly into the rectum by using fingers or any mechanical device or applicator
Stop use and ask a doctor if
- condition worsens, symptoms persist for more than 7 days or clear up and occur again within a few days, and do not begin use of any other hydrocortisone product unless you have asked a doctor
- rectal bleeding occurs
Keep out of reach of children. If swallowed, get medical help or contact a Poison Control Center right away.

Directions:
- **for itching of skin irritation, inflammation, and rashes:**
  - adults and children 2 years of age and older: apply to affected area not more than 3 to 4 times daily
  - children under 2 years of age: ask a doctor
- **for external anal and genital itching, adults:**
  - when practical, clean the affected area with mild soap and warm water and rinse thoroughly

- gently dry by patting or blotting with toilet tissue or a soft cloth before applying
- apply to affected area not more than 3 to 4 times daily
- children under 12 years of age: ask a doctor

Other Information:
- store at 20° to 25°C (68° to 77°F)
- contents filled by weight, not volume

Inactive Ingredients: aloe barbadensis gel, aluminum sulfate, calcium acetate, cetearyl alcohol, cetyl alcohol, cholecalciferol, corn oil, glycerin, isopropyl palmitate, light mineral oil, maltodextrin, methylparaben, potato dextrin, propylene glycol, propylparaben, purified water, sodium cetearyl sulfate, sodium lauryl sulfate, vitamin A palmitate, vitamin E, white petrolatum, and white wax

Questions? call **1-800-223-0182**, weekdays, 9 AM - 5 PM EST

How Supplied: CORTIZONE•10® Plus creme: 1 oz. and 2 oz. tubes.

CORTIZONE•10® MAXIMUM STRENGTH QUICK SHOT™ SPRAY

Drug Facts

Active Ingredient: **Purpose:**
Hydrocortisone 1% .... Anti-itch

Uses:
- temporarily relieves itching of minor skin irritations, inflammation, and rashes due to:
  - eczema
  - insect bites
  - cosmetics
  - psoriasis
  - detergents
  - soaps
  - poison ivy, oak, sumac
  - jewelry
  - seborrheic dermatitis
- other uses of this product should be only under the advice and supervision of a doctor

Warnings:
For external use only
Flammable - keep away from fire or flame
Do not use
- for the treatment of diaper rash. Consult a doctor.
When using this product
- avoid contact with the eyes
Stop use and ask a doctor if condition worsens, or if symptoms persist for more than 7 days or clear up and occur again within a few days, and do not begin use of any other hydrocortisone product unless you have asked a doctor
Keep out of reach of children. If swallowed, get medical help or contact a Poison Control Center right away.

Directions:
- adults and children 2 years of age and older: apply to affected area not more than 3 to 4 times daily
- children under 2 years of age: do not use; ask a doctor
Other Information:
- store at 15° to 30°C (59° to 86°F)
- store away from heat and protect from freezing

Inactive Ingredients: benzyl alcohol, propylene glycol, purified water, and SD alcohol 40-2 (60% v/v)
Questions? call **1-800-223-0182**, Monday to Friday, 9 AM - 5 PM EST

How Supplied: CORTIZONE•10® Quick Shot Spray: 1.5 oz. pump bottle

---

DESITIN® CREAMY WITH ALOE and VITAMIN E
Zinc Oxide Diaper Rash Ointment

Drug Facts:

Active Ingredient: **Purpose:**
Zinc oxide 10% .... Skin protectant

Uses:
- helps treat and prevent diaper rash
- protects chafed skin due to diaper rash and helps seal out wetness

Warnings:
For external use only
When using this product
- avoid contact with the eyes
Stop use and ask a doctor if:
- condition worsens or does not improve within 7 days
Keep out of reach of children. If swallowed, get medical help or contact a Poison Control Center right away.

Directions:
- change wet and soiled diapers promptly
- cleanse the diaper area
- allow to dry
- apply ointment liberally as often as necessary, with each diaper change, especially at bedtime or any time when exposure to wet diapers may be prolonged

Other Information:
- store at 20° to 25°C (68° to 77°F)

Inactive Ingredients: aloe barbadensis leaf juice, cyclomethicone, dimethicone, fragrance, methylparaben, microcrystalline wax, mineral oil, propylparaben, purified water, sodium borate, sorbitan sesquioleate, vitamin E, white petrolatum, and white wax

Questions? Call **1-800-223-0182**, Monday to Friday, 9 AM–5 PM EST

How Supplied: Desitin Creamy with Aloe and Vitamin E is available in 2 oz. (57g) and 4 oz. (113g) tubes.

DESITIN® OINTMENT
Zinc Oxide Diaper Rash Ointment

Drug Facts:

Active Ingredient: **Purpose:**
Zinc oxide 40% .... Skin protectant

Uses:
- helps treat and prevent diaper rash
- protects chafed skin due to diaper rash and helps seal out wetness

Warnings:
For external use only.
When using this product
- avoid contact with the eyes

Stop use and ask a doctor if
• condition worsens or does not improve within 7 days
Keep out of reach of children. If swallowed, get medical help or contact a Poison Control Center right away.

Directions:
• change wet and soiled diapers promptly
• cleanse the diaper area
• allow to dry
• apply ointment liberally as often as necessary, with each diaper change, especially at bedtime or any time when exposure to wet diapers may be prolonged

Other Information:
• store at 15° to 30°C (59° to 86°F)

Inactive Ingredients: BHA, cod liver oil, fragrance, lanolin, methylparaben, petrolatum, talc, and water

Questions? call **1-800-223-0182,** Monday to Friday, 9 AM - 5 PM EST

How Supplied: Desitin Ointment is available in 1 ounce (28g), 2 ounce (57g), and 4 ounce (114g) tubes, and 9 ounce (255g) and 16 ounce (454g) jars.

KAOPECTATE® Anti-Diarrheal/ Upset stomach reliever

Description: KAOPECTATE®, is a pleasant tasting oral suspension for use in the control of diarrhea. Each 15 mL of KAOPECTATE® Anti-Diarrheal contains bismuth subsalicylate 262 mg, contributing 130 mg total salicylates. KAOPECTATE® Anti-Diarrheal is low sodium, with each 15 mL tablespoonful containing 10 mg sodium.
Drug Facts

Active Ingredient
(per 15 mL):   **Purpose:**
Bismuth subsalicylate .. Anti-diarrheal/
262 mg   Upset stomach reliever

Uses:
• relieves diarrhea
• relieves nausea and upset stomach associated with this symptom

Warnings: Reye's syndrome: Children and teenagers who have or are recovering from chicken pox or flu-like symptoms should not use this product. When using this product, if changes in behavior with nausea and vomiting occur, consult a doctor because these symptoms could be an early sign of Reye's syndrome, a rare but serious illness.
Allergy Alert: Contains salicylate. Do not take if you are • allergic to salicylates (including aspirin) • taking other salicylate products
Do not use if you have • bloody or black stool • an ulcer • a bleeding problem
Ask a doctor before use if you have • fever • mucus in the stool **Ask a doctor or pharmacist before use if you are** taking any drug for • anticoagulation (thinning the blood) • diabetes • gout

• arthritis **When using this product** a temporary, but harmless, darkening of the stool and/or tongue may occur **Stop use and ask a doctor if** • symptoms get worse • ringing in the ears or loss of hearing occurs • diarrhea lasts more than 2 days **If pregnant or breast-feeding,** ask a health professional before use.
Keep out of reach of children. In case of overdose, get medical help or contact a Poison Control Center right away.

Directions: KAOPECTATE® Anti-Diarrheal • shake well immediately before each use • adults and children 12 years of age and older: 30 mL or 2 tablespoonfuls • for accurate dosing, use convenient pre-measured dose cup • repeat dose every ½ hour to 1 hour as needed • do not exceed 8 doses in 24 hours • use until diarrhea stops but not more than 2 days • drink plenty of clear fluids to help prevent dehydration caused by diarrhea

Dosing Chart—Regular Strength
KAOPECTATE®

Age	Dose
adults and children 12 years and over	30 mL or 2 tablespoonfuls

Inactive Ingredients:
KAOPECTATE® Anti-Diarrheal — Peppermint: caramel, carboxymethylcellulose sodium, FD&C red no. 40, flavor, microcrystalline cellulose, purified water, sodium salicylate, sorbic acid, sucrose, titanium dioxide, xanthan gum
KAOPECTATE® Anti-Diarrheal Regular Flavor (vanilla): caramel, carboxymethylcellulose sodium, flavor, microcrystalline cellulose, purified water, sodium salicylate, sorbic acid, sucrose, titanium dioxide, xanthan gum

How Supplied: KAOPECTATE® Anti-Diarrheal 262 mg Peppermint and **262 mg Regular Flavor (vanilla):** available in 8 and 12 oz bottles; Store at room temperature 20° to 25C (68° to 77°F). Avoid excessive heat. **Do not use if inner seal is broken or missing.**

EXTRA STRENGTH KAOPECTATE® Anti-Diarrheal

Description: EXTRA STRENGTH KAOPECTATE® is a pleasant tasting oral suspension for use in the control of diarrhea. Each 15 mL of **EXTRA STRENGTH KAOPECTATE® Anti-Diarrheal** contains bismuth subsalicylate 525 mg, contributing 236 mg total salicylates. **EXTRA STRENGTH KAOPECTATE®** is low sodium. Each 15 mL tablespoonful contains **sodium 11 mg.**
Drug Facts

Active Ingredient
(per 15 mL):   **Purpose:**
Bismuth subsalicylate .. Anti-diarrheal/
525 mg   Upset stomach reliever

Uses:
• relieves diarrhea
• relieves nausea and upset stomach associated with this symptom

Warnings: Reye's syndrome: Children and teenagers who have or are recovering from chicken pox or flu-like symptoms should not use this product. When using this product, if changes in behavior with nausea and vomiting occur, consult a doctor because these symptoms could be an early sign of Reye's syndrome, a rare but serious illness.
Allergy Alert: Contains salicylate. Do not take if you are • allergic to salicylates (including aspirin) • taking other salicylate products
Do not use if you have • bloody or black stool • an ulcer • a bleeding problem
Ask a doctor before use if you have • fever • mucus in the stool **Ask a doctor or pharmacist before use if you are** taking any drug for • anticoagulation (thinning the blood) • diabetes • gout • arthritis **When using this product** a temporary, but harmless, darkening of the stool and/or tongue may occur **Stop use and ask a doctor if** • symptoms get worse • ringing in the ears or loss of hearing occurs • diarrhea lasts more than 2 days **If pregnant or breast-feeding,** ask a health professional before use.
Keep out of reach of children. In case of overdose, get medical help or contact a Poison Control Center right away.

Directions: EXTRA STRENGTH KAOPECTATE® Anti-Diarrheal • shake well immediately before each use • adults and children 12 years of age and older: 30 mL or 2 tablespoonfuls • for accurate dosing, use convenient pre-measured dose cup • repeat dose every hour as needed • do not exceed 4 doses in 24 hours • use until diarrhea stops but not more than 2 days • drink plenty of clear fluids to help prevent dehydration caused by diarrhea

Dosing Chart—Extra Strength
KAOPECTATE®

Age	Dose
adults and children 12 years and over	30 mL or 2 tablespoonfuls

Inactive Ingredients: caramel, carboxymethylcellulose sodium, FD&C red no. 40, flavor, microcrystalline cellulose, purified water, sodium salicylate, sorbic

Continued on next page

This product information was prepared in November 2003. On these and other Pfizer Consumer Healthcare Products, detailed information may be obtained by addressing Pfizer Consumer Healthcare, Pfizer, Inc., Morris Plains, NJ 07950

Kaopectate—Cont.

acid, sucrose, titanium dioxide, xanthan gum

How Supplied: EXTRA STRENGTH KAOPECTATE® Anti-Diarrheal 525 mg - Peppermint: available in 8 oz bottles. Store at room temperature 20° to 25C (68° to 77°F). Avoid excessive heat. Also available in caplets.

KAOPECTATE®
[kā-ō-pĕk-tāt]
Stool Softener

Drug Facts

Active Ingredient
(in each softgel): **Purpose:**
Docusate calcium
240 mg .... Stool softener laxative

Use: • relieves occasional constipation (irregularity), generally produces a bowel movement in 12 to 72 hours

Warnings:
Do not use
• when stomach pain, nausea, or vomiting are present unless directed by a doctor.
Ask a doctor before use if you have
• stomach pain, nausea, or vomiting
• a sudden change in bowel habits that lasts over 2 weeks
Ask a doctor or pharmacist before use if you are presently taking mineral oil.
Stop use and ask a doctor if
• you have rectal bleeding or failure to have a bowel movement after use. These could be signs of a serious condition.
• you need to use a laxative for more than 1 week
If pregnant or breast-feeding, ask a health professional before use.
Keep out of reach of children. In case of overdose, get medical help or contact a Poison Control Center right away.

Directions:
• adults and children 12 years of age or over: one softgel daily
• children under 12 years of age: ask a doctor
Other Information: • store at 59° to 77°F • protect from heat, humidity, and light

Inactive Ingredients: corn oil, FD&C blue no. 1, FD&C red no. 40, gelatin, glycerin, methylparaben, propylparaben, and sorbitol. Printed with edible white ink.
Questions? call toll-free **1-800-717-2824**
LIQUI-GELS® is a registered trademark of Cardinal Health, Inc. or one of its subsidiaries

How Supplied: 30 Liqui-Gels® Softgels

LUBRIDERM® Advanced Therapy Moisturizing Lotion
[lū brĭ dĕrm]

Description: Developed by dermatologists for healthier skin, Lubriderm provides essential moisturizing elements that your skin needs. Lubriderm Advanced Therapy, with its unique combination of nutrient-enriched moisturizers, helps heal even severely dry skin. Its nourishing, rich and creamy formula leaves you with soft, smooth and comfortable skin.

Directions: Smooth Lubriderm on hands and body every day. Particularly effective when used after showering or bathing.
For external use only.

Ingredients: Water, Cetyl Alcohol, Glycerin, Mineral Oil, Cyclomethicone, Propylene Glycol Dicaprylate/Dicaprate, PEG-40 Stearate, Isopropyl Isostearate, Emulsifying Wax, Lecithin, Carbomer, Diazolidinyl Urea, Titanium Dioxide, Sodium Benzoate, BHT, Tri(PPG-3 Myristyl Ether) Citrate, Disodium EDTA, Retinyl Palmitate, Tocopheryl Acetate, Sodium Pyruvate, Fragrance, Sodium Hydroxide, Xanthan Gum, and Iodopropynyl Butylcarbamate.
Made in Canada
How Supplied: Available in 6, 10, 16, and 19.6 fl. oz plastic bottles and a 3.3 fl. oz. tube.

LUBRIDERM® SKIN NOURISHING MOISTURIZING LOTION
[lū-brĭ-dĕrm]
with Premium Oat extract

Description: Lubriderm Skin Nourishing Moisturizing Lotion is an oat extract formula from the makers of Lubriderm, the brand you know and trust to keep your skin healthy. Lubriderm Skin Nourishing Lotion is enriched with premium oat extract to provide soothing relief to your dry skin. This unique, nourshing, non-greasy formula absorbs quickly and enhances your skin's ability to draw in and retain moisture, leaving it looking and feeling healthier.
• Enriched with premium oat extract
• Non-comedogenic (won't clog pores)
• Hypoallergenic
• Moisturizes dry skin for 24 hours
Directions: Smooth Lubriderm on hands and body every day. Particularly effective when used after showering or bathing.
For external use only.

Ingredients: Water, Glycerin, Petrolatum, Caprylic/Capric Triglyceride, Glyceryl Stearate SE, Cetyl Alcohol, Cocoa Butter, Caster Oil, Cetearyl Alcohol, Polysorbate 60, Oat Kernel Extract, Glyceryl Stearate, PEG-100 Stearate, Diazolidinyl Urea, Xanthum Gum, Disodium EDTA, Fragrance, and Iodopropynyl Butylcarbamate.

Questions? call toll-free 1-800-223-0182
Made in Canada
How Supplied: 16 fl oz bottle

NEOSPORIN® Ointment
[nē "uh-spō' rŭn]

Drug Facts

Active Ingredients
(in each gram): **Purpose:**
Bacitracin
400 units .... First aid antibiotic
Neomycin 3.5 mg ..... First aid antibiotic
Polymyxin B
5,000 units .... First aid antibiotic

Use: first aid to help prevent infection in minor:
• cuts • scrapes • burns
Warnings:
For external use only.
Do not use
• if you are allergic to any of the ingredients
• in the eyes
• over large areas of the body
Ask a doctor before use if you have
• deep or puncture wounds
• animal bites
• serious burns
Stop use and ask a doctor if
• you need to use longer than 1 week
• condition persists or gets worse
• rash or other allergic reaction develops
Keep out of reach of children. If swallowed, get medical help or contact a Poison Control Center right away.

Directions:
• clean the affected area
• apply a small amount of this product (an amount equal to the surface area of the tip of a finger) on the area 1 to 3 times daily
• may be covered with a sterile bandage
Other Information:
• store at 20° to 25°C (68° to 77° F)

Inactive Ingredients: cocoa butter, cottonseed oil, olive oil, sodium pyruvate, vitamin E, and white petrolatum
Questions? call **1-800-223-0182,** weekdays, 9 AM - 5 PM EST

How Supplied: Tubes, $\frac{1}{2}$ oz (14.2 g), 1 oz (28.3 g), $\frac{1}{32}$ oz (0.9 g) foil packets packed 10 per box (Neo To Go®) or 144 per box.

NEOSPORIN® SCAR SOLUTION®
[nē"uh-spō'run]
Silicone Scar Sheets

Uses: • Significantly improves the appearance of existing scars • Helps prevent the formation of scars on newly healed wounds

What is Neosporin® Scar Solution®?
Neosporin Scar Solution Silicone Scar Sheets are indicated for use on raised and discolored scars. Silicone sheet technology is clinically proven to significantly improve the appearance of scars and has been used by burn centers and

plastic surgeons for years. Each sheet is thin, self-adhesive and fabric-backed, which makes Neosporin Scar Solution convenient to wear under clothing.

How does Neosporin Scar Solution work?

Neosporin Scar Solution sheets use patented Silon® technology, and are believed to mimic the natural barrier function of normal skin... improving the appearance of scars, both new and old. Silicone sheets have been shown to improve the appearance of scars, even those that are years old.

One package of Neosporin Scar Solution provides the full, 12-week supply recommended to improve the appearance of scars.

What types of scars does Neosporin Scar Solution work on?

Neosporin Scar Solution sheets are effective on keloids and hypertrophic scars, which are distinguished by a raised and discolored appearance. These scars may result from burns, surgical procedures and minor skin injuries.

Are Neosporin Scar Solution sheets effective on both existing and new scars?

Neosporin Scar Solution sheets are effective on existing scars and may help prevent the formation of scars on newly closed, dry wounds.

Can Neosporin Scar Solution sheets be used anywhere on the body?

When used as directed, Neosporin Scar Solution sheets can be used on any part of the body. For certain body parts (such as flexible joints), medical tape may be used to hold sheets in place.

Can I wear Neosporin Scar Solution sheets at the gym or in the shower?

Although Neosporin Scar Solution sheets may be worn while exercising or bathing, it is recommended that sheets be removed.

Can Neosporin Scar Solution sheets be used for various sizes of scars?

Yes, Neosporin Scar Solution sheets can be used for various sizes of scars; however, the sheet should extend completely around the scarred area.

How do I apply Neosporin Scar Solution?

Step 1

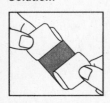

Wash and dry existing scar or newly healed wound area to remove dirt, make-up, moisturizers, etc. Do not use on open wounds.

Step 2

Tear open packet and peel off liner from adhesive side of sheet.

Step 3

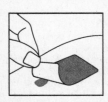

Apply sheet with adhesive side directly on scar. Sheet should cover beyond the scarred area on all sides.

Step 4

Remove and wash sheet daily to improve adhesion. Each sheet can be worn for 3-4 days days. After 3-4 days, discard old sheet in trash and replace with new one.

Usage Tips

• Each sheet should be worn for a minimum of 12 hours per day.
• Gradual improvements may be seen in 4–8 weeks.
• Sheets can be cut to fit the size of smaller scars, or applied side by side for larger scars. Trim sheet prior to removing from liner.
• Wash sheet with mild soap and water to improve adhesion before wearing. To dry, pat fabric side of sheet.
• Medical tape may be used to hold sheets in place, if necessary.

Cautions

• This product is not sterile and does not contain antibiotics.
• Do not use on open wounds or un-healed skin.
• If a rash or other allergic reaction occurs, stop use and consult a doctor.
• Keep out of reach of children under age 3 and pets, as sheets may present a choking hazard.
• Do not place adhesive side of sheet on fabrics or furniture.

Questions or Comments?

Call **1-800-223-0182**, weekdays, 9 AM - 5 PM EST.
Dist: **PFIZER CONSUMER HEALTH-CARE**
Morris Plains, NJ 07950 USA
© 2004 Pfizer www.prodhelp.com
Licensed under U.S. Patent Nos. 4,832,009 and 5,980,923
Silon® is a registered trademark of Bio Med Sciences, Inc

07-0654-05

How Supplied: Neosporin Scar Solution contains 28 sheets per carton.

NEOSPORIN® + PAIN RELIEF MAXIMUM STRENGTH Cream
[nē "uh-spō'rŭn]

Drug Facts

Active Ingredients

(in each gram):	Purpose:
Neomycin 3.5 mg	First aid antibiotic
Polymyxin B 10,000 units	First aid antibiotic
Pramoxine HCl 10 mg	External analgesic

Uses: first aid to help prevent infection and for temporary relief of pain or discomfort in minor:
• cuts • scrapes • burns

Warnings:
For external use only.
Do not use
• if you are allergic to any of the ingredients
• in the eyes
• over large areas of the body
Ask a doctor before use if you have
• deep or puncture wounds
• animal bites • serious burns
Stop use and ask a doctor if
• you need to use longer than 1 week
• condition persists or gets worse

• symptoms persist for more than 1 week, or clear up and occur again within a few days
• rash or other allergic reaction develops
Keep out of reach of children. If swallowed, get medical help or contact a Poison Control Center right away.

Directions:
• adults and children 2 years of age and older
  • clean the affected area
  • apply a small amount of this product (an amount equal to the surface area of the tip of a finger) on the area 1 to 3 times daily
  • may be covered with a sterile bandage
• children under 2 years of age: ask a doctor

Other Information:
• store at 20° to 25°C (68° to 77° F)

Inactive Ingredients: emulsifying wax, methylparaben, mineral oil, propylene glycol, purified water, and white petrolatum
Questions? call **1-800-223-0182**, weekdays, 9 AM–5 PM EST

How Supplied: ½ oz (14.2 g) tubes

NEOSPORIN® + PAIN RELIEF MAXIMUM STRENGTH Ointment
[nē "uh-spō 'rŭn]

Drug Facts

Active Ingredients

(in each gram):	Purpose:
Bacitracin 500 units	First aid antibiotic
Neomycin 3.5 mg	First aid antibiotic
Polymyxin B 10,000 units	First aid antibiotic
Pramoxine HCl 10 mg	External analgesic

Uses: first aid to help prevent infection and for temporary relief of pain or discomfort in minor:
• cuts • scrapes • burns

Warnings:
For external use only.
Do not use
• if you are allergic to any of the ingredients
• in the eyes
• over large areas of the body
Ask a doctor before use if you have
• deep or puncture wounds
• animal bites
• serious burns

Continued on next page

This product information was prepared in November 2003. On these and other Pfizer Consumer Healthcare Products, detailed information may be obtained by addressing Pfizer Consumer Healthcare, Pfizer, Inc., Morris Plains, NJ 07950

Neosporin Plus Ointment—Cont.

Stop use and ask a doctor if
- you need to use longer than 1 week
- condition persists or gets worse
- symptoms persist for more than 1 week, or clear up and occur again within a few days
- rash or other allergic reaction develops

Keep out of reach of children. If swallowed, get medical help or contact a Poison Control Center right away.

Directions:
- adults and children 2 years of age and older
  - clean the affected area
  - apply a small amount of this product (an amount equal to the surface area of the tip of a finger) on the area 1 to 3 times daily
  - may be covered with a sterile bandage
- children under 2 years of age: ask a doctor

Other Information:
- store at 20° to 25°C (68° to 77° F)

Inactive Ingredient: white petrolatum

Questions? call **1-800-223-0182**, weekdays, 9 AM - 5 PM EST

How Supplied: $1/2$ oz (14.2 g) and 1 oz (28.3 g) tubes

PEDIACARE®
Multi-Symptom Cold Liquid
[pē′dē-uh-kar]

Drug Facts

Active Ingredients
(in each 5 mL):   **Purpose:**
Chlorpheniramine
  maleate 1 mg .... Antihistamine
Dextromethorphan
  HBr 5 mg .... Cough suppressant
Pseudoephedrine
  HCl 15 mg .... Nasal decongestant

Uses: • temporarily relieves these symptoms due to the common cold:
• sneezing • runny nose • cough • nasal congestion

Warnings:
Do not use in a child who is taking a prescription monoamine oxidase inhibitor (MAOI) (certain drugs for depression, psychiatric, or emotional conditions, or Parkinson's disease), or for 2 weeks after stopping the MAOI drug. If you do not know if your child's prescription drug contains an MAOI, ask a doctor or pharmacist before giving this product.
Ask a doctor before use if the child has
- a breathing problem such as chronic bronchitis
- persistent or chronic cough such as occurs with asthma or a cough accompanied by excessive phlegm (mucus)
- glaucoma • heart disease • diabetes
- thyroid disease • high blood pressure

Ask a doctor or pharmacist before use if the child is taking sedatives or tranquilizers

When using this product
- **do not exceed recommended dosage**
- excitability may occur
- drowsiness may occur
- sedatives and tranquilizers may increase drowsiness

Stop use and ask a doctor if
- nervousness, dizziness, or sleeplessness occur
- cough persists for more than 1 week, tends to recur or is accompanied by fever, rash, or persistent headache. These could be signs of a serious condition.
- symptoms do not improve within 7 days, or are accompanied by fever

Keep out of reach of children. In case of overdose, get medical help or contact a Poison Control Center right away.

Directions:
- children 6 to under 12 years: 2 teaspoonfuls (10 mL).
  If needed, repeat dose every 4 hours. Do not exceed 4 doses in 24 hours.
- children under 6 years: consult a doctor.

Other Information:
- protect from light. Store in outer carton until contents are used.
- store at 20°–25°C (68°–77°F)

Inactive Ingredients: citric acid, corn syrup, FD&C red no. 40, flavors, glycerin, propylene glycol, purified water, sodium benzoate, and sorbitol

Questions? call toll-free **1-888-474-3099**
Do not use if carton is opened, or if imprinted plastic bottle wrap or imprinted foil inner seal is broken or missing

How Supplied: Pediacare® Multi-Symptom Cold Liquid is available in a 4 fl oz bottle.

PEDIACARE® Long-Acting Cough Plus Cold Liquid
[pē′dē-uh-kār]

Drug Facts

Active Ingredients
(in each 5 mL):   **Purpose:**
Dextromethorphan
  HBr 7.5 mg .... Cough suppressant
Pseudoephedrine
  HCl 15 mg .... Nasal decongestant

Uses: • temporarily relieves these symptoms due to the common cold, hay fever, or other upper respiratory allergies:
• cough • nasal congestion

Warnings:
Do not use in a child who is taking a prescription monoamine oxidase inhibitor (MAOI) (certain drugs for depression, psychiatric, or emotional conditions, or Parkinson's disease), or for 2 weeks after stopping the MAOI drug. If you do not know if your child's prescription drug contains an MAOI, ask a doctor or pharmacist before giving this product.
Ask a doctor before use if the child has
- a persistent or chronic cough such as occurs with asthma
- a cough accompanied by excessive phlegm (mucus)
- heart disease • diabetes
- thyroid disease • high blood pressure

When using this product • do not exceed recommended dosage
Stop use and ask a doctor if
- nervousness, dizziness, or sleeplessness occur
- cough persists for more than 1 week, tends to recur or is accompanied by fever, rash, or persistent headache. These could be signs of a serious condition.
- symptoms do not improve within 7 days, or are accompanied by fever

Keep out of reach of children. In case of overdose, get medical help or contact a Poison Control Center right away.

Directions:
- find the right dose on the chart below
- if needed, repeat dose every 6 hours
- do not exeed 4 doses in 24 hours

Children 6 to under 12 years	2 teapoonfuls (10 mL)
Children 2 to under 6 years	1 teaspoonful (5 mL)
Children under 2 years	consult a doctor

Other Information:
- protect from light. Store in outer carton until contents are used.
- store at 20°–25°C (68°–77°F)

Inactive Ingredients: citric acid, corn syrup, FD&C blue no. 1, FD&C red no. 40, flavor, glycerin, propylene glycol, purified water, sodium benzoate, and sorbitol

Questions? call toll-free **1-888-474-3099**
Do not use if carton is opened, or if imprinted plastic bottle wrap or imprinted foil inner seal is broken or missing

How Supplied: Pediacare Long-Acting Cough Plus Cold Liquid is available in a 4 fl oz bottle.

PEDIACARE® NightRest Cough & Cold Liquid
[pē′dē-uh-kār]

Drug Facts

Active Ingredients
(in each 5 mL):   **Purpose:**
Chlorpheniramine maleate
  1 mg .... Antihistamine
Dextromethorphan HBr
  7.5 mg .... Cough suppressant
Pseudoephedrine HCl
  15 mg .... Nasal decongestant

Uses: • temporarily relieves these symptoms due to the common cold, hay fever, or other upper respiratory allergies:
• sneezing • runny nose • cough • nasal congestion

Warnings:
Do not use in a child who is taking a prescription monoamine oxidase inhibitor (MAOI) (certain drugs for depression, psychiatric, or emotional conditions, or Parkinson's disease), or for 2 weeks after stopping the MAOI drug. If you do not

know if your child's prescription drug contains an MAOI, ask a doctor or pharmacist before giving this product.

Ask a doctor before use if the child has
- a breathing problem such as chronic bronchitis
- persistent or chronic cough such as occurs with asthma or a cough accompanied by excessive phlegm (mucus)
- glaucoma • heart disease • diabetes
- thyroid disease • high blood pressure

Ask a doctor or pharmacist before use if the child is taking sedatives or tranquilizers

When using this product
- **do not exceed recommended dosage**
- excitability may occur
- drowsiness may occur
- sedatives and tranquilizers may increase drowsiness

Stop use and ask a doctor if
- nervousness, dizziness, or sleeplessness occur
- cough persists for more than 1 week, tends to recur or is accompanied by fever, rash, or persistent headache. These could be signs of a serious condition.
- symptoms do not improve within 7 days, or are accompanied by fever

Keep out of reach of children. In case of overdose, get medical help or contact a Poison Control Center right away.

Directions:
- children 6 to under 12 years: 2 teaspoonfuls (10 mL).
  If needed, repeat dose every 6 hours. Do not exceed 4 doses in 24 hours.
- children under 6 years: consult a doctor.

Other Information:
- protect from light. Store in outer carton until contents are used.
- store at 20°–25°C (68°–77°F)

Inactive Ingredients: citric acid, corn syrup, FD&C red no. 40, flavors, glycerin, propylene glycol, purified water, sodium benzoate, and sorbitol

Questions? call toll-free **1-888-474-3099**
Do not use if carton is opened, or if imprinted plastic bottle wrap or imprinted foil inner seal is broken or missing

How Supplied: Pediacare® NightRest Cough & Cold Liquid is available in a 4 fl oz bottle.

PEDIACARE®
Long-Acting Cough Infant Drops
[pē′dē-uh-kār]
(7.5 mg/0.8 ml)

Drug Facts

Active Ingredients
(in each 0.8 mL):   **Purpose:**
Dextromethorphan HBr
7.5 mg .... Cough suppressant

Uses: temporarily relieves cough associated with the common cold

Warnings:
Do not use in a child who is taking a prescription monoamine oxidase inhibitor (MAOI) (certain drugs for depression, psychiatric, or emotional conditions, or Parkinson's disease), or for 2 weeks after

stopping the MAOI drug. If you do not know if your child's prescription drug contains an MAOI, ask a doctor or pharmacist before giving this product.

Ask a doctor before use if the child has
- a persistent or chronic cough such as occurs with asthma
- a cough accompanied by excessive phlegm (mucus)

When using this product
- **do not exceed recommended dosage.**

Stop use and ask a doctor if
- cough persists for more than 1 week, tends to recur or is accompanied by fever, rash, or persistent headache. These could be signs of a serious condition.

Keep out of reach of children. In case of overdose, get medical help or contact a Poison Control Center right away.

Directions:
- to be taken by mouth only. Not for nasal use.
- children 2 to under 6 years of age: 1 dropperful (0.8 ml). If needed, repeat dose every 6–8 hours. Do not exceed 4 doses in 24 hours.
- children under 2 years of age: Consult a doctor

Other Information:
- protect from light. Store in outer carton until contents are used.
- store at 20°–25°C (68°–77°F)

Inactive Ingredients: citric acid, flavor, glycerin, purified water, sodium benzoate, and sorbital

Questions? call toll-free **1-888-474-3099**
Do not use if carton is opened, or if imprinted plastic bottle wrap is broken or missing

How Supplied: Available in 1/2 fl oz liquid

PEDIACARE®
Decongestant Infant Drops
[pē′dē-uh-kār]

Drug Facts

Active Ingredient
(in each 0.8 mL):   **Purpose:**
Pseudoephedrine
HCl 7.5 mg .... Nasal decongestant

Use: temporarily relieves nasal congestion due to the common cold, hay fever, or other upper respiratory allergies

Warnings:
Do not use in a child who is taking a prescription monoamine oxidase inhibitor (MAOI) (certain drugs for depression, psychiatric, or emotional conditions, or Parkinson's disease), or for 2 weeks after stopping the MAOI drug. If you do not know if your child's prescription drug contains an MAOI, ask a doctor or pharmacist before giving this product.

Ask a doctor before use if the child has
- heart disease
- high blood pressure
- diabetes
- thyroid disease

When using this product
- **do not exceed recommended dosage.**

Stop use and ask a doctor if
- nervousness, dizziness, or sleeplessness occur

- symptoms do not improve within 7 days, or are accompanied by fever

Keep out of reach of children. In case of overdose, get medical help or contact a Poison Control Center right away.

Directions:
- to be taken by mouth only. Not for nasal use.
- children 2 to under 6 years of age: 2 dropperfuls. If needed, repeat dose every 4–6 hours. Do not exceed 4 doses in 24 hours.
- children under 2 years of age: Consult a doctor

Other Information:
- protect from light. Store in outer carton until contents are used.
- store at 20°–25°C (68°–77°F)

Inactive Ingredients: benzoic acid, citric acid, flavors, glycerin, polyethylene glycol, propylene glycol, purified water, sodium benzoate, sorbitol, and sucrose

Questions? call toll-free **1-888-474-3099**
Do not use if carton is opened, or if imprinted plastic bottle wrap is broken or missing

How Supplied: PediaCare® Decongestant Infant Drops are available in fruit flavor in ½ fl oz dropper.

PEDIACARE®
Decongestant & Cough Infant Drops
[pē′dē-uh-kār]

Drug Facts

Active Ingredients
(in each 0.8 mL):   **Purpose:**
Dextromethorphan
HBr 2.5 mg .... Cough suppressant
Pseudoephedrine
HCl 7.5 mg .... Nasal decongestant

Uses:
- temporarily relieves these symptoms due to the common cold, hay fever, or other upper respiratory allergies:
  - cough • nasal congestion

Warnings: **Do not use** in a child who is taking a prescription monoamine oxidase inhibitor (MAOI) (certain drugs for depression, psychiatric, or emotional conditions, or Parkinson's disease), or for 2 weeks after stopping the MAOI drug. If you do not know if your child's prescription drug contains an MAOI, ask a doctor or pharmacist before giving this product.

Ask a doctor before use if the child has
- a persistent or chronic cough such as occurs with asthma
- a cough accompanied by excessive phlegm (mucus)

Continued on next page

This product information was prepared in November 2003. On these and other Pfizer Consumer Healthcare Products, detailed information may be obtained by addressing Pfizer Consumer Healthcare, Pfizer, Inc., Morris Plains, NJ 07950

PediaCare—Cont.

- heart disease • high blood pressure
- diabetes
- thyroid disease

When using this product • do not exceed recommended dosage.
Stop use and ask a doctor if
- nervousness, dizziness, or sleeplessness occur
- cough persists for more than 1 week, tends to recur or is accompanied by fever, rash, or persistent headache. These could be signs of a serious condition.
- symptoms do not improve within 7 days, or are accompanied by fever

Keep out of reach of children. In case of overdose, get medical help or contact a Poison Control Center right away.

Directions:
- to be taken by mouth only. Not for nasal use.
- children 2 to under 6 years of age: 2 dropperfuls (1.6 mL). If needed, repeat dose every 4 hours. Do not exceed 4 doses in 24 hours
- children under 2 years: Consult a doctor

Other Information:
- protect from light. Store in outer carton until contents are used.
- store at 20°–25°C (68°–77°F)

Inactive Ingredients: citric acid, flavor, glycerin, purified water, sodium benzoate, and sorbitol
Questions? call toll-free **1-888-474-3099**
Do not use if carton is opened, or if imprinted plastic bottle wrap is broken or missing

How Supplied: Pediacare® Decongestant and Cough is available in 1/2 fl oz liquid bottle.

PEDIACARE® Freezer Pops
Long-Acting Cough: Glacier Grape Flavor and Polar Berry Blue Flavor
[pe'dē-uh-kār]

Drug Facts

Active Ingredient
(per freezer pop): **Purpose:**
Dextromethorphan HBr
7.5 mg .... Cough suppressant

Use: • temporarily relieves cough associated with the common cold

Warnings:
Do not use in a child who is taking a prescription monoamine oxidase inhibitor (MAOI) (certain drugs for depression, psychiatric, or emotional conditions, or Parkinson's disease), or for 2 weeks after stopping the MAOI drug. If you do not know if your child's prescription drug contains an MAOI, ask a doctor or pharmacist before giving this product.
Ask a doctor before use if the child has
- a persistent or chronic cough such as occurs with asthma
- a cough accompanied by excessive phlegm (mucus)

When using this product • do not exceed recommended dosage
Stop use and ask a doctor if
- cough persists for more than 1 week, tends to recur or is accompanied by fever, rash, or persistent headache. These could be signs of a serious condition.

Keep out of reach of children. In case of overdose, get medical help or contact a Poison Control Center right away.

Directions:
- to use: cut off top of freezer pop sleeve with scissors. Push up freezer pop from sleeve bottom
- if needed, repeat dose every 6–8 hours
- do not exceed 4 doses in 24 hours

Children 6 to under 12 years	2 freezer pops (50 mL as liquid)
Children 2 to under 6 years	1 freezer pop (25 mL as liquid)
Children under 2 years	consult a doctor

Other Information:
- protect from light. Store in outer carton until contents are used.
- store at 25°C (77°F) or less

Inactive Ingredients: Glacier Grape Flavor: citric acid, corn syrup, ethyl maltol, FD&C blue no. 1, FD&C red no. 40, flavor, pectin, potassium sorbate, propylene glycol, sodium alginate, sodium benzoate, sodium chloride, sodium citrate, sucralose, and water. Polar Berry Blue Flavor: benzyl alcohol, citric acid, corn syrup, ethyl maltol, FD&C blue no. 1, flavor, pectin, potassium sorbate, propylene glycol, sodium alginate, sodium benzoate, sodium chloride, sodium citrate, soybean oil, sucralose, tocopherols, and water
Questions? call toll-free **1-888-474-3099**

How Supplied: Each flavor available in boxes of 8 freezer pops.

POLYSPORIN® Ointment
[pŏl 'ē-spō 'rŭn]

Drug Facts

Active Ingredients
(in each gram): **Purpose:**
Bacitracin
500 units .... First aid antibiotic
Polymyxin B
10,000 units .... First aid antibiotic

Use: first aid to help prevent infection in minor:
- cuts • scrapes • burns

Warnings:
For external use only.
Do not use
- if you are allergic to any of the ingredients
- in the eyes
- over large areas of the body
Ask a doctor before use if you have
- deep or puncture wounds
- animal bites
- serious burns

Stop use and ask a doctor if
- you need to use longer than 1 week
- condition persists or gets worse
- rash or other allergic reaction develops
Keep out of reach of children. If swallowed, get medical help or contact a Poison Control Center right away.

Directions:
- clean the affected area
- apply a small amount of this product (an amount equal to the surface area of the tip of a finger) on the area 1 to 3 times daily
- may be covered with a sterile bandage

Other Information:
- store at 20° to 25°C (68° to 77° F)

Inactive Ingredient: white petrolatum base
Questions? call **1-800-223-0182**, weekdays, 9 AM - 5 PM EST

How Supplied: Tubes, $1/2$ oz (14.2 g), 1 oz (28.3 g); $1/32$ oz (0.9 g) foil packets packed in cartons of 144.

MEN'S ROGAINE® EXTRA STRENGTH
(5% Minoxidil Topical Solution)
Hair Regrowth Treatment
Ocean Rush™ Scent

Drug Facts

Active Ingredient: Minoxidil 5% w/v

Use: to regrow hair on the top of the scalp (vertex only)

Warnings:
For external use only. For use by men only.
Flammable Keep away from fire or flame
Do not use if
- you are a woman
- your amount of hair loss is different than that shown on the side of the product carton or your hair loss is on the front of the scalp. 5% minoxidil topical solution is not intended for frontal baldness or receding hairline.
- you have no family history of hair loss
- your hair loss is sudden and/or patchy
- you do not know the reason for your hair loss
- you are under 18 years of age. Do not use on babies and children.
- your scalp is red, inflamed, infected, irritated, or painful
- you use other medicines on the scalp
Ask a doctor before use if you have heart disease
When using this product
- do not apply on other parts of the body
- avoid contact with the eyes. In case of accidental contact, rinse eyes with large amounts of cool tap water.
- some people have experienced changes in hair color and/or texture
- it takes time to regrow hair. Results may occur at 2 months with twice a day usage. For some men, you may need to use this product for at least 4 months before you see results.
- the amount of hair regrowth is different for each person. This product will not work for all men.

Stop use and ask a doctor if
- chest pain, rapid heartbeat, faintness, or dizziness occurs
- sudden, unexplained weight gain occurs
- your hands or feet swell
- scalp irritation or redness occurs
- unwanted facial hair growth occurs
- you do not see hair regrowth in 4 months

May be harmful if used when pregnant or breast-feeding. Keep out of reach of children. If swallowed, get medical help or contact a Poison Control Center right away.

Directions:
- apply one mL with dropper 2 times a day directly onto the scalp in the hair loss area
- using more or more often will not improve results
- continued use is necessary to increase and keep your hair regrowth, or hair loss will begin again.

Other Information See hair loss pictures on side of product carton. Before use, read all information on product carton and enclosed booklet. Keep the product carton. It contains important information. Hair regrowth has not been shown to last longer than 48 weeks in large clinical trials with continuous treatment with 5% minoxidil topical solution for men. In clinical studies with mostly white men aged 18–49 years with moderate degrees of hair loss, 5% minoxidil topical solution for men provided more hair regrowth than 2% minoxidil topical solution. Store at controlled room temperature 20° to 25°C (68° to 77° F)

Inactive Ingredients: Alcohol, fragrance, propylene glycol, and purified water.

How Supplied: Men's Rogaine Extra Strength Ocean Rush™ Scent is available in one 60 mL bottle. Men's Rogaine Extra Strength Original Formula Unscented is available in packs of three or four 60 mL bottles. (One 60 mL bottle is a one month supply.)

Women's ROGAINE®
(2% Minoxidil Topical Solution)
Hair Regrowth Treatment
Spring Bloom™ Scent

Drug Facts

Active Ingredient: Minoxidil 2% w/v

Use: to regrow hair on the scalp

Warnings:
For external use only
Flammable: Keep away from fire or flame
Do not use if
- your degree of hair loss is more than that shown on the side of the product carton, because this product may not work for you
- you have no family history of hair loss
- your hair loss is sudden and/or patchy
- your hair loss is associated with childbirth
- you do not know the reason for your hair loss

- you are under 18 years of age. Do not use on babies and children.
- your scalp is red, inflamed, infected, irritated, or painful
- you use other medicines on the scalp

Ask a doctor before use if you have heart disease

When using this product
- do not apply on other parts of the body
- avoid contact with the eyes. In case of accidental contact, rinse eyes with large amounts of cool tap water.
- some people have experienced changes in hair color and/or texture
- it takes time to regrow hair. You may need to use this product 2 times a day for at least 4 months before you see results.
- the amount of hair regrowth is different for each person. This product will not work for everyone

Stop use and ask a doctor if
- chest pain, rapid heartbeat, faintness, or dizziness occurs
- sudden, unexplained weight gain occurs
- your hands or feet swell
- scalp irritation or redness occurs
- unwanted facial hair growth occurs
- you do not see hair regrowth in 4 months

May be harmful if used when pregnant or breast-feeding.

Keep out of reach of children. If swallowed, get medical help or contact a Poison Control Center right away.

Directions:
- apply one mL with dropper 2 times a day directly onto the scalp in the hair loss area
- using more or more often will not improve results
- continued use is necessary to increase and keep your hair regrowth, or hair loss will begin again

Other Information: See hair loss pictures on side of product carton. Before use, read all information on product carton and enclosed booklet. Keep the product carton. It contains important information. In clinical studies of mostly white women aged 18–45 years with mild to moderate degrees of hair loss, the following response to 2% minoxidil topical solution was reported: 19% of women reported moderate hair regrowth after using 2% minoxidil topical solution for 8 months (19% had moderate regrowth; 40% had minimal regrowth). This compares with 7% of women reporting moderate hair regrowth after using the placebo, the liquid without minoxidil in it, for 8 months (7% had moderate regrowth; 33% had minimal regrowth). Store at controlled room temperature 20° to 25°C (68° to 77° F)

Inactive Ingredients: Alcohol, fragrance, propylene glycol, and purified water.

How Supplied: Women's ROGAINE Spring Bloom™ Scent is available in one 60 mL bottle. Women's Rogaine Original Unscented is available in packs of three or four 60 mL bottles. (One 60 mL bottle is a one-month supply.)

ROLAIDS® Antacid Tablets
Original Peppermint, Spearmint, and Cherry

Drug Facts:

Active Ingredients
(in each tablet):	Purpose:
Calcium carbonate 550 mg	Antacid
Magnesium hydroxide 110 mg	Antacid

Uses: relieves: • heartburn • sour stomach • acid indigestion • upset stomach due to these symptoms

Warnings:
Ask a doctor or pharmacist before use if you are presently taking a prescription drug. Antacids may interact with certain prescription drugs.
Do not take more than 12 tablets in a 24-hour period, or use the maximum dosage for more than 2 weeks, except under the advice and supervision of a physician.
Keep out of reach of children.

Directions
- chew 2 to 4 tablets, hourly if needed

Other Information:
- each tablet contains: calcium 220 mg and magnesium 45 mg
- store at 59° to 77°F in a dry place

Inactive Ingredients: Peppermint and Spearmint Flavors: dextrose, flavoring, magnesium stearate, polyethylene glycol, pregelatinized starch and sucrose
Cherry Flavor: dextrose, flavoring, magnesium stearate, polyethylene glycol, pregelatinized starch, D&C red no. 27 aluminum lake, and sucrose

Questions? call **1-800-223-0182** weekdays, 9 AM – 5 PM EST

How Supplied: Rolaids® is available in 12-tablet rolls, 3-packs containing three 12-tablet rolls and in bottles containing 150 tablets.

EXTRA STRENGTH ROLAIDS®
Antacid Tablets
Freshmint, Fruit, Cool Strawberry, and Tropical Punch Flavors

Drug Facts:

Active Ingredients:
(in each tablet):	Purpose:
Calcium carbonate 675 mg	Antacid
Magnesium hydroxide 135 mg	Antacid

Continued on next page

This product information was prepared in November 2003. On these and other Pfizer Consumer Healthcare Products, detailed information may be obtained by addressing Pfizer Consumer Healthcare, Pfizer, Inc., Morris Plains, NJ 07950

Rolaids Extra Strength—Cont.

Uses: relieves: • heartburn • sour stomach • acid indigestion • upset stomach due to these symptoms

Warnings: Ask a doctor or pharmacist before use if you are presently taking a prescription drug. Antacids may interact with certain prescription drugs. Do not take more than 10 tablets in a 24-hour period, or use the maximum dosage for more than 2 weeks, except under the advice and supervision of a physician. **Keep out of reach of children.**

Directions:
• chew 2 to 4 tablets, hourly if needed

Other Information:
• each tablet contains: calcium 271 mg and magnesium 56 mg
• store at 59° to 77° F in a dry place

Inactive Ingredients: Freshmint Flavor: dextrose, flavoring, magnesium stearate, polyethylene glycol, pregelatinized starch and sucrose
Fruit Flavor: dextrose, flavoring, magnesium stearate, polyethylene glycol, pregelatinized starch, sucrose and FD&C yellow no. 5 aluminum lake (tartrazine)
Cool Strawberry and Tropical Punch: carmine, dextrose, flavoring, magnesium stearate, polyethylene glycol, pregelatinized starch and sucrose
Questions? call **1-800-223-0182**, weekdays, 9 AM–5 PM EST

How Supplied: Extra Strength Rolaids® is available in 10-tablet rolls, 3-packs containing three 10-tablet rolls and in bottles containing 100 tablets.

Extra Strength ROLAIDS® Softchews Antacid
[rō-lāds]
Vanilla Creme and Wild Cherry

Drug Facts

Active Ingredient:
(in each chew) **Purpose:**
Calcium carbonate
1177mg .... Antacid

Uses: relieves:
• heartburn
• sour stomach
• acid indigestion
• upset stomach due to these symptoms

Warnings:
Ask a doctor or pharmacist before use if you are now taking a prescription drug. Antacids may interact with certain prescription drugs.
Do not take more than 6 chews in a 24-hour period, or use the maximum dosage for more than 2 weeks, except under the advice and supervision of a physician.
Keep out of reach of children.

Directions: chew 2 to 3 chews, hourly if needed

Other Information:
• **Each chew contains:** calcium 471 mg
• store at 59° to 77°F in a dry place

Inactive Ingredients:
Vanilla Creme: corn starch, corn syrup, corn syrup solids, flavoring, glycerin, hydrogenated coconut oil, nonfat dry milk, sodium chloride, soy lecithin, and sucrose
Wild Cherry: corn starch, corn syrup, corn syrup solids, FD&C red no. 40 aluminum lake, flavoring, glycerin, hydrogenated coconut oil, nonfat dry milk, sodium chloride, soy lecithin, and sucrose
Questions? call **1-800-223-0182**, weekdays, 9 AM -5 PM EST

How Supplied: Extra Strength Rolaids Softchews are available in 6 chew sticks, 3-packs containing 6-chew sticks, and in 7-packs containing 6-chew sticks

---

ROLAIDS® MULTI-SYMPTOM ANTACID & ANTIGAS TABLETS
Berry and Cool Mint

Drug Facts

Active Ingredients **Purpose:**
(in each tablet):
Calcium carbonate 675 mg ...... Antacid
Magnesium hydroxide
135 mg .... Antacid
Simethicone 60 mg .... Antigas

Uses: relieves: • heartburn • acid indigestion • pressure, bloating and discomfort commonly referred to as gas

Warnings:
Ask a doctor or pharmacist before use if you are presently taking a prescription drug. Antacids may interact with certain prescription drugs.
Do not take more than 8 tablets in a 24-hour period, or use the maximum dosage for more than 2 weeks, except under the advice and supervision of a physician.
Keep out of reach of children.

Directions: chew 2 to 4 tablets, hourly if needed

Other Information:
• **each tablet contains:** calcium 271 mg and magnesium 56 mg
• store at 59° to 77°F in a dry place

Inactive Ingredients: Berry Flavor: corn starch, dextrose, FD&C blue #1, FD&C red #3, flavoring, magnesium stearate, polyethylene glycol, pregelatinized starch, and sucrose

Inactive Ingredients: Cool Mint Flavor: corn starch, dextrose, FD&C blue #1, flavoring, magnesium stearate, polyethylene glycol, pregelatinized starch, and sucrose
Questions? call, **1-800-223-0182**, weekdays, 9 AM–5 PM EST

How Supplied: Rolaids Multi-Symptom is available in 10-tablet rolls, 3-packs containing three 10-tablet rolls and in bottles containing 100 tablets.

SUDAFED® Non-Drowsy 12 Hour Nasal Decongestant Tablets
[sū 'duh-fĕd]
*Capsule-shaped Tablets

Drug Facts:

Active Ingredient:
(in each tablet) **Purpose:**
Pseudoephedrine
HCl 120 mg .... Nasal decongestant

Uses:
• temporarily relieves nasal congestion due to the common cold, hay fever or other upper respiratory allergies, and nasal congestion associated with sinusitis
• temporarily relieves sinus congestion and pressure

Warnings:
Do not use if you are now taking a prescription monoamine oxidase inhibitor (MAOI) (certain drugs for depression, psychiatric, or emotional conditions, or Parkinson's disease), or for 2 weeks after stopping the MAOI drug. If you do not know if your prescription drug contains an MAOI, ask a doctor or pharmacist before taking this product.
Ask a doctor before use if you have
• heart disease
• high blood pressure
• thyroid disease
• diabetes
• trouble urinating due to an enlarged prostate gland
When using this product
• do not use more than directed
Stop use and ask a doctor if
• you get nervous, dizzy, or sleepless
• symptoms do not improve within 7 days or are accompanied by fever
If pregnant or breast-feeding, ask a health professional before use.
Keep out of reach of children. In case of overdose, get medical help or contact a Poison Control Center right away.

Directions:
• adults and children 12 years of age and over: one tablet every 12 hours not to exceed two tablets in 24 hours
• children under 12 years of age: use of product not recommended

Other Information:
• store at 59° to 77°F in a dry place
• protect from light

Inactive Ingredients: hypromellose, magnesium stearate, microcrystalline cellulose, polyethylene glycol, povidone, and titanium dioxide. May also contain: candelilla wax or carnauba wax. Printed with edible blue ink.

Questions? call **1-800-524-2624** (English/Spanish), weekdays, 9 AM–5 PM EST

How Supplied: Boxes of 10 and 20.

SUDAFED® Non-Drowsy 24 Hour Nasal Decongestant Tablets
[sū 'duh-fěd]

Drug Facts:

Active Ingredient:
(in each tablet)   **Purpose:**
Pseudoephedrine
  HCl 240 mg .... Nasal decongestant

Uses:
- temporarily relieves nasal congestion due to the common cold, hay fever or other upper respiratory allergies, and nasal congestion associated with sinusitis
- reduces swelling of nasal passages
- relieves sinus pressure

Warnings:
Do not use if you are now taking a prescription monoamine oxidase inhibitor (MAOI) (certain drugs for depression, psychiatric, or emotional conditions, or Parkinson's disease), or for 2 weeks after stopping the MAOI drug. If you do not know if your prescription drug contains an MAOI, ask a doctor or pharmacist before taking this product.
Ask a doctor before use if you have
- heart disease
- high blood pressure
- thyroid disease
- trouble urinating due to an enlarged prostate gland
- diabetes
- had obstruction or narrowing of the bowel. Rarely, tablets of this kind may cause bowel obstruction (blockage), usually in people with severe narrowing of the bowel (esophagus, stomach or intestine).
When using this product
- do not use more than directed
Stop use and ask a doctor if
- you get nervous, dizzy, or sleepless
- symptoms do not improve within 7 days or are accompanied by fever
- you experience persistent abdominal pain or vomiting
If pregnant or breast-feeding, ask a health professional before use.
Keep out of reach of children. In case of overdose, get medical help or contact a Poison Control Center right away.

Directions:
- adults and children 12 years of age and over: **swallow one** whole tablet with fluid every 24 hours
- **do not exceed one tablet in 24 hours**
- **do not divide, crush, chew or dissolve the tablet**
- the tablet does not completely dissolve and may be seen in the stool (this is normal)
- not for use in children under 12 years of age

Other Information:
- store at 59° to 77°F in a dry place

Inactive Ingredients: Cellulose, cellulose acetate, hydroxypropyl cellulose, hypromellose, magnesium stearate, polyethylene glycol, polysorbate 80, povidone, sodium chloride, and titanium dioxide

Questions? call **1-800-524-2624** (English/Spanish), weekdays, 9 AM – 5 PM EST

How Supplied: Box of 5 tablets and 10 tablets. **BLISTER PACKAGED FOR YOUR PROTECTION. DO NOT USE IF INDIVIDUAL SEALS ARE BROKEN.**

SUDAFED® Non-Drowsy Nasal Decongestant 30-mg Tablets
[sū 'duh-fěd]

Drug Facts:

Active Ingredient:
(in each tablet)   **Purpose:**
Pseudoephedrine HCl
  30 mg .... Nasal decongestant

Uses:
- temporarily relieves nasal congestion due to the common cold, hay fever or other upper respiratory allergies, and nasal congestion associated with sinusitis
- temporarily relieves sinus congestion and pressure

Warnings:
Do not use if you are now taking a prescription monoamine oxidase inhibitor (MAOI) (certain drugs for depression, psychiatric, or emotional conditions, or Parkinson's disease), or for 2 weeks after stopping the MAOI drug. If you do not know if your prescription drug contains an MAOI, ask a doctor or pharmacist before taking this product.
Ask a doctor before use if you have
- heart disease
- high blood pressure
- thyroid disease
- diabetes
- trouble urinating due to an enlarged prostate gland
When using this product
- do not use more than directed
Stop use and ask a doctor if
- you get nervous, dizzy, or sleepless
- symptoms do not improve within 7 days or are accompanied by fever
If pregnant or breast-feeding, ask a health professional before use.
Keep out of reach of children. In case of overdose, get medical help or contact a Poison Control Center right away.

Directions:
- take every 4 to 6 hours
- do not take more than 4 doses in 24 hours

adults and children 12 years of age and over	2 tablets
children 6 to under 12 years of age	1 tablet
children under 6 years of age	ask a doctor

Other Information:
- store at 59° to 77°F in a dry place

Inactive Ingredients: Acacia, candelilla wax, corn starch, FD&C red no. 40 aluminum lake, FD&C yellow no. 6 aluminum lake, hypromellose, lactose monohydrate, magnesium stearate, pharmaceutical glaze, poloxamer 407, polyethylene glycol, polyethylene oxide, polysorbate 60, povidone, sodium benzoate, sodium lauryl sulfate, stearic acid, sucrose, talc, and titanium dioxide. Printed with edible black ink.

Questions? call **1-800-524-2624** (English/Spanish), weekdays, 9 AM – 5 PM EST

How Supplied: Boxes of 24, 48 and 96.

SUDAFED® NON-DROWSY NON-DRYING SINUS, LIQUID CAPS
[sū 'duh-fěd]

Drug Facts:

Active Ingredients: **Purpose:**
(in each liquid cap)
Guaifenesin 200 mg .... Expectorant
Pseudoephedrine
  HCl 30 mg .... Nasal decongestant

Uses:
- temporarily relieves nasal congestion associated with sinusitis
- promotes nasal and/or sinus drainage
- temporarily relieves sinus congestion and pressure
- helps loosen phlegm (mucus) and thin bronchial secretions to rid the bronchial passageways of bothersome mucus and make coughs more productive

Warnings:
Do not use if you are now taking a prescription monoamine oxidase inhibitor (MAOI) (certain drugs for depression, psychiatric, or emotional conditions, or Parkinson's disease), or for 2 weeks after stopping the MAOI drug. If you do not know if your prescription drug contains an MAOI, ask a doctor or pharmacist before taking this product.
Ask a doctor before use if you have
- heart disease
- high blood pressure
- thyroid disease
- diabetes
- trouble urinating due to an enlarged prostate gland
- cough that occurs with too much phlegm (mucus)
- persistent or chronic cough such as occurs with smoking, asthma, chronic bronchitis, or emphysema
When using this product
- do not use more than directed
Stop use and ask a doctor if
- you get nervous, dizzy, or sleepless
- symptoms do not improve within 7 days or are accompanied by fever
- cough persists for more than 1 week, tends to recur, or is accompanied by a fever, rash, or persistent headache. These could be signs of a serious condition.

Continued on next page

This product information was prepared in November 2003. On these and other Pfizer Consumer Healthcare Products, detailed information may be obtained by addressing Pfizer Consumer Healthcare, Pfizer, Inc., Morris Plains, NJ 07950

Sudafed Non-Drowsy—Cont.

If pregnant or breast-feeding, ask a health professional before use.

Keep out of reach of children. In case of overdose, get medical help or contact a Poison Control Center right away.

Directions:
- adults and children 12 years of age and over: swallow 2 liquid caps
- take every 4 hours
- do not exceed 8 liquid caps in 24 hours
- children under 12 years of age: ask a doctor

Other Information:
- store at 59° to 77°F
- protect from heat, humidity, and light

Inactive Ingredients: FD&C blue no. 1, gelatin, glycerin, polyethylene glycol 400, povidone, propylene glycol, and sorbitol. Printed with edible white ink.

Questions? call **1-800-524-2624** (English/Spanish), weekdays, 9 AM - 5 PM EST

How Supplied: Sudafed Non-Drying Sinus is supplied in boxes of 24 liquid caps.

SUDAFED® Non-drowsy Severe Cold Caplets
[sū 'duh-fĕd]

Drug Facts:

Active Ingredients: **Purposes:**
(in each caplet)
Acetaminophen
  500 mg ...... Pain reliever-fever reducer
Dextromethorphan HBr
  15 mg .... Antitussive
Pseudoephedrine HCl
  30 mg .... Nasal decongestant

Uses:
- temporarily relieves these symptoms due to the common cold:
  - nasal congestion
  - headache
  - minor aches and pains
  - cough
  - sore throat
- temporarily reduces fever

Warnings:

Alcohol warning: If you consume 3 or more alcoholic drinks every day, ask your doctor whether you should take acetaminophen or other pain relievers/fever reducers. Acetaminophen may cause liver damage.

Do not use:
- with another product containing any of these active ingredients
- if you are now taking a prescription monoamine oxidase inhibitor (MAOI) (certain drugs for depression, psychiatric, or emotional conditions, or Parkinson's disease), or for 2 weeks after stopping the MAOI drug. If you do not know if your prescription drug contains an MAOI, ask a doctor or pharmacist before taking this product.

Ask a doctor before use if you have:
- heart disease
- thyroid disease
- diabetes
- high blood pressure

- trouble urinating due to an enlarged prostate gland
- cough accompanied by excessive phlegm (mucus)
- persistent or chronic cough as occurs with smoking, asthma, or emphysema

When using this product:
- **do not use more than directed**

Stop use and ask a doctor if:
- new symptoms occur
- sore throat is severe
- you get nervous, dizzy, or sleepless
- pain, cough or nasal congestion gets worse or lasts more than 7 days
- cough comes back or occurs with rash or headache that lasts. These could be signs of a serious condition.
- redness or swelling is present
- fever gets worse or lasts more than 3 days
- sore throat lasts for more than 2 days, is accompanied or followed by fever, headache, rash, swelling, nausea, or vomiting

If pregnant or breast-feeding, ask a health professional before use.

Keep out of reach of children.

Overdose warning: Taking more than the recommended dose may cause liver damage. In case of overdose, get medical help or contact a Poison Control Center right away. Quick medical attention is critical for adults as well as for children even if you do not notice any signs or symptoms.

Directions:
- do not use more than directed (see overdose warning)
- adults and children 12 years of age and over: 2 caplets
- children under 12 years of age: ask a doctor
- take every 6 hours while symptoms persist
- do not take more than 8 caplets in 24 hours or as directed by a doctor

Other Information:
- store at 59° to 77°F in a dry place

Inactive Ingredients: candelilla wax, crospovidone, hypromellose, magnesium stearate, microcrystalline cellulose poloxamer 407, polyethylene glycol, polyethylene oxide, povidone, pregelatinized starch, silicon dioxide, sodium lauryl sulfate, stearic acid, and titanium dioxide

Questions? call toll free **1-800-524-2624**, Monday to Friday, 9 AM – 5 PM EST

How Supplied: Boxes of 12 and 24 caplets; boxes of 12 tablets.

SUDAFED® Sinus & Allergy Tablets
[sū 'duh-fĕd]

Drug Facts:

Active Ingredients: **Purpose:**
(in each tablet)
Chlorpheniramine maleate
  4 mg .... Antihistamine
Pseudoephedrine HCl
  60 mg .... Nasal decongestant

Uses:
- temporarily relieves these symptoms due to hay fever (allergic rhinitis) or other upper respiratory allergies:

  - runny nose
  - sneezing
  - itchy, watery eyes
  - nasal congestion
  - itching of the nose or throat
- temporarily relieves these symptoms due to the common cold:
  - runny nose
  - sneezing
  - nasal congestion

Warnings:

Do not use if you are now taking a prescription monoamine oxidase inhibitor (MAOI) (certain drugs for depression, psychiatric, or emotional conditions, or Parkinson's disease), or for 2 weeks after stopping the MAOI drug. If you do not know if your prescription drug contains an MAOI, ask a doctor or pharmacist before taking this product.

Ask a doctor before use if you have
- high blood pressure
- thyroid disease
- heart disease
- glaucoma
- diabetes
- trouble urinating due to an enlarged prostate gland
- a breathing problem such as emphysema or chronic bronchitis

Ask a doctor or pharmacist before use if you are taking sedatives or tranquilizers

When using this product
- **do not use more than directed**
- drowsiness may occur
- excitability may occur, especially in children
- avoid alcoholic drinks
- alcohol, sedatives, and tranquilizers may increase drowsiness
- be careful when driving a motor vehicle or operating machinery

Stop use and ask a doctor if
- you get nervous, dizzy, or sleepless
- symptoms do not improve within 7 days or are accompanied by fever

If pregnant or breast-feeding, ask a health professional before use.

Keep out of reach of children. In case of overdose, get medical help or contact a Poison Control Center right away.

Directions:
- take every 4 to 6 hours
- do not take more than 4 doses in 24 hours

adults and children 12 years of age and over	1 tablet
children 6 to under 12 years of age	½ tablet
children under 6 years of age	ask a doctor

Other Information:
- store at 59° to 77°F in a dry place

Inactive Ingredients: Lactose, magnesium stearate, potato starch, and povidone

Questions? call **1-800-524-2624** (English/Spanish), weekdays, 9 AM–5 PM EST

How Supplied: Boxes of 24 tablets.

SUDAFED® Non-drowsy Sinus Headache Caplets and Tablets
[sū 'duh-fĕd]

Drug Facts:

Active Ingredients:
(in each caplet)   Purposes:
Acetaminophen 500 mg .... Pain reliever
Pseudoephedrine
    HCl 30 mg .... Nasal decongestant

Uses:
- temporarily relieves nasal congestion associated with sinusitis
- temporarily relieves headache, minor aches, and pains

Warnings:
Alcohol warning: If you consume 3 or more alcoholic drinks every day, ask your doctor whether you should take acetaminophen or other pain relievers/fever reducers. Acetaminophen may cause liver damage.
Do not use
- with another product containing any of these active ingredients.
- if you are now taking a prescription monoamine oxidase inhibitor (MAOI) (certain drugs for depression, psychiatric, or emotional conditions, or Parkinson's disease), or for 2 weeks after stopping the MAOI drug. If you do not know if your prescription drug contains an MAOI, ask a doctor or pharmacist before taking this product.
Ask a doctor before use if you have
- heart disease
- thyroid disease
- diabetes
- high blood pressure
- trouble urinating due to an enlarged prostate gland
When using this product
- do not use more than directed
Stop use and ask a doctor if
- you get nervous, dizzy, or sleepless
- new symptoms occur
- redness or swelling is present
- pain or nasal congestion gets worse or lasts more than 7 days
- fever gets worse or lasts more than 3 days
If pregnant or breast-feeding, ask a health professional before use.
Keep out of reach of children.
Overdose warning: Taking more than the recommended dose may cause liver damage. In case of overdose, get medical help or contact a Poison Control Center right away. Quick medical attention is critical for adults as well as for children even if you do not notice any signs or symptoms.

Directions:
- do not use more than directed (see overdose warning)
- children under 12 years of age: ask a doctor
- adults and children 12 years of age and over: 2 caplets every 6 hours while symptoms persist
- do not take more than 8 caplets in 24 hours or as directed by a doctor

Other Information:
- store at 59° to 77°F in a dry place

Inactive Ingredients: calcium stearate, candelilla wax, croscarmellose sodium, crospovidone, FD&C yellow no. 6 aluminum lake, hypromellose, microcrystalline cellulose, polyethylene glycol, polysorbate 80, povidone, pregelatinized starch, stearic acid and titanium dioxide.

Questions? call **1-800-524-2624** (English/Spanish), weekdays, 9 AM–5 PM EST

How Supplied: Boxes of 24 and 48 caplets; boxes of 24 tablets.

SUDAFED® PE NON-DROWSY NASAL DECONGESTANT
[sū'duh-fĕd]

Drug Facts
Active Ingredient
(in each tablet):   Purpose:
Phenylephrine HCl   Nasal
    10 mg .... decongestant

Uses:
- temporarily relieves nasal congestion due to the common cold, hay fever or other upper respiratory allergies, and nasal congestion associated with sinusitis
- temporarily relieves sinus congestion and pressure

Warnings:
Do not use if you are now taking a prescription monoamine oxidase inhibitor (MAOI) (certain drugs for depression, psychiatric, or emotional conditions, or Parkinson's disease), or for 2 weeks after stopping the MAOI drug. If you do not know if your prescription drug contains an MAOI, ask a doctor or pharmacist before taking this product.
Ask a doctor before use if you have
- heart disease • high blood pressure
- thyroid disease • diabetes • trouble urinating due to an enlarged prostate gland
When using this product • do not use more than directed
Stop use and ask a doctor if • you get nervous, dizzy, or sleepless
- symptoms do not improve within 7 days or are accompanied by fever
If pregnant or breast-feeding, ask a health professional before use.
Keep out of reach of children. In case of overdose, get medical help or contact a Poison Control Center right away.

Directions:
- take every 4 hours
- do not take more than 6 doses in 24 hours
- adults and children 12 years of age and over: 1 tablet
- children under 12 years of age: ask a doctor
Other Information:
- store at 59° to 77°F in a dry place

Inactive Ingredients: acesulfame potassium, candelilla wax, colloidal silicon dioxide, crospovidone, FD&C red no. 40 aluminum lake, FD&C yellow no. 6 aluminum lake, hypromellose, magnesium stearate, microcrystalline cellulose, polydextrose, polyethylene glycol, pregelatinized starch, stearic acid, titanium dioxide and triacetin.

Questions?
call **1-800-524-2624** (English/Spanish), weekdays, 9 AM–5 PM EST

How Supplied: Available in boxes of 18 tablets

TUCKS®
[tuks]
Hemorrhoidal Ointment

Drug Facts

Active Ingredients: Purpose:
Mineral oil 46.6% .... Protectant
Pramoxine HCl 1% .... Pain reliever
Zinc oxide 12.5% .... Protectant

Uses:
- temporarily relieves these local symptoms associated with hemorrhoids and other anorectal disorders:
  - pain • soreness • burning • itching
- temporarily forms a protective coating over inflamed tissues to help prevent drying of tissues

Warnings:
For external use only.
When using this product
- do not use more than directed unless told to do so by a doctor
- do not put into the rectum by using fingers or any mechanical device or applicator
Stop use and ask a doctor if
- allergic reaction occurs
- rectal bleeding occurs
- redness, irritation, swelling, pain, or other symptoms begin or increase
- condition worsens or does not improve within 7 days
Keep out of reach of children. If swallowed, get medical help or contact a Poison Control Center right away.

Directions:
- adults: apply externally to the affected area up to 5 times daily
  - when practical, clean the affected area with mild soap and warm water and rinse thoroughly
  - gently dry by patting or blotting with toilet tissue or a soft cloth before applying
  - to use dispensing cap
    - attach it to tube, lubricate well, then gently insert part way into anus
    - squeeze tube to deliver medication
    - thoroughly cleanse dispensing cap after use
- children under 12 years of age: ask a doctor
Other Information: • store at 20° to 25°C (68° to 77°F)

Inactive Ingredients: benzyl benzoate, calcium phosphate dibasic, cocoa

Continued on next page

This product information was prepared in November 2003. On these and other Pfizer Consumer Healthcare Products, detailed information may be obtained by addressing Pfizer Consumer Healthcare, Pfizer, Inc., Morris Plains, NJ 07950

Tucks Ointment—Cont.

butter, glyceryl monooleate, glyceryl monostearate, kaolin, peruvian balsam, and polyethylene wax

Questions? call **1-800-223-0182**, weekdays, 9 AM - 5 PM EST

How Supplied:
Available in 1 oz tube

TUCKS®
[tuks]
HYDROCORTISONE ANTI-ITCH OINTMENT

Drug Facts
Active Ingredient: **Purpose:**
Hydrocortisone acetate 1.12% (equivalent to hydrocortisone 1%) . Anti-itch

Uses:
- temporarily relieves external anal itching and itching associated with minor skin irritations and rashes
- other uses of this product should be only under the advice and supervision of a doctor

Warnings:
For external use only.
Do not use
- for the treatment of diaper rash. Consult a doctor.
When using this product
- avoid contact with the eyes
- do not use more than directed unless told to do so by a doctor
- do not put into the rectum by using fingers or any mechanical device or applicator
Stop use and ask a doctor if
- rectal bleeding occurs
- condition worsens, or if symptoms persist for more than 7 days or clear up and occur again within a few days, and do not begin use of any other hydrocortisone product unless you have asked a doctor
Keep out of reach of children. If swallowed, get medical help or contact a Poison Control Center right away.

Directions:
- adults: apply externally to the affected area not more than 3 to 4 times daily
  - when practical, clean the affected area with mild soap and warm water and rinse thoroughly
  - gently dry by patting or blotting with toilet tissue or a soft cloth before applying
- children under 12 years of age: ask a doctor
Other Information: • store at 20° to 25°C (68° to 77°F)

Inactive Ingredients: diazolidinyl urea, methylparaben, microcrystalline wax, mineral oil, propylene glycol, propylparaben, sorbitan sesquioleate, and white petrolatum

Questions? call **1-800-223-0182**, weekdays, 9 AM - 5 PM EST

How Supplied: Available in 0.7oz tube

TUCKS®
[tuks]
Topical Starch Hemorrhoidal Suppositories

Drug Facts
Active Ingredient: **Purpose:**
Topical starch 51% .... Protectant

Uses:
- temporarily relieves these local symptoms associated with hemorrhoids and other anorectal disorders:
  - itching • burning • discomfort
- temporarily forms a protective coating over inflamed tissues to help prevent drying of tissues

Warnings:
For rectal use only.
When using this product
- do not use more than directed unless told to do so by a doctor
Stop use and ask a doctor if
- rectal bleeding occurs
- condition worsens or does not improve within 7 days
If pregnant or breast-feeding, ask a health professional before use.
Keep out of reach of children. If swallowed, get medical help or contact a Poison Control Center right away.

Directions:
- see bottom panel for directions for opening suppository wrapper
- adults: insert one (1) suppository rectally up to 6 times daily or after each bowel movement by following these steps:
  - when practical, clean the affected area with mild soap and warm water and rinse thoroughly
  - gently dry by patting or blotting with toilet tissue or a soft cloth before applying
  - detach one (1) suppository from the strip of suppositories
  - remove wrapper before inserting into the rectum
- children under 12 years of age: ask a doctor
Other Information:
- store at 20° to 25°C (68° to 77° F) to avoid melting

Inactive Ingredients: benzyl alcohol, hydrogenated vegetable oil, and vitamin E

Question? call **1-800-223-0182**, weekdays, 9 AM – 5 PM EST

How Supplied:
Available in 12 count and 24 count Blister Pack

TUCKS®
[tuks]
Witch Hazel Hemorrhoidal Pad

Drug Facts:
Active Ingredient: **Purpose:**
Witch hazel 50% .... Astringent

Uses:
- temporarily relieves the local itching and discomfort associated with hemorrhoids
- aids in protecting irritated anorectal areas
- temporarily relieves irritation and burning

Warnings:
For external use only.
When using this product
- do not use more than directed unless told to do so by a doctor
- do not put directly in the rectum by using fingers or any mechanical device or applicator
Stop use and ask a doctor if
- rectal bleeding occurs
- condition worsens or does not improve within 7 days
Keep out of reach of children. If swallowed, get medical help or contact a Poison Control Center right away.

Directions:
- adults:
  - when practical, clean the affected area with mild soap and warm water, and rinse thoroughly
  - gently dry by patting or blotting with toilet tissue or a soft cloth before applying
  - apply externally to the affected area up to 6 times daily or after each bowel movement
  - after application, discard pad
- children under 12 years of age: ask a doctor
Other Information:
- store at 20° to 25°C (68° to 77°F)

Inactive Ingredients: water, glycerin, alcohol, propylene glycol, sodium citrate, diazolidinyl urea, citric acid, methylparaben, propylparaben
Questions? call **1-800-223-0182**, weekdays, 9 AM - 5 PM EST

How Supplied: Available in 40's, 100's, and Take Along 12's.

MAXIMUM STRENGTH UNISOM SLEEPGELS®
Nighttime Sleep Aid

Drug Facts

Active Ingredient
(in each softgel)   **Purpose:**
Diphenhydramine HCl
50 mg .... Nighttime sleep-aid

Use:
- helps to reduce difficulty falling asleep
Warnings:
Do not use
- for children under 12 years of age
- with any other product containing diphenhydramine, even one used on skin.
Ask a doctor before use if you have
- a breathing problem such as emphysema or chronic bronchitis
- glaucoma
- trouble urinating due to an enlarged prostate gland
Ask a doctor or pharmacist before use if you are taking sedatives or tranquilizers
When using this product avoid alcoholic drinks
Stop use and ask a doctor if sleeplessness persists continuously for more than 2 weeks. Insomnia may be a symptom of serious underlying medical illness.
If pregnant or breast-feeding, ask a health professional before use.
Keep out of reach of children. In case of overdose, get medical help or contact a Poison Control Center right away.

Directions:
- adults and children 12 years of age and over: 1 softgel (50 mg) at bedtime if needed, or as directed by a doctor

Other Information:
- store at 59° to 86°F (15° to 30°C)

Inactive Ingredients: FD&C blue no. 1, gelatin, glycerin, polyethylene glycol, polyvinyl acetate phthalate, propylene glycol, purified water, sorbitol, and titanium dioxide

Questions? call **1-800-223-0182**, weekdays, 9 AM – 5 PM EST

How Supplied: Boxes of 8 (non-child resistant), 16, 32 and 64 softgels.

UNISOM® SleepTabs™
[*yu 'na-som*]
Nighttime Sleep Aid
(doxylamine succinate)

Drug Facts

Active Ingredient:　　　　**Purpose:**
(in each tablet)
Doxylamine succinate
　25 mg .... Nighttime sleep-aid

Use:
- helps to reduce difficulty in falling asleep

Warnings:
Ask a doctor before use if you have
- a breathing problem such as asthma, emphysema or chronic bronchitis
- glaucoma
- trouble urinating due to an enlarged prostate gland

Ask a doctor or pharmacist before use if you are taking any other drugs
When using this product
- avoid alcoholic beverages
- take only at bedtime

Stop use and ask a doctor if sleeplessness persists continuously for more than two weeks. Insomnia may be a symptom of serious underlying medical illness.

If pregnant or breast-feeding, ask a health professional before use.

Keep out of reach of children. In case of overdose, get medical help or contact a Poison Control Center right away.

Directions:
- adults: take one tablet 30 minutes before going to bed; take once daily or as directed by a doctor
- do not give to children under 12 years of age

Other Information:
- store at 59° to 86°F (15° to 30°C)

Inactive Ingredients: dibasic calcium phosphate, FD&C blue no. 1 aluminum lake, magnesium stearate, microcrystalline cellulose, and sodium starch glycolate

Questions?
call **1-800-223-0182**, Monday to Friday, 9 AM - 5 PM EST

How Supplied: Boxes of 8, 32, 48 and 64 tablets in child resistant packaging. Boxes of 16 tablets in non-child resistant packaging.

VISINE® ORIGINAL
Redness Reliever Eye Drops

Drug Facts:

Active Ingredient:　　　　**Purpose:**
Tetrahydrozoline
　HCl 0.05% .... Redness reliever

Use:
- for the relief of redness of the eye due to minor eye irritations

Warnings:
Ask a doctor before use if you have narrow angle glaucoma
When using this product
- pupils may become enlarged temporarily
- overuse may cause more eye redness
- remove contact lenses before using
- do not use if this solution changes color or becomes cloudy
- do not touch tip of container to any surface to avoid contamination
- replace cap after each use
Stop use and ask a doctor if
- you feel eye pain
- changes in vision occur
- redness or irritation of the eye lasts
- condition worsens or lasts more than 72 hours
If pregnant or breast-feeding, ask a health professional before use.
Keep out of reach of children. If swallowed, get medical help or contact a Poison Control Center right away.

Directions:
- put 1 to 2 drops in the affected eye(s) up to 4 times daily
- children under 6 years of age: ask a doctor

Other Information:
- store at 15° to 25°C (59° to 77°F)

Inactive Ingredients: benzalkonium chloride, boric acid, edetate disodium, purified water, sodium borate, and sodium chloride
Questions? call **1-800-223-0182**, weekdays, 9 AM – 5 PM EST

Caution: Do not use if Visine imprinted neckband on bottle is broken or missing.

How Supplied: In ½ FL OZ and 1 FL OZ plastic dispenser bottle and ½ FL OZ plastic bottle with eye dropper.

VISINE-A®
Antihistamine & Redness Reliever Eye Drops

Drug Facts:

Active Ingredients:　　　　**Purpose:**
Naphazoline hydrochloride
　0.025% .... Redness reliever
Pheniramine maleate
　0.3% .... Antihistamine

Uses: Temporarily relieves itchy, red eyes due to:
- pollen
- ragweed
- grass
- animal hair and dander

Warnings:
Do not use
- if you are sensitive to any ingredient in this product
Ask a doctor before use if you have:
- heart disease
- high blood pressure
- narrow angle glaucoma
- trouble urinating due to an enlarged prostate gland
When using this product:
- pupils may become enlarged temporarily
- do not touch tip of container to any surface to avoid contamination
- replace cap after each use
- remove contact lenses before using
- do not use if this solution changes color or becomes cloudy
- overuse may cause more eye redness
Stop use and ask a doctor if:
- you feel eye pain
- changes in vision occur
- redness or irritation of the eye lasts
- condition worsens or lasts more than 72 hours
Keep out of reach of children. If swallowed, get medical help or contact a Poison Control Center right away. Accidental swallowing by infants and children may lead to coma and marked reduction in body temperature.

Directions:
- adults and children 6 years of age and over: put 1 or 2 drops in the affected eye(s) up to 4 times a day
- children under 6 years of age: consult a doctor

Other Information:
- some users may experience a brief tingling sensation
- store between 15° and 25°C (59° and 77°F)

Inactive Ingredients: boric acid and sodium borate buffer system preserved with benzalkonium chloride (0.01%) and edetate disodium (0.1%), sodium hydroxide and/or hydrochloric acid (to adjust pH), and purified water

Questions? call **1-800-223-0182**, weekdays 9 AM – 5 PM EST

Caution: Do not use if Pfizer imprinted neckband on bottle is broken or missing.

How Supplied: In ½ FL OZ plastic dispenser bottle.

Continued on next page

This product information was prepared in November 2003. On these and other Pfizer Consumer Healthcare Products, detailed information may be obtained by addressing Pfizer Consumer Healthcare, Pfizer, Inc., Morris Plains, NJ 07950

VISINE A.C.®
Astringent/Redness Reliever Eye Drops

Drug Facts:

Active Ingredients: **Purpose:**
Tetrahydrozoline
  HCl 0.05% .... Redness reliever
Zinc sulfate 0.25% .... Astringent

Use:
- for temporary relief of discomfort and redness of the eye due to minor eye irritations

Warnings:
Ask a doctor before use if you have narrow angle glaucoma
When using this product:
- pupils may become enlarged temporarily
- overuse may cause more eye redness
- remove contact lenses before using
- do not use if this solution changes color or becomes cloudy
- do not touch tip of container to any surface to avoid contamination
- replace cap after each use

Stop use and ask a doctor if:
- you feel eye pain
- changes in vision occur
- redness or irritation of the eye lasts
- condition worsens or lasts more than 72 hours

If pregnant or breast-feeding, ask a health professional before use.
Keep out of reach of children. If swallowed, get medical help or contact a Poison Control Center right away.

Directions:
- put 1 to 2 drops in the affected eye(s) up to 4 times daily
- children under 6 years of age: ask a doctor

Other Information:
- some users may experience a brief tingling sensation
- store at 15° to 25°C (59° to 77°F)

Inactive Ingredients: benzalkonium chloride, boric acid, edetate disodium, purified water, sodium chloride, and sodium citrate

Questions? call **1-800-223-0182**, Weekdays, 9 AM – 5 PM EST

Caution: Do not use if Visine imprinted neckband on bottle is broken or missing.

How Supplied: In ½ FL OZ and 1 FL OZ plastic dispenser bottle.

VISINE ADVANCED RELIEF®
Lubricant/Redness Reliever Eye Drops

Drug Facts:

Active Ingredients: **Purpose:**
Dextran 70 0.1% .... Lubricant
Polyethylene glycol
  400 1% .... Lubricant
Povidone 1% .... Lubricant
Tetrahydrozoline
  HCl 0.05% .... Redness reliever

Uses:
- for the relief of redness of the eye due to minor eye irritations
- for use as a protectant against further irritation or to relieve dryness of the eye

Warnings:
Ask a doctor before use if you have narrow angle glaucoma
When using this product:
- pupils may become enlarged temporarily
- overuse may cause more eye redness
- remove contact lenses before using
- do not use if this solution changes color or becomes cloudy
- do not touch tip of container to any surface to avoid contamination
- replace cap after each use

Stop use and ask a doctor if:
- you feel eye pain
- changes in vision occur
- redness or irritation of the eye lasts
- condition worsens or lasts more than 72 hours

If pregnant or breast-feeding, ask a health professional before use.
Keep out of reach of children. If swallowed, get medical help or contact a Poison Control Center right away.

Directions:
- put 1 or 2 drops in the affected eye(s) up to 4 times daily
- children under 6 years of age: ask a doctor

Other Information:
- store at 15° to 25°C (59° to 77°F)

Inactive Ingredients: benzalkonium chloride, boric acid, edetate disodium, purified water, sodium borate, and sodium chloride
Questions? call **1-800-223-0182**, weekdays, 9 AM – 5 PM EST

Caution: Do not use if Visine imprinted neckband on bottle is broken or missing.

How Supplied: In ½ FL OZ and 1 FL OZ plastic dispenser bottle.

VISINE L.R.®
Redness Reliever Eye Drops

Drug Facts:

Active Ingredient: **Purpose:**
Oxymetazoline HCl
  0.025% .... Redness reliever

Use:
- for the relief of redness of the eye due to minor eye irritations

Warnings:
Ask a doctor before use if you have narrow angle glaucoma
When using this product:
- overuse may cause more eye redness
- remove contact lenses before using
- do not use if this solution changes color or becomes cloudy
- do not touch tip of container to any surface to avoid contamination
- replace cap after each use

Stop use and ask a doctor if:
- you feel eye pain
- changes in vision occur
- redness or irritation of the eye lasts
- condition worsens or lasts more than 72 hours

If pregnant or breast-feeding, ask a health professional before use.
Keep out of reach of children. If swallowed, get medical help or contact a Poison Control Center right away.

Directions:
- adults and children 6 years of age and over: put 1 or 2 drops in the affected eye(s)
- this may be repeated as needed every 6 hours or as directed by a doctor
- children under 6 years of age: ask a doctor

Other Information:
- store at 15° to 25°C (59° to 77°F)

Inactive Ingredients: benzalkonium chloride, boric acid, edetate disodium, purified water, sodium borate, and sodium chloride

Questions? call **1-800-223-0182**, weekdays, 9 AM – 5 PM EST

Caution: Do not use if Visine imprinted neckband on bottle is broken or missing.

How Supplied: In ½ FL OZ and 1 FL OZ plastic dispenser bottle.

VISINE TEARS®
Lubricant Eye Drops

Drug Facts

Active Ingredients: **Purpose:**
Glycerin 0.2% .... Lubricant
Hypromellose 0.2% .... Lubricant
Polyethylene glycol 400 1% ... Lubricant

Uses:
- for the temporary relief of burning and irritation due to dryness of the eye
- for protection against further irritation

Warnings:
When using this product
- remove contact lenses before using
- do not use if this solution changes color or becomes cloudy
- do not touch tip of container to any surface to avoid contamination
- replace cap after each use

Stop use and ask a doctor if
- you feel eye pain
- changes in vision occur
- redness or irritation of the eye lasts
- condition worsens or lasts more than 72 hours

If pregnant or breast-feeding, ask a health professional before use.
Keep out of reach of children. If swallowed, get medical help or contact a Poison Control Center right away.

Directions:
- put 1 or 2 drops in the affected eye(s) as needed
- children under 6 years of age: ask a doctor

Other Information:
- store at 15° to 25°C (59° to 77°F)

Inactive Ingredients: ascorbic acid, benzalkonium chloride, boric acid, dextrose, disodium phosphate, glycine, magnesium chloride, potassium chloride, purified water, sodium borate, sodium chloride, sodium citrate, and sodium lactate

Questions? call **1-800-223-0182**, weekdays, 9 AM – 5 PM EST

Caution: Do not use if Visine imprinted neckband on bottle is broken or missing.

How Supplied: In ½ FL OZ and 1 FL OZ plastic dispenser bottle.

VISINE TEARS®
Preservative Free, Single-Use Containers
Lubricant Eye Drops

Drug Facts:

Active Ingredients: Purpose:
Glycerin 0.2% .... Lubricant
Hypromellose 0.2% .... Lubricant
Polyethylene glycol 400 1% ... Lubricant

Uses:
• for the temporary relief of burning and irritation due to dryness of the eye
• for protection against further irritation

Warnings:
When using this product
• remove contact lenses before using
• do not use if this solution changes color or becomes cloudy
• do not touch tip of container to any surface to avoid contamination
• do not reuse; once opened, discard
Stop use and ask a doctor if:
• you feel eye pain
• changes in vision occur
• redness or irritation of the eye lasts
• condition worsens or lasts more than 72 hours
If pregnant or breast-feeding, ask a health professional before use.
Keep out of reach of children. If swallowed, get medical help or contact a Poison Control Center right away.

Directions:
• put 1 or 2 drops in the affected eye(s) as needed
• children under 6 years of age: ask a doctor

Other Information:
• store at 15° to 25°C (59° to 77°F)

Inactive Ingredients: ascorbic acid, dextrose, disodium phosphate, glycine, magnesium chloride, potassium chloride, purified water, sodium chloride, sodium citrate, sodium lactate, and sodium phosphate

Questions? call **1-800-223-0182**, weekdays, 9 AM - 5 PM EST

Caution: Use only if single use container is intact.

How Supplied: 1 box contains 28 single-use containers, 0.01 FL OZ (0.4 mL) each

---

ZANTAC 75®
Ranitidine Tablets 75 mg
Acid Reducer
[*zan ' tak*]

Drug Facts:

Active Ingredient:
(in each tablet) Purpose:
Ranitidine 75 mg
(as ranitidine
hydrochloride 84 mg) .... Acid reducer

Uses:
• relieves heartburn associated with acid indigestion and sour stomach
• prevents heartburn associated with acid indigestion and sour stomach brought on by certain foods and beverages

Warnings:
Allergy alert: Do not use if you are allergic to ranitidine or other acid reducers
Do not use:
• if you have trouble swallowing
• with other acid reducers
Stop use and ask a doctor if:
• stomach pain continues
• you need to take this product for more than 14 days
If pregnant or breast-feeding, ask a health professional before use.
Keep out of reach of children. In case of overdose, get medical help or contact a Poison Control Center right away.

Directions:
• adults and children 12 years and over:
  • to **relieve** symptoms, swallow 1 tablet with a glass of water
  • to **prevent** symptoms, swallow 1 tablet with a glass of water **30 to 60 minutes before** eating food or drinking beverages that cause heartburn
  • can be used up to twice daily (up to 2 tablets in 24 hours)
• children under 12 years: ask a doctor

Other Information:
• do not use if foil under bottle cap or individual blister unit is open or torn
• store at 20°–25°C (68°–77°F)
• avoid excessive heat or humidity
• this product is sodium and sugar free

Inactive Ingredients: hypromellose, magnesium stearate, microcrystalline cellulose, synthetic red iron oxide, titanium dioxide, triacetin

Read the Label: Read the directions, consumer information leaflet and warnings before use. Keep the carton. It contains important information.

Questions? call **1-800-223-0182**, weekdays, 9 AM – 5 PM EST.

How Supplied: Zantac 75 is available in convenient blister packs in boxes of 4, 10, 20 and 30 tablets, and in bottles of 60, and 80 count.

MAXIMUM STRENGTH
ZANTAC 150®
Ranitidine Tablets 150 mg/Acid Reducer

Drug Facts

Active Ingredient
(in each tablet): Purpose:
Ranitidine 150 mg .... Acid reducer
(as ranitidine hydrochloride 168 mg)

Uses:
• relieves heartburn associated with acid indigestion and sour stomach
• prevents heartburn associated with acid indigestion and sour stomach brought on by certain foods and beverages

Warnings:
Allergy alert: Do not use if you are allergic to ranitidine or other acid reducers
Do not use
• if you have trouble or pain swallowing food, vomiting with blood, or bloody or black stools. These may be signs of a serious condition. See your doctor.
• with other acid reducers
• if you have kidney disease, except under the advice and supervision of a doctor
Ask a doctor before use if you have
• had heartburn over 3 months. This may be a sign of a more serious condition.
• heartburn with **lightheadedness, sweating or dizziness**
• chest pain or shoulder pain with shortness of breath; sweating; pain spreading to arms, neck or shoulders; or lightheadedness
• frequent **chest pain** • frequent wheezing, particularly with heartburn
• unexplained weight loss • nausea or vomiting
• stomach pain
Stop use and ask a doctor if
• your heartburn continues or worsens
• you need to take this product for more than 14 days
If pregnant or breast-feeding, ask a health professional before use.
Keep out of reach of children. In case of overdose, get medical help or contact a Poison Control Center right away.

Directions:
• adults and children 12 years and over:
  • to **relieve** symptoms, swallow 1 tablet with a glass of water
  • to **prevent** symptoms, swallow 1 tablet with a glass of water **30 to 60 minutes before** eating food or drinking beverages that cause heartburn
  • can be used up to twice daily (do not take more than 2 tablets in 24 hours)
• children under 12 years: ask a doctor

Continued on next page

This product information was prepared in November 2003. On these and other Pfizer Consumer Healthcare Products, detailed information may be obtained by addressing Pfizer Consumer Healthcare, Pfizer, Inc., Morris Plains, NJ 07950

Zantac Max. Strength—Cont.

Other Information: • do not use if foil under bottle cap or individual blister unit is open or torn • store at 20°–25°C (68°–77°F) • avoid excessive heat or humidity • this product is sugar free

Inactive Ingredients: hypromellose, magnesium stearate, microcrystalline cellulose, synthetic red iron oxide, titanium dioxide, triacetin

How Supplied: Available in boxes of 8 and 50 tablets.

Questions? call **1-800-223-0182**, weekdays, 9 AM–5 PM EST

The Procter & Gamble Company

P. O. BOX 599
CINCINNATI, OH 45201

Direct Inquiries to:
Consumer Relations
(800) 832–3064

HEAD & SHOULDERS CLASSIC CLEAN DANDRUFF SHAMPOO

Head & Shoulders Classic Clean Dandruff Shampoo for normal/oily hair offers effective control of persistent dandruff and beautiful hair from a pleasant-to-use formula. Double-blind, expert-graded testing have proven that it reduces dandruff very effectively. It is also gentle enough to use every day for clean, manageable hair.

The formula ingredients below are for Classic Clean version. Head & Shoulders is also available in a Classic Clean 2-in-1 version for increased manageability and hair damage prevention. The key formula difference is increased dimethicone conditioner and substitution of Polyquaternium-10 polymer instead of Guar Hydroxypropyltrimonium Chloride.

Drug Facts

Active Ingredient: **Purpose:**
Pyrithione zinc 1%   Anti-dandruff

Uses: helps prevent recurrence of flaking and itching associated with dandruff

Warnings:
For external use only
When using this product
• avoid contact with eyes. If contact occurs, rinse eyes thoroughly with water.
Stop use and ask a doctor if
• condition worsens or does not improve after regular use of this product as directed.
Keep this and all drugs out of reach of children. If swallowed, get medical help or contact a Poison Control Center right away.

Directions:
• for maximum dandruff control, use every time you shampoo.
• wet hair.
• massage onto scalp
• rinse.
• repeat if desired.
• for best results use at least twice a week or as directed by a doctor.

Inactive Ingredients: Water, Ammonium laureth sulfate, Ammonium lauryl sulfate, Glycol distearate, Dimethicone, Cetyl alcohol, Cocamide MEA, Fragrance, Sodium chloride, Guar hydroxypropyltrimonium chloride, Hydrogenated polydecene, Sodium citrate, Sodium benzoate, Trimethylolpropane tricaprylate/tricaprate, Citric acid, Benzyl alcohol, Methylchloroisothiazolinone, Methylisothiazolinone, Ext. D&C violet no. 2, FD&C blue no. 1, Ammonium xylenesulfonate

How Supplied: Head & Shoulders Classic Clean Dandruff Shampoo is available in 2.0 FL, 6.8 FL OZ, 13.5 FL OZ, 25.4 FL OZ, 33.9 FL OZ unbreakable plastic bottles.

Questions [or comments]? **1-800-723-9569**

HEAD & SHOULDERS DRY SCALP CARE DANDRUFF SHAMPOO

Head & Shoulders Dry Scalp Care Dandruff Shampoo offers effective control of persistent dandruff and beautiful hair from a pleasant-to-use formula. Double-blind, expert-graded testing have proven that it reduces dandruff very effectively. It is also gentle enough to use every day for clean, manageable hair.

The formula ingredients below are for Dry Scalp version. Head & Shoulders is also available in a conditioning Smooth & Silky 2-in-1 version whose primary formula difference is a lower level of the moisturizing and protective conditioning ingredient Dimethicone and substitution of Polyquarternium-10 polymer for a portion of the Guar Hydroxypropyltrimonium Chloride.

Drug Facts

Active Ingredient: **Purpose:**
Pyrithione zinc 1%   Anti-dandruff

Uses: Helps prevent recurrence of flaking and itching associated with dandruff

Warnings:
For external use only
When using this product
• avoid contact with eyes. If contact occurs, rinse eyes thoroughly with water.
Stop use and ask a doctor if
• condition worsens or does not improve after regular use of this product as directed.

Keep this and all drugs out of reach of children. If swallowed, get medical help or contact a Poison Control Center right away.

Directions:
• for maximum dandruff control, use every time you shampoo.
• wet hair.
• massage onto scalp.
• rinse.
• repeat if desired.
• for best results use at least twice a week or as directed by a doctor.

Inactive Ingredients: Water, Ammonium laureth sulfate, Ammonium lauryl sulfate, Dimethicone, Glycol distearate, Cetyl alcohol, Cocamide MEA, Fragrance, Sodium chloride, Polyquaternium-10, Hydrogenated polydecene, Sodium citrate, Sodium benzoate, Trimethylolpropane tricaprylate/tricaprate, Citric acid, Benzyl alcohol, Methylchloroisothiazolinone, Methylisothiazolinone, Ext. D&C violet no. 2, FD&C blue no. 1, Ammonium xylenesulfonate

How Supplied: Head & Shoulders Dry Scalp Care Dandruff Shampoo is available in 6.8 FL OZ, 13.5 FL OZ, 25.4 FL OZ, 33.9 FL OZ unbreakable plastic bottles.

Questions [or comments]? **1-800-723-9569**

HEAD & SHOULDERS® INTENSIVE TREATMENT DANDRUFF AND SEBORRHEIC DERMATITIS SHAMPOO

Head & Shoulders Intensive Treatment Dandruff and Seborrheic Dermatitis Shampoo offers effective control of persistent dandruff and beautiful hair from a pleasant-to-use formula. Double-blind, expert-graded testing have proven that it reduces dandruff very effectively. It is also gentle enough to use every day for clean, manageable hair.

Drug Facts

Active Ingredient: **Purpose:**
Selenium Sulfide 1%   Anti-dandruff
                            Anti-seborrheic dermatitis

Uses: Helps stop itching, flaking, scaling, irritation and redness associated with dandruff and seborrheic dermatitis.

Warnings:
For external use only
Ask a doctor before use if you have a condition that covers a large portion of the body.
When using this product
• avoid contact with eyes. If contact occurs, rinse eyes thoroughly with water.
Stop use and ask a doctor if
• condition worsens or does not improve after regular use of this product as directed.

Keep this and all drugs out of reach of children. If swallowed, get medical help or contact a Poison Control Center right away.

Directions:
• wet hair.
• massage onto scalp
• rinse thoroughly
• for best results use at least twice a week or as directed by a doctor.
• caution: if used on bleached, tinted, grey, or permed hair, rinse for 5 minutes
• for maximum dandruff control, use every time you shampoo

Inactive Ingredients: Water, Ammonium laureth sulfate, Ammonium lauryl sulfate, Glycol distearate, Cocamide MEA, Fragrance, Dimethicone, Tricetylmonium chloride, Ammonium xylenesulfonate, Cetyl alcohol, DMDM hydantoin, Sodium chloride, Stearyl alcohol, Hydroxypropyl methylcellulose, FD&C red no. 4

How Supplied: Head & Shoulders Intensive Treatment Dandruff and Seborrheic Dermatitis Shampoo is available in 13.5 FL OZ unbreakable plastic bottles.

Questions [or comments]? 1-800-723-9569

METAMUCIL® FIBER LAXATIVE
[met uh-mü sil]
(psyllium husk)

*Also see **Metamucil Dietary Fiber Supplement** in PDR for Nonprescription Drugs*

Description: Metamucil contains psyllium husk (from the plant *Plantago ovata*), a bulk forming, natural therapeutic fiber for restoring and maintaining regularity when recommended by a physician. Metamucil contains no chemical stimulants and does not disrupt normal bowel function. Each dose of Metamucil powder and Metamucil Fiber Wafers contains approximately 3.4 grams of psyllium husk (or 2.4 grams of soluble fiber). Each dose of Metamucil capsules fiber laxative (5 capsules) contains approximately 2.6 grams of psyllium husk (or 2.0 grams of soluble fiber). Inactive ingredients, sodium, calcium, potassium, calories, carbohydrate, dietary fiber, and phenylalanine content are shown in the following table for all versions and flavors. Metamucil Smooth Texture Sugar-Free unflavored and Metamucil capsules contains no sugar and no artificial sweeteners; Metamucil Smooth Texture Sugar-Free Orange Flavor contains aspartame (phenylalanine content per dose is 25 mg). Metamucil powdered products and Metamucil capsules are gluten-free. Metamucil Fiber Wafers contain gluten: Apple contains 0.7g/dose, Cinnamon contains 0.5g/dose. Each two-wafer dose contains 5 grams of fat.

Actions: The active ingredient in Metamucil is psyllium husk, a natural fiber which promotes elimination due to its bulking effect in the colon. This bulking effect is due to both the water-holding capacity of undigested fiber and the increased bacterial mass following partial fiber digestion. These actions result in enlargement of the lumen of the colon, and softer stool, thereby decreasing intraluminal pressure and straining, and speeding colonic transit in constipated patients.

Indications: Metamucil is indicated for the treatment of occasional constipation, and when recommended by a physician, for chronic constipation and constipation associated with irritable bowel syndrome, diverticulosis, hemorrhoids, convalescence, senility and pregnancy. Pregnancy: Category B. If considering use of Metamucil as part of a cholesterol-lowering program, see **Metamucil Dietary Fiber Supplement** in Dietary Supplement Section.

Drug Facts

Active Ingredient: **Purpose:**
(in each DOSE)
Psyllium husk
  approximately 3.4 g ..... Fiber therapy
                                      for regularity
For Metamucil capsules each dose of 5 capsules contains approximately 2.6 gm of psyllium husk.

Uses:
• effective in treating occasional constipation and restoring regularity

Warnings:

Choking: Taking this product without adequate fluid may cause it to swell and block your throat or esophagus and may cause choking. Do not take this product if you have difficulty in swallowing. If you experience chest pain, vomiting, or difficulty in swallowing or breathing after taking this product, seek immediate medical attention.

Allergy alert: This product may cause allergic reaction in people sensitive to inhaled or ingested psyllium.

Ask a doctor before use if you have:
• a sudden change in bowel habits persisting for 2 weeks
• abdominal pain, nausea or vomiting

Stop use and ask a doctor if:
• constipation lasts more than 7 days
• rectal bleeding occurs
These may be signs of a serious condition.

Keep out of reach of children. In case of overdose, get medical help or contact a Poison Control Center right away.

Directions: For Powders: Put one dose into an empty glass. Fill glass with at least 8 oz of water or your favorite beverage. Stir briskly and drink promptly. If mixture thickens, add more liquid and stir. Mix this product (child or adult dose) with at least 8 ounces (a full glass) of water or other fluid. For capsules: Take product with 8 oz of liquid (swallow 1 capsule at a time) up to 3 times daily. Take this product with at least 8 oz (a full glass) of liquid. For Wafers: Take this product (child or adult dose) with at least 8 ounces (a full glass) of liquid. Taking these products without enough liquid may cause choking. See choking warning.

Adults 12 yrs. & older	Powders: 1 dose in 8 oz of liquid. Capsules: 5 capsules with 8 oz of liquid (swallow one capsule at a time). Wafers: 1 dose with 8 oz of liquid. Take at the first sign of irregularity; can be taken up to 3 times daily. Generally produces effect in 12 – 72 hours.
6 – 11 yrs.	Powders: ½ adult dose in 8 oz of liquid. Wafers: 1 wafer with 8 oz of liquid. Can be taken up to 3 times daily. Capsules: consider use of powder or wafer products
Under 6 yrs.	consult a doctor

Laxatives, including bulk fibers, may affect how well other medicines work. If you are taking a prescription medicine by mouth, take this product at least 2 hours before or 2 hours after the prescribed medicine. As your body adjusts to increased fiber intake, you may experience changes in bowel habits or minor bloating. **New Users:** Start with 1 dose per day; gradually increase to 3 doses per day as necessary.

Other Information:
• **Each product contains:** Potassium; sodium (See table for amount/dose)
• **PHENYLKETONURICS:** Smooth Texture Sugar Free Orange product contains phenylalanine 25 mg per dose
• Each product contains a 100% natural, therapeutic fiber

Inactive Ingredients: See table Notice to Health Care Professionals:
To minimize the potential for allergic reaction, health care professionals who frequently dispense powdered psyllium products should avoid inhaling airborne dust while dispensing these products.

Handling and Dispensing: To minimize generating airborne dust, spoon product from the canister into a glass according to label directions.

How Supplied: Powder: canisters and cartons of single-dose packets. Capsules: 100, 160 and 300 count bottles. Wafers: cartons of single dose packets. (See table) [See table at top of next page]

Continued on next page

Metamucil Fiber Laxative/Dietary Fiber Supplement

Versions/Flavors	Ingredients (alphabetical order)	Sodium mg/dose	Calcium mg/dose	Potassium mg/dose	Calories kcal/dose	Total Carbohydrate g/dose	Dietary Fiber (Soluble) g/dose	Dosage (Weight in gms)	How Supplied
Smooth Texture Orange Flavor Metamucil Powder	Citric Acid, FD&C Yellow #6, Natural and Artificial Flavor, Psyllium Husk, Sucrose	5	7	30	45	12	3 (2.4)	1 rounded tablespoon ~12g	Canisters: Doses: 48, 72, 114; Cartons: 30 single-dose packets.
Smooth Texture Sugar-Free Orange Flavor Metamucil Powder	Aspartame, Citric Acid, FD&C Yellow #6, Maltodextrin, Natural and Artificial Flavor, Psyllium Husk	5	7	30	20	5	3 (2.4)	1 rounded teaspoon ~5.8g	Canisters: Doses: 30, 48, 72, 114, 180; Cartons: 30 single-dose packets.
Smooth Texture Sugar-Free Unflavored Metamucil Powder	Citric Acid, Maltodextrin, Psyllium Husk	4	7	30	20	5	3 (2.4)	1 rounded teaspoon ~5.4g	Canisters: Doses: 48, 72 114.
Coarse Milled Unflavored Metamucil Powder	Psyllium Husk, Sucrose	3	6	30	25	7	3 (2.4)	1 rounded teaspoon ~7g	Canisters: Doses: 48, 72 114.
Coarse Milled Orange Flavor Metamucil Powder	Citric Acid, FD&C Yellow #6, Natural and Artificial Flavor, Psyllium Husk, Sucrose	5	6	30	40	11	3 (2.4)	1 rounded tablespoon ~11g	Canisters: Doses: 48,72 114.
Metamucil Capsules	Caramel color, FD&C Blue No. 1 Aluminum Lake, FD&C Red No. 40 Aluminum Lake, FD&C Yellow No. 6 Aluminum Lake, gelatin, polysorbate 80, psyllium husk	0	5	30	10	3	3 (2.4)	6 capsules 3.2g	Bottles: 100 ct, 160 ct, 300 ct
**Fiber Laxative Wafers**									
Apple Metamucil Wafers	(1)	20	14	60	120	17	6	2 wafers 24 g	Cartons: 12 doses
Cinnamon Metamucil Wafers	(2)	20	14	60	120	17	6	2 wafers 24 g	Cartons: 12 doses

(1) ascorbic acid, brown sugar, cinnamon, corn oil, corn starch, fructose, lecithin, molasses, natural and artificial flavors, oat hull fiber, psyllium husk, sodium bicarbonate, sucrose, water, wheat flour
(2) ascorbic acid, cinnamon, corn oil, corn starch, fructose, lecithin, molasses, natural and artificial flavors, nutmeg, oat hull fiber, oats, psyllium husk, sodium bicarbonate, sucrose, water, wheat flour

Metamucil—Cont.

**Questions?** **1-800-983-4237**
Shown in Product Identification Guide, page 514

PEPTO-BISMOL® ORIGINAL LIQUID, MAXIMUM STRENGTH LIQUID, ORIGINAL AND CHERRY FLAVOR CHEWABLE TABLETS AND EASY-TO-SWALLOW CAPLETS
For upset stomach, indigestion, heartburn, nausea and diarrhea.

Multi-symptom Pepto-Bismol® contains bismuth subsalicylate and is the only leading OTC stomach remedy clinically proven effective for both upper and lower GI symptoms. It has been clinically proven in double-blind placebo-controlled trials for relief of upset stomach symptoms and diarrhea.

Active Ingredient:
(per tablespoon/per tablet/per caplet)
Original Liquid/Tablets/Caplets
Bismuth subsalicylate 262 mg
Maximum Strength Liquid
Bismuth subsalicylate 525 mg

Inactive Ingredients:
[Original Liquid] benzoic acid, flavor, magnesium aluminum silicate, methylcellulose, red 22, red 28, saccharin sodium, salicylic acid, sodium salicylate, sorbic acid, water

[Maximum Strength Liquid] benzoic acid, flavor, magnesium aluminum silicate, methylcellulose, red 22, red 28, saccharin sodium, salicylic acid, sodium salicylate, sorbic acid, water

[Original Tablets] calcium carbonate, flavor, magnesium stearate, mannitol, povidone, red 27 aluminum lake, saccharin sodium, talc

[Cherry Tablets] adipic acid, calcium carbonate, flavor, magnesium stearate, mannitol, povidone, red 27 aluminum lake, red 40 aluminum lake, saccharin sodium, talc

[Caplets] calcium carbonate, magnesium stearate, mannitol, microcrystalline cellulose, polysorbate 80, povidone, red 27 aluminum lake, silicon dioxide, sodium starch glycolate.

Other Information:
Sodium Content
Original Liquid—each Tbsp contains: sodium 6 mg • low sodium
Maximum Strength Liquid—each Tbsp contains: sodium 6 mg • low sodium
Chewable Tablets—each Original or Cherry Flavor Tablet contains: sodium less than 1 mg • very low sodium
Caplets—each Caplet contains: sodium 2 mg • low sodium
Salicylate Content
Original Liquid—each Tbsp contains: salicylate 130 mg
Maximum Strength Liquid—each Tbsp contains: salicylate 236 mg
Chewable Tablets—each tablet contains: [original] salicylate 102 mg
[cherry] salicylate 99 mg
Caplets—each caplet contains: salicylate 99 mg
All Forms are sugar free.

Indications:
• relieves upset stomach symptoms (i.e., indigestion, heartburn, nausea and fullness caused by over-indulgence in food and drink) without constipating; and,
• controls diarrhea.

Actions: For upset stomach symptoms, the active ingredient is believed to work via a topical effect on the stomach mucosa. For diarrhea, it is believed to work by several mechanisms in the gastrointestinal tract, including: 1) normalizing fluid movement via an antisecretory merchanism, 2) binding bacterial toxins and 3) antimicrobial activity.

Warnings:
Reye's syndrome: Children and teenagers who have or are recovering from chicken pox or flu-like symptoms should not use this product. When using this product, if changes in behavior with nausea and vomiting occur, consult a doctor because these symptoms could be an early sign of Reye's syndrome, a rare but serious illness.
Allergy alert: Contains salicylate. Do not take if you are
• allergic to salicylates (including aspirin)
• taking other salicylate products
Do not use if you have
• an ulcer
• a bleeding problem
• bloody or black stool
Ask a doctor before use if you have
• fever
• mucus in the stool
Ask a doctor or pharmacist before use if you are taking any drug for
• anticoagulation (thinning the blood)
• diabetes
• gout
• arthritis
When using this product a temporary, but harmless, darkening of the stool and/or tongue may occur
Stop use and ask a doctor if
• symptoms get worse
• ringing in the ears or loss of hearing occurs
• diarrhea lasts more than 2 days
If pregnant or breast feeding, ask a health professional before use.

Keep out of reach of children. In case of overdose, get medical help or contact a Poison Control Center right away.
Notes: May cause a temporary and harmless darkening of the tongue or stool. Stool darkening should not be confused with melena.
While no lead is intentionally added to Pepto-Bismol, this product contains certain ingredients that are mined from the ground and thus contain small amounts of naturally occurring lead. For example, bismuth, contained in the active ingredient of Pepto-Bismol, is mined and therefore contains some naturally occurring lead. The small amounts of naturally occurring lead in Pepto-Bismol are low in comparison to average daily lead exposure; this is for the information of healthcare professionals. Pepto-Bismol is indicated for treatment of acute upset stomach symptoms and diarrhea. It is not intended for chronic use.

Overdosage: In case of overdose, patients are advised to contact a physician or Poison Control Center. Emesis induced by ipecac syrup is indicated in large ingestions provided ipecac can be administered within one hour of ingestion. Activated charcoal should be administered after gastric emptying. Patients should be evaluated for signs and symptoms of salicylate toxicity.

Directions:
Pepto-Bismol® Original Liquid, Original & Cherry Flavor Chewable Tablets, and Caplets
[Original Liquid]
• shake well before using
• for accurate dosing, use dose cup
[Original Tablet, Cherry Tablets]
• chew or dissolve in mouth
[Caplets]
• swallow with water, do not chew

• adults and children 12 years and over: 1 dose (2 Tbsp or 30 ml; 2 tablets or 2 caplets) every 1/2 to 1 hour as needed
• do not exceed 8 doses (16 Tbsp or 240 ml); 16 tablets or capsules in 24 hours
• use until diarrhea stops but not more than 2 days
• children under 12 years: ask a doctor
• drink plenty of clear fluids to help prevent dehydration caused by diarrhea

---

Pepto-Bismol® Maximum Strength Liquid
• shake well before use
• for accurate dosing, use dose cup
• adults and children 12 years and over: 1 dose (2 Tbsp 30 ml) every 1 hour as needed
• do not exceed 4 doses (8 Tbsp or 120 ml) in 24 hours
• use until diarrhea stops but not more than 2 days
• children under 12 years: ask a doctor
• drink plenty of clear fluids to help prevent dehydration caused by diarrhea

How Supplied: Pepto-Bismol® Original and Maximum Strength Liquids are

pink. Pepto-Bismol® Original Liquid is available in: 4, 8, 12 and 16 fl oz bottles. Pepto-Bismol® Maximum Strength Liquid is available in: 4, 8 and 12 fl oz bottles. Pepto-Bismol® Original and Cherry Flavor Tablets are pink, round, chewable tablets imprinted with a debossed triangle and "Pepto-Bismol" on one side. Tablets are available in: boxes of 30 and 48. Pepto-Bismol® Caplets are pink and imprinted with "Pepto-Bismol" on one side. Caplets are available in bottles of 24 and 40.
• avoid excessive heat (over 104°F or 40°C)
• protect liquids from freezing
Questions: 1-800-717-3786
www.pepto-bismol.com
Shown in Product Identification Guide, page 514

PRILOSEC OTC® TABLETS
[prī-lō-sĕk]

Drug Facts:

Active Ingredient:
(in each tablet) 　　　　　　**Purpose:**
Omeprazole magnesium
　delayed-release tablet
　20.6 mg (equivalent to 20 mg
　omeprazole) .... Acid reducer

Use:
• treats frequent heartburn (occurs ***2 or more*** days a week)
• not intended for immediate relief of heartburn; this drug may take 1 to 4 days for full effect

Warnings:
Allergy alert: Do not use if you are allergic to omeprazole
Do not use if you have
• trouble or pain swallowing food
• vomiting with blood
• bloody or black stools
These may be signs of a serious condition. See your doctor.
Ask a doctor before use if you have
• had heartburn over 3 months. This may be a sign of a more serious condition.
• heartburn with **lightheadedness, sweating or dizziness**
• chest pain or shoulder pain with shortness of breath; sweating; pain spreading to arms, neck or shoulders; or lightheadedness
• frequent **chest pain**
• frequent wheezing, particularly with heartburn
• unexplained weight loss
• nausea or vomiting
• stomach pain
Ask a doctor or pharmacist before use if you are taking
• warfarin (blood-thinning medicine)
• prescription antifungal or anti-yeast medicines
• diazepam (anxiety medicine)
• digoxin (heart medicine)
Stop use and ask a doctor if
• your heartburn continues or worsens
• you need to take this product for more than 14 days
• you need to take more than 1 course of treatment every 4 months

Continued on next page

Prilosec OTC—Cont.

If pregnant or breast-feeding, ask a health professional before use.

Keep out of reach of children. In case of overdose, get medical help or contact a Poison Control Center right away.

Directions:
- adults 18 years of age and older
- this product is to be used once a day (every 24 hours), every day for 14 days
- it may take 1 to 4 days for full effect, although some people get complete relief of symptoms within 24 hours

14-Day Course of Treatment
- swallow 1 tablet with a glass of water before eating in the morning
- take every day for 14 days
- do not take more than 1 tablet a day
- do not chew or crush the tablets
- do not crush tablets in food
- do not use for more than 14 days unless directed by your doctor

Repeated 14-Day Courses (if needed)
- you may repeat a 14-day course every 4 months
- **do not take for more than 14 days or more often than every 4 months unless directed by a doctor**
- children under 18 years of age: ask a doctor

Other Information:
- read the directions, warnings and package insert before use
- keep the carton and package insert. They contain important information.
- store at 20–25°C (68–77°F)
- keep product out of high heat and humidity
- protect product from moisture

How Prilosec OTC Works For Your Frequent Heartburn

Prilosec OTC works differently from other OTC heartburn products, such as antacids and other acid reducers. Prilosec OTC stops acid production at the source – the **acid pump** that produces stomach acid. Prilosec OTC is to be used once a day (every 24 hours), every day for 14 days.

What to Expect When Using Prilosec OTC

Prilosec OTC is a different type of medicine from antacids and other acid reducers. Prilosec OTC may take 1 to 4 days for full effect, although some people get complete relief of symptoms within 24 hours. Make sure you take the entire 14 days of dosing to treat your frequent heartburn.

Safety Record

For years, doctors have prescribed Prilosec to treat acid-related conditions in millions of people safely.

Who Should Take Prilosec OTC

This product is for adults (18 years and older) with **frequent heartburn**-when you have heartburn 2 or more days a week.
- Prilosec OTC is **not** intended for those who have heartburn infrequently, one episode of heartburn a week or less, or for those who want immediate relief of heartburn.

Tips for Managing Heartburn
- Do not lie flat or bend over soon after eating.
- Do not eat late at night or just before bedtime.
- Certain foods or drinks are more likely to cause heartburn, such as rich, spicy, fatty and fried foods, chocolate, caffeine, alcohol and even some fruits and vegetables.
- Eat slowly and do not eat big meals.
- If you are overweight, lose weight.
- If you smoke, quit smoking.
- Raise the head of your bed.
- Wear loose-fitting clothing around your stomach.

Inactive Ingredients: glyceryl monostearate, hydroxypropyl cellulose, hypromellose, iron oxide, magnesium stearate, methacrylic acid copolymer, microcrystalline cellulose, paraffin, polyethylene glycol 6000, polysorbate 80, polyvinylpyrrolidone, sodium stearyl fumarate, starch, sucrose, talc, titanium dioxide, triethyl citrate

How Supplied: Prilosec OTC is available in 14 tablet, 28 tablet and 42 tablet sizes. These sizes contain one, two and three 14-day courses of treatment, respectively. Do not use for more than 14 days in a row unless directed by your doctor. For the 28 count (two 14-day courses) and the 42 count (three 14-day courses), you may repeat a 14-day course every 4 months.

Safety Feature – Do not use if tablet blister unit is open or torn.

Questions? 1-800-289-9181

Shown in Product Identification Guide, page 514

THERMACARE®
[thərm' ă-kār]
Therapeutic Heat Wraps with Air-Activated Heat Discs

Uses:
Back/Hip Wrap: Provides temporary relief of minor muscular and joint aches & pains associated with overexertion, strains, sprains, and arthritis.
Neck to Arm Wrap: Provides temporary relief of minor muscular and joint aches and pains associated with overexertion, strains, sprains and arthritis.
Menstrual Patch: Provides temporary relief of minor menstrual cramps and associated back ache.

Warnings:
Do not microwave or attempt to reheat this product to avoid risk of fire. This product has the potential to cause skin irritation or burns. Heat discs contain iron (~2 grams) which can be harmful if ingested. If ingested, rinse mouth with water and call a Poison Control Center right away. If the heat discs contents contact your skin or eyes, rinse right away with water.
Do not use:
- on broken or damaged skin
- with medicated lotions, creams, or ointments
- on areas of bruising or swelling that have occurred within 48 hours
- on people unable to remove the product, including children and infants
- on areas of the body where heat cannot be felt
- with other forms of heat

Ask a doctor before use if you have diabetes, poor circulation, rheumatoid arthritis or are pregnant.

When using this product: it is normal to experience temporary skin redness after removing the wrap. If your skin is still red after a few hours, stop using ThermaCare until the redness goes away completely. To reduce the risk of prolonged redness in the future, we recommend you: (a) wear for a shorter period of time, (b) wear looser clothing over wrap, (c) wear over a thin layer of clothing • Periodically check your skin: (a) if your skin is sensitive to heat, (b) if your tolerance to heat has decreased over the years, (c) when wearing a tight fitting belt or waistband • Consider wearing during the day before deciding to use during sleep.

Stop use and ask a doctor: if after 7 days (4 days for menstrual product) your pain gets worse or remains unchanged. This may be a sign of a more serious condition.
- if you experience any discomfort, swelling, rash or other changes on your skin that persist where the wrap is worn.

Keep out of reach of children and pets.

Directions: Tear open the pouch when ready to use. It may take up to 30 minutes for ThermaCare to reach its therapeutic temperature. Place on pain area on lower back or hip with darker discs toward skin. Attach firmly.

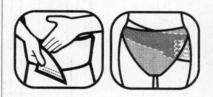

Peel away paper to reveal adhesive side. Place on pain area with adhesive side toward skin. Attach firmly.

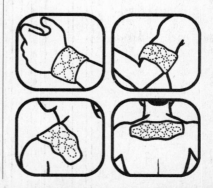

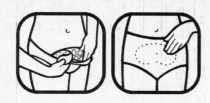

Peel away paper to reveal adhesive side. Place on pain area with adhesive side toward panties. Attach firmly.

For maximum effectiveness, we recommend you wear for 8 hours. Do not use for more than 8 hours in any 24 hour period.

DO NOT MICROWAVE

How Supplied:
Back/Hip Wrap: Available in trial size of 1 L/XL or in boxes of 2 S/M or L/XL wraps.

Neck to Arm: Available in boxes of 3 wraps.

Menstrual: Available in boxes of 3 patches.

Shown in Product Identification Guide, page 514

VICKS® 44® COUGH RELIEF
Dextromethorphan HBr/ Cough Suppressant
Alcohol 5%

- Maximum Strength
- Non-Drowsy
- For Adults & Children

Drug Facts:

Active Ingredient:
(per 15 ml tablespoon)   **Purpose:**
Dextromethorphan HBr
  30 mg .... Cough suppressant

Uses: Temporarily relieves cough due to minor throat and bronchial irritation associated with a cold

Warnings:
Do not use if you are now taking a prescription monoamine oxidase inhibitor (MAOI) (certain drugs for depression, psychiatric or emotional conditions, or Parkinson's disease), or for 2 weeks after stopping the MAOI drug. If you do not know if your prescription drug contains an MAOI, ask a doctor or pharmacist before taking this product.

Ask a doctor before use if you have:
- cough that occurs with too much phlegm (mucus)
- persistent or chronic cough such as occurs with smoking, asthma, or emphysema

Stop use and ask a doctor if:
- cough lasts more than 7 days, comes back, or occurs with fever, rash, or headache that lasts. These could be signs of a serious condition.

If pregnant or breast feeding, ask a health professional before use.

Keep out of reach of children. In case of overdose, get medical help or contact a Poison Control Center right away.

Directions:
- use teaspoon (tsp), tablespoon (TBSP) or dose cup
- do not exceed 4 doses per 24 hours
  Under 6 yrs. .... ask a doctor
  6–11 yrs. .... 1½ tsp (7½ ml) every 6-8 hours
  12 yrs. & older .... 1 TBSP (15 ml) every 6-8 hours

Other Information:
- **each tablespoon contains** sodium 31 mg
- store at room temperature

Inactive Ingredients: Alcohol, FD&C blue no.1, FD&C red 40, carboxymethylcellulose sodium, citric acid, flavor, high fructose corn syrup, polyethylene oxide, polyoxyl 40 stearate, propylene glycol, purified water, saccharin sodium, sodium benzoate, sodium citrate.

How Supplied: Available in 4 FL OZ (118 ml) 6 FL OZ (177 ml) plastic bottle. A calibrated dose cup accompanies each bottle.

TAMPER EVIDENT: Do not use if imprinted shrinkband is missing or broken.
Questions? 1-800-342-6844
Dist. by Procter & Gamble, Cincinnati, OH 45202.
US Pat 5,458,879   42434792
Shown in Product Identification Guide, page 515

VICKS® 44D®
COUGH & HEAD CONGESTION RELIEF
Cough Suppressant/ Nasal Decongestant
Alcohol 5%

- Maximum Strength
- Non-Drowsy
- For Adults & Children

Drug Facts:

Active Ingredients:
(per 15 ml tablespoon)   **Purpose:**
Dextromethorphan HBr
  30 mg .... Cough suppressant
Pseudoephedrine HCl
  60 mg .... Nasal decongestant

Uses: Temporarily relieves these cold symptoms
- cough
- nasal congestion

Warnings:
Failure to follow these warnings could result in serious consequences.
Do not use if you are now taking a prescription monoamine oxidase inhibitor (MAOI) (certain drugs for depression, psychiatric or emotional conditions, or Parkinson's disease), or for 2 weeks after stopping the MAOI drug. If you do not know if your prescription drug contains an MAOI, ask a doctor or pharmacist before taking this product.

Ask a doctor before use if you have:
- heart disease
- cough that lasts or is chronic such as occurs with smoking, asthma, or emphysema
- thyroid disease
- diabetes

- high blood pressure
- cough that occurs with too much phlegm (mucus)
- trouble urinating due to enlarged prostate gland

When using this product do not take more than directed.

Stop use and ask a doctor if:
- symptoms do not get better within 7 days or are accompanied by fever.
- you get nervous, dizzy or sleepless
- cough lasts more than 7 days, comes back, or occurs with fever, rash, or headache that lasts.
  These could be signs of a serious condition.

If pregnant or breast-feeding, ask a health professional before use.

Keep out of reach of children. In case of overdose, get medical help or contact a Poison Control Center right away.

Directions:
- use teaspoon (tsp), tablespoon (TBSP) or dose cup
- do not exceed 4 doses in a 24 hour period
  Under 6 yrs. .... ask a doctor
  6–11 yrs. .... $1^1/_2$ tsp ($7^1/_2$ ml) every 6 hours
  12 yrs. & older .... 1 TBSP (15 ml) every 6 hours

Other Information:
- **each tablespoonful contains** sodium 31 mg
- store at room temperature

Inactive Ingredients: Alcohol, FD&C blue no. 1, carboxymethylcellulose sodium, citric acid, flavor, high fructose corn syrup, polyethylene oxide, polyoxyl 40 stearate, propylene glycol, purified water, FD&C red no. 40, saccharin sodium, sodium benzoate, sodium citrate.

How Supplied: Available in 1 FL OZ (30 ml) 4 FL OZ (118 ml) 6 FL OZ (177 ml) and 8 FL OZ (236 ml) plastic bottles. A calibrated dose cup accompanies each bottle.

TAMPER EVIDENT: Do not use if imprinted shrinkband is missing or broken.
Question? 1-800-342-6844
Dist. by Procter & Gamble, Cincinnati OH 45202.
US Pat 5,458,879   42434796
Shown in Product Identification Guide, page 515

VICKS® 44E®
Cough & Chest Congestion Relief
Cough Suppressant/Expectorant
Alcohol 5%

- Non-Drowsy
- For Adults & Children

Drug Facts:

Active Ingredients:
(per 15 ml tablespoon)   **Purpose:**
Dextromethorphan HBr
  20 mg .... Cough suppressant
Guaifenesin
  200 mg .... Expectorant

Continued on next page

Vicks 44E—Cont.

Uses:
- temporarily relieves cough due to the common cold
- helps loosen phlegm and thin bronchial secretions to rid the bronchial passageways of bothersome mucus

Warnings:

Do not use
- if you are now taking a prescription monoamine oxidase inhibitor (MAOI) (certain drugs for depression, psychiatric or emotional conditions, or Parkinson's disease), or for 2 weeks after stopping the MAOI drug. If you do not know if your prescription drug contains an MAOI, ask a doctor or pharmacist before taking this product.

Ask a doctor before use if you have:
- a sodium restricted diet
- persistent or chronic cough such as occurs with smoking, asthma, chronic bronchitis or emphysema
- cough that occurs with too much phlegm (mucus)

Stop use and ask a doctor if:
- cough lasts more than 7 days, comes back, or occurs with fever, rash, or headache that lasts. These could be signs of a serious condition.

If pregnant or breast-feeding, ask a health professional before use.

Keep out of reach of children. In case of overdose, get medical help or contact a Poison Control Center right away.

Directions:
- use teaspoon (tsp), tablespoon (TBSP) or dose cup
- do not exceed 6 doses per 24 hours

Under 6 yrs.	ask a doctor
6–11 yrs.	1½ tsp (7½ ml) every 4 hours
12 yrs. & older.	1 TBSP (15 ml) every 4 hours

Other Information:
- **each tablespoon contains** sodium 31 mg
- store at room temperature

Inactive Ingredients: Alcohol, FD&C blue 1, carboxymethylcellulose sodium, citric acid, flavor, high fructose corn syrup, polyethylene oxide, polyoxyl 40 stearate, propylene glycol, purified water, FD&C red no. 40, saccharin sodium, sodium benzoate, sodium citrate.

How Supplied: Available in 4 FL OZ (118 ml) 6 FL OZ (177 ml) and 8 FL OZ (236 ml) plastic bottles. A calibrated dose cup accompanies each bottle.

TAMPER EVIDENT: Do not use if imprinted shrinkband is missing or broken.

Questions? 1-800-342-6844

Dist. by Procter & Gamble, Cincinnati OH 45202.

US Pat 5,458,879   42434800

Shown in Product Identification Guide, page 515

VICKS® 44M®
COUGH, COLD & FLU RELIEF
Cough Suppressant/Nasal
Decongestant/Antihistamine/
Pain Reliever–Fever Reducer
Alcohol 10%

Maximum strength cough formula

Drug Facts:

Active Ingredients:
(per 5 ml teaspoon) **Purpose:**
Acetaminophen
  162.5 mg ... Pain reliever/fever reducer
Chlorpheniramine maleate
  1 mg .... Antihistamine
Dextromethorphan HBr
  7.5 mg .... Cough suppressant
Pseudoephedrine HCl
  15 mg .... Nasal decongestant

Uses: Temporarily relieves cough/cold/flu symptoms
- cough
- sneezing
- headache
- sore throat
- fever
- runny nose
- nasal congestion

Warnings:

Failure to follow these warnings could result in serious consequences.

Alcohol warning If you consume 3 or more alcoholic drinks every day, ask your doctor whether you should take acetaminophen or other pain relievers/fever reducers. Acetaminophen may cause liver damage.

Sore throat warning If sore throat is severe, persists more than two days, is accompanied or followed by a fever, headache, rash, nausea or vomiting, consult a doctor promptly.

Do not use • with other medicines containing acetaminophen if you are now taking a prescription monoamine oxidase inhibitor (MAOI) (certain drugs for depression, psychiatric or emotional conditions, or Parkinson's disease), or for 2 weeks after stopping the MAOI drug. If you do not know if your prescription drug contains an MAOI, ask a doctor or pharmacist before taking this product.

Ask a doctor before use if you have:
- heart disease
- breathing problems or chronic cough such as occurs with smoking, asthma, chronic bronchitis or emphysema
- thyroid disease
- diabetes
- glaucoma
- high blood pressure
- cough that occurs with too much phlegm (mucus)
- trouble urinating due to enlarged prostate gland

Ask a doctor or pharmacist before use if you are taking sedatives or tranquilizers.

When using this product:
- **do not use more than directed**
- excitability may occur, especially in children
- drowsiness may occur
- avoid alcoholic drinks

- be careful when driving a motor vehicle or operating machinery
- alcohol, sedatives, and tranquilizers may increase drowsiness

Stop use and ask a doctor if:
- you get nervous, dizzy or sleepless
- fever gets worse or lasts more than 3 days
- new symptoms occur
- redness or swelling is present
- symptoms do not get better within 7 days or are accompanied by fever
- cough lasts more than 7 days, comes back, or occurs with fever, rash, or headache that lasts.
  These could be signs of a serious condition.

If pregnant or breast-feeding, ask a health professional before use.

Keep out of reach of children.

Overdose Warning: Taking more than recommended dose can cause serious health problems. In case of overdose, get medical help or contact a Poison Control Center right away. Quick medical attention is critical for adults as well as for children even if you do not notice any signs or symptoms.

Directions:
- take only as recommended—see **Overdose Warning**
- use teaspoon or dose cup
- do not exceed 4 doses per 24 hours
- children 12 and under: ask a doctor.
- 12 yrs. & older: take 4 teaspoons (20 ml) every 6 hours.

Other Information:
- **each teaspoon contains** sodium 8 mg
- store at room temperature

Inactive Ingredients: Alcohol, FD&C blue 1, carboxymethylcellulose sodium, citric acid, flavor, high fructose corn syrup, polyethylene glycol, polyethylene oxide, propylene glycol, purified water, FD&C red 40, saccharin sodium, sodium citrate.

How Supplied: Available in 4 FL OZ (118 ml) 6 FL OZ (177 ml) and 8 FL OZ (236 ml) plastic bottles. A calibrated dose cup accompanies each bottle.

TAMPER EVIDENT: Do not use if imprinted shrinkband is missing or broken. Not recommended for children.

Questions? 1-800-342-6844

Dist. by Procter & Gamble, Cincinnati OH 45202.

US Pat 5,458,879   42434741

Shown in Product Identification Guide, page 515

CHILDREN'S VICKS® NYQUIL®
COLD/COUGH RELIEF
Antihistamine/Nasal Decongestant/
Cough Suppressant

Children's NyQuil was specially formulated with three effective ingredients to relieve nighttime cough, nasal congestion, and runny nose so children can rest. Children's NyQuil® is alcohol free and analgesic free and has a pleasant cherry flavor.

Drug Facts:

Active Ingredients: Purpose:
(per tablespoon, 15 ml)
Chlorpheniramine maleate
  2 mg .... Antihistamine
Dextromethorphan HBr
  15 mg .... Cough suppressant
Pseudoephedrine HCl
  30 mg .... Nasal decongestant

Uses: Temporarily relieves cold symptoms:
- cough due to minor throat and bronchial irritation
- sneezing
- runny nose
- nasal congestion

Warnings:
Failure to follow these warnings could result in serious consequences.
Do not use
- if you are now taking a prescription monoamine oxidase inhibitor (MAOI) (certain drugs for depression, psychiatric or emotional conditions, or Parkinson's disease), or for 2 weeks after stopping the MAOI durg. If you do not know if your prescription drug contains an MAOI, ask a doctor or pharmacist before taking this product.

Ask a doctor before use if you have:
- heart disease
- a breathing problem or chronic cough that lasts or as occurs with smoking, asthma, chronic bronchitis or emphysema
- thyroid disease
- diabetes
- glaucoma
- high blood pressure
- cough that occurs with too much phlegm (mucus)
- a sodium-restricted diet
- trouble urinating due to enlarged prostate gland

Ask a doctor or pharmacist before use if you are taking sedatives or tranquilizers.

When using this product:
- do not use more than directed
- excitability may occur, especially in children
- drowsiness may occur
- avoid alcoholic drinks
- be careful when driving a motor vehicle or operating machinery
- alcohol, sedatives, and tranquilizers may increase drowsiness

Stop use and ask a doctor if:
- you get nervous, dizzy or sleepless
- symptoms do not get better within 7 days or are accompanied by a fever
- cough lasts more than 7 days, comes back, or occurs with fever, rash, or headache that lasts.
  These could be signs of a serious condition.

If pregnant or breast-feeding, ask a health professional before use.

Keep out of reach of children. In case of overdose, get medical help or contact a Poison Control Center right away. Quick medical attention is critical for adults as well as for children even if you do not notice any signs or symptoms.

Directions:
- use tablespoon (TBSP) or dose cup
- do not exceed 4 doses per 24 hours
  under 6 yrs. .... ask a doctor

6–11 yrs. .... 1 TBSP or 15 ml
                                every 6 hours
12 yrs. & older .... 2 TBSP or 30 ml
                                every 6 hours

Other Information:
- **each tablespoon contains** sodium 71 mg
- store at room temperature

Inactive Ingredients: Citric acid, flavor, potassium sorbate, propylene glycol, purified water, FD&C red 40, sodium citrate, sucrose.

How Supplied: Available in 4 FL OZ (118 ml) 6 FL OZ (177 ml) plastic bottles with child-resistant, tamper-evident cap and a calibrated medicine cup.
Questions? 1-800-362-1683
Exp. Date: See Bottom.   42434744
Dist. by Procter & Gamble, Cincinnati OH 45202.

Shown in Product Identification Guide, page 514

VICKS® Cough Drops
Menthol Cough Suppressant/
Oral Anesthetic
Menthol and Cherry Flavors

CONSUMER INFORMATION: Vicks Cough Drops provide fast and effective relief. Each drop contains effective medicine to suppress your impulse to cough as it dissolves into a soothing syrup to relieve your sore throat.

Drug Facts:

Active Ingredient:
Menthol:
Active Ingredient: Purpose:
(per drop)
Menthol 3.3 mg ...... Cough suppressant/
                                oral anesthetic
Cherry:
Active Ingredient: Purpose:
(per drop)
Menthol 1.7 mg ...... Cough suppressant/
                                oral anesthetic

Uses: Temporarily relieves:
- sore throat
- coughs due to colds or inhaled irritants

Warnings:
Ask a doctor before use if you have:
- cough associated with excessive phlegm (mucus)
- persistent or chronic cough such as those caused by asthma, emphysema, or smoking
- a severe sore throat accompanied by difficulty in breathing or that lasts more than 2 days
- a sore throat accompanied or followed by fever, headache, rash, swelling, nausea or vomiting

Stop use and ask a doctor if:
- you need to use more than 7 days
- cough lasts more than 7 days, comes back, or occurs with fever, rash, or headache that lasts. These could be the signs of a serious condition.

If pregnant or breast-feeding, ask a health professional before use.
Keep out of reach of children.

Directions:
- under 5 yrs.: ask a doctor (menthol)
- adults & children 5 yrs & older: allow 2 drops to dissolve slowly in mouth (cherry)
- adults & children 5 yrs & older: allow 3 drops to dissolve slowly in mouth
Cough: may be repeated every hour.
Sore Throat: may be repeated every 2 hours.

Other Information:
- store at room temperature

Inactive Ingredients:
Menthol: Ascorbic acid, caramel, corn syrup, eucalyptus oil, sucrose.
Cherry: Ascorbic acid, citric acid, corn syrup, eucalyptus oil, FD&C blue 1, flavor, FD&C red 40, sucrose.

How Supplied: Vicks® Cough Drops are available in boxes of 20 triangular drops. Each red or green drop is debossed with "V."
Questions? 1-800-707-1709
Made in Mexico by Procter & Gamble Manufactura S. de R.I. de C.V. Dist. by Procter & Gamble
Cincinnati OH 45202
50144381

VICKS® DAYQUIL® LIQUID
VICKS® DAYQUIL® LIQUICAPS®
Multi-Symptom Cold/Flu Relief
Nasal Decongestant/
Pain Reliever/Cough
Suppressant/Fever Reducer
Non-drowsy

Drug Facts:

Active Ingredients:

LIQUID:

Active Ingredients: Purpose:
(per 15 ml tablespoon)
Acetaminophen
  325 mg ...... Pain reliever/fever reducer
Dextromethorphan HBr
  15 mg .... Cough suppressant
Pseudoephedrine HCl
  30 mg .... Nasal decongestant

LIQUICAP®:

Active Ingredients: Purpose:
(per softgel)
Acetaminophen
  325 mg ...... Pain reliever/fever reducer
Dextromethorphan HBr
  15 mg .... Cough suppressant
Pseudoephedrine HCl
  30 mg .... Nasal decongestant

Uses: Temporarily relieves common cold/flu symptoms:
- nasal congestion
- cough due to minor throat and bronchial irritation
- sore throat
- headache
- minor aches and pains
- fever

Continued on next page

Vicks DayQuil—Cont.

Warnings:
Failure to follow these warnings could result in serious consequences.
Alcohol warning: If you consume 3 or more alcoholic drinks every day, ask your doctor whether you should take acetaminophen or other pain relievers/fever reducers. Acetaminophen may cause liver damage.
Sore throat warning: If sore throat is severe, persists more than 2 days, is accompanied by fever, nausea, rash or vomiting, consult a doctor promptly.
Do not use • with other medicines containing acetaminophen • if you are now taking a prescription monoamine oxidase inhibitor (MAOI) (certain drugs for depression, psychiatric or emotional conditions, or Parkinson's disease), or for 2 weeks after stopping the MAOI drug. If you do not know if your prescription drug contains an MAOI, ask a doctor or pharmacist before taking this product.
Ask a doctor before use if you have:
• heart disease
• thyroid disease
• diabetes
• persistent or chronic cough such as occurs with smoking, asthma, or emphysema
• high blood pressure
• cough that occurs with too much phlegm (mucus)
• trouble urinating due to enlarged prostate gland
• sodium-restricted diet (Specific to DayQuil Liquid only)
When using this product:
• **do not use more than directed**
Stop use and ask a doctor if:
• you get nervous, dizzy or sleepless
• fever gets worse or lasts more than 3 days
• new symptoms occur
• symptoms do not get better within 7 days or are accompanied by a fever
• redness or swelling is present
• cough lasts more than 7 days, comes back, or occurs with fever, rash, or headache that lasts. These could be the signs of a serious condition.
If pregnant or breast-feeding, ask a health professional before use.
Keep out of reach of children. Overdose warning: Taking more than the recommended dose can cause serious health problems. In case of overdose, get medical help or contact a Poison Control Center right away. Quick medical attention is critical for adults as well as for children even if you do not notice any signs or symptoms.

Directions:
• take only as recommended – see Overdose warning
LIQUID:
• use tablespoon (TBSP) or dose cup
• do not exceed 4 doses per 24 hours
  under 6 yrs. .... ask a doctor
  6–11 yrs. .... 1 TBSP or 15 ml every 6 hours
  12 yrs. & older .... 2 TBSP or 30 ml every 6 hours
• If taking NyQuil® and DayQuil, limit total to 4 doses per 24 hours.

LIQUICAP:
• take only as recommended – see **Overdose Warning**
• do not exceed 4 doses per 24 hours
  under 6 yrs. .... ask a doctor
  6–11 yrs. .... 1 softgel with water every 6 hours
  12 yrs. & older .. 2 softgels with water every 6 hours
• If taking NyQuil® and DayQuil, limit total to 4 doses per 24 hours.

Other Information:
LIQUID:
• **each tablespoon contains** sodium 71 mg
• store at room temperature
LIQUICAP:
• store at room temperature

Inactive Ingredients:
LIQUID: Citric acid, FD&C yellow 6, flavor, glycerin, polyethylene glycol, propylene glycol, purified water, saccharin sodium, sodium citrate, sucrose.
LIQUICAP: FD&C red 40, FD&C yellow 6, gelatin, glycerin, polyethylene glycol, povidone, propylene glycol, purified water, sorbitol special, titanium dioxide.

How Supplied: Available in: **LIQUID** 6 FL OZ (177 ml) and 10 FL OZ (295 ml) plastic bottles with child-resistant, tamper-evident cap and a calibrated medicine cup.
LIQUICAP: in 2-count, 12-count and 36- 40- and 60-count child-resistant packages and 20- nonchild-resistant packages. Each softgel is imprinted: "DayQ."
LIQUID:
TAMPER EVIDENT: Do not use if imprinted shrinkband is missing or broken.
LIQUICAP, 12- and 36- 40- and 60-count:
TAMPER EVIDENT: This package is safety sealed and child resistant. Use only if blisters are intact. If difficult to open, use scissors.
LIQUICAP, 20-count:
This Package for households without young children.
TAMPER EVIDENT: Use only if blisters are intact. If difficult to open, use scissors.

Questions? **1-800-251-3374**
Made in Canada
Dist. by Procter & Gamble
Cincinnati OH 45202
42435018
Shown in Product Identification Guide, page 515

VICKS® NYQUIL® COUGH
Antihistamine
Cough Suppressant
All Night Cough Relief
Cherry Flavor

alcohol 10%

Drug Facts:

Active Ingredients: **Purpose:**
(per 15 ml tablespoon)
Dextromethorphan HBr
  15 mg .... Cough suppressant
Doxylamine succinate
  6.25 mg .... Antihistamine

Uses:
Temporarily relieves cold symptoms
• cough
• runny nose and sneezing

Warnings:
Do not use if you are now taking a prescription monoamine oxidase inhibitor (MAOI) (certain drugs for depression, psychiatric or emotional conditions, or Parkinson's disease), or for 2 weeks after stopping the MAOI drug. If you do not know if your prescription drug contains an MAOI, ask a doctor or pharmacist before taking this product.
Ask a doctor before use if you have:
• asthma
• emphysema
• breathing problems
• excessive phlegm (mucus)
• glaucoma
• chronic bronchitis
• persistent or chronic cough
• cough associated with smoking
• trouble urinating due to enlarged prostate gland
Ask a doctor or pharmacist before use if you are:
taking sedatives or tranquilizers.
When using this product:
• **do not use more than directed**
• marked drowsiness may occur
• avoid alcoholic drinks
• excitability may occur, especially in children
• be careful when driving a motor vehicle or operating machinery
• alcohol, sedatives, and tranquilizers may increase drowsiness
Stop use and ask a doctor if:
• cough lasts more than 7 days, comes back, or occurs with fever, rash, or headache that lasts.
These could be signs of a serious condition.
If pregnant or breast-feeding, ask a health professional before use.
Keep out of reach of children. In case of overdose, get medical help or contact a Poison Control Center right away.

Directions: [1 oz bottle] use tablespoon (TBSP)
Use tablespoon (TBSP) or dose cup
• do not exceed 4 doses per 24 hours
Under 12 yrs. .... ask a doctor
12 yrs. and older .... 2 TBSP or 30 ml every 6 hours
[6 & 10 oz bottle, twin, quad pack]
• if taking NyQuil and DayQuil®, limit total to 4 doses per day.
Other Information:
• **each tablespoon contains** sodium 17 mg
• store at room temperature

Inactive Ingredients: Alcohol, F&C blue no. 1, citric acid, flavor, high fructose corn syrup, polyethylene glycol, propylene glycol, purified water, FD&C red no. 40, saccharin sodium, sodium citrate

How Supplied: Available in 1 FL OZ (30 ml) 6 FL OZ (177 ml), 10 FL OZ (295 ml) plastic bottles with child-resistant, tamper-evident cap and calibrated Medicine cup.

TAMPER EVIDENT: Do not use if imprinted shrinkband is missing or broken. *Questions?* 1-800-362-1683
Dist. by Procter & Gamble, Cincinnati OH 45202. 42437885
Shown in Product Identification Guide, page 515

**VICKS® NYQUIL® LIQUICAPS®
VICKS® NYQUIL® LIQUID
(Original and Cherry)
Multi-Symptom Cold/Flu Relief
Antihistamine/Cough
Suppressant/Pain Reliever/
Nasal Decongestant/
Fever Reducer**

Liquid (Original and Cherry)—alcohol 10%

Drug Facts:

Active Ingredients:
LiquiCaps®:

Active Ingredients: (per softgel)	**Purpose:**
Acetaminophen 325 mg	Pain reliever/fever reducer
Dextromethorphan HBr 15 mg	Cough suppressant
Doxylamine succinate 6.25 mg	Antihistamine
Pseudoephedrine HCl 30 mg	Nasal decongestant

Liquid (Original and Cherry):

Active Ingredients: (per 15 ml tablespoon)	**Purpose:**
Acetaminophen 500 mg	Pain reliever/fever reducer
Dextromethorphan HBr 15 mg	Cough suppressant
Doxylamine succinate 6.25 mg	Antihistamine
Pseudoephedrine HCl 30 mg	Nasal decongestant

Uses:
LiquiCaps® Liquid (Original and Cherry):
Temporarily relieves these common cold/flu symptoms:
• nasal congestion
• cough due to minor throat & bronchial irritation
• sore throat
• headache
• minor aches and pains
• fever
• runny nose and sneezing

Warnings:
Failure to follow these warnings could result in serious consequences.
Alcohol warning If you consume 3 or more alcoholic drinks every day, ask your doctor whether you should take acetaminophen or other pain relievers/ fever reducers. Acetaminophen may cause liver damage.
Sore throat warning If sore throat is severe, persists more than 2 days, is accompanied or followed by fever, rash, nausea, or vomiting, consult a doctor promptly.

Do not use • with other medications containing acetaminophen • if you are now taking a prescription monoamine oxidase inhibitor (MAOI) (certain drugs for depression, psychiatric or emotional conditions, or Parkinson's disease), or for 2 weeks after stopping the MAOI drug. If you do not know if your prescription drug contains an MAOI, ask a doctor or pharmacist before taking this product.

Ask a doctor before use if you have:
• heart disease
• a breathing problem or chronic cough such as occurs with smoking, asthma, chronic bronchitis, or emphysema
• thyroid disease
• diabetes
• glaucoma
• high blood pressure
• cough that occurs with too much phlegm (mucus)
• chronic bronchitis

Ask a doctor or pharmacist before use if you are taking sedatives or tranquilizers.

When using this product
• **do not use more than directed**
• excitability may occur, especially in children
• marked drowsiness may occur
• avoid alcoholic drinks
• be careful when driving a motor vehicle or operating machinery
• alcohol, sedatives, and tranquilizers may increase drowsiness

Stop use and ask a doctor if:
• symptoms do not get better within 7 days or are accompanied by fever.
• you get nervous, dizzy or sleepless
• fever gets worse or lasts more than 3 days
• new symptoms occur
• swelling or redness is present.
• cough lasts more than 7 days, comes back, or occurs with fever, rash, or headache that lasts. These could be signs of a serious condition.

If pregnant or breast-feeding, ask a health professional before use.

Keep out of reach of children.

Overdose warning: Taking more than the recommended dose can cause serious health problems. In case of overdose, get medical help or contact a Poison Control Center right away. Quick medical attention is critical for adults as well as for children even if you do not notice any signs or symptoms.

Directions:
LiquiCaps®:
• take only as recommended – see **Overdose warning**
• children under 12 yrs.: ask a doctor.
• do not exceed 4 doses per 24 hours
• 12 yrs and older . . . . 2 softgels with water every 6 hours
• If taking NyQuil and DayQuil®, limit total to 4 doses per 24 hours.

Liquid (Original and cherry):

AGE	DOSAGE

take only as recommended – see **Overdose warning**

use tablespoon (TBSP) or dose cup

do not exceed 4 doses per 24 hours

children under 12	ask a doctor
adults and children 12 years and over	2 TBSP (30 ml) every 6 hours

If taking NyQuil and DayQuil®, limit total to 4 doses per 24 hours.

Other Information:
LiquiCaps®:
• store at room temperature
Liquid (Original and Cherry):
• **each tablespoon contains** sodium 17 mg
• store at room temperature

Inactive Ingredients:
LiquiCaps®: FD&C Blue no. 1, gelatin, glycerin, polyethylene glycol, povidone, propylene glycol, purified water, sorbitol special, D&C Yellow no. 10, tilanium dioxide.
Liquid (Original): Alcohol, citric acid, flavor, FD&C Green no. 3, high fructose corn syrup, polyethylene glycol, propylene glycol, purified water, saccharin sodium, sodium citrate, yellow 6, D&C Yellow 10.
Liquid (Cherry): Alcohol, FD&C Blue 1, citric acid, flavor, high fructose corn syrup, polyethylene glycol, propylene glycol, purified water, FD&C Red 40, saccharin sodium, sodium citrate.

How Supplied:
LiquiCaps®: Available in 2-count 12- 20-, 40-, 60-count and 36-count child-resistant blister packages and 20-count non-child resistant blister packages. Each softgel is imprinted: "NyQ".
Liquid: Available in 1 FL OZ (30 ml) 6 and 10 FL OZ (177 ml and 295 ml, respectively) 16 FL OZ (473 ml) plastic bottles with child-resistant, tamper-evident cap and calibrated medicine cup.
LiquiCaps®: 12- and 36-ct 20-, 40-, 60-count
TAMPER EVIDENT: This package is safety sealed and child resistant. Use only if blisters are intact. If difficult to open, use scissors.
Liquid (Original and cherry):
TAMPER EVIDENT: Do not use if imprinted shrinkband is missing or broken.
Questions? 1-800-362-1683
Liqui Caps®:
Made in Canada
Dist. by Procter & Gamble, Cincinnati OH 45202.
©2001   42435017
Liquid (Original): Dist. by Procter & Gamble Cincinnati OH 45202   42434786
Liquid (Cherry): Dist. by Procter & Gamble Cincinnati OH 45202   42434789
Shown in Product Identification Guide, page 515

Continued on next page

PEDIATRIC VICKS® 44e®
Cough & Chest Congestion Relief
Cough suppressant/Expectorant

- Non-drowsy
- Alcohol-free
- Aspirin-free

Drug Facts:

Active Ingredients:
(per 15 ml tablespoon) **Purpose:**
Dextromethorphan
  HBr 10 mg .... Cough suppressant
Guaifenesin 100mg .... Expectorant

Uses:
- temporarily relieves cough due to the common cold
- helps loosen phlegm and thin bronchial secretions to rid bronchial passageways of bothersome mucus

Warnings:
Do not use
- if you are now taking a prescription monoamine oxidase inhibitor (MAOI) (certain drugs for depression, psychiatric or emotional conditions, or Parkinson's disease), or for 2 weeks after stopping the MAOI drug. If you do not know if your prescription drug contains an MAOI, ask a doctor or pharmacist before taking this product.
Ask a doctor before use if you have:
- a sodium restricted diet
- cough that occurs with too much phlegm (mucus)
- persistent or chronic cough such as occurs with smoking, asthma, chronic bronchitis or emphysema
Stop use and ask a doctor if:
- cough lasts more than 7 days, comes back, or occurs with fever, rash, or headache that lasts. These could be signs of a serious condition.
If pregnant or breast-feeding, ask a health professional before use.
Keep out of reach of children. In case of overdose, get medical help or contact a Poison Control Center right away.

Directions:
- use tablespoon (TBSP) or dose cup
- do not exceed 6 doses per 24 hours
  Under 2 yrs. .... ask a doctor
  2–5 yrs. .... ½ TBSP (7½ ml)
  every 4 hours
  6–11 yrs. .... 1 TBSP (15 ml)
  every 4 hours
  12 yrs.&
  older .... 2 TBSP (30 ml)
  every 4 hours

Other Information:
- **each tablespoon contains** sodium 30 mg
- store at room temperature

Inactive Ingredients: Carboxymethylcellulose sodium, citric acid, FD&C red no. 40, flavor, high fructose corn syrup, polyethylene oxide, polyoxyl 40 stearate, propylene glycol, purified water, saccharin sodium, sodium benzoate, sodium citrate.

How Supplied: 4 FL OZ (118 ml) plastic bottles. A calibrated dose cup accompanies each bottle.
TAMPER EVIDENT: Do not use if imprinted shrinkband is missing or broken.
Questions? 1-800-342-6844

Dist. by Procter & Gamble, Cincinnati OH 45202.
US Pat 5,458,879   42434802
Shown in Product Identification Guide, page 515

PEDIATRIC VICKS® 44m®
Cough & Cold Relief
Cough Suppressant/Nasal Decongestant/Antihistamine

- Alcohol-free
- Aspirin-free

Drug Facts:

Active Ingredients:
(per 15 ml tablespoon) **Purpose:**
Chlorpheniramine maleate
  2 mg .... Antihistamine
Dextromethorphan HBr
  15 mg .... Cough suppressant
Pseudoephedrine HCl
  30 mg .... Nasal decongestant

Uses: Temporarily relieves cough/cold symptoms
- cough
- sneezing
- runny nose
- nasal congestion

Warnings:
Failure to follow these warnings could result in serious consequences.
Do not use:
- if you are now taking a prescription monoamine oxidase inhibitor (MAOI) (certain drugs for depression, psychiatric or emotional conditions, or Parkinson's disease), or for 2 weeks after stopping the MAOI drug. If you do not know if your prescription drug contains an MAOI, ask a doctor or pharmacist before taking this product.
Ask a doctor before use if you have:
- heart disease
- a sodium restricted diet
- a breathing problem or chronic cough that lasts or occurs with smoking, asthma, chronic bronchitis or emphysema
- thyroid disease
- diabetes
- glaucoma
- high blood pressure
- cough that occurs with too much phlegm (mucus)
- trouble urinating due to enlarged prostate gland
Ask a doctor or pharmicist before use if you are taking sedatives or tranquilizers.
When using this product:
- **do not use more than directed**
- excitability may occur, especially in children
- drowsiness may occur
- avoid alcoholic drinks
- be careful when driving a motor vehicle or operating machinery
- alcohol, sedatives, and tranquilizers may increase drowsiness
Stop use and ask a doctor if:
- you get nervous, dizzy or sleepless
- symptoms do not get better within 7 days or are accompanied by a fever.
- cough last more than 7 days, comes back, or occurs with fever, rash, or headache that lasts
  These could be signs of a serious condition.

If pregnant or breast-feeding, ask a health professional before use.
Keep out of reach of children. In case of overdose, get medical help or contact a Poison Control Center right away.

Directions:
- use tablespoon (TBSP) or dose cup
- do not exceed 4 doses per 24 hours
  Under 6 yrs. .... ask a doctor
  6–11 yrs. .... 1 TBSP (15 ml)
  every 6 hours
  12 yrs. & older .... 2 TBSP (30 ml)
  every 6 hours

Other Information:
- **each tablespoon contains** sodium 30 mg
- store at room temperature

Inactive Ingredients: Carboxymethylcellulose sodium, citric acid, FD&C red 40, flavor, high fructose corn syrup, polyethylene oxide, polyoxyl 40 stearate, propylene glycol, purified water, saccharin sodium, sodium benzoate, sodium citrate.

How Supplied: 4 FL OZ (118 ml) plastic bottles. A calibrated dose cup accompanies each bottle.
TAMPER EVIDENT: Do not use if imprinted shrinkband is missing or broken.
Questions? 1-800-342-6844
Dist. by Procter & Gamble, Cincinnati OH 45202.
US Pat 5,458,879   42434743
Shown in Product Identification Guide, page 515

VICKS® SINEX® [NASAL SPRAY]
[Ultra Fine Mist] for Sinus Relief
[sĭ 'nĕx]
Phenylephrine HCl Nasal Decongestant

Drug Facts:

Active Ingredients: **Purpose:**
Phenylephrine
  HCl 0.5% .... Nasal decongestant

Uses: Temporarily relieves sinus/nasal congestion due to
- colds
- hay fever
- upper respiratory allergies
- sinusitis

Warnings:
Ask a doctor before use if you have:
- heart disease
- thyroid disease
- diabetes
- high blood pressure
- trouble urinating due to enlarged prostate gland
When using this product:
- **do not exceed recommended dosage**
- use of this container by more than one person may cause infection
- temporary burning, stinging, sneezing, or increased nasal discharge may occur
- frequent or prolonged use may cause nasal congestion to recur or worsen
Stop use and ask a doctor if:
- symptoms persist for more than 3 days
If pregnant or breast-feeding, ask a health professional before use.

Keep out of reach of children. In case of accidental ingestion, get medical help or contact a poison control center right away.

Directions:
Nasal Spray:
- under 12 yrs. ask a doctor
- adults & children 12 yrs. & older: 2 or 3 sprays in each nostril without tilting your head, not more often than every 4 hours.

Ultra Fine Mist: Remove protective cap. Before using for the first time, prime the pump by firmly depressing its rim several times. Hold container with thumb at base and nozzle between first and second fingers. Without tilting your head, insert nozzle into nostril. Fully depress rim with a firm, even stroke and inhale deeply.
- under 12 yrs.: ask a doctor
- adults & children 12 yrs. & older: 2 or 3 sprays in each nostril, not more often than every 4 hours.

Other Information:
- store at room temperature

Inactive Ingredients: Benzalkonium chloride, camphor, chlorhexidine gluconate, citric acid, disodium EDTA, eucalyptol, menthol, purified water, tyloxapol

How Supplied: Available in $\frac{1}{2}$ FL OZ (14.7 ml) plastic squeeze bottle and $\frac{1}{2}$ FL OZ (14.7 ml) measured dose Ultra Fine mist pump. Note: This container is properly filled when approximately half full. Air space equal to one half of volume is necessary to propel the fine spray.
TAMPER EVIDENT:
Do not use if imprinted shrinkband is missing or broken.
Questions? 1-800-873-8276
Nasal Spray 42436771
Ultra Fine Mist 42436765
Dist. by Procter & Gamble
Cincinnati OH 45202

VICKS® SINEX®
[sī 'něx]
12-HOUR [Nasal Spray]
[Ultra Fine Mist] for Sinus Relief
Oxymetazoline HCl
Nasal Decongestant

Drug Facts:
Active Ingredients:	**Purpose:**
Oxymetazoline HCl 0.05%	Nasal decongestant

Uses: Temporarily relieves sinus/nasal congestion due to
- colds
- hay fever
- upper respiratory allergies
- sinusitis

Warnings:
Ask a doctor before use if you have:
- heart disease
- thyroid disease
- diabetes
- high blood pressure
- trouble urinating due to enlarged prostate gland

When using this product:
- **do not exceed recommended dosage**
- temporary burning, stinging, sneezing, or increased nasal discharge may occur
- frequent or prolonged use may cause nasal congestion to recur or worsen
- use of this container by more than one person may cause infection

Stop use and ask a doctor if:
- symptoms persist for more than 3 days

If pregnant or breast-feeding, ask a health professional before use.

Keep out of reach of children. In case of accidental ingestion, get medical help or contact a poison control center right away.

Directions:
Nasal Spray:
- under 6 yrs: ask a doctor
- adults & children 6 yrs. & older (with adult supervision): 2 or 3 sprays in each nostril without tilting your head, not more often than every 10 to 12 hours. Do not exceed 2 doses in 24 hours.

Ultra Fine Mist: Remove protective cap. Before using for the first time, prime the pump by firmly depressing its rim several times. Hold container with thumb at base and nozzle between first and second fingers. Without tilting your head, insert nozzle into nostril. Fully depress rim with a firm, even stroke and inhale deeply.
- under 6 yrs.: ask a doctor
- adults & children 6 yrs. & older (with adult supervision): 2 or 3 sprays in each nostril, not more often than every 10 to 12 hours. Do not exceed 2 doses in 24 hours.

Other Information:
- store at room temperature

Inactive Ingredients: Benzalkonium chloride, camphor, chlorhexidine gluconate, disodium EDTA, eucalyptol, menthol, potassium phosphate, purified water, sodium chloride, sodium phosphate, tyloxapol.

How Supplied: Available in ½ FL OZ (14.7 ml) plastic squeeze bottle and ½ FL OZ (14.7 ml) measured-dose Ultra Fine mist pump.
TAMPER EVIDENT: Do not use if imprinted shrinkband is missing or broken.
Nasal Spray 42436768
Ultra Fine Mist 42436763
Questions? 1-800-873-8276
Dist. by
Procter & Gamble,
Cincinnati OH 45202

VICKS® VAPOR INHALER
Levmetamfetamine/Nasal
Decongestant

Drug Facts:
Active Ingredients:	**Purpose:**
(per inhaler)	
Levmetamfetamine 50 mg	Nasal decongestant

Uses: Temporarily relieves nasal congestion due to:
- a cold
- hay fever or other upper respiratory allergies
- sinusitis

Warnings:
When using this product:
- **do not exceed recommended dosage**
- temporary burning, stinging, sneezing, or increased nasal discharge may occur
- frequent or prolonged use may cause nasal congestion to recur or worsen
- do not use for more than 7 days
- do not use container by more than one person as it may spread infection
- use only as directed

Stop use and ask a doctor if:
- symptoms persist

If pregnant or breast-feeding, ask a health professional before use.

Keep out of reach of children. If swallowed, get medical help or contact a poison control center right away.

Directions:
The product delivers in each 800 ml air 0.04 to 0.15 mg of levmetamfetamine.
- do not use more often than every 2 hours
- under 6 yrs.: ask a doctor
- 6–11 yrs.: with adult supervision, 1 inhalation in each nostril.
- 12 yrs. & older: 2 inhalation in each nostril.

Other Information:
- store at room temperature
- keep inhaler tightly closed.
- This inhaler is effective for a minimum of 3 months after first use.

Inactive Ingredients: Bornyl acetate, camphor, lavender oil, menthol, methyl salicylate.

How Supplied: Available as a cylindrical plastic nasal inhaler.
Net weight: 0.007 OZ (204 mg).
TAMPER EVIDENT: Use only if imprinted wrap is intact.
***Questions?* 1-800-873-8276**
Dist. by Procter & Gamble, Cincinnati OH 45202. ©2001 42438038

VICKS® VAPORUB®
VICKS® VAPORUB® CREAM
(greaseless)
[vā 'pō-rub]
Cough
Suppressant/Topical Analgesic

Drug Facts:

Active Ingredients:
Vicks® VapoRub®:
Active Ingredients:	**Purpose:**
Camphor 4.8%	Cough suppressant, & topical analgesic
Eucalyptus oil 1.2%	Cough suppressant &
Menthol 2.6%	Cough suppressant, & topical analgesic

Vicks® VapoRub® Cream:
Active Ingredients:	**Purpose:**
Camphor 5.2%	Cough suppressant, & topical analgesic
Eucalyptus oil 1.2%	Cough suppressant

Continued on next page

Vicks VapoRub—Cont.

Menthol 2.8% .... Cough suppressant, & topical analgesic

Uses: • On chest & throat, temporarily relieves cough due to the common cold
• on aching muscles and joints, temporarily relieves minor aches & pains

Warnings:
Failure to follow these warnings could result in serious consequences.
For external use only; avoid contact with eyes.
Do not use:
• by mouth
• with tight bandages
• in nostrils
• on wounds or damaged skin
Ask a doctor before use if you have:
• cough that occurs with too much phlegm (mucus)
• persistent or chronic cough such as occurs with smoking, asthma or emphysema
When using this product do not:
• **heat**
• **microwave**
• **use near an open flame**
• **add to hot water or any container where heating water. May cause splattering and result in burns.**
Stop use and ask a doctor if:
• muscle aches/pains persist more than 7 days or come back
• cough lasts more than 7 days, comes back, or occurs with fever, rash, or headache that lasts.
These could be signs of a serious condition.
If pregnant or breast-feeding, ask a health professional before use.
Keep out of reach of children. In case of accidental ingestion, get medical help or contact a Poison Control Center right away.

Directions: • **See important warnings under "When using this product"**
• under 2 yrs.: ask a doctor
• adults and children 2 yrs. & older: Rub a thick layer on chest & throat or rub on sore aching muscles. If desired, cover with a soft cloth. Keep clothing loose about throat/chest to help vapors reach the nose/mouth. Repeat up to three times per 24 hours or as directed by a doctor.

Other Information:
• store at room temperature
Inactive Ingredients:
Vicks® VapoRub®: Cedarleaf oil, nutmeg oil, special petrolatum, thymol, turpentine oil
Vicks® VapoRub® Cream: Carbomer 954, cedarleaf oil, cetyl alcohol, cetyl palmitate, cyclomethicone copolyol, dimethicone copolyol, dimethicone, EDTA, glycerin, imidazolidinyl urea, isopropyl palmitate, methylparaben, nutmeg oil, peg-100 stearate, propylparaben, purified water, sodium hydroxide, stearic acid, stearyl alcohol, thymol, titanium dioxide, turpentine oil

How Supplied:
Vicks® VapoRub®: Available in 1.76 oz (50 g) 3.53 oz (100 g) and 6 oz (170 g) plastic jars 0.45 oz (12 g) tin.

Vicks® VapoRub® Cream: Available in 2 oz (60 g) 2.99 oz (85 g) tube $^1/_6$ oz pouch.
Questions? 1-800-873-8276
www.vicks.com
Vicks® VapoRub® 50142932
Vicks® VapoRub® Cream 50117758
US Pat. 5,322,689
Made in Mexico by Procter & Gamble Manufactura, S. de R.L. de C.V.
Dist. by Procter & Gamble, Cincinnati OH 45202

VICKS® VAPOSTEAM®

[$vā\,'p\bar{o}\,"st\bar{e}m$]
Liquid Medication for Hot Steam Vaporizers.
Camphor/Cough Suppressant

Drug Facts:

Active Ingredient: **Purpose:**
Camphor 6.2% .... Cough suppressant

Uses: Temporarily relieves cough associated with a cold.

Warnings:
Failure to follow these warnings could result in serious consequences.
For external use only
Flammable Keep away from fire or flame. For steam inhalation only at room temperature.
Ask a doctor before use if you have:
• a persistent or chronic cough such as occurs with smoking, emphysema or asthma
• cough that occurs with too much phlegm (mucus)
When using this product do not
• **heat**
• **microwave**
• **use near an open flame**
• **take by mouth**
• **direct steam from the vaporizer too close to the face**
• **add to hot water or any container where heating water except when adding to cold water only in a hot steam vaporizer. May cause splattering and result in burns.**
Stop use and ask a doctor if:
• cough lasts more than 7 days, comes back, or occurs with fever, rash, or headache that lasts.
These could be signs of a serious condition.
Keep out of reach of children. In case of eye exposure (flush eyes with water); or in case of accidental ingestion; seek medical help or contact a Poison Control Center right away.

Directions:
see important warnings under "When using this product"
• under 2 yrs.: ask a doctor
• adults & children 2 yrs. & older: use 1 tablespoon of solution for each quart of water or 1½ teaspoonsful of solution for each pint of water
• add solution directly to cold water only in a hot steam vaporizer
• follow manufacturer's directions for using vaporizer. Breathe in medicated vapors. May be repeated up to 3 times a day.

Inactive Ingredients: Alcohol 78%, cedarleaf oil, eucalyptus oil, laureth-7, menthol, nutmeg oil, poloxamer 124, silicone.

How Supplied: Available in 4 FL OZ (118 ml) and 8 FL OZ (235 ml) bottles.
Questions? 1-800-873-8276
Made in Mexico by Procter & Gamble Manufactura S. de R.L. de C.V.
Dist. by Procter & Gamble Cincinnati OH 45202
50144018

The Purdue Frederick Company
(See Purdue Products L.P.)

Purdue Products L.P.
ONE STAMFORD FORUM
STAMFORD, CT 06901-3431

For Medical Information Contact:
(888) 726-7535
Adverse Drug Experiences:
(888) 726-7535
Customer Service:
(800) 877-5666
FAX: (800) 877-3210

BETADINE® SOLUTION
(povidone-iodine, 10%)
BETADINE ® SKIN CLEANSER
(povidone-iodine, 7.5%)
Topical Antiseptic
Bactericide/Virucide

Action: Topical microbicides active against organisms commonly encountered in minor skin wounds and burns.

Uses: **Solution**—Kills microorganisms in minor burns, cuts and scrapes.

Skin Cleanser—Disinfectant hand wash and skin cleanser significantly reduces bacteria on the skin.

Directions: Solution—For minor cuts, scrapes and burns, apply directly to affected area as needed. May be covered with gauze or adhesive bandage. If bandaged, let dry first. **Skin Cleanser**—For handwashing, wet skin and apply a sufficient amount to work up a rich, golden lather. Wash for at least 15 seconds.

Warnings: For External Use Only. Do not use in the eyes. Do not use if you are sensitive to iodine or other product ingredients. Do not use longer than one week unless directed by a doctor. In case of deep or puncture wounds, animal bites, or serious burns, consult physician. If redness, irritation, swelling or pain persists or increases, or if infection occurs, discontinue use and consult physician. If swallowed, get medical help or contact a Poison Control Center right away. Keep out of reach of children.

How Supplied:
Solution: 1/2 oz., 4 oz., 8 oz., 16 oz. (1 pt.), 32 oz. (1 qt.), and 1 gal. plastic bottles.
Skin Cleanser: 4 fl. oz. plastic bottles
Avoid storing at excessive heat.
Copyright 1991, 2004, Purdue Products L.P.

Shown in Product Identification Guide, page 515

COLACE® CAPSULES, COLACE® LIQUID 1% SOLUTION, COLACE® SYRUP

[kō' lās]
docusate sodium

Actions: Colace® (docusate sodium) is a stool softener. It helps moisten and soften hard, dry stools and facilitates natural defecation.
Uses: Relieves occasional constipation (irregularity). Generally produces a bowel movement in 12 to 72 hours.

Directions:
Colace Capsules, 50 mg:
• doses may be taken as a single daily dose or in divided doses
• adults and children 12 years of age and over: take 1–6 capsules daily
• children 2 to under 12 years of age: take 1–3 capsules daily
• children under 2 years of age: ask a doctor
Colace Capsules, 100 mg:
• doses may be taken as a single daily dose or in divided doses
• adults and children 12 years of age and over: take 1–3 capsules daily
• children 2 to under 12 years of age: take 1 capsule daily
• children under 2 years of age: ask a doctor
Colace Liquid 1% Solution:
• doses must be given in a 6–8 oz glass of milk or fruit juice, or in infant's formula to prevent throat irritation
• adults and children 12 years of age and over: take 5–15 ml once or twice a day

• children 2 to under 12 years of age: take 5–15 ml once a day
• children under 2 years of age: ask a doctor
Colace Syrup:
• give in a 6 oz to 8 oz glass of milk or fruit juice to prevent throat irritation
• adults and children 12 years of age and over: 1–6 tablespoons daily or as directed by a doctor
• children 2 to under 12 years of age: 1–2½ tablespoons daily or as directed by a doctor
• children under 2 years of age: ask a doctor

Warnings: Do not use if you are presently taking mineral oil, unless told to do so by a doctor. **Do not use Colace Syrup** if you are on a sodium-restricted diet unless told to do so by a doctor. **Ask a doctor before use if you need** to take laxative products for longer than 1 week. **Ask a doctor before use if you have** stomach pain, nausea, vomiting, noticed a sudden change in bowel habits that lasts over 2 weeks. **Stop use and ask a doctor if** you have rectal bleeding or fail to have a bowel movement after use of a laxative. These could be signs of a serious condition. **If pregnant or breast-feeding,** ask a health professional before use. **Keep out of reach of children.** In case of overdose, get medical help or contact a Poison Control Center right away.

Other Information: Colace® Capsules: Sodium content: 3 mg/50 mg capsule; 5 mg/100 mg capsule. VERY LOW SODIUM. Store at 25°C (77°F). Excursions permitted between 15–30°C (59–86°F). Keep bottle tightly closed.
Colace® Liquid 1% Solution: Each milliliter contains 10 mg of docusate sodium. Sodium content 1 mg/mL. VERY LOW SODIUM. Supplied in 30 mL bottle with calibrated medicine dropper.
Colace® Syrup: Each tablespoon (15 mL) contains 60 mg of docusate sodium. Sodium content: 36 mg/15 mL. Store at 20°–25°C (68°–77°F). Contains no sugar or alcohol.

How Supplied: Colace Capsules **50 mg:** In boxes of 10 capsules. Bottles of 30 and 60 capsules. Colace Capsules **100 mg:** In boxes of 10 capsules. Bottles of 30, 60 and 250 capsules.
Colace Liquid 1% Solution: 1 fl. oz. (30 mL) bottles.
Colace Syrup: 16 oz. (473 mL) bottles.
Copyright 2003, Purdue Products L.P., Stamford, CT 06901-3431
Shown in Product Identification Guide, page 515

COLACE® GLYCERIN SUPPOSITORIES USP 1.2 GRAMS

[kō' lās]
glycerin
(Laxative for infants & children)
COLACE® GLYCERIN SUPPOSITORIES USP 2.1 GRAMS
glycerin
(Laxative for adults & children)

Action & Uses: Colace® suppositories are a laxative that relieves occasional

constipation (irregularity). Generally produces a bowel movement in 1/4 to 1 hour.

Directions:
Colace® Glycerin Suppositories USP 2.1 grams (laxative for adults and children)
• adults and children 6 years of age and over: Insert 1 suppository well into the rectum and retain for 15 minutes; it need not melt to produce laxative action. Do not exceed 1 suppository daily or as directed by a doctor.
• children under 6 years: Use Colace® Suppositories for infants and children
Colace® Glycerin Suppositories USP 1.2 grams (laxative for infants and children)
• children 2 to under 6 years of age: Insert 1 suppository well into the rectum and retain for 15 minutes; it need not melt to produce laxative action. Do not exceed 1 suppository daily or as directed by a doctor.
• children under 2 years: ask a doctor

Warnings: For rectal use only. Do not use laxative products for longer than 1 week unless told to do so by a doctor. **Ask a doctor before use if there is** stomach pain, nausea, vomiting, or a sudden change in bowel habits that lasts over 2 weeks. **When using this** product, there may be rectal discomfort or a burning sensation. **Stop use and ask a doctor if** there is rectal bleeding or a failure to have a bowel movement after use of a laxative. These could be signs of a serious condition. **If pregnant or breast-feeding,** ask a health professional before use. **Keep out of reach of children.** If swallowed, get medical help or contact a Poison Control Center right away.
Other Information: Avoid excessive heat. Keep jar tightly closed.

How Supplied: Infants and children suppositories: Jars of 12 and 24. Adults and children suppositories: Jars of 12, 24, 48 and 100.
Copyright 2003, Purdue Products L.P., Stamford, CT 06901-3431
Shown in Product Identification Guide, page 515

MINERAL OIL

Description: Intestinal lubricant laxative. Odorless, tasteless, crystal clear liquid.

Action & Uses: Relieves occasional constipation (irregularity). Generally produces a bowel movement in 6 to 8 hours.

Directions:
• adults and children 12 years of age or over take 1–3 tablespoonfuls at bedtime or as directed by a doctor

Warnings: Take only at bedtime and do not take with meals. **Do not use** for longer than 1 week, if you are presently taking a stool-softener laxative, if you are pregnant, in children under 12 years

Continued on next page

Mineral Oil—Cont.

of age, in bedridden patients, in persons with difficulty swallowing. **Ask a doctor before use if you have** stomach pain, nausea, vomiting, noticed a sudden change in bowel habits that lasts over 2 weeks. **Stop use and ask a doctor if** you have rectal bleeding or fail to have a bowel movement after use of a laxative. These could be signs of a serious condition. **If pregnant or breast-feeding,** ask a health professional before use. **Keep out of reach of children.** In case of overdose, get medical help or contact a Poison Control Center right away.
Other Information: Store between 20°–25°C (68°–77°F). Keep bottle tightly closed. Protect from sunlight.

How Supplied: Bottles of 6 oz. and 16 oz.
Copyright 2003, Purdue Products L.P., Stamford, CT 06901-3431

PERI-COLACE® TABLETS
docusate sodium and standardized senna concentrate

Actions: This combination stool softener and natural stimulant laxative ingredient helps moisten and soften hard, dry stools and stimulates defecation.

Uses: Relieves occasional constipation (irregularity). Generally produces a bowel movement in 6 to 12 hours.

Directions:
- doses may be taken as a single daily dose or in divided doses preferably in the evening
- adults and children 12 years of age and over: take 2–4 tablets daily
- children 6 to under 12 years of age: take 1–2 tablets daily
- children 2 to under 6 years of age: take up to 1 tablet daily
- children under 2 years of age: ask a doctor

Warnings: Do not use laxative products for longer than 1 week unless told to do so by a doctor; if you are presently taking mineral oil, unless told to do so by a doctor. **Ask a doctor before use if you have** stomach pain, nausea, vomiting, noticed a sudden change in bowel habits that lasts over 2 weeks. **Stop use and ask a doctor if** you have rectal bleeding or fail to have a bowel movement after use of a laxative. These could be signs of a serious condition. **If pregnant or breast-feeding,** ask a health professional before use. **Keep out of reach of children.** In case of overdose, get medical help or contact a Poison Control Center right away.
Other Information: Sodium content: 4 mg/tablet. VERY LOW SODIUM. Store at 25°C (77°F). Keep bottle tightly closed.

How Supplied: In boxes of 10 tablets. Bottles of 30 and 60 tablets.
Copyright 2003, Purdue Products L.P., Stamford, CT 06901-3431

Shown in Product Identification Guide, page 515

SENOKOT® Tablets
(standardized senna concentrate)

SENOKOT-S® Tablets
(standardized senna concentrate and docusate sodium)

<u>Natural Vegetable Laxative Ingredient</u>

Actions: Senna provides a colon-specific action which is gentle, effective, and predictable, generally producing bowel movement in 6 to 12 hours. Senokot-S Tablets also contain a stool softener for smoother, easier evacuation.

Uses: For the relief of occasional constipation. Senokot Products generally produce bowel movement in 6 to 12 hours.

Directions:
- take preferably at bedtime or as directed by a doctor
- adults and children 12 years of age or older: starting dosage 2 tablets once a day; maximum dosage 4 tablets twice a day
- children 6 to under 12 years of age: starting dosage 1 tablet once a day; maximum dosage 2 tablets twice a day
- children 2 to under 6 years of age: starting dosage ½ tablet once a day; maximum dosage 1 tablet twice a day
- children under 2 years of age: ask a doctor

Warnings: Ask a doctor before use if you have stomach pain, nausea or vomiting. If you have noticed a sudden change in bowel movements that persists over a period of 2 weeks, consult a doctor before using a laxative. Do not use laxative products for longer than 1 week unless directed by a doctor; with Senokot-S, if you are presently taking mineral oil, unless told to do so by a doctor. Stop use and ask a doctor if you have rectal bleeding or failure to have a bowel movement after the use of a laxative. This may indicate a serious condition. Discontinue use and consult your doctor. As with any drug, if you are pregnant or nursing a baby, seek the advice of a health professional before using this product. In case of accidental overdose, seek professional assistance or contact a Poison Control Center right away. Keep out of children's reach.

How Supplied: Senokot Tablets: Boxes of 20; bottles of 50 and 100; Unit Strip Packs in boxes of 100 individually sealed tablets. Each Senokot Tablet contains 8.6 mg sennosides.

Senokot-S Tablets: Packages of 10; bottles of 30, 60 and 1000; Unit Strip boxes of 100. Each Senokot-S Tablet contains 8.6 mg sennosides and 50 mg docusate sodium.

Copyright 1991, 2004, Purdue Products L.P.

Shown in Product Identification Guide, page 515

EDUCATIONAL MATERIAL

Up-to-date Information:
www.senokot.com provides dosing information for the Senokot® Products family of laxatives, as well as patient education about constipation and its causes. A special section on toilet training, written by a pediatrician, describes the popular child-centered approach.

Reese Pharmaceutical Company
**10617 FRANK AVENUE
CLEVELAND, OH 44106**

Direct Inquiries to:
Voice: (800) 321-7178
FAX: (216) 231-6444

REESE'S PINWORM TREATMENTS
[rēsĭs]

Directions for Use: For the treatment of pinworms. Read package insert carefully before taking this medication. Take according to directions. Do not exceed recommended dosage unless directed by a doctor. Medication should be taken only one time as a single dose: do not repeat treatment unless directed by a doctor. When one individual in a household has pinworms, the entire household should be treated unless otherwise advised. These products can be taken any time of day, with or without food. If you are pregnant, nursing a baby, or have liver disease, do not take this product unless directed by a doctor.

DOSAGE GUIDE		
under 25 lbs or 2 yrs of age, consult a doctor		
WEIGHT LBS.	**DOSAGE**	
	Teaspoons	Caplets
25–37	1/2	2
38–62	1	4
63–87	1-1/2	6
88–112	2	8
113–137	2-1/2	10
138–162	3	12
163–187	3-1/2	14
188 & over	4	16

Warnings: Keep this and all drugs out of the reach of children. In case of accidental overdose, seek professional assistance or contact a poison control center immediately.

How Supplied:
Oral Suspension Liquid
NDC: 10956-618-01
Each 1 mL contains: pyrantel pamoate 144mg
(equivalent of 50 mg pyrantel base)
Pre-Measured Caplet
NDC: 10956-658-24
Packaged in boxes of 24 caplets.
Each caplet contains: pyrantel pamoate 180mg
(equivalent of 62.5 mg pyrantel base)
Shown in Product Identification Guide, page 516

Schering-Plough HealthCare Products

3 CONNELL DRIVE
BERKELEY HEIGHTS, NJ 07922

Direct Product Requests to:
Schering-Plough HealthCare Products
3 Connell Drive
Berkeley Heights, NJ 07922

For Medical Emergencies Contact:
Consumer Relations Department
P.O. Box 377
Memphis, TN 38151
(901) 320-2998 (Business Hours)
(901) 320-2364 (After Hours)

CLARITIN® NON-DROWSY 24 HOUR TABLETS
Brand of Loratadine

Drug Facts:

Active Ingredient
(in each tablet): **Purpose:**
Loratadine 10 mg .... Antihistamine

Uses: temporarily relieves these symptoms due to hay fever or other upper respiratory allergies:
• runny nose • itchy, watery eyes
• sneezing • itching of the nose or throat

Warnings:
Do not use if you have ever had an allergic reaction to this product or any of its ingredients.
Ask a doctor before use if you have liver or kidney disease. Your doctor should determine if you need a different dose.
When using this product do not take more than directed. Taking more than directed may cause drowsiness.
Stop use and ask a doctor if an allergic reaction to this product occurs. Seek medical help right away.
If pregnant or breast-feeding, ask a health professional before use.
Keep out of reach of children. In case of overdose, get medical help or contact a Poison Control Center right away.

Directions:

adults and children 6 years and over	1 tablet daily; not more than 1 tablet in 24 hours
children under 6 years of age	ask a doctor
consumers with liver or kidney disease	ask a doctor

Other Information:
• safety sealed: do not use if the individual blister unit imprinted with Claritin® is open or torn
• store between 20°C to 25°C (68°F to 77°F)
• protect from excessive moisture

Inactive Ingredients: corn starch, lactose monohydrate, magnesium stearate

How Supplied: Boxes of 5, 10, 20, and 30 tablets
Questions or comments?
1-800-CLARITIN (1-800-252-7484) or **www.claritin.com**
Shown in Product Identification Guide, page 516

CLARITIN-D NON-DROWSY 12 HOUR TABLETS

Drug Facts:

Active Ingredients
(in each tablet): **Purpose:**
Loratadine 5 mg .... Antihistamine
Pseudoephedrine sulfate
  120 mg .... Nasal decongestant

Uses:
• temporarily relieves these symptoms due to hay fever or other upper respiratory allergies:
  • runny nose
  • sneezing • itchy, watery eyes
  • itching of the nose or throat
• temporarily relieves nasal congestion due to the common cold, hay fever, or other upper respiratory allergies
• reduces swelling of nasal passages
• temporarily relieves sinus congestion and pressure
• temporarily restores freer breathing through the nose

Warnings:
Do not use
• if you have ever had an allergic reaction to this product or any of its ingredients
• if you are now taking a prescription monoamine oxidase inhibitor (MAOI) (certain drugs for depression, psychiatric, or emotional conditions, or Parkinson's disease), or for 2 weeks after stopping the MAOI drug. If you do not know if your prescription drug contains an MAOI, ask a doctor or pharmacist before taking this product.
Ask a doctor before use if you have
• heart disease • thyroid disease
• high blood pressure • diabetes
• trouble urinating due to an enlarged prostate gland

• liver or kidney disease. Your doctor should determine if you need a different dose.
When using this product do not take more than directed. Taking more than directed may cause drowsiness.
Stop use and ask a doctor if
• an allergic reaction to this product occurs. Seek medical help right away.
• symptoms do not improve within 7 days or are accompanied by a fever
• nervousness, dizziness or sleeplessness occurs
If pregnant or breast-feeding, ask a health professional before use.
Keep out of reach of children. In case of overdose, get medical help or contact a Poison Control Center right away.

Directions:
• do not divide, crush, chew or dissolve the tablet

adults and children 12 years and over	1 tablet every 12 hours; not more than 2 tablets in 24 hours
children under 12 years of age	ask a doctor
consumers with liver or kidney disease	ask a doctor

Other Information:
• each tablet contains: calcium 30 mg
• safety sealed: do not use if the individual blister unit imprinted with Claritin-D® 12 Hr. is open or torn
• store between 15°C to 25°C (59°F to 77°F)
• keep in a dry place

Inactive Ingredients: croscarmellose sodium, dibasic calcium phosphate, hypromellose, lactose monohydrate, magnesium stearate, pharmaceutical ink, povidone, titanium dioxide

How Supplied: Boxes of 10, 20, and 30 tablets
Questions or comments?
1-800-CLARITIN (1-800-252-7484) or **www.claritin.com**
Shown in Product Identification Guide, page 516

CLARITIN-D NON–DROWSY 24 HOUR TABLETS

Drug Facts:

Active Ingredients
(in each tablet): **Purpose:**
Loratadine 10 mg .... Antihistamine
Pseudoephedrine
  sulfate 240 mg .... Nasal decongestant

Uses:
• temporarily relieves these symptoms due to hay fever or other upper respiratory allergies:

Continued on next page

Information on Schering-Plough HealthCare Products appearing on these pages is effective as of November 2003.

Claritin-D 24 hour—Cont.

- runny nose
- sneezing • itchy, watery eyes
- itching of the nose or throat
- temporarily relieves nasal congestion due to the common cold, hay fever or other upper respiratory allergies
- reduces swelling of nasal passages
- temporarily relieves sinus congestion and pressure
- temporarily restores freer breathing through the nose

Warnings:
Do not use
- if you have ever had an allergic reaction to this product or any of its ingredients
- if you are now taking a prescription monoamine oxidase inhibitor (MAOI) (certain drugs for depression, psychiatric, or emotional conditions, or Parkinson's disease), or for 2 weeks after stopping the MAOI drug. If you do not know if your prescription drug contains an MAOI, ask a doctor or pharmacist before taking this product.

Ask a doctor before use if you have
- heart disease
- thyroid disease
- high blood pressure
- diabetes
- trouble urinating due to an enlarged prostate gland
- liver or kidney disease. Your doctor should determine if you need a different dose.

When using this product do not take more than directed. Taking more than directed may cause drowsiness.

Stop use and ask a doctor if
- an allergic reaction to this product occurs. Seek medical help right away.
- symptoms do not improve within 7 days or are accompanied by a fever
- nervousness, dizziness or sleeplessness occurs

If pregnant or breast-feeding, ask a health professional before use.

Keep out of reach of children. In case of overdose, get medical help or contact a Poison Control Center right away.

Directions:
- do not divide, crush, chew or dissolve the tablet

adults and children 12 years and over	1 tablet daily with a full glass of water; not more than 1 tablet in 24 hours
children under 12 years of age	ask a doctor
consumers with liver or kidney disease	ask a doctor

Other Information:
- safety sealed: do not use if the individual blister unit imprinted with Claritin-D® 24 hour is open or torn
- store between 20° C to 25° C (68° F to 77° F)
- protect from light and store in a dry place

Inactive Ingredients: carnauba wax, dibasic calcium phosphate, ethylcellulose, hydroxypropyl cellulose, hypromel-lose, magnesium stearate, pharmaceutical ink, polyethylene glycol, povidone, silicon dioxide, sugar, titanium dioxide, white wax

How Supplied: Boxes of 5, 10, and 15 Tablets

Questions or comments?
1-800-CLARITIN (1-800-252-7484) or **www.claritin.com**
Shown in Product Identification Guide, page 516

CHILDREN'S CLARITIN® 24 HOUR NON-DROWSY ALLERGY SYRUP

Drug Facts:

Active Ingredient
(in each 5 mL): **Purpose:**
Loratadine 5 mg .... Antihistamine

Uses: temporarily relieves these symptoms due to hay fever or other upper respiratory allergies:
- runny nose • itchy, watery eyes
- sneezing • itching of the nose or throat

Warnings:
Do not use if you have ever had an allergic reaction to this product or any of its ingredients.

Ask a doctor before use if you have liver or kidney disease. Your doctor should determine if you need a different dose.

When using this product do not take more than directed. Taking more than directed may cause drowsiness.

Stop use and ask a doctor if an allergic reaction to this product occurs. Seek medical help right away.

If pregnant or breast-feeding, ask a health professional before use.

Keep out of reach of children. In case of overdose, get medical help or contact a Poison Control Center right away.

Directions:

adults and children 6 years and over	2 teaspoonfuls daily; do not take more than 2 teaspoonfuls in 24 hours
children 2 to under 6 years of age	1 teaspoonful daily; do not take more than 1 teaspoonful in 24 hours
consumers with liver or kidney disease	ask a doctor

Other Information:
- safety sealed; do not use if Schering-Plough HealthCare imprinted bottle wrap is torn or missing
- store between 20°C to 25°C (68°F to 77°F)

Inactive Ingredients: citric acid, edetate disodium, flavor, glycerin, propylene glycol, sodium benzoate, sugar, water

How Supplied: 2 fl oz and 4 fl oz bottle
Questions or comments?
1-800-CLARITIN (1-800-252-7484) or **www.claritin.com**
Shown in Product Identification Guide, page 516

CLARITIN® REDITABS 24 HOUR NON-DROWSY ORALLY DISINTEGRATING TABLETS
Brand of Loratadine

Drug Facts:

Active Ingredient
(in each tablet): **Purpose:**
Loratadine 10 mg .... Antihistamine

Uses: temporarily relieves these symptoms due to hay fever or other upper respiratory allergies:
- runny nose • itchy, watery eyes
- sneezing • itching of the nose or throat

Warnings: Do not use if you have ever had an allergic reaction to this product or any of its ingredients.

Ask a doctor before use if you have liver or kidney disease. Your doctor should determine if you need a different dose.

When using this product do not take more than directed. Taking more than directed may cause drowsiness.

Stop use and ask a doctor if an allergic reaction to this product occurs. Seek medical help right away.

If pregnant or breast-feeding, ask a health professional before use.

Keep out of reach of children. In case of overdose, get medical help or contact a Poison Control Center right away.

Directions:
- place 1 tablet on tongue; tablet disintegrates, with or without water

adults and children 6 years and over	1 tablet daily; not more than 1 tablet in 24 hours
children under 6 years of age	ask a doctor
consumers with liver or kidney disease	ask a doctor

Other Information:
- safety sealed: do not use if interior foil pouch or individual blister unit imprinted with Claritin® RediTabs® inside the foil pouch is open or torn
- store between 20°C to 25°C (68°F to 77°F)
- keep in a dry place
- use within 6 months of opening foil pouch
- use tablet immediately after opening individual blister

Inactive Ingredients: citric acid, gelatin, mannitol, mint flavor

How Supplied: Boxes of 4, 10, and 20 tablets

Questions or comments?

1-800-CLARITIN (1-800-252-7484) or **www.claritin.com**
Shown in Product Identification Guide, page 516

ONCE DAILY/NON-DROWSY CLARITIN Hives Relief™
Loratadine 10mg/Antihistamine

Drug Facts

Active Ingredient: **Purpose:**
(in each tablet)
Loratadine 10 mg   Antihistamine

Use:
- relieves itching due to hives (urticaria). This product will not prevent hives or an allergic skin reaction from occurring.

Warnings:
Severe Allergy Warning: Get emergency help **immediately** if you have hives along with any of the following symptoms:
- trouble swallowing
- swelling of tongue
- trouble speaking
- wheezing or problems breathing
- dizziness or loss of consciousness
- swelling in or around mouth
- drooling

These symptoms may be signs of anaphylactic shock. This condition can be life threatening if not treated by a health professional **immediately**. Symptoms of anaphylactic shock may occur when hives first appear or up to a few hours later.

Not a Substitute for Epinephrine. If your doctor has prescribed an epinephrine injector for "anaphylaxis" or severe allergy symptoms that could occur with your hives, never use this product as a substitute for the epinephrine injector. If you have been prescribed an epinephrine injector, you should carry it with you at all times.

Do not use
- to **prevent** hives from any known cause such as:
  - foods
  - medicines
  - insect stings
  - latex or rubber gloves

because this product will not stop hives from occurring. Avoiding the cause of your hives is the only way to prevent them. Hives can sometimes be serious. If you do not know the cause of your hives, see your doctor for a medical exam. Your doctor may be able to help you find a cause.
- if you have ever had an allergic reaction to this product (loratadine) or any of its ingredients

Ask a doctor before use if you have
- liver or kidney disease. Your doctor should determine if you need a different dose.
- hives that are an unusual color, look bruised or blistered
- hives that do not itch

When using this product do not take more than directed. Taking more than directed may cause drowsiness.

Stop use and ask a doctor if
- an allergic reaction to this product occurs. Get medical help right away.
- symptoms don't improve after 3 days of treatment
- the hives have lasted more than 6 weeks.

If pregnant or breast-feeding, ask a health professional before use.

Keep out of reach of children. In case of overdose, get medical help or contact a Poison Control Center right away.

Directions:

adults and children 6 years and over	1 tablet daily; not more than 1 tablet in 24 hours
consumers with liver or kidney disease	ask a doctor

Other Information:
- safety sealed: do not use if individual blister unit imprinted with Claritin® is open or torn
- Store between 20° to 25°C (68° to 77° F)
- protect from excessive moisture.

Inactive Ingredients: corn starch, lactose monohydrate, magnesium stearate

How Supplied: Boxes of 10 tablets
Questions or comments?
1-800-CLARITIN (1-800-252-7484) or www.claritin.com
©2003 Distributed by Schering-Plough HealthCare Products, Inc.
Memphis, TN 38151 USA. All rights reserved.   26143-00

LOTRIMIN ULTRA®
[lo-tre-min]
Butenafine Hydrochloride Cream 1%
Antifungal
Athlete's Foot Cream
Jock Itch Cream

Drug Facts:

Active Ingredient: **Purpose:**
Butenafine hydrochloride 1% .... Antifungal

Uses:
Athlete's Foot Cream:
- cures most athlete's foot between the toes. Effectiveness on the bottom or sides of foot is unknown.
- cures most jock itch and ringworm
- relieves itching, burning, cracking, and scaling which accompany these conditions

Jock Itch Cream:
- cures most jock itch
- relieves itching, burning, cracking, and scaling which accompany this condition

Warnings:
For external use only
Do not use
- on nails or scalp
- in or near the mouth or the eyes
- for vaginal yeast infections

When using this product do not get into the eyes. If eye contact occurs, rinse thoroughly with water.

Stop use and ask a doctor if too much irritation occurs or gets worse

Keep out of reach of children. If swallowed, get medical help or contact a Poison Control Center right away.

Directions:
Athlete's Foot Cream:
- adults and children 12 years and older
  - use the tip of the cap to break the seal and open the tube
  - wash the affected skin with soap and water and dry completely before applying

Apply between and around the toes

1 week twice a day or
4 weeks once a day

- **for athlete's foot between the toes:** apply to affected skin between and around the toes twice a day for 1 week (morning and night), or once a day for 4 weeks, or as directed by a doctor. Wear well-fitting, ventilated shoes. Change shoes and socks at least once daily.
- **for jock itch and ringworm** apply once a day to affected skin for 2 weeks or as directed by a doctor
  - wash hands after each use
- children under 12 years: ask a doctor

Jock Itch Cream:
- adults and children 12 years and over
  - use the tip of the cap to break the seal and open the tube
  - wash the affected skin with soap and water and dry completely before applying
  - apply once a day to affected skin for 2 weeks or as directed by a doctor
  - wash hands after each use
- children under 12 years: ask a doctor

Other Information:
- do not use if seal on tube is broken or is not visible
- store between 20° to 25°C (68° to 77°F)

Inactive Ingredients: benzyl alcohol, cetyl alcohol, diethanolamine, glycerin, glyceryl monostearate SE, polyoxyethylene (23) cetyl ether, propylene glycol dicaprylate, purified water, sodium benzoate, stearic acid, white petrolatum

How Supplied: Available in 0.42 oz (12 gram) tubes for both athlete's foot and jock itch. Also available in a 0.85 oz (24 gram) tube for athlete's foot.
Shown in Product Identification Guide, page 516

Standard Homeopathic Company
210 WEST 131st STREET
BOX 61067
LOS ANGELES, CA 90061

Direct Inquiries to:
Jay Borneman
(800) 624-9659 x20

HYLAND'S BACKACHE WITH ARNICA

Active Ingredients: BENZOICUM ACIDUM 3X HPUS, COLCHICUM AUTUMNALE 3X HPUS, SULPHUR 3X

Continued on next page

Hyland's Backache—Cont.

HPUS, ARNICA MONTANA 6X HPUS, RHUS TOXICODENDRON 6X HPUS.

Inactive Ingredients: Lactose, N.F.

Indications: A homeopathic medicine for the temporary relief of symptoms of low back pain due to strain or overexertion.

Directions: Adults and children over 12 years of age: Take 1–2 caplets with water every 4 hours or as needed.

Warnings: Do not use if imprinted cap band is broken or missing. If symptoms persist for more than seven days or worsen, contact a licensed health care professional. As with any drug, if you are pregnant or nursing a baby, seek the advice of a licensed health care professional before using this product. Keep this and all medications out of the reach of children. In case of accidental overdose, contact a poison control center immediately. In case of emergency, the manufacturer may be reached 24 hours a day, 7 days a week at 800/624-9659.

How Supplied: Bottles of 40 5.5 grain caplets (NDC 54973-2965-2). Store at room temperature.

HYLAND'S BUMPS 'N BRUISES™ TABLETS

Active Ingredients: Arnica Montana 6X HPUS, Hypericum Perforatum 6X HPUS, Bellis Perennis 6X HPUS, Ruta Graveolens 6X HPUS.

Inactive Ingredients: Lactose, N.F.

Indications: A homeopathic medicine for the temporary relief of symptoms of bruising and swelling from falls, trauma or overexertion. Easy to take soft tablets dissolve instantly in the mouth.

Directions: For over 1 year of age: Dissolve 3–4 tablets in a teaspoon of water or on the tongue at the time of injury. May be repeated as needed every 15 minutes until relieved.

Warnings: Do not use if imprinted cap band is broken or missing. If symptoms persist for more than 7 days or worsen, consult a licensed health care professional. As with any drug, if you are pregnant or nursing a baby, consult a health care professional before using this product. Keep this and all medications out of the reach of children. In case of accidental overdose, contact a poison control center immediately. In case of emergency, the manufacturer may be reached 24 hours a day, 7 days a week at 800/624-9659.

How Supplied: Bottles of 125 1-grain sublingual tablets (NDC 54973-7508-1). Store at room temperature.

HYLAND'S CALMS FORTÉ™

Active Ingredients: *Passiflora* (Passion Flower) 1X triple strength HPUS, *Avena Sativa* (Oat) 1X double strength HPUS, *Humulus Lupulus* (Hops) 1X double strength HPUS, *Chamomilla* (Chamomile) 2X HPUS, *Calcarea Phosphorica* (Calcium Phosphate) 3X HPUS, *Ferrum Phosphorica* (Iron Phosphate) 3X HPUS, *Kali Phosphoricum* (Potassium Phosphate) 3X HPUS, *Natrum Phosphoricum* (Sodium Phosphate) 3X HPUS, *Magnesia Phosphoricum* (Magnesium Phosphate) 3X HPUS.

Inactive Ingredients: Lactose, N.F., Calcium Sulfate, Starch (Corn and Tapioca), Magnesium Stearate.

Indications: Temporary symptomatic relief of simple nervous tension and sleeplessness.

Directions: Adults: As a relaxant: Swallow 1–2 tablets with water as needed, three times daily, preferably before meals. For insomnia: 1 to 3 tablets ½ to 1 hour before retiring. Repeat as needed without danger of side effects. Children: As a relaxant: Swallow 1 tablet with water as needed, three times daily, preferably before meals. For insomnia: 1 to 2 tablets ½ to 1 hour before retiring. Repeat as needed without danger of side effects.

Warning: Do not use if imprinted cap band is broken or missing. If symptoms persist for more than seven days or worsen, consult a licensed health care professional. As with any drug, if you are pregnant or nursing a baby, seek the advice of a licensed health care professional before using this product. Keep this and all medications out of the reach of children. In case of accidental overdose, contact a Poison Control Center immediately. In case of emergency, the manufacturer may be reached 24 hours a day, 7 days a week by calling 800/624-9659.

How Supplied: Bottles of 100 4-grain tablets (NDC 54973-1121-02), 50 4-grain tablets (NDC 54973-1121-01) and 32 5.5-grain caplets (NDC 54973-1121-48). Store at room temperature.

HYLAND'S COMPLETE FLU CARE TABLETS

Active Ingredients: Eupatorium Perfoliatum 3X, HPUS; Bryonia Alba 3X, HPUS; Gelsemium Sempervirens 3X, HPUS; Euphrasia Officinalis 3X, HPUS; Kali Iodatum 3X, HPUS; Anas Barbariae Hepatis Et Cordis Extractum 200C HPUS.

Inactive Ingredients: Lactose N.F.

Indications: Temporarily relieves the symptoms of fever, chills, body aches, headache, cough and congestion from the flu or common cold.

Directions: Adults: Take 2–3 Quick Dissolving Tablets under tongue every 4 hours or as needed.
Children 6–12 years old: ½ adult does.

Warnings: Ask a doctor before use if you are pregnant or nursing a baby. Stop use and ask a doctor if symptoms persist for more than 7 days or worsen. Keep out of the reach of children. Do not use if imprinted tamper band is broken or missing.
In case of accidental overdoes, contact a poison control center immediately. In case of emergency, the manufacturer may be contacted 24 hours a day, 7 days a week at 800/624-9659.

How Supplied: 2 Bottles of 60 Tablets (NDC 54973-3015-02)

HYLAND'S EARACHE DROPS

Active Ingredients: Pulsatilla 30C HPUS, Chamomilla 30C HPUS, Sulphur 30C HPUS, Calc Carb 30C HPUS, Belladonna 30C HPUS, Lycopodium 30C HPUS.

Inactive Ingredients: Citric Acid USP, Purified Water, Sodium Benzoate USP, Vegetable Glycerin USP.

Indications: Temporarily relieves the symptoms of fever, pain, irritability and sleeplessness associated with earaches after diagnosis by a physician. Relieves common pain and itching of "swimmer's ear." If symptoms persist for more than 48 hours, or if there is a discharge from the ear, discontinue use and contact your physician.

Directions: Adults and children of all ages: Tilt head sideways and apply 3–4 drops into involved ear 4 times daily or as needed. Tilt ear upward for at least 2 minutes after application or gently place cotton in ear to keep drops in.

Warnings: Keep away from eyes. Do not take by mouth. Earache drops are only to be used in the ears. Tip of applicator should not enter ear canal. Ask a doctor before use if pregnant or nursing. Consult a physician if symptoms persist for more than 48 hours or if there is discharge from the ear. Keep this and all medications out of reach of children. Do not use if imprinted tamper band is broken or missing. In case of accidental overdose, contact a poison control center immediately. In case of emergency, the manufacturer may be contacted 24 hours a day, 7 days a week at 800/624-9659.

How Supplied: Bottle of .33 ounce (NDC 54973-7516-1)

HYLAND'S EARACHE TABLETS

Active Ingredients: Pulsatilla (Wind Flower) 30C, HPUS; Chamomilla (Chamomile) 30C, HPUS; Sulphur 30C, HPUS; Calcarea Carbonica (Carbonate of Lime) 30C, HPUS; Belladonna 30C, HPUS; $(3 \times 10^{-60}$ % Alkaloids) and Lycopodium (Club Moss) 30C, HPUS.

Inactive Ingredients: Lactose NF

Indications: For the relief of symptoms of fever, pain, irritability and sleeplessness associated with earaches in children after diagnosis by a physician. If symptoms persist for more than 48 hours or if there is a discharge from the ear, discontinue use and contact your health care professional.

Directions: Dissolve 4 tablets under the tongue 3 times per day for 48 hours or until symptoms subside. If you prefer, tablets may be dissolved in a teaspoon of water and then given to the child. Earache Tablets are very soft and dissolve almost instantly under the tongue.

Warnings: Do not use if imprinted blisters are broken or damaged. If symptoms persist for more than 48 hours, or if there is a discharge from the ear, discontinue use and consult a licensed health care professional. As with any drug, if you are pregnant or nursing a baby, seek the advice of a licensed health care professional before using this product. Keep this and all medications out of the reach of children. In case of accidental overdose, contact a poison control center immediately. In cases of emergency, the manufacturer may be contacted 24 hours a day, 7 days a week at 800/624-9659.

How Supplied: Blister pack of 40 tablets (NDC 54973-7507-1). Store at room temperature.

HYLAND'S LEG CRAMPS OINTMENT

Formula: Aconitum Nap. 3X HPUS, Arnica Montana 3X HPUS, Ledum Pal. 3X HPUS, Mag. Phos. 10X HPUS, Rhus Tox. 6X HPUS, Viscum Alb. 3X HPUS.

Indications: Temporarily relieves the symptoms of cramps and pains in legs and calves.

Directions: Apply liberally to affected area. Hyland's Leg Cramps Ointment will warm the area while easing the symptoms.

Warnings: For external use only. Do not use if tube seal is broken or missing. If symptoms persist for more than seven days or worsen, contact a licensed health care provider. Keep this and all medications out of reach of children.

How Supplied: Tube of 2.5 ounces (NDC 54973-75143-3).

HYLAND'S LEG CRAMPS WITH QUININE

Active Ingredients: Cinchona Officinalis 3X, HPUS (Quinine), Viscum Album 3X, HPUS; Gnaphalium Polycephalum 3X, HPUS; Rhus Toxicodendron 6X, HPUS; Aconitum Napellus 6X, HPUS; Ledum Palustre 6X, HPUS; Magnesia Phosphorica 6X, HPUS.

Inactive Ingredients: Lactose, N.F.

Indications: Hyland's Leg Cramps is a traditional homeopathic formula for the relief of symptoms of cramps and pains in lower back and legs often made worse by damp weather. Working without contraindications or side effects, Hyland's Leg Cramps stimulates your body's natural healing response to relieve symptoms. Hyland's Leg Cramps is safe for adults and can be used in conjuction with other medications.

Directions: Adults: Dissolve 2–3 tablets under tongue every 4 hours as needed.

Warnings: Do not use if imprinted cap band is missing or broken. If symptoms persist for more than seven days or worsen, contact a licensed health care professional. As with any drug, if you are pregnant or nursing a baby, seek the advice of a licensed health care professional before using this product. Do not use if pregnant, sensitive to quinine or under 12 years of age. Keep this and all medications out of the reach of children. In case of accidental overdose, contact a poison control center immediately. In case of emergency, the manufacturer may be reached 24 hours a day, 7 days a week at 800-624-9659.

How Supplied: Bottles of 100 three-grain sublingual tablets (NDC 54973-2956-02), Bottles of 50 three-grain sublingual tablets (NDC 54973-2956-01), Bottles of 40 5.5 grain caplets (NDC 54973-2956-68). Store at room temperature.

HYLAND'S NERVE TONIC

Active Ingredients: Calcarea Phosphorica (Calcium Phosphate) 3X HPUS; Ferrum Phosphorica (Iron Phosphate) 3X HPUS; Kali Phosphoricum (Potassium Phosphate) 3X HPUS; Natrum Phosphoricum (Sodium Phosphate) 3X HPUS; Magnesia Phosphoricum (Magnesium Phosphate) 3X HPUS.

Inactive Ingredients: Lactose, N.F.

Indications: Temporary symptomatic relief of simple nervous tension and stress.

Directions: Adults take 2–6 tablets before each meal and at bedtime. Children: 2 tablets. In severe cases take 3 tablets every 2 hours.

Warnings: Do not use if imprinted cap band is broken or missing. If symptoms persist for more than seven days or worsen, contact a licensed health care professional. As with any drug, if you are pregnant or nursing a baby, seek the advice of a licensed health care professional before using this product. Keep this and all medications out of the reach of children. In case of accidental overdose, contact a poison control center immediately. In cases of emergency, the manufacturer

may be contacted 24 hours a day, 7 days a week at 800/624-9659.

How Supplied: Bottles of 32 caplets (NDC 54973-1129-68), Bottles of 500 tablets (NDC 54973-1129-1), Bottles of 1000 tablets (NDC 54973-1129-2), Bottles of 100 tablets (NDC 54973-3014-02)

HYLAND'S SEASONAL ALLERGY TABLETS

Formula: Allium Cepa 6X HPUS, Natrum Muriaticum 6X HPUS Histaminum Hydrochloricum 12X HPUS, Luffa Operculata 12X HPUS, Galphimia Glauca 12X HPUS, Nux Vomica 6X HPUS.

Indications: Temporarily relieves the runny eyes and nose symptoms of allergy from pollen, ragweed, grasses, mold and animal dander.

Directions: Adults and Children over 12 years of age: Dissolve 1 to 2 tablets on tongue every 4 hours as needed.

Warnings: Ask a doctor before use if pregnant or nursing. If symptoms persist for more than seven days or worsen, contact a licensed health care provider. Keep this and all medications out of reach of children. Do not use if imprinted tamper band is broken or missing. In case of accidental overdose, contact a poison control center immediately. In case of emergency, the manufacturer may be contacted 24 hours a day, 7 days a week at 800/624-9659.

How Supplied: Bottles of 60 tablets. (NDC 54973-3012-01).

SMILE'S PRID®

Contains: Acidum Carbolicum 2X HPUS, Ichthammol 2X HPUS, Arnica Montana 3X HPUS, Calendula Off 3X HPUS, Echinacea Ang 3X HPUS, Sulphur 12X HPUS, Hepar Sulph 12X HPUS, Silicea 12X HPUS, Rosin, Beeswax, Petrolatum, Stearyl Alcohol, Methyl & Propyl Paraben.

Indications: Temporary topical relief of pain symptoms associated with boils, minor skin eruptions, redness and irritation. Also aids in relieving the discomfort of superficial cuts, scratches and wounds.

Directions: Wash affected parts with hot water, dry and apply PRID® twice daily on clean bandage or gauze. Do not squeeze or pressure irritated skin area. After irritation subsides, repeat application once a day for several days. Children under two years: consult a physician. CAUTION: If symptoms persist for more than seven days or worsen, or if fever occurs, contact a licensed health care professional. Do not use on broken skin. Keep out of reach of children. In case of accidental ingestion, seek professional

Continued on next page

Smile's Prid—Cont.

assistance or contact a poison control center. For external use only. Avoid contact with eyes.

How Supplied: 18GM tin (NDC 0619-4202-54). Keep in a cool dry place.

HYLAND'S TEETHING GEL

Active Ingredients: Calcarea Phosphorica (Calcium Phosphate) 12X, HPUS; Chamomilla (Chamomile) 6X, HPUS; Coffea Cruda (Coffee) 6X, HPUS; and Belladonna 6X, HPUS (Alkaloids 0.0000003%)

Inactive Ingredients: Deionized water, Vegetable Glycerin, Hydroxyethyl Cellulose, Methyl Paraben and Propyl Paraben.

Indications: A homeopathic combination for the temporary relief of symptoms of simple restlessness and wakeful irritability due to cutting teeth.

Directions: Apply to gums as necessary. If symptoms persist for more than seven days or worsen, discontinue use and contact your health care professional. Please note, if your baby has been crying or has been very upset, your baby may fall asleep after using this product because the pain has been relieved and your child can rest.

Warnings: Do not use if tube tip is broken or missing. If symptoms persist for more than seven days or if irritation persists, inflammation develops or fever or infection develop, discontinue use and consult a licensed health care professional. As with any drug, if you are pregnant or nursing a baby, seek the advice of a licensed health care professional before using this product. Keep this and all medications out of the reach of children. In case of accidental overdose, contact a poison control center immediately. In case of emergency, the manufacturer may be contacted 24 hours a day, 7 days a week at 800/624-9659.

How Supplied: Tubes of 1/3 OZ. (NDC 54973-7504-3). Store at room temperature.

HYLAND'S TEETHING TABLETS

Active Ingredients: *Calcarea Phosphorica* (Calcium Phosphate) 3X HPUS, *Chamomilla* (Chamomile) 3X HPUS, *Coffea Cruda* (Coffee) 3X HPUS, *Belladonna* 3X HPUS (Alkaloids 0.0003%).

Inactive Ingredients: Lactose N.F.

Indications: A homeopathic combination for the temporary relief of symptoms of simple restlessness and wakeful irritability due to cutting teeth.

Directions: Dissolve 2 to 3 tablets under the tongue 4 times per day. If you

prefer, tablets may first be dissolved in a teaspoon of water and then given to the child. If the child is restless or wakeful, 2 tablets every hour for 6 doses or as recommended by a licensed health care professional. Teething Tablets are very soft and dissolve almost instantly under the tongue. Please note, if your baby has been crying or has been very upset, your baby may fall asleep after using this product because the pain has been relieved and your child can rest.

Warning: Do Not use if imprinted cap band is broken or missing. If symptoms persist for more than seven days, or if irritation persist, inflammation develops or fever or infection develop, discontinue use and consult a licensed health care professional. As with any drug, if you are pregnant or nursing a baby, seek the advice of a health care professional before using this product. Keep this and all medications out of the reach of children. In case of accidental overdose, contact a poison control center immediately. In case of emergency, the manufacturer may be contacted 24 hours a day, 7 days a week at 800/624-9659.

How Supplied: Bottles of 125—one grain sublingual tablets (NDC 54973-7504-01). Store at room temperature.

UAS Laboratories
**9953 VALLEY VIEW RD
EDEN PRAIRIE, MN 55344**

Direct Inquiries To:
Dr. S.K. Dash: (952) 935-1707
(952) 935-1650

Medical Emergency Contact:
Dr. S.K. Dash: (952) 935-1707
Fax: (952) 935-1650

DDS®-ACIDOPHILUS
Capsule, Tablet & Powder free of dairy products, corn, soy, and preservatives

Description: DDS®-Acidophilus is the source of a special strain of Lactobacillus acidophilus free of dairy products, corn, soy and preservatives. Each capsule or tablet contains one billion viable DDS®-1 L.acidophilus at the time of manufacturing. One gram of powder contains two billion viable DDS®-1 L.acidophilus.

Indications and Usages: An aid in implanting the gut with beneficial Lactobacillus acidophilus under conditions of digestive disorders, acne, yeast infections, and following antibiotic therapy.

Administration: One to two capsules or tablets twice daily before meals. One-fourth teaspoon powder can be substituted for two capsules or tablets.

How Supplied: Bottles of 100 capsules or tablets. 12 bottles per case. Powder is available in 2 oz. bottle; 12 bottles per case.

Storage: Keep refrigerated under 40°F.

DDS®-Acidophilus
Booklet describing superior-strain Acidophilus without dairy products, corn, soy, or preservatives. Two billion viable DDS®-1. L.acidopohilus per gram.

Upsher-Smith Laboratories, Inc.
**6701 EVENSTAD DRIVE
MAPLE GROVE, MN 55369**

Direct Inquiries to:
Professional Services
(800) 654-2299
(763) 315-2001

AMLACTIN® 12% Moisturizing Lotion and Cream
[ăm-lăk-tĭn]
Cosmetic Lotion and Cream

Description: AMLACTIN® Moisturizing Lotion and Cream are special formulations of 12% lactic acid neutralized with ammonium hydroxide to provide a lotion or cream pH of 4.5–5.5. Lactic acid, an alpha-hydroxy acid, is a naturally occurring humectant for the skin. AMLACTIN® moisturizes and softens rough, dry skin.

How Supplied: 225g (8oz) plastic bottle: List No. 0245-0023-22
400g (14oz) plastic bottle: List No. 0245-0023-40
140g (4.9oz) tube: List No. 0245-0024-14

AMLACTIN AP® Anti-Itch Moisturizing Cream
[ăm-lăk'-tĭn]
1% Pramoxine HCl

Description: AMLACTIN AP® Anti-Itch Moisturizing Cream is a special formulation containing 12% lactic acid neutralized with ammonium hydroxide to provide a cream pH of 4.5–5.5 with pramoxine HCl. Lactic acid, an alpha-hydroxy acid, is a naturally occurring humectant which moisturizes and softens rough, dry skin. Pramoxine HCl, USP, 1% is an effective antipruritic ingredient used to relieve itching associated with dry skin.

How Supplied: 140g (4.9oz) tube: NDC No. 0245-0025-14

AMLACTIN® *XL*™
Moisturizing Lotion
ULTRAPLEX™ Formulation
[ăm-lăk'-tĭn]

Description: AmLactin® *XL*™ Moisturizing Lotion is a clinically proven moisturizer which provides powerful mosturizing for rough, dry skin. AmLactin® *XL*™ Moisturizing Lotion contains ULTRAPLEX™ formulation, a proprietary blend of alpha-hydroxy moisturizing compounds.

How Supplied: 160g (5.6oz) tube: List No. 0245-0022-16

Wyeth Consumer Healthcare
Wyeth
FIVE GIRALDA FARMS
MADISON, NJ 07940

Direct Inquiries to:
Wyeth Consumer Healthcare Product Information 800-322-3129

ADVIL®
Ibuprofen Tablets, USP
Ibuprofen Caplets (Oval-Shaped Tablets)
Ibuprofen Gel Caplets (Oval-Shaped Gelatin Coated Tablets)
Ibuprofen Liqui-Gel Capsules
Fever reducer/Pain reliever

Active Ingredient: Each tablet, caplet, gel caplet, or liquigel capsule contains Ibuprofen 200 mg

Uses: temporarily relieves minor aches and pains due to the common cold, headache, toothache, muscular aches, backache, minor pain of arthritis, menstrual cramps; and temporarily reduces fever.

Warnings
Allergy alert: ibuprofen may cause a severe allergic reaction which may include:
• hives
• facial swelling
• asthma (wheezing)
• shock
Stomach bleeding warning: Taking more than recommended may cause stomach bleeding.
Alcohol warning: if you consume 3 or more alcoholic drinks every day, ask your doctor whether you should take ibuprofen or other pain relievers/fever reducers. Ibuprofen may cause stomach bleeding.

Do not use if you have ever had an allergic reaction to any other pain reliever/fever reducer
Ask a doctor before use if you have
• problems or serious side effects from taking pain relievers or fever reducers
• stomach problems that last or come back, such as heartburn, upset stomach, or pain
• ulcers
• bleeding problems
• high blood pressure, heart or kidney disease, are taking a diuretic, or are over 65 years of age
Ask a doctor or pharmacist before use if you are
• under a doctor's care for any serious condition
• taking any other product containing ibuprofen, or any other pain reliever/fever reducer
• taking a prescription drug for anticoagulation (blood thinning)
• taking any other drug
• taking aspirin for cardioprotection
When using this product take with food or milk if stomach upset occurs
Stop use and ask a doctor if
• an allergic reaction occurs. Seek medical help right away.
• pain gets worse or lasts more than 10 days
• fever gets worse or lasts more than 3 days
• stomach pain or upset gets worse or lasts
• redness or swelling is present in the painful area
• any new symptoms appear
If pregnant or breast-feeding, ask a health professional before use. It is especially important not to use ibuprofen during the last 3 months of pregnancy unless definitely directed to do so by a doctor because it may cause problems in the unborn child or complications during delivery.
Keep out of reach of children. In case of overdose, get medical help or contact a Poison Control Center right away.

Dosage and Administration:
Directions—Do not take more than directed
Adults and children 12 years and over:
• take 1 tablet, caplet, gelcap or liquigel capsule every 4 to 6 hours while symptoms persist
• if pain or fever does not respond to 1 tablet, caplet, gelcap, or liquigel capsule, 2 tablets, caplets, gelcaps or liquigel capsules may be used • do not exceed 6 tablets, caplets, gelcaps or liquigel capsules in 24 hours, unless directed by a doctor
• the smallest effective dose should be used
Children under 12 years: ask a doctor

Inactive Ingredients:
Tablets and Caplets: acetylated monoglyceride, beeswax and/or carnauba wax, croscarmellose sodium, iron oxides, lecithin, methylparaben, microcrystalline cellulose, pharmaceutical glaze, povidone, propylparaben, silicon dioxide, simethicone, sodium benzoate, sodium lauryl sulfate, starch, stearic acid, sucrose, titanium dioxide.

Gel Caplets: croscarmellose sodium, FD&C red no. 40, FD&C yellow no. 6, gelatin, glycerin, hypromellose, iron oxides, medium chain triglycerides, pharmaceutical ink, propyl gallate, silicon dioxide, sodium lauryl sulfate, starch, stearic acid, titanium dioxide, triacetin
Liqui-Gels: FD&C green no. 3, gelatin, light mineral oil, pharmaceutical ink, polyethylene glycol, potassium hydroxide, purified water, sorbitan, sorbitol.
Other Information
• **each Liqui-gel capsule contains:** potassium 20 mg
• read all warnings and directions before use. Keep carton.
• store at 20–25°C (68–77°F)
• avoid excessive heat 40°C (above 104°F)

How Supplied:
Coated tablets in a 10 ct. vial and bottles of 24, 50, 100, 165 (non-child resistant), and 225. Coated caplets in bottles of 24, 50, 100, 165 (non-child resistant), and 225.
Gel caplets in bottles of 24, 50, 100, 165 (non-child resistant) and 225.
Liqui-Gels in bottles of 20, 40, 80, 135 (non-child resistant) and 180.

ADVIL® ALLERGY SINUS CAPLETS
Pain Reliever/Fever Reducer
Nasal Decongestant
Antihistamine

Active Ingredients (in each caplet):
Chlorpheniramine maleate 2 mg
Ibuprofen 200 mg
Pseudoephedrine HCl 30 mg

Uses:
• temporarily relieves these symptoms associated with hay fever or other upper respiratory allergies, and the common cold:
  • runny nose • sneezing • headache
  • itchy, watery eyes
  • nasal congestion • minor aches and pains • itching of the nose or throat
  • sinus pressure • fever

Warnings:
Allergy alert: Ibuprofen may cause a severe allergic reaction which may include:
• hives • facial swelling • asthma (wheezing) • shock
Stomach bleeding warning: Taking more than recommended may cause stomach bleeding.
Alcohol warning: If you consume 3 or more alcoholic drinks every day, ask your doctor whether you should take ibuprofen or other pain relievers/fever reducers. Ibuprofen may cause stomach bleeding.
Do not use
• if you have ever had an allergic reaction to any other pain reliever/fever reducer
• if you are now taking a prescription monoamine oxidase inhibitor (MAOI

Continued on next page

Advil Allergy Sinus—Cont.

(certain drugs for depression, psychiatric, or emotional conditions, or Parkinson's disease), or for 2 weeks after stopping the MAOI drug. If you do not know if your prescription drug contains an MAOI, ask a doctor or pharmacist before taking this product.

Ask a doctor before use is you have
- a breathing problem such as emphysema or chronic bronchitis
- heart disease • high blood pressure • thyroid disease • diabetes • kidney disease • ulcers • bleeding problems • glaucoma
- problems or serious side effects from taking pain relievers or fever reducers
- stomach problems that last or come back, such as heartburn, upset stomach, or pain
- trouble urinating due to an enlarged prostate gland

Ask a doctor or pharmacist before use if you are
- under a doctor's care for any serious condition
- taking sedatives or tranquilizers
- over 65 years of age
- taking any other product that contains ibuprofen, or any other pain reliever/fever reducer
- taking any other product that contains pseudoephedrine, chlorpheniramine or any other nasal decongestant or antihistamine
- taking a prescription drug for anticoagulation (blood thinning), or a diuretic
- taking any other drug
- taking aspirin for cardio protection

When using this product
- **do not use more than directed**
- avoid alcoholic drinks
- be careful when driving a motor vehicle or operating machinery
- drowsiness may occur
- take with food or milk if stomach upset occurs
- alcohol, sedatives, and tranquilizers may increase drowsiness

Stop use and ask a doctor if
- an allergic reaction occurs. Seek medical help right away.
- nasal congestion lasts for more than 7 days
- fever lasts for more than 3 days
- you get nervous, dizzy, or sleepless
- symptoms continue or get worse
- stomach pain occurs with the use of this product even if mild pain persists
- any new symptoms appear

If pregnant or breast-feeding, ask a health professional before use. It is especially important not to use this product during the last 3 months of pregnancy unless definitely directed to do so by a doctor because it may cause problems in the unborn child or complications during delivery.

Keep out of reach of children. In case of overdose, get medical help or contact a Poison Control Center right away.

Directions:
- adults: take 1 caplet every 4–6 hours while symptoms persist.
- do not take more than 6 caplets in any 24-hour period, unless directed by a doctor
- children under 12 years of age: consult a doctor

Other Information:
- read all warnings and directions before use. Keep carton.
- store in a dry place 20–25°C (68–77°F)
- avoid excessive heat above 40°C (104°F)

Inactive Ingredients: carnauba wax, croscarmellose sodium, FD&C red no. 40 aluminum lake, FD&C yellow no. 6 aluminum lake, glyceryl behenate, hypromellose, iron oxide black, microcrystalline cellulose, polydextrose, polyethylene glycol, pregelatinized starch, propylene glycol, silicon dioxide, starch, titanium dioxide

How Supplied: Packages of 10 and 20 caplets

ADVIL® MULTI-SYMPTOM COLD CAPLETS
Pain Reliever/Fever Reducer
Nasal Decongestant
Antihistamine

Drug Facts
Active Ingredients (in each caplet):
Chlorpheniramine maleate 2 mg
Ibuprofen 200 mg
Pseudoephedrine HCl 30 mg

Uses: temporarily relieves these symptoms associated with hay fever or other upper respiratory allergies, and the common cold:
- runny nose
- sneezing
- headache
- itchy, watery eyes
- nasal congestion
- minor aches and pains
- itching of the nose or throat
- sinus pressure
- fever

Warnings:
Allergy alert: Ibuprofen may cause a severe allergic reaction which may include:
- hives
- facial swelling
- asthma (wheezing)
- shock

Stomach bleeding warning: Taking more than recommended may cause stomach bleeding.

Alcohol warning: If you consume 3 or more alcoholic drinks every day, ask your doctor whether you should take ibuprofen or other pain relievers/fever reducers. Ibuprofen may cause stomach bleeding.

Do not use
- if you have ever had an allergic reaction to any other pain reliever/fever reducer
- if you are now taking a prescription monoamine oxidase inhibitor (MAOI) (certain drugs for depression, psychiatric, or emotional conditions, or Parkinson's disease), or for 2 weeks after stopping the MAOI drug. If you do not know if your prescription drug contains an MAOI, ask a doctor or pharmacist before taking this product

Ask a doctor before use if you have
- a breathing problem such as emphysema or chronic bronchitis

- heart disease • high blood pressure
- thyroid disease • diabetes
- kidney disease • ulcers • bleeding problems • glaucoma
- problems or serious side effects from taking pain relievers or fever reducers
- stomach problems that last or come back, such as heartburn, upset stomach, or pain
- trouble urinating due to an enlarged prostate gland

Ask a doctor or pharmacist before use if you are
- under a doctor's care for any serious condition
- taking sedatives or tranquilizers
- over 65 years of age
- taking any other product that contains ibuprofen, or any other pain reliever/fever reducer
- taking any other product that contains pseudoephedrine, chlorpheniramine or any other nasal decongestant or antihistamine
- taking a prescription drug for anticoagulation (blood thinning), or a diuretic
- taking any other drug
- taking aspirin for cardioprotection

When using this product
- **do not use more than directed**
- avoid alcoholic drinks
- be careful when driving a motor vehicle or operating machinery
- drowsiness may occur
- take with food or milk if stomach upset occurs
- alcohol, sedatives, and tranquilizers may increase drowsiness

Stop use and ask a doctor if
- an allergic reaction occurs. Seek medical help right away.
- nasal congestion lasts for more than 7 days
- fever lasts for more than 3 days
- you get nervous, dizzy, or sleepless
- symptoms continue or get worse
- stomach pain occurs with the use of this product even if mild pain persists
- any new symptoms appear

If pregnant or breast-feeding, ask a health professional before use. It is especially important not to use this product during the last 3 months of pregnancy unless definitely directed to do so by a doctor because it may cause problems in the unborn child or complications during delivery.

Keep out of reach of children. In case of overdose, get medical help or contact a Poison Control Center right away.

Directions:
- adults: take 1 caplet every 4–6 hours while symptoms persist.
- do not take more than 6 caplets in any 24-hour period, unless directed by a doctor
- children under 12 years of age: consult a doctor

Other Information:
- read all warnings and directions before use. Keep carton.
- store in a dry place 20–25°C (68–77°F)
- avoid excessive heat above 40°C (104°F)

Inactive Ingredients: carnauba wax, croscarmellose sodium, FD&C red no. 40 aluminum lake, FD&C yellow no. 6 aluminum lake, glyceryl behenate, hypromellose, iron oxide black, microcrystalline cellulose, polydextrose, polyethylene glycol, pregelatinized starch, propylene glycol, silicon dioxide, starch, titanium dioxide

How Supplied: Packages of 10 and 30 caplets.

ADVIL® COLD & SINUS
Caplets, Tablets and Liqui-Gels
Pain Reliever/Fever Reducer/Nasal Decongestant

Active Ingredients (in each tablet or caplet):
Ibuprofen 200 mg
Pseudoephedrine HCl 30 mg

Active Ingredients (in each Liqui-Gel):
Solubilized Ibuprofen equal to 200 mg ibuprofen (present as the free acid and potassium salt)
Pseudoephedrine HCl 30 mg

Uses: Temporarily relieves these symptoms associated with the common cold, sinusitis or flu:
• headache • fever • nasal congestion
• minor body aches and pains

Warnings:
Allergy Alert: Ibuprofen may cause a severe allergic reaction which may include: • hives • facial swelling • asthma (wheezing) • shock
Stomach bleeding warning: Taking more than recommended may cause stomach bleeding

Alcohol warning: If you consume 3 or more alcoholic drinks every day, ask your doctor whether you should take ibuprofen or other pain relievers/fever reducers. Ibuprofen may cause stomach bleeding.
Do not use
• if you have ever had an allergic reaction to any other pain reliever/fever reducer
• if you are now taking a prescription monoamine oxidase inhibitor (MAOI) (certain drugs for depression, psychiatric, or emotional conditions, or Parkinson's disease), or for 2 weeks after stopping the MAOI drug. If you do not know if your prescription drug contains an MAOI, ask a doctor or pharmacist before taking this product
Ask a doctor before use if you have
• heart disease • high blood pressure
• thyroid disease • diabetes
• trouble urinating due to an enlarged prostate gland
• had problems or serious side effects from taking pain relievers or fever reducers
• kidney disease
• ulcers
• bleeding problems
• stomach problems that last or come back, such as heartburn, upset stomach or pain
Ask a doctor or pharmacist before use if you are
• taking any other product that contains ibuprofen or any other pain reliever/fever reducer
• taking any other product that contains pseudoephedrine or any other nasal decongestant
• under a doctor's care for any continuing medical condition

• over 65 years of age
• taking a prescription product for anticoagulation (blood thinning) or a diuretic
• taking any other drug
• taking aspirin for cardioprotection
When using this product
• do not use more than directed
• take with food or milk if stomach upset occurs
Stop use and ask a doctor if
• an allergic reaction occurs. Seek medical help right away.
• you get nervous, dizzy, or sleepless
• nasal congestion lasts for more than 7 days
• fever lasts for more than 3 days
• symptoms continue or get worse
• any new symptoms appear
• stomach pain occurs with use of this product or if even mild pain persists
If pregnant or breast-feeding, ask a health professional before use. It is especially important not to use this product during the last 3 months of pregnancy unless definitely directed to do so by a doctor because it may cause problems in the unborn child or complications during delivery.
Keep out of reach of children. In case of overdose, get medical help or contact a Poison Control Center right away.

Directions:
• adults and children 12 years of age and over:
  • take 1 tablet, caplet or liqui-gel every 4 to 6 hours while symptoms persist. If symptoms do not respond to 1 tablet, caplet or liqui-gel, 2 tablets, caplets or liqui-gels may be used.
  • do not use more than 6 tablets, caplets or liqui-gels in any 24-hour period unless directed by a doctor
  • the smallest effective dose should be used
• children under 12 years of age: consult a doctor

Other Information:
• store at 20–25°C (68–77°F). Avoid excessive heat above 40°C (104°F).
• read all warnings and directions before use. Keep carton.
• **each Liqui-gel contains:** potassium 20 mg

Inactive Ingredients (tablets and caplets): carnauba or equivalent wax, croscarmellose sodium, iron oxides, methylparaben, microcrystalline cellulose, propylparaben, silicon dioxide, sodium benzoate, sodium lauryl sulfate, starch, stearic acid, sucrose, titanium dioxide

Inactive Ingredients (liqui-gels): D&C yellow no. 10, FD&C red no. 40, fractionated coconut oil, gelatin, pharmaceutical ink, polyethylene glycol, potassium hydroxide, purified water, sorbitan, sorbitol

How Supplied: Advil® Cold and Sinus is an oval-shaped, tan-colored caplet, a tan-colored tablet or a liqui-gel. The caplet is supplied in blister packs of 20 and 40. The tablet is available in blister packs of 20. The liqui-gel is available in blister packs of 16 and 32.

ADVIL®
FLU & BODY ACHE Caplets
Pain Reliever/Fever Reducer/Nasal Decongestant

Active Ingredients (in each caplet):
Ibuprofen 200 mg
Pseudoephedrine HCl 30 mg
Uses:
• temporarily relieves these symptoms associated with the common cold, sinusitis, or flu
  • headache
  • fever
  • nasal congestion
  • minor body aches and pains

Warnings:
Allergy alert: Ibuprofen may cause a severe allergic reaction which may include: • hives • facial swelling • asthma (wheezing) • shock
Stomach bleeding warning: Taking more than recommended may cause stomach bleeding
Alcohol warning: If you consume 3 or more alcoholic drinks every day, ask your doctor whether you should take ibuprofen or other pain relievers/fever reducers. Ibuprofen may cause stomach bleeding.
Do not use
• if you have ever had an allergic reaction to any other pain reliever/fever reducer
• if you are now taking a prescription monoamine oxidase inhibitor (MAOI) (certain drugs for depression, psychiatric, or emotional conditions, or Parkinson's disease), or for 2 weeks after stopping the MAOI drug. If you do not know if your prescription drug contains an MAOI, ask a doctor or pharmacist before taking this product
Ask a doctor before use if you have
• heart disease • high blood pressure
• thyroid disease • diabetes
• ulcers • kidney disease
• bleeding problems
• stomach problems that last or come back, such as heartburn, upset stomach or pain
• trouble urinating due to an enlarged prostate gland
• had problems or serious side effects from taking pain relievers or fever reducers
Ask a doctor or pharmacist before use if you are
• taking any other product that contains ibuprofen or any other pain reliever/fever reducer
• taking any other product that contains pseudoephedrine or any other nasal decongestant
• under a doctor's care for any continuing medical condition
• over 65 years of age
• taking any other drug
• taking a prescription product for anticoagulation (blood thinning) or a diuretic
• taking aspirin for cardioprotection
When using this product
• do not use more than directed
• take with food or milk if stomach upset occurs
Stop use and ask a doctor if
• an allergic reaction occurs. Seek medical help right away.

Continued on next page

Advil Flu/Body Ache—Cont.

- you get nervous, dizzy, or sleepless
- nasal congestion lasts for more than 7 days
- fever lasts for more than 3 days
- symptoms continue or get worse
- any new symptoms appear
- stomach pain occurs with use of this product or if even mild pain persists

If pregnant or breast-feeding, ask a health professional before use. It is especially important not to use this product during the last 3 months of pregnancy unless definitely directed to do so by a doctor because it may cause problems in the unborn child or complications during delivery.

Keep out of reach of children. In case of overdose, get medical help or contact a Poison Control Center right away.

Directions:
- adults and children 12 years of age and over: Take 1 caplet every 4 to 6 hours while symptoms persist. If symptoms do not respond to 1 caplet, 2 caplets may be used.
- do not use more than 6 caplets in any 24-hour period unless directed by a doctor
- the smallest effective dose should be used
- children under 12 years of age: consult a doctor

Other Information:
- store at 20–25°C (68–77°F). Avoid excessive heat above 40°C (104°F).
- read all warnings and directions before use. Keep carton.

Inactive Ingredients: carnauba or equivalent wax, croscarmellose sodium, iron oxide, methylparaben, microcrystalline cellulose, propylparaben, silicon dioxide, sodium benzoate, sodium lauryl sulfate, starch, stearic acid, sucrose, titanium dioxide

How Supplied:
Blister packs of 20 caplets.

ADVIL®
MIGRAINE Liquigels

Use: Treats migraine

Active Ingredient:
Each brown, oval capsule contains solubilized ibuprofen, a pain reliever, equal to 200 mg ibuprofen (present as the free acid and potassium salt)

Warnings:
Allergy alert: Ibuprofen may cause a severe allergic reaction which may include:
- hives
- facial swelling
- asthma (wheezing)
- shock

Stomach bleeding warning: Taking more than recommended may cause stomach bleeding.

Alcohol warning: If you consume 3 or more alcoholic drinks every day, ask your doctor whether you should take ibuprofen or other pain relievers/fever reducers. Ibuprofen may cause stomach bleeding.

Do not use if you have ever had an allergic reaction to any other pain reliever/fever reducer

Ask a doctor before use if you have
- never had migraines diagnosed by a health professional
- a headache that is different from your usual migraines
- the worse headache of your life
- fever and stiff neck
- headaches beginning after, or caused by head injury, exertion, coughing or bending
- experienced your first headache after the age of 50
- daily headaches
- a migraine so severe as to require bed rest
- problems or serious side effects from taking pain relievers or fever reducers
- stomach problems that last or come back, such as heartburn, upset stomach, or pain
- ulcers
- bleeding problems
- high blood pressure, heart or kidney disease, are taking a diuretic, or are over 65 years of age

Ask a doctor or pharmacist before use if you are
- under a doctor's care for any serious condition
- taking another product containing ibuprofen, or any other pain reliever/fever reducer
- taking a prescription drug for anticoagulation (blood thinning)
- taking any other drug
- taking aspirin for cardioprotection

When using this product take with food or milk of stomach upset occurs.

Stop use and ask a doctor if
- an allergic reaction occurs. Seek medical help right away.
- migraine headache pain is not relieved or gets worse after first dose
- stomach pain occurs with the use of this product
- any new symptoms appear

If pregnant or breast-feeding, ask a health professional before use. It is especially important not to use ibuprofen during the last 3 months of pregnancy unless definitely directed to do so by a doctor because it may cause problems in the unborn child or complications during delivery.

Keep out of reach of children. In case of overdose, get medical help or contact a Poison Control Center right away.

Directions:

Adults:	• take 2 capsules with a glass of water • if symptoms persist or worsen, ask your doctor • do not take more than 2 capsules in 24 hours, unless directed by a doctor
Under 18 years of age:	• ask a doctor

Other Information:
- **each capsule contains:** potassium 20 mg
- read all directions and warnings before use. Keep carton.
- store at 20–25°C (68–77°F)
- avoid excessive heat 40°C (above 104°F)

Inactive Ingredients:
D&C yellow no. 10, FD&C green no. 3, FD&C red no. 40, gelatin, light mineral oil, pharmaceutical ink, polyethylene glycol, potassium hydroxide, purified water, sorbitan, sorbitol

How Supplied: Bottles of 20, & 40 liquigels.

JUNIOR STRENGTH ADVIL®
SWALLOW TABLETS
Fever Reducer/Pain Reliever

Active Ingredient:
(in each tablet)
Ibuprofen 100 mg

Uses: temporarily:
- reduces fever
- relieves minor aches and pains due to the common cold, flu, sore throat, headaches and toothaches

Warnings:
Allergy alert: Ibuprofen may cause a severe allergic reaction which may include:
- hives • asthma (wheezing)
- facial swelling • shock

Stomach bleeding warning: Taking more than recommended may cause stomach bleeding

Sore throat warning: Severe or persistent sore throat or sore throat accompanied by high fever, headache, nausea, and vomiting may be serious. Consult doctor promptly. Do not use more than 2 days or administer to children under 3 years of age unless directed by doctor.

Do not use if the child has ever had an allergic reaction to any other fever reducer/pain reliever

Ask a doctor before use if the child has
- not been drinking fluids • ulcers
- bleeding problems
- stomach problems that last or come back, such as heartburn, upset stomach or pain
- high blood pressure, heart or kidney disease or is taking a diuretic
- lost a lot of fluid due to continued vomiting or diarrhea
- problems or serious side effects from taking fever reducers or pain relievers

Ask a doctor or pharmacist before use if the child is
- under a doctor's care for any serious condition
- taking any other drug
- taking any other product that contains ibuprofen, or any other pain reliever/fever reducer
- taking a prescription product for anticoagulation (blood thinning)

When using this product give with food or milk if stomach upset occurs

Stop use and ask a doctor if
- an allergic reaction occurs. Seek medical help right away.

- fever or pain gets worse or lasts more than 3 days
- the child does not get any relief within first day (24 hours) of treatment
- stomach pain or upset gets worse or lasts
- redness or swelling is present in the painful area
- any new symptoms appear

Keep out of reach of children. In case of overdose, get medical help or contact a Poison Control Center right away.

Directions:
- **do not give more than directed**
- find right dose on chart below. If possible, use weight to dose; otherwise use age.
- repeat dose every 6–8 hours, if needed
- do not use more than 4 times a day

Dosing Chart		
Weight (lb)	Age (yr)	Dose (tablets)
under 48 lb	under 6 yr	ask a doctor
48–71 lb	6–10 yr	2 tablets
72–95 lb	11 yr	3 tablets

Other Information:
- one dose lasts 6–8 hours
- store at 20–25°C (68–77°F)

Inactive Ingredients: acetylated monoglycerides, carnauba wax, colloidal silicon dioxide, croscarmellose sodium, iron oxides, methylparaben, microcrystalline cellulose, povidone, pregelatinized starch, propylene glycol, propylparaben, shellac, sodium benzoate, starch, stearic acid, sucrose, titanium dioxide

How Supplied: Coated Tablets in bottles of 24.

CHILDREN'S ADVIL® CHEWABLE TABLETS
Fever Reducer/Pain Reliever

Active Ingredient:
(in each tablet)
Ibuprofen 50 mg

Uses: temporarily:
- reduces fever
- relieves minor aches and pains due to the common cold, flu, sore throat, headaches and toothaches

Warnings:
Allergy alert: Ibuprofen may cause a severe allergic reaction which may include:
- hives • asthma (wheezing)
- facial swelling • shock

Stomach bleeding warning: Taking more than recommended may cause stomach bleeding

Sore throat warning: Severe or persistent sore throat or sore throat accompanied by high fever, headache, nausea, and vomiting may be serious. Consult doctor promptly. Do not use more than 2 days or administer to children under 3 years of age unless directed by doctor.

Dosing Chart		
Weight (lb)	Age (yr)	Dose (tablets)
under 24 lb	under 2 yr	ask a doctor
24–35 lb	2–3 yr	2 tablets
36–47 lb	4–5 yr	3 tablets
48–59 lb	6–8 yr	4 tablets
60–71 lb	9–10 yr	5 tablets
72–95 lb	11 yr	6 tablets

Do not use if the child has ever had an allergic reaction to any other fever reducer/pain reliever

Ask a doctor before use if the child has
- not been drinking fluids
- lost a lot of fluid due to continued vomiting or diarrhea
- ulcers
- bleeding problems
- stomach problems that last or come back, such as heartburn, upset stomach or pain
- high blood pressure, heart or kidney disease or is taking a diuretic
- problems or serious side effects from taking other fever reducers or pain relievers

Ask a doctor or pharmacist before use if the child is
- under a doctor's care for any serious condition
- taking any other drug
- taking a prescription product for anticoagulation (blood thinning)
- taking any other product that contains ibuprofen, or any other pain reliever/fever reducer

When using this product give with food or milk if stomach upset occurs

Stop use and ask a doctor if
- an allergic reaction occurs. Seek medical help right away.
- fever or pain gets worse or lasts more than 3 days
- the child does not get any relief within first day (24 hours) of treatment
- stomach pain or upset gets worse or lasts
- redness or swelling is present in the painful area
- any new symptoms appear

Keep out of reach of children. In case of overdose, get medical help or contact a Poison Control Center right away.

Directions:
- **do not give more than directed**
- find right dose on chart below. If possible, use weight to dose; otherwise use age.
- repeat dose every 6–8 hours, if needed
- do not use more than 4 times a day

[See table above]

Other Information:
- **Phenylketonurics:** contains phenylalanine 2.1 mg per tablet
- one dose lasts 6–8 hours
- store in a dry place at 20–25°C (68–77°F)

Inactive Ingredients: (GRAPE FLAVOR) artificial flavor, aspartame, cellulose acetate phthalate, D&C red no. 30 lake, FD&C blue no. 2 lake, gelatin, magnasweet, magnesium stearate, manni-

tol, microcrystalline cellulose, silicon dioxide, sodium starch glycolate

How Supplied: Blister of 24 (grape flavor).

CHILDREN'S ADVIL® COLD SUSPENSION
Pain Reliever/Fever Reducer/Nasal Decongestant

Active Ingredients:
(in each 5mL teaspoon)
Ibuprofen 100 mg
Pseudoephedrine HCl 15mg

Uses: temporarily relieves these cold, sinus and flu symptoms:
- nasal and sinus congestion • headache
- stuffy nose • sore throat
- minor aches and pains • fever

Warnings:
Allergy alert: Ibuprofen may cause a severe allergic reaction which may include: • hives • facial swelling • asthma (wheezing) • shock

Stomach bleeding warning: Taking more than recommended may cause stomach bleeding

Sore throat warning: Severe or persistent sore throat or sore throat accompanied by high fever, headache, nausea, and vomiting may be serious. Consult a doctor right away. Do not use more than 2 days or give to children under 3 years of age unless directed by a doctor.

Do not use:
- if the child has ever had an allergic reaction to any pain reliever, fever reducer or nasal decongestant
- in a child who is taking a prescription monoamine oxidase inhibitor (MAOI) (certain drugs for depression, psychiatric, or emotional conditions, or Parkinson's disease), or for 2 weeks after stopping the MAOI drug. If you do not know if your child's prescription drug contains an MAOI, ask a doctor or pharmacist before giving this product.

Ask a doctor before use if the child has
- not been drinking fluids
- lost a lot of fluid due to continued vomiting or diarrhea
- problems or serious side effects from taking any pain reliever, fever reducer or nasal decongestant
- stomach problems that last or come back, such as heartburn, upset stomach or pain • diabetes

Continued on next page

Children's Advil Cold—Cont.

- high blood pressure, heart or kidney disease or is taking a diuretic
- thyroid disease • ulcers • bleeding problems

Ask a doctor or pharmacist before use if the child is

- under a doctor's care for any serious condition
- taking any other drug
- taking any other product that contains ibuprofen or any other pain reliever/fever reducer
- taking any other product that contains pseudoephedrine or any other nasal decongestant
- taking a prescription product for anti-coagulation (blood thinning)

When using this product

- do not use more than directed
- give with food or milk if stomach upset occurs

Stop use and ask a doctor if

- an allergic reaction occurs. Seek medical help right away.
- the child does not get any relief within first day (24 hours) of treatment
- fever or pain or nasal congestion gets worse or lasts for more than 3 days
- stomach pain or upset gets worse or lasts
- symptoms continue or get worse
- redness or swelling is present in the painful area
- the child gets nervous, dizzy, sleepless or sleepy
- any new symptoms appear

Keep out of reach of children. In case of overdose, get medical help or contact a Poison Control Center right away.

Directions:

- do not give more than directed
- shake well before using
- find right dose on chart below. If possible, use weight to dose; otherwise use age.
- if needed, repeat dose every **6 hours**
- do not use more than **4 times a day**
- replace original bottle cap to maintain child resistance
- measure only with dosing cup provided. Dosing cup to be used with Children's Advil Cold Suspension only. Do not use with other products. Dose lines account for product remaining in cup due to thickness of suspension.

Dosing Chart

Weight (lb)	Age (yr)	Dose (teaspoons)
under 24	under 2 yr	ask a doctor
24–47	2–5 yr	1 teaspoon
48–95	6–11 yr	2 teaspoons

Other Information:

- **each teaspoon contains:** sodium 3 mg
- store at room temperature 20–25°C (68–77°F)
- alcohol free

Inactive Ingredients: acetic acid, artificial flavor, butylated hydroxy toluene, carboxymethylcellulose sodium, citric acid, edetate disodium, FD&C blue no. 1, FD&C red no. 40, glycerin, microcrystalline cellulose, polysorbate 80, propylene glycol, purified water, sodium benzoate, sorbitol solution, sucrose, xanthan gum

How Supplied: Bottles of 4 fl. oz. in grape flavor.

CHILDREN'S ADVIL® SUSPENSION
Fever Reducer/Pain Reliever

Active Ingredient:
(in each 5 mL)
Ibuprofen 100 mg

Uses: temporarily:
- reduces fever
- relieves minor aches and pains due to the common cold, flu, sore throat, headaches and toothaches

Warnings:

Allergy alert: Ibuprofen may cause a severe allergic reaction which may include:
- hives • asthma (wheezing)
- facial swelling • shock

Stomach bleeding warning: Taking more than recommended may cause stomach bleeding.

Sore throat warning: Severe or persistent sore throat or sore throat accompanied by high fever, headache, nausea, and vomiting may be serious. Consult doctor promptly. Do not use more than 2 days or administer to children under 3 years of age unless directed by doctor.

Do not use if the child has ever had an allergic reaction to any other fever reducer/pain reliever

Ask a doctor before use if the child has
- ulcers
- bleeding problems
- stomach problems that last or come back, such as heartburn, upset stomach or pain
- high blood pressure, heart or kidney disease or is taking a diuretic
- not been drinking fluids
- lost a lot of fluid due to continued vomiting or diarrhea
- problems or serious side effects from taking fever reducers or pain relievers

Ask a doctor or pharmacist before use if the child is
- under a doctor's care for any serious condition
- taking a prescription product for anti-coagulation (blood thinning)
- taking any other drug
- taking any other product that contains ibuprofen, or any other pain reliever/fever reducer

When using this product give with food or milk if stomach upset occurs

Stop use and ask a doctor if
- an allergic reaction occurs. Seek medical help right away.
- fever or pain gets worse or lasts more than 3 days
- the child does not get any relief within first day (24 hours) of treatment
- stomach pain or upset gets worse or lasts
- redness or swelling is present in the painful area
- any new symptoms appear

Keep out of reach of children. In case of overdose, get medical help or contact a Poison Control Center right away.

Directions:
- do not give more than directed
- shake well before using
- find right dose on chart below. If possible, use weight to dose; otherwise use age.
- repeat dose every 6–8 hours, if needed
- do not use more than 4 times a day
- measure only with the blue dosing cup provided. Blue dosing cup to be used with Children's Advil Suspension only. Do not use with other products. Dose lines account for product remaining in cup due to thickness of suspension.

[See table below]

Other Information:
- one dose lasts 6–8 hours
- store at 20–25°C (68–77°F)

Inactive Ingredients: (FRUIT FLAVOR) artifical flavors, carboxymethylcellulose sodium, citric acid, edetate disodium, FD&C red no. 40, glycerin, microcrystalline cellulose, polysorbate 80, purified water, sodium benzoate, sorbitol solution, sucrose, xanthan gum

Each teaspoon contains: sodium 3 mg

Inactive Ingredients: (GRAPE FLAVOR) acetic acid, artifical flavor, butylated hydroxytoluene, carboxymethylcellulose sodium, citric acid, edetate disodium, FD&C blue no. 1, FD&C red no. 40, glycerin, microcrystalline cellulose, polysorbate 80, propylene glycol, purified water, sodium benzoate, sorbitol solution, sucrose, xanthan gum

Each teaspoon contains: sodium 3 mg

Inactive Ingredients: (BLUE RASPBERRY FLAVOR) carboxymethylcellulose sodium, citric acid, edetate disodium, FD&C blue no. 1, glycerin, microcrystalline cellulose, natural and artificial flavors, polysorbate 80, propylene glycol, purified water, sodium benzoate, sodium citrate, sorbitol solution, sucrose, xanthan gum

Dosing Chart

Weight (lb)	Age (yr)	Dose (tsp)
under 24 lb	under 2 yr	ask a doctor
24–35 lb	2–3 yr	1 tsp
36–47 lb	4–5 yr	1½ tsp
48–59 lb	6–8 yr	2 tsp
60–71 lb	9–10 yr	2½ tsp
72–95 lb	11 yr	3 tsp

Each teaspoon contains: sodium 10 mg

How Supplied: Bottles of 4 fl. oz. in grape, fruit, and blue raspberry flavors.

INFANTS' ADVIL® CONCENTRATED DROPS
Fever Reducer/Pain Reliever

Active Ingredient:
(in each 1.25 mL)
Ibuprofen 50 mg

Uses: temporarily:
- reduces fever
- relieves minor aches and pains due to the common cold, flu, headaches and toothaches

Warnings:
Allergy Allert: Ibuprofen may cause a severe allergic reaction which may include:
- hives • asthma (wheezing)
- facial swelling • shock

Stomach bleeding warning: Taking more than recommended may cause stomach bleeding.

Do not use if the child has ever had an allergic reaction to any other fever reducer/pain reliever

Ask a doctor before use if the child has
- not been drinking fluids
- lost a lot of fluid due to continued vomiting or diarrhea
- problems or serious side effects from taking fever reducers or pain relievers
- ulcers
- bleeding problems
- stomach problems that last or come back, such as heartburn, upset stomach or pain
- high blood pressure, heart or kidney disease or is taking a diuretic

Ask a doctor or pharmacist before use if the child is
- under a doctor's care for any serious condition
- taking any other drug
- taking any other product that contains ibuprofen, or any other pain reliever/fever reducer
- taking a prescription product for anticoagulation (blood thinning)

When using this product give with food or milk if upset stomach occurs

Stop use and ask a doctor if
- an allergic reaction occurs. Seek medical help right away.
- fever or pain gets worse or lasts more than 3 days
- the child does not get any relief within first day (24 hours) of treatment
- stomach pain or upset gets worse or lasts

- redness or swelling is present in the painful area
- any new symptoms appear

Keep out of reach of children. In case of overdose, get medical help or contact a Poison Control Center right away.

Directions:
- **do not give more than directed**
- **shake well before using**
- find right dose on chart below. If possible, use weight to dose; otherwise use age.
- repeat dose every 6–8 hours, if needed
- do not use more than 4 times a day
- measure with the dosing device provided. Do not use with any other device.

[See table below]

Other Information:
- one dose lasts 6–8 hours
- store at 20–25°C (68–77°F)

Inactive   Ingredients: (WHITE GRAPE FLAVOR) artificial flavor, carboxymethylcellulose sodium, citric acid, edetate disodium, glycerin, microcrystalline cellulose, polysorbate 80, propylene glycol, purified water, sodium benzoate, sorbitol solution, sucrose, xanthan gum
Inactive Ingredients: (GRAPE FLAVOR) artificial flavor, caroboxymethylcellulose sodium, citric acid, edetate disodium, FD&C blue no. 1, FD&C red no. 40, glycerin, microcrystalline cellulose, polysorbate 80, purified water, sodium benzoate, sorbitol solution, sucrose, xanthan gum

How Supplied: Bottles of ½ fl. oz. in grape and white grape flavors.

ALAVERT
Loratadine orally disintegrating tablets
Loratadine swallow tablets
Antihistamine

Active Ingredient (in each tablet):
Loratadine 10 mg

Uses:
- temporarily relieves these symptoms due to hay fever or other upper respiratory allergies:
  - runny nose • sneezing • itchy, watery eyes
  - itching of the nose or throat

Warnings:
Do not use if you have ever had an allergic reaction to this product or any of its ingredients
Ask a doctor before use if you have liver or kidney disease. Your doctor should determine if you need a different dose.
When using this product do not use more than directed. Taking more than recommended may cause drowsiness.

Stop use and ask a doctor if an allergic reaction to this product occurs. Seek medical help right away.
If pregnant or breast-feeding, ask a health professional before use.
Keep out of reach of children. In case of overdose, get medical help or contact a Poison Control Center right away.

Directions:
- (orally disintegrating tablet) tablet melts in mouth. Can be taken with or without water.

Age	Dose
adults and children 6 years and over	1 tablet daily; do not use more than 1 tablet in 24 hours
children under 6	ask a doctor
consumers who have liver or kidney disease	ask a doctor

Other Information:
- (orally disintegrating tablet) Phenylketonurics: Contains Phenylalanine 8.4 mg per tablet
- store at 20–25°C (68–77°F)
- keep in a dry place

Inactive Ingredients (Loratadine orally disintegrating tablets): artificial & natural flavor, aspartame, citric acid, colloidal silicon dioxide, corn syrup solids, crospovidone, magnesium stearate, mannitol, microcrystalline cellulose, modified food starch, sodium bicarbonate

Inactive Ingredients (Loratadine swallow tablets): lactose monohydrate, magnesium stearate, microcrystalline cellulose, sodium starch glycolate

How Supplied: Loratadine orally disintegrating tablets in packages of 6, 12, 24 & 48

How Supplied: Loratadine swallow tablets in packages of 15 and 30 tablets

---

ALAVERT ALLERGY & SINUS D-12 HOUR TABLETS
Loratadine/Pseudoephedrine Sulfate Extended Release Tablets
Antihistamine/Nasal Decongestant

Active Ingredients (in each tablet):
Loratadine 5 mg
Pseudoephedrine sulfate 120 mg

Uses:
- temporarily relieves these symptoms due to hay fever or other upper respiratory allergies:
  - runny nose
  - sneezing • itchy, watery eyes
  - itching of the nose or throat
- temporarily relieves nasal congestion due to the common cold, hay fever or other respiratory allergies
- reduces swelling of nasal passages

Dosing Chart		
Weight (lb)	Age (mos)	Dose (mL)
under 6 mos		ask a doctor
12–17 lb	6–11 mos	1.25 mL
18–23 lb	12–23 mos	1.875 mL

Continued on next page

Alavert D-12—Cont.

- temporarily relieves sinus congestion and pressure
- temporarily restores freer breathing through the nose

Warnings:

Do not use
- if you have ever had an allergic reaction to this product or any of its ingredients
- if you are now taking a prescription monoamine oxidase inhibitor (MAOI) (certain drugs for depression, psychiatric, or emotional conditions, or Parkinson's disease), or for 2 weeks after stopping the MAOI drug. If you do not know if your prescription drug contains an MAOI, ask a doctor or pharmacist before taking this product.

Ask a doctor before use if you have
- heart disease • high blood pressure
- thyroid disease • diabetes
- trouble urinating due to an enlarged prostate gland
- liver or kidney disease. Your doctor should determine if you need a different dose.

When using this product do not take more than directed. Taking more than directed may cause drowsiness.

Stop use and ask a doctor if
- an allergic reaction to this product occurs. Seek medical help right away.
- symptoms do not improve within 7 days or are accompanied by a fever
- nervousness, dizziness or sleeplessness occurs

If pregnant or breast-feeding, ask a health professional before use.

Keep out of reach of children. In case of overdose, get medical help or contact a Poison Control Center right away.

Directions:
- do not divide, crush, chew or dissolve the tablet

Age	Dose
adults and children 12 years and over	1 tablet every 12 hours; not more than 2 tablets in 24 hours
children under 12 years of age	ask a doctor
consumers with liver or kidney disease	ask a doctor

Other Information:
- store between 15° and 25°C (59° and 77°F)
- keep in a dry place

Inactive Ingredients: croscarmellose sodium, dibasic calcium phosphate, hypromellose, lactose monohydrate, magnesium stearate, pharmaceutical ink, povidone, titanium dioxide

How Supplied: Blister packs of 12 and 24 tablets.

MAXIMUM STRENGTH
ANBESOL® Gel and Liquid
Oral Anesthetic

ANBESOL JUNIOR® Gel
Oral Anesthetic

BABY ANBESOL® Gel
Grape Flavor
Oral Anesthetic

Active Ingredients: Anbesol is an oral anesthetic which is available in a Maximum Strength gel and liquid. Anbesol Junior, available in a gel, is an oral anesthetic. Baby Anbesol, available in a grape-flavored gel, is an oral anesthetic and is alcohol-free.
Maximum Strength Anbesol Gel and Liquid contain Benzocaine 20%.
Anbesol Junior Gel contains Benzocaine 10%.
Baby Anbesol Gel contains Benzocaine 7.5%.

Uses: Maximum Strength Anbesol temporarily relieves pain associated with toothache, canker sores, minor dental procedures, sore gums, braces, and dentures. **Anbesol Junior** temporarily relieves pain associated with braces, sore gums, canker sores, toothaches, and minor dental procedures. **Baby Anbesol Gel** temporarily relieves sore gums due to teething in infants and children 4 months of age and older.

Warnings: Allergy alert: Do not use these products if you have a history of allergy to local anesthetics such as procaine, butacaine, benzocaine, or other "caine" anesthetics.
Baby Anbesol: Do not use to treat fever and nasal congestion. These are not symptoms of teething and may indicate the presence of infection. If these symptoms persist, consult your doctor.
Maximum Strength Anbesol, Anbesol Junior and Baby Anbesol:
When using this product
- avoid contact with the eyes
- do not exceed recommended dosage
- do not use for more than 7 days unless directed by a doctor/dentist
Stop use and ask a doctor if
- sore mouth symptoms do not improve in 7 days
- irritation, pain, or redness persists or worsens
- swelling, rash, or fever develops
Keep out of reach of children. If more than used for pain is accidentally swallowed, get medical help or contact a Poison Control Center right away.

Directions: Maximum Strength Anbesol: Gel—
- to open tube, cut tip of the tube on score mark with scissors
- adults and children 2 years of age and older: apply to the affected area up to 4 times daily or as directed by a doctor/dentist
- children under 12 years of age: adult supervision should be given in the use of this product
- children under 2 years of age: consult a doctor/dentist
- for denture irritation:
  - apply thin layer to the affected area

- do not reinsert dental work until irritation/pain is relieved
- rinse mouth well before reinserting
Do not refrigerate.
Tamper-Evident: Safety Sealed Tube. Do Not Use if tube tip is cut prior to opening.
Liquid—
- adults and children 2 years of age and older:
  - wipe liquid on with cotton, or cotton swab, or fingertip
  - apply to the affected area up to 4 times daily or as directed by a doctor/dentist
- children under 12 years of age: adult supervision should be given in the use of this product
- children under 2 years of age; consult a doctor/dentist
Tamper-Evident: Do Not Use if plastic blister or backing material is broken or if backing material is separated from the plastic.
Anbesol Junior Gel:
- to open tube, cut tip of the tube on score mark with scissors
- adults and children 2 years of age and older: apply to the affected area up to 4 times daily or as directed by a doctor/dentist
- children under 12 years of age: adult supervision should be given in the use of this product
- children under 2 years of age: consult a doctor/dentist
Tamper-Evident: Safety Sealed Tube. Do Not Use if tube tip is cut prior to opening.
Grape Baby Anbesol Gel:
- to open tube, cut tip of the tube on score mark with scissors
- children 4 months of age and older: apply to the affected area not more than 4 times daily or as directed by a doctor/dentist
- infants under 4 months of age: no recommended dosage or treatment except under the advice and supervision of a doctor/dentist
Tamper-Evident: Safety Sealed Tube. Do Not Use if tube tip is cut prior to opening.

Inactive Ingredients:
Maximum Strength Gel: benzyl alcohol, carbomer 934P, D&C yellow no. 10, FD&C blue no. 1, FD&C red no. 40, flavor, glycerin, methylparaben, polyethylene glycol, propylene glycol, saccharin.
Maximum Strength Liquid: benzyl alcohol, D&C yellow no. 10, FD&C blue no. 1, FD&C red no. 40, flavor, methylparaben, polyethylene glycol, propylene glycol, saccharin.
Junior Gel: artificial flavor, benzyl alcohol, carbomer 934P, D&C red no. 33, glycerin, methylparaben, polyethylene glycol, potassium acesulfame
Grape Baby Gel: benzoic acid, carbomer 934P, D&C red no. 33, edetate disodium, FD&C blue no. 1, flavor, glycerin, methylparaben, polyethylene glycol, propylparaben, saccharin, water

Storage: Store at 20–25°C (68–77°F)

How Supplied: Gels in .25 oz (7.1 g) or .33 oz (9.4 g) tubes, Maximum Strength Liquid in .31 fl oz (9 mL) tube.

ANBESOL COLD SORE THERAPY
Fever blister/Cold sore treatment

Active Ingredients:
Allantoin 1%,
Benzocaine 20%,
Camphor 3%,
White petrolatum 64.9%

Uses:
- temporarily relieves pain associated with fever blisters and cold sores
- relieves dryness and softens fever blisters and cold sores

Warnings: For external use only
Allergy alert: Do not use this product if you have a history of allergy to local anesthetics such as procaine, butacaine, benzocaine, or other "caine" anesthetics.
Do not use over deep or puncture wounds, infections, or lacerations. Consult a doctor.
When using this product • avoid contact with the eyes
- do not exceed recommended dosage
Stop use and ask a doctor if
- condition worsens
- symptoms persist for more than 7 days
- symptoms clear up and occur again within a few days
Keep out of reach of children. If swallowed, get medical help or contact a Poison Control Center right away.

Directions:
- to open tube, cut tip of the tube on score mark with scissors
- adults and children 2 years of age and older: apply to the affected area not more than 3 to 4 times daily
- children under 12 years of age: adult supervision should be given in the use of this product
- children under 2 years of age: consult a doctor
Tamper-Evident:
Safety Sealed Tube.
Do Not Use if tube tip is cut prior to opening.

Inactive Ingredients: aloe extract, benzyl alcohol, butylparaben, glyceryl stearate, isocetyl stearate, menthol, methylparaben, propylparaben, sodium lauryl sulfate, vitamin E, white wax
Other Information:
- store at 20–25°C (68–77°F)

How Supplied: 0.33 oz Tube

CHILDREN'S DIMETAPP® Cold & Allergy Elixir
Nasal Decongestant, Antihistamine

Active Ingredients:
Each 5 mL (1 teaspoonful) contains:
Brompheniramine Maleate, USP 1 mg
Pseudoephedrine Hydrochloride, USP 15 mg
Uses:
- temporarily relieves nasal congestion due to the common cold, hay fever or other upper respiratory allergies, or associated with sinusitis
- temporarily relieves these symptoms due to hay fever (allergic rhinitis):
  - runny nose
  - sneezing
  - itchy, watery eyes
  - itching of the nose or throat
- temporarily restores freer breathing through the nose

Warnings:
Do not use if you are now taking a prescription monoamine oxidase inhibitor (MAOI) (certain drugs for depression, psychiatric, or emotional conditions, or Parkinson's disease), or for 2 weeks after stopping the MAOI drug. If you do not know if your prescription drug contains an MAOI, ask a doctor or pharmacist before taking this product.
Ask a doctor before use if you have
- heart disease
- high blood pressure
- thyroid disease
- diabetes
- trouble urinating due to an enlarged prostate gland
- glaucoma
- a breathing problem such as emphysema or chronic bronchitis
Ask a doctor or pharmacist before use if you are taking sedatives or tranquilizers.
When using this product
- do not use more than directed
- drowsiness may occur
- avoid alcoholic beverages
- alcohol, sedatives, and tranquilizers may increase drowsiness
- be careful when driving a motor vehicle or operating machinery
- excitability may occur, especially in children
Stop use and ask a doctor if
- you get nervous, dizzy, or sleepless
- symptoms do not get better within 7 days or are accompanied by fever
If pregnant or breast-feeding, ask a health professional before use.
Keep out of reach of children. In case of overdose, get medical help or contact a Poison Control Center right away.

Directions:
- do not take more than 4 doses in any 24-hour period

age	dose
adults and children 12 years and over	4 tsp every 4 hours
children 6 to under 12 years	2 tsp every 4 hours
children under 6 years	ask a doctor

Each teaspoon contains: sodium 3 mg.
Store at 20–25°C (68–77°F).
Dosage cup provided.

Inactive Ingredients: artificial flavor, citric acid, FD&C blue no. 1, FD&C red no. 40, glycerin, propylene glycol, purified water, sodium benzoate, sodium citrate, sorbitol solution, sucralose

How Supplied: Purple, grape-flavored liquid in bottles of 4 fl oz, 8 fl oz, and 12 fl oz. Not a USP elixir.

CHILDREN'S DIMETAPP® DM COLD & COUGH Elixir
Nasal Decongestant, Antihistamine, Cough Suppressant

Active Ingredients: Each 5 mL (1 teaspoonful) contains

Brompheniramine Maleate, USP 1 mg
Dextromethorphan Hydrobromide, USP 5 mg
Pseudoephedrine Hydrochloride, USP 15 mg
Uses:
- temporarily relieves cough due to minor throat and bronchial irritation occurring with a cold, and nasal congestion due to the common cold, hay fever or other upper respiratory allergies, or associated with sinusitis
- temporarily relieves these symptoms due to hay fever (allergic rhinitis):
  - runny nose
  - sneezing
  - itchy, watery eyes
  - itching of the nose or throat
- temporarily restores freer breathing through the nose

Warnings:
Do not use if you are now taking a prescription monoamine oxidase inhibitor (MAOI) (certain drugs for depression, psychiatric, or emotional conditions, or Parkinson's disease), or for 2 weeks after stopping the MAOI drug. If you do not know if your prescription drug contains an MAOI, ask a doctor or pharmacist before taking this product.
Ask a doctor before use if you have
- heart disease
- high blood pressure
- thyroid disease
- diabetes
- trouble urinating due to an enlarged prostate gland
- glaucoma
- cough that occurs with too much phlegm (mucus)
- a breathing problem or persistent or chronic cough that lasts such as occurs with smoking, asthma, chronic bronchitis, or emphysema
Ask a doctor or pharmacist before use if you are taking sedatives or tranquilizers.
When using this product
- do not use more than directed
- may cause marked drowsiness
- avoid alcoholic beverages
- alcohol, sedatives, and tranquilizers may increase drowsiness
- be careful when driving a motor vehicle or operating machinery
- excitability may occur, especially in children
Stop use and ask a doctor if
- you get nervous, dizzy, or sleepless
- symptoms do not get better within 7 days or are accompanied by fever
- cough lasts more than 7 days, comes back, or is accompanied by fever, rash, or persistent headache. These could be signs of a serious condition
If pregnant or breast-feeding, ask a health professional before use.

Continued on next page

Dimetapp DM—Cont.

Keep out of reach of children. In case of overdose, get medical help or contact a Poison Control Center right away.

Directions:
• do not take more than 4 doses in any 24-hour period

Age	Dose
adults and children 12 years and over	4 tsp every 4 hours
children 6 to under 12 years	2 tsp every 4 hours
children under 6 years	ask a doctor

Each teaspoon contains: sodium 3 mg Store at 20–25°C (68–77°F). Dosage cup provided.

Inactive Ingredients: artificial flavor, citric acid, FD&C blue no. 1, FD&C red no. 40, glycerin, propylene glycol, purified water, sodium benzoate, sodium citrate, sorbitol solution, sucralose

How Supplied: Red, grape-flavored liquid in bottles of 4 fl oz and 8 fl oz. Not a USP Elixir.

CHILDREN'S DIMETAPP® LONG ACTING COUGH PLUS COLD SYRUP
Cough suppressant/Nasal decongestant

Active Ingredients (in each 5 mL tsp):
Dextromethorphan HBr, USP 7.5 mg
Pseudoephedrine HCl, USP 15 mg

Uses:
• temporarily relieves these symptoms occurring with a cold:
  • nasal congestion
  • cough due to minor throat and bronchial irritation

Warnings:
Do not use if you are now taking a prescription monoamine oxidase inhibitor (MAOI) (certain drugs for depression, psychiatric, or emotional conditions, or Parkinson's disease), or for 2 weeks after stopping the MAOI drug. If you do not know if your prescription drug contains an MAOI, ask a doctor or pharmacist before taking this product.
Ask a doctor before use if you have
• heart disease • high blood pressure
• thyroid disease • diabetes
• trouble urinating due to an enlarged prostate gland
• cough that occurs with too much phlegm (mucus)
• cough that lasts or is chronic such as occurs with smoking, asthma, or emphysema
When using this product do not use more than directed.
Stop use and ask a doctor if
• you get nervous, dizzy, or sleepless
• symptoms do not get better within 7 days or are accompanied by fever

• cough lasts more than 7 days, comes back, or is accompanied by fever, rash, or persistent headache. These could be signs of a serious condition.
If pregnant or breast-feeding, ask a health professional before use.
Keep out of reach of children. In case of overdose, get medical help or contact a Poison Control Center right away.

Directions:
• do not take more than 4 doses in any 24-hour period

age	dose
12 years and older	4 tsp every 6 hours
6 to under 12 years	2 tsp every 6 hours
2 to under 6 years	1 tsp every 6 hours
under 2 years	ask a doctor

Other Information: • each teaspoon contains: sodium 5 mg
• store at 20–25°C (68–77°F)
• dosage cup provided

Inactive Ingredients: citric acid, FD&C red no. 40, glycerin, high fructose corn syrup, natural flavor, propylene glycol, purified water, saccharin sodium, sodium benzoate, sodium chloride, sodium citrate

How Supplied: Bottles of 4 fl. oz.

CHILDREN'S DIMETAPP® ND
Non-Drowsy Allergy Syrup
Loratadine Syrup
Antihistamine

Drug Facts

Active Ingredient (in each 5 mL teaspoon):
Loratadine 5 mg

Uses: temporarily relieves these symptoms due to hay fever or other upper respiratory allergies:
• runny nose • sneezing • itchy, watery eyes
• itching of the nose or throat

Warnings:
Do not use if you have ever had an allergic reaction to this product or any of its ingredients
Ask a doctor before use if you have liver or kidney disease. Your doctor should determine if you need a different dose.
When using this product do not take more than directed. Taking more than directed may cause drowsiness.
Stop use and ask a doctor if an allergic reaction to this product occurs. Seek medical help right away.
If pregnant or breast-feeding, ask a health professional before use.
Keep out of reach of children. In case of overdose, get medical help or contact a

Poison Control Center right away.
Directions:

adults and children 6 years and over	2 teaspoonfuls daily; do not take more than 2 teaspoonfuls in 24 hours
children 2 to under 6 years of age	1 teaspoonful daily; do not take more than 1 teaspoonful in 24 hours
consumers with liver or kidney disease	ask a doctor

Other Information:
• store at 2–25°C (36–77°F)

Inactive Ingredients: artificial flavor, citric acid, glycerin, propylene glycol, purified water, sodium benzoate, sucrose

How Supplied: Bottles of 4 fl oz.

DIMETAPP®
Infant Drops Decongestant Plus Cough
Nasal decongestant/cough suppressant
Alcohol-Free

Active Ingredients: Each 0.8 mL contains: 2.5 mg Dextromethorphan Hydrobromide, USP; 7.5 mg Pseudoephedrine Hydrochloride, USP.

Indications: Temporarily relieves cough occurring with the common cold and temporarily relieves nasal congestion due to the common cold, hay fever, or other upper respiratory allergies, or associated with sinusitis

Warnings:
Do not use in a child who is taking a prescription monoamine oxidase inhibitor (MAOI) (certain drugs for depression, psychiatric, or emotional conditions, or Parkinson's disease), or for 2 weeks after stopping the MAOI drug. If you do not know if your child's prescription drug contains an MAOI, ask a doctor or pharmacist before giving this product.
Ask a doctor before use if your child has
• heart disease
• high blood pressure
• thyroid disease
• diabetes
• cough that occurs with too much phlegm (mucus)
• cough that lasts or is chronic such as occurs with asthma
When using this product
• do not use more than directed
Stop use and ask a doctor if
• your child gets nervous, dizzy, or sleepless
• symptoms do not get better within 7 days or are accompanied by fever
• cough lasts more than 7 days, comes back, or is accompanied by fever, rash, or persistent headache. These could be signs of a serious condition.
Keep out of reach of children. In case of overdose, get medical help or contact a Poison Control Center right away.

Directions: do not give more than 4 doses in any 24-hour period
- children 2–3 years: 1.6 mL every 4–6 hours or as directed by a physician
- children under 2 years: ask a doctor
- measure with the dosing device provided. Do not use with any other device.

Storage: Store at 20–25°C (68–77°F).

Inactive Ingredients: citric acid, flavors, glycerin, high fructose corn syrup, maltol, menthol, polyethylene glycol, propylene glycol, sodium benzoate, sorbitol, sucrose, water.

How Supplied: ½ oz bottle with oral dosing device.

FIBERCON® Caplets
Calcium Polycarbophil
Bulk-Forming Laxative

Active Ingredient
(in each caplet):
Calcium polycarbophil 625 mg (equivalent to 500 mg polycarbophil)

Uses:
- relieves constipation to help restore and maintain regularity
- this product generally produces bowel movement in 12 to 72 hours

Warnings:
Choking: Taking this product without adequate fluid may cause it to swell and block your throat or esophagus and may cause choking. Do not take this product if you have difficulty in swallowing. If you experience chest pain, vomiting, or difficulty in swallowing or breathing after taking this product, seek immediate medical attention.

Ask a doctor before use if you have
- abdominal pain, nausea, or vomiting
- a sudden change in bowel habits that persists over a period of 2 weeks

Ask a doctor or pharmacist before use if you are taking any other drug. Take this product 2 or more hours before or after other drugs. All laxatives may affect how other drugs work.

When using this product
- do not use for more than 7 days unless directed by a doctor
- do not take caplets more than 4 times in a 24 hour period unless directed by a doctor

Stop use and ask a doctor if rectal bleeding occurs or if you fail to have a bowel movement after use of this or any other laxative These could be signs of a serious condition.

Keep out of reach of children. In case of overdose, get medical help or contact a Poison Control Center right away.

Directions:
- take each dose of this product with at least 8 ounces (a full glass) of water or other fluid. Taking this product without enough liquid may cause choking. See choking warning.
- FiberCon works naturally so continued use for one to three days is normally required to provide full benefit. Dosage may vary according to diet, exercise, previous laxative use or severity of constipation.

Age	Recommended dose	Daily maximum
adults & children 12 years of age and over	2 caplets once a day	up to 4 times a day
children under 12 years	consult a physician	

[See table above]

Inactive Ingredients: calcium carbonate, caramel, crospovidone, hypromellose, light mineral oil, magnesium stearate, microcrystalline cellulose, povidone, silicon dioxide, sodium lauryl sulfate

Each caplet contains: 122 mg calcium.
Storage Protect contents from moisture. Store at 20–25°C (68–77°F)

How Supplied: Film-coated scored caplets.
Package of 36 caplets, and
Bottles of 60, 90 and 140 caplets.

PREPARATION H®
Hemorrhoidal Ointment and Maximum Strength Cream
PREPARATION H®
Hemorrhoidal Suppositories
PREPARATION H®
Hemorrhoidal Cooling Gel

Active Ingredients: Preparation H is available in ointment, cream, gel, and suppository product forms. The **Ointment** contains Petrolatum 71.9%, Mineral Oil 14%, Shark Liver Oil 3% and Phenylephrine HCl 0.25%.
The **Maximum Strength Cream** contains White Petrolatum 15%, Glycerin 14.4%, Pramoxine HCl 1% and Phenylephrine HCl 0.25%.
The **Suppositories** contain Cocoa Butter 85.5%, Shark Liver Oil 3%, and Phenylephrine HCl 0.25%.
The **Cooling Gel** contains Phenylephrine HCl 0.25% and Witch Hazel 50%.

Uses: **Preparation H Ointment and Suppositories**
- help relieve the local itching and discomfort associated with hemorrhoids
- temporarily shrink hemorrhoidal tissue and relieve burning
- temporarily provide a coating for relief of anorectal discomforts
- temporarily protect the inflamed, irritated anorectal surface to help make bowel movements less painful

Maximum Strength Cream
- for temporary relief of pain, soreness and burning
- helps relieve the local itching and discomfort associated with hemorrhoids
- temporarily shrinks hemorrhoidal tissue
- temporarily provides a coating for relief of anorectal discomforts
- temporarily protects the inflamed, irritated anorectal surface to help make bowel movements less painful

Cooling Gel
- helps relieve the local itching and discomfort associated with hemorrhoids
- temporarily relieves irritation and burning
- temporarily shrinks hemorrhoidal tissue

- aids in protecting irritated anorectal areas

Warnings:
For all product forms:
Ask a doctor before use if you have
- heart disease
- high blood pressure
- thyroid disease
- diabetes
- difficulty in urination due to enlargement of the prostate gland

Ask a doctor or pharmacist before use if you are presently taking a prescription drug for high blood pressure or depression.

When using this product do not exceed the recommended daily dosage unless directed by a doctor.

Stop use and ask a doctor if
- bleeding occurs
- condition worsens or does not improve within 7 days

If pregnant or breast-feeding, ask a health professional before use.

Keep out of reach of children. If swallowed, get medical help or contact a Poison Control Center right away.

Ointment: For external and/or intrarectal use only. Stop use and ask a doctor if introduction of applicator into the rectum causes additional pain.

Maximum Strength Cream: For external use only. Stop use and ask a doctor if an allergic reaction develops; or if the symptom being treated does not subside or if redness, irritation, swelling, pain, or other symptoms develop or increase.

Cooling Gel: For external use only.
When using this product do not put into the rectum by using fingers or any mechanical device or applicator.

Suppositories: For rectal use only.

Directions:
Ointment—
- adults: when practical, cleanse the affected area by patting or blotting with an appropriate cleansing wipe. Gently dry by patting or blotting with a tissue or a soft cloth before applying ointment.
- when first opening the tube, puncture foil seal with top end of cap
- apply to the affected area up to 4 times daily, especially at night, in the morning or after each bowel movement
- intrarectal use:
  - remove cover from applicator, attach applicator to tube, lubricate applicator well and gently insert applicator into the rectum
  - thoroughly cleanse applicator after each use and replace cover
- also apply ointment to external area
- regular use provides continual therapy for relief of symptoms
- children under 12 years of age: ask a doctor

Tamper-Evident: Do Not Use if tube seal under cap embossed with "H" is broken or missing.

Continued on next page

Preparation H—Cont.

Maximum Strength Cream—

- adults: when practical, cleanse the affected area by patting or blotting with an appropriate cleansing wipe. Gently dry by patting or blotting with a tissue or a soft cloth before applying cream.
- when first opening the tube, puncture foil seal with top end of cap
- apply externally or in the lower portion of the anal canal only
- apply externally to the affected area up to 4 times daily, especially at night, in the morning or after each bowel movement
- for application in the lower anal canal: remove cover from dispensing cap. Attach dispensing cap to tube. Lubricate dispensing cap well, then gently insert dispensing cap partway into the anus.
- thoroughly cleanse dispensing cap after each use and replace cover
- children under 12 years of age: ask a doctor

Tamper-Evident: Do Not Use if tube seal under cap embossed with "H" is broken or missing.

Suppositories—

- adults: when practical, cleanse the affected area by patting or blotting with an appropriate cleansing wipe. Gently dry by patting or blotting with a tissue or a soft cloth before insertion of this product.
- detach one suppository from the strip; remove the foil wrapper before inserting into the rectum as follows:
  - hold suppository with rounded end up
  - carefully separate foil tabs by inserting tip of fingernail at end marked "peel down"
  - slowly and evenly peel apart (do not tear) foil by pulling tabs down both sides, to expose the suppository
  - remove exposed suppository from wrapper
  - insert one suppository into the rectum up to 4 times daily, especially at night, in the morning or after each bowel movement
- children under 12 years of age: ask a doctor

Tamper-Evident: Individually quality sealed for your protection. Do Not Use if foil imprinted "PREPARATION H" is torn or damaged.

Cooling Gel—

- adults: when practical, cleanse the affected area by patting or blotting with an appropriate cleansing wipe. Gently dry by patting or blotting with a tissue or a soft cloth before applying gel.
- when first opening the tube, puncture foil seal with top end of cap
- apply externally to the affected area up to 4 times daily, especially at night, in the morning or after each bowel movement
- children under 12 years of age: ask a doctor

Tamper-Evident: Do Not Use if tube seal under cap embossed with "H" is broken or missing.

Inactive Ingredients: Ointment—
benzoic acid, BHA, BHT, corn oil, glycerin, lanolin, lanolin alcohol, methylparaben, paraffin, propylparaben, thyme oil, tocopherol, water, wax

Maximum Strength Cream—aloe barbadensis leaf extract, BHA, carboxymethylcellulose sodium, cetyl alcohol, citric acid, edetate disodium, glyceryl stearate, laureth-23, methylparaben, mineral oil, panthenol, propyl gallate, propylene glycol, propylparaben, purified water, sodium benzoate, steareth-2, steareth-20, stearyl alcohol, tocopherol, vitamin E, xanthan gum
Suppositories—methylparaben, propylparaben, starch
Cooling Gel—aloe barbadensis gel, benzophenone-4, edetate disodium, hydroxyethylcellulose, methylparaben, polysorbate 80, propylene glycol, propylparaben, sodium citrate, vitamin E, water

Storage: Store at 20–25°C (68–77°F).

How Supplied: Ointment: Net Wt. 1 oz and 2 oz **Cream:** Net Wt. 0.9 oz and 1.8 oz **Suppositories:** 12's, 24's and 48's. **Cooling Gel:** Net Wt. 0.9 oz and 1.8 oz

---

PREPARATION H® HYDROCORTISONE CREAM
Anti-itch cream

Active Ingredient:
Hydrocortisone 1%

Uses:
- temporary relief of external anal itching
- temporary relief of itching associated with minor skin irritations and rashes
- other uses of this product should be only under the advice and supervision of a doctor

Warnings:
For external use only
Do not use for the treatment of diaper rash. Consult a doctor.
When using this product
- avoid contact with the eyes
- do not exceed the recommended daily dosage unless directed by a doctor
- do not put into the rectum by using fingers or any mechanical device or applicator

Stop use and ask a doctor if
- bleeding occurs
- condition worsens
- symptoms persist for more than 7 days or clear up and occur again within a few days. Do not begin use of any other hydrocortisone product unless you have consulted a doctor.
Keep out of reach of children. If swallowed, get medical help or contact a Poison Control Center right away.

Directions:
- adults: when practical, cleanse the affected area by patting or blotting with an appropriate cleansing wipe. Gently dry by patting or blotting with a tissue or soft cloth before application of this product.
- when first opening the tube, puncture foil seal with top end of cap
- adults and children 12 years of age and older: apply to the affected area not more than 3 to 4 times daily
- children under 12 years of age: do not use, consult a doctor

Tamper-Evident: Do Not Use if tube seal under cap embossed with "H" is broken or missing.

Inactive Ingredients: BHA, carboxymethylcellulose sodium, cetyl alcohol, citric acid, edetate disodium, glycerin, glyceryl oleate, glyceryl stearate, lanolin, methylparaben, petrolatum, propyl gallate, propylene glycol, propylparaben, simethicone, sodium benzoate, sodium lauryl sulfate, stearyl alcohol, water, xanthan gum.
Storage: Store at 20–25 °C (68–77 °F)

How Supplied: 0.9 oz. tubes

PREPARATION H®
MEDICATED WIPES

Active Ingredient: Witch Hazel 50%.
Uses:
- helps relieve the local itching and discomfort associated with hemorrhoids
- temporary relief of irritation and burning
- aids in protecting irritated anorectal areas
- **for vaginal care**—cleanse the area by gently wiping, patting or blotting. Repeat as needed.
- **for use as a moist compress**—if necessary, first cleanse the area as described below. Fold wipe to desired size and place in contact with tissue for a soothing and cooling effect. Leave in place for up to 15 minutes and repeat as needed.

Warnings:
For external use only
When using this product
- do not exceed the recommended daily dosage unless directed by a doctor
- do not put this product into the rectum by using fingers or any mechanical device or applicator
Stop use and ask a doctor if
- bleeding occurs
- condition worsens or does not improve within 7 days
If pregnant or breast-feeding, ask a health professional before use. **Keep out of reach of children.** If swallowed, get medical help or contact a Poison Control Center right away.

Directions:
Container and Refill:
- remove tab on right side of wipes pouch label and peel back to open
- grab the top wipe at the edge of the center fold and pull out of pouch
- carefully reseal label on pouch after each use to retain moistness
Travel Pack, Container and Refill:
- adults: unfold wipe and cleanse the area by gently wiping, patting or blotting. If necessary, repeat until all matter is removed from the area.
- use up to 6 times daily or after each bowel movement and before applying topical hemorrhoidal treatments, and then discard
- children under 12 years of age: consult a doctor
- store at 20–25°C (68–77°F)
- for best results, flush only one or two wipes at a time

Tamper-Evident (Container & Refill): Pouch quality sealed for your protection. Do Not Use if tear strip imprinted "Safety Sealed" is torn or missing Tamper-Evident (Travel Pack): Each wipe is enclosed in a sealed foil pouch. Do Not Use if the pouch is broken or torn.

Inactive Ingredients: aloe barbadensis gel, capryl/capramidopropyl betaine, citric acid, diazolidinyl urea, glycerin, methylparaben, propylene glycol, propylparaben, sodium citrate, water.

How Supplied: Containers of 48 wipes. Refills of 48 wipes. 8 count travel pack. 10 count portable pack.

PRIMATENE® Mist
Epinephrine Inhalation Aerosol Bronchodilator

Active Ingredient: (in each inhalation)
Epinephrine 0.22 mg

Uses:
- temporarily relieves shortness of breath, tightness of chest, and wheezing due to bronchial asthma
- eases breathing for asthma patients by reducing spasms of bronchial muscles

Warnings:
For inhalation only
Do not use
- unless a doctor has said you have asthma
- if you are now taking a prescription monoamine oxidase inhibitor (MAOI) (certain drugs for depression, psychiatric, or emotional conditions, or Parkinson's disease), or for 2 weeks after stopping the MAOI drug If you do not know if your prescription drug contains an MAOI, ask a doctor or pharmacist before taking this product
Ask a doctor before use if you have
- heart disease • thyroid disease
- diabetes • high blood pressure
- ever been hospitalized for asthma
- trouble urinating due to an enlarged prostate gland
Ask a doctor or pharmacist before use if you are taking any prescription drug for asthma
When using this product
- overuse may cause nervousness, rapid heart beat, and heart problems
- do not continue to use, but seek medical assistance immediately if symptoms are not relieved within 20 minutes or become worse
- do not puncture or throw into incinerator. Contents under pressure.
- do not use or store near open flame or heat above 120°F (49°C). May cause bursting.
Contains CFC 12, 114, substances which harm public health and environment by destroying ozone in the upper atmosphere
If pregnant or breast-feeding, ask a health professional before use.
Keep out of reach of children. In case of overdose, get medical help or contact a Poison Control Center right away.

Directions:
- **do not use more often or at higher doses unless directed by a doctor**
- supervise children using this product
- adults and children 4 years and over: start with one inhalation, then wait at least 1 minute. If not relieved, use once more. Do not use again for at least 3 hours.
- children under 4 years of age: ask a doctor

Directions For Use of Mouthpiece:
The Primatene Mist mouthpiece, which is enclosed in the Primatene Mist 15 mL size (not the refill size), should be used for inhalation only with Primatene Mist.
1. Take plastic cap off mouthpiece. (For refills, use mouthpiece from previous purchase.)
2. Take plastic mouthpiece off bottle.
3. Place other end of mouthpiece on bottle.
4. Turn bottle upside down. Place thumb on bottom of mouthpiece over circular button and forefinger on top of vial. Empty the lungs as completely as possible by exhaling.
5. Place mouthpiece in mouth with lips closed around opening. Inhale deeply while squeezing mouthpiece and bottle together. Release immediately and remove unit from mouth. Complete taking the deep breath, drawing the medication into your lungs and holding breath as long as comfortable.
6. Exhale slowly keeping lips nearly closed. This helps distribute the medication in the lungs.
7. Replace plastic cap on mouthpiece.

Care of the Mouthpiece:
The Primatene Mist mouthpiece should be washed once daily with soap and hot water, and rinsed thoroughly. Then it should be dried with a clean, lint-free cloth.

Other Information:
- store at room temperature, between 20–25°C (68–77°F) • contains no sulfites

Inactive Ingredients: ascorbic acid, dehydrated alcohol (34%), dichlorodifluoromethane (CFC 12), dichlorotetrafluoroethane (CFC 114), hydrochloric acid, nitric acid, purified water

How Supplied:
$1/2$ Fl oz (15 mL) With Mouthpiece.
$1/2$ Fl oz (15 mL) Refill
$3/4$ Fl oz (22.5 mL) Refill

PRIMATENE® Tablets
Bronchodilator, Expectorant

Active Ingredients (in each tablet):

Ephedrine HCl, USP	12.5 mg
Guaifenesin, USP	200 mg

Uses:
- temporarily relieves shortness of breath, tightness of chest, and wheezing due to bronchial asthma
- eases breathing for asthma patients by reducing spasms of bronchial muscles
- helps loosen phlegm (mucus) and thin bronchial secretions to rid bronchial passageways of bothersome mucus, and to make coughs more productive

Warnings:
Do not use
- unless a diagnosis of asthma has been made by a doctor
- if you are now taking a prescription monoamine oxidase inhibitor (MAOI) (certain drugs for depression, psychiatric, or emotional conditions, or Parkinson's disease), or for 2 weeks after stopping the MAOI drug If you do not know if your prescription drug contains an MAOI, ask a doctor or pharmacist before taking this product
Ask a doctor before use if you have
- heart disease • high blood pressure
- thyroid disease • diabetes
- trouble urinating due to an enlarged prostate gland
- ever been hospitalized for asthma
- cough that occurs with too much phlegm (mucus)
- cough that lasts or is chronic such as occurs with smoking, asthma, chronic bronchitis, or emphysema
Ask a doctor or pharmacist before use if you are taking any prescription drug for asthma
When using this product some users may experience nervousness, tremor, sleeplessness, nausea, and loss of appetite
Stop use and ask a doctor if
- symptoms are not relieved within 1 hour or become worse
- nervousness, tremor, sleeplessness, nausea, and loss of appetite persist or become worse
- cough lasts more than 7 days, comes back, or occurs with fever, rash, or persistent headache These could be signs of a serious condition
If pregnant or breast-feeding, ask a health professional before use.
Keep out of reach of children. In case of overdose, get medical help or contact a Poison Control Center right away.

Directions:
- do not use more than dosage below unless directed by a doctor
- adults and children 12 years and over: take 2 tablets initially, then 2 tablets every 4 hours, as needed, not to exceed 12 tablets in 24 hours
- children under 12 years: ask a doctor

Other Information:
- store at 20–25°C (68–77°F)

Inactive Ingredients: crospovidone, D&C yellow no. 10 aluminum lake, FD&C yellow no. 6 aluminum lake, magnesium stearate, microcrystalline cellulose, povidone, silicon dioxide (colloidal)

How Supplied: Available in 24 and 60 tablet blister cartons.

ROBITUSSIN® Expectorant

Active Ingredient: (in each 5 mL tsp) Guaifenesin, USP 100 mg

Use: helps loosen phlegm (mucus) and thin bronchial secretions to make coughs more productive

Continued on next page

Robitussin—Cont.

Warnings:
Ask a doctor before use if you have
- cough that occurs with too much phlegm (mucus)
- cough that lasts or is chronic such as occurs with smoking, asthma, chronic bronchitis, or emphysema

Stop use and ask a doctor if cough lasts more than 7 days, comes back, or is accompanied by fever, rash, or persistent headache. These could be signs of a serious condition.

If pregnant or breast-feeding, ask a health professional before use.

Keep out of reach of children. In case of overdose, get medical help or contact a Poison Control Center right away.

Directions:
- do not take more than 6 doses in any 24-hour period
- adults and children 12 yrs and over: 2–4 tsp every 4 hours
- children 6 to under 12 yrs: 1–2 tsp every 4 hours
- children 2 to under 6 yrs: ½–1 tsp every 4 hours
- children under 2 yrs: ask a doctor

Other Information:
- store at 20–25°C (68–77°F)
- alcohol-free
- dosage cup provided

Inactive Ingredients: caramel, citric acid, FD&C red no. 40, flavors, glucose, glycerin, high fructose corn syrup, menthol, saccharin sodium, sodium benzoate, water.

How Supplied: Bottles of 4 fl oz, 8 fl oz.

ROBITUSSIN® ALLERGY & COUGH SYRUP
Nasal Decongestant, Cough Suppressant, Antihistamine

Active Ingredients: (in each 5 mL tsp)
Brompheniramine maleate, USP 2 mg
Dextromethorphan HBr, USP 10 mg
Pseudoephedrine HCl, USP 30 mg

Uses:
- temporarily relieves these symptoms due to hay fever (allergic rhinitis):
  - runny nose • sneezing • itchy, watery eyes • itching of the nose or throat
  - nasal congestion
- temporarily controls cough due to minor throat and bronchial irritation associated with inhaled irritants
- temporarily restores freer breathing through the nose

Warnings:
Do not use if you are now taking a prescription monoamine oxidase inhibitor (MAOI) (certain drugs for depression, psychiatric, or emotional conditions, or Parkinson's disease), or for 2 weeks after stopping the MAOI drug. If you do not know if your prescription drug contains an MAOI, ask a doctor or pharmacist before taking this product.

Ask a doctor before use if you have
- heart disease • high blood pressure
- thyroid disease • diabetes
- trouble urinating due to an enlarged prostate gland • glaucoma
- cough that occurs with too much phlegm (mucus)
- cough that lasts or is chronic such as occurs with smoking, asthma, chronic bronchitis or emphysema

Ask a doctor or pharmacist before use if you are taking sedatives or tranquilizers

When using this product
- **do not use more than directed**
- marked drowsiness may occur
- avoid alcoholic beverages
- alcohol, sedatives, and tranquilizers may increase drowsiness
- be careful when driving a motor vehicle or operating machinery
- excitability may occur, especially in children

Stop use and ask a doctor if
- you get nervous, dizzy, or sleepless
- symptoms do not get better within 7 days or are accompanied by fever
- cough lasts more than 7 days, comes back, or is accompanied by fever, rash, or persistent headache. These could be signs of a serious condition.

If pregnant or breast-feeding, ask a health professional before use.

Keep out of reach of children. In case of overdose, get medical help or contact a Poison Control Center right away.

Directions:
- do not take more than 4 doses in any 24-hour period
- adults and children 12 yrs and over: 2 tsp every 4 hours
- children 6 to under 12 yrs: 1 tsp every 4 hours
- children under 6 yrs: ask a doctor

Other Information:
- store at 20–25°C (68–77°F)
- alcohol free
- dosage cup provided

Inactive Ingredients: artificial flavor, citric acid, glycerin, propylene glycol, saccharin sodium, sodium benzoate, sorbitol, water

How Supplied: Bottles of 4 fl. oz.

ROBITUSSIN® COUGH & COLD
Liquid-filled Capsules
Nasal Decongestant, Expectorant, Cough Suppressant

Active Ingredients (in each capsule):
Dextromethorphan HBr, USP 10 mg
Guaifenesin, USP 200 mg
Pseudoephedrine HCl, USP 30 mg

Uses:
- temporarily relieves nasal congestion, and cough due to minor throat and bronchial irritation occurring with the common cold
- helps loosen phlegm (mucus) and thin bronchial secretions to drain bronchial tubes
- temporarily relieves nasal congestion associated with hay fever or other upper respiratory allergies, or associated with sinusitis

Warnings:
Do not use if you are now taking a prescription monoamine oxidase inhibitor (MAOI) (certain drugs for depression, psychiatric, or emotional conditions, or Parkinson's disease), or for 2 weeks after stopping the MAOI drug. If you do not know if your prescription drug contains an MAOI, ask a doctor or pharmacist before taking this product.

Ask a doctor before use if you have
- heart disease • high blood pressure
- thyroid disease • diabetes
- trouble urinating due to an enlarged prostate gland
- cough that occurs with too much phlegm (mucus)
- cough that lasts or is chronic such as occurs with smoking, asthma, chronic bronchitis, or emphysema

When using this product do not use more than directed.

Stop use and ask a doctor if
- you get nervous, dizzy, or sleepless
- symptoms do not get better within 7 days or are accompanied by fever
- cough lasts more than 7 days, comes back, or is accompanied by fever, rash, or persistent headache. These could be signs of a serious condition.

If pregnant or breast-feeding, ask a health professional before use.

Keep out of reach of children. In case of overdose, get medical help or contact a Poison Control Center right away.

Directions:
- do not use more than 4 doses in any 24-hr period
- adults and children 12 yrs and over: 2 capsules every 4 hours
- children 6 to under 12 yrs: 1 capsule every 4 hours
- children under 6 years: ask a doctor

Other Information:
- store at 20–25°C (68–77°F)

Inactive Ingredients (Capsules): FD&C blue no. 1, FD&C red no. 40, gelatin, glycerin, mannitol, pharmaceutical glaze, polyethylene glycol, povidone, propylene glycol, sorbitan, sorbitol, titanium dioxide, water

How Supplied: Capsules in packages of 12 (individually packaged).

ROBITUSSIN® COUGH, COLD & FLU Liquid-filled Capsules
Pain Reliever/Fever Reducer, Cough Suppressant, Nasal Decongestant, Expectorant

Active Ingredients (in each capsule):
Acetaminophen, USP 250 mg
Dextromethorphan HBr, USP 10 mg
Guaifenesin, USP 100 mg
Pseudoephedrine HCl, USP 30 mg

Uses:
- temporarily relieves these symptoms associated with a cold, or flu:
  - headache • fever
  - minor aches and pains
- temporarily relieves nasal congestion, and cough due to minor throat and bronchial irritation occurring with a cold
- helps loosen phlegm (mucus) and thin bronchial secretions to drain bronchial tubes

Warnings:

Alcohol warning: If you consume 3 or more alcoholic drinks every day, ask your doctor whether you should take acetaminophen or other pain relievers/fever reducers. Acetaminophen may cause liver damage.

Taking more than the recommended dose (overdose) may cause serious liver damage.

Do not use

- if you are now taking a prescription monoamine oxidase inhibitor (MAOI) (certain drugs for depression, psychiatric, or emotional conditions, or Parkinson's disease), or for 2 weeks after stopping the MAOI drug. If you do not know if your prescription drug contains an MAOI, ask a doctor or pharmacist before taking this product.
- with any other product containing acetaminophen as this may lead to an overdose. Overdose requires prompt medical attention even if you do not notice any signs or symptoms.

Ask a doctor before use if you have

- heart disease • high blood pressure
- thyroid disease • diabetes
- trouble urinating due to an enlarged prostate gland
- cough that occurs with too much phlegm (mucus)
- cough that lasts or is chronic such as occurs with smoking, asthma, chronic bronchitis, or emphysema

Ask a doctor or pharmacist before use if you are taking any other product containing acetaminophen, or any other pain reliever/fever reducer.

When using this product do not use more than directed.

Stop use and ask a doctor if

- you get nervous, dizzy, or sleepless
- pain, cough, or nasal congestion gets worse or lasts more than 7 days
- fever gets worse or lasts more than 3 days
- redness or swelling is present
- new symptoms occur
- cough comes back or occurs with rash or headache that lasts. These could be signs of a serious condition.

If pregnant or breast-feeding, ask a health professional before use.

Keep out of reach of children. In case of overdose, get medical help or contact a Poison Control Center right away. Prompt medical attention is critical for adults as well as for children, even if you do not notice any signs or symptoms.

Directions:

- do not use more than 4 doses in any 24-hour period.
- do not exceed recommended dosage. Taking more than the recommended dose (overdose) may cause serious liver damage.
- adults and children 12 yrs and over: 2 capsules every 4 hours
- children under 12 years: ask a doctor

Other Information:

- **each capsule contains:** sodium 3mg
- store at 20–25°C (68–77°F)
- avoid excessive heat above 40°C (104°F). Protect from light.

Inactive Ingredients: D&C yellow no. 10, FD&C red no. 40, fractionated coconut oil, gelatin, glycerin, mannitol, pharmaceutical ink, polyethylene glycol, povidone, propylene glycol, purified water, sorbitol, sorbitol anhydrides

How Supplied: In blister packs of 12 liquid-filled capsules.

ROBITUSSIN® SEVERE CONGESTION Liquid-filled Capsules
Nasal Decongestant, Expectorant

Active Ingredients:
(in each capsule)

Guaifenesin, USP 200 mg
Pseudoephedrine HCl USP 30 mg

Uses:

- temporarily relieves nasal congestion associated with
  - the common cold
  - hay fever
  - upper respiratory allergies
  - sinusitis
- helps loosen phlegm (mucus) and thin bronchial secretions to make coughs more productive

Warnings:

Do not use if you are now taking a prescription monoamine oxidase inhibitor (MAOI) (certain drugs for depression, psychiatric, or emotional conditions, or Parkinson's disease), or for 2 weeks after stopping the MAOI drug. If you do not know if your prescription drug contains an MAOI, ask a doctor or pharmacist before taking this product.

Ask a doctor before use if you have

- heart disease • high blood pressure
- thyroid disease • diabetes
- trouble urinating due to an enlarged prostate gland
- cough that occurs with too much phlegm (mucus)
- cough that lasts or is chronic such as occurs with smoking, asthma, chronic bronchitis, or emphysema

When using this product do not use more than directed.

Stop use and ask a doctor if

- you get nervous, dizzy, or sleepless
- symptoms do not get better within 7 days or are accompanied by fever
- cough lasts more than 7 days, comes back, or is accompanied by fever, rash, or persistent headache. These could be signs of a serious condition.

If pregnant or breast-feeding, ask a health professional before use.

Keep out of reach of children. In case of overdose, get medical help or contact a Poison Control Center right away.

Directions:

- do not use more than 4 doses in any 24-hr period
- adults and children 12 yrs and over: 2 capsules every 4 hours
- children 6 to under 12 yrs: 1 capsule every 4 hours
- children under 6 yrs: ask a doctor

Other Information: store at 20–25°C (68–77°F).

Inactive Ingredients: FD&C green no. 3, gelatin, glycerin, mannitol, pharmaceutical glaze, polyethylene glycol, povidone, propylene glycol, sorbitan, sorbitol, titanium dioxide, water

How Supplied: Blister Packs of 12's.

ROBITUSSIN® COUGH DROPS
Menthol Eucalyptus, Cherry, and Honey-Lemon Flavors

Active Ingredient: (in each drop)
Menthol Eucalyptus:
Menthol, USP 10 mg
Cherry and Honey-Lemon:
Menthol, USP 5 mg

Uses:

- temporarily relieves
  - occasional minor irritation, pain, sore mouth, and sore throat
  - cough associated with a cold or inhaled irritants

Warnings:

Sore throat warning: Severe or persistent sore throat or sore throat accompanied by high fever, headache, nausea, and vomiting may be serious. Consult a doctor right away. Do not use more than 2 days or give to children under 3 years of age unless directed by a doctor

Ask a doctor before use if you have

- cough that occurs with too much phlegm (mucus)
- cough that lasts or is chronic such as occurs with smoking, asthma, or emphysema

Stop use and ask a doctor if cough lasts more than 7 days, comes back, or is accompanied by fever, rash, or persistent headache. These could be signs of a serious condition.

If pregnant or breast-feeding, ask a health professional before use.

Keep out of reach of children.

Directions:

- adults and children 4 years and over: allow 1 drop to dissolve slowly in the mouth
  - for sore throat: may be repeated every 2 hours, as needed, or as directed by a doctor
  - for cough: may be repeated every 2 hours, as needed, or as directed by a doctor
- children under 4 years of age: ask a doctor

Other Information: store at 20–25°C (68–77°F).

Inactive Ingredients:

Menthol Eucalyptus: corn syrup, eucalyptus oil, flavor, sucrose
Cherry: corn syrup, FD&C red no. 40, flavor, methylparaben, propylparaben, sodium benzoate, sucrose
Honey-Lemon: citric acid, corn syrup, D&C yellow no. 10, FD&C yellow no. 6, honey, lemon oil, methylparaben, povidone, propylparaben, sodium benzoate, sucrose

How Supplied: All 3 flavors of Robitussin Cough Drops are available in bags of 25 drops.

Continued on next page

ROBITUSSIN® FLU
Pain Reliever/Fever Reducer, Nasal Decongestant, Cough Suppressant, Antihistamine

Active Ingredients: (in each 5 mL tsp)
Acetaminophen, USP 160 mg
Chlorpheniramine maleate, USP 1 mg
Dextromethorphan HBr, USP 5 mg
Pseudoephedrine HCl, USP 15 mg

Uses:
- temporarily relieves these symptoms occurring with a cold or flu, hay fever, or other upper respiratory allergies:
- headache • cough • runny nose • itching of the nose or throat • nasal congestion • sneezing • minor aches and pains • itchy, watery eyes • fever

Warnings:
Alcohol warning: If you consume 3 or more alcoholic drinks every day, ask your doctor whether you should take acetaminophen or other pain relievers/fever reducers. Acetaminophen may cause liver damage.
Taking more than the recommended dose (overdose) may cause serious liver damage.
Do not use:
- if you are now taking a prescription monoamine oxidase inhibitor (MAOI) (certain drugs for depression, psychiatric, or emotional conditions, or Parkinson's disease), or for 2 weeks after stopping the MAOI drug. If you do not know if your prescription drug contains an MAOI, ask a doctor or pharmacist before taking this product.
- with any other product containing acetaminophen as this may lead to an overdose. Overdose requires prompt medical attention even if you do not notice any signs or symptoms.
Ask a doctor before use if you have
- heart disease • thyroid disease
- trouble urinating due to an enlarged prostate gland • diabetes
- cough that occurs with too much phlegm (mucus) • glaucoma
- a breathing problem or chronic cough that lasts or as occurs with smoking, asthma, chronic bronchitis, or emphysema • high blood pressure
Ask a doctor or pharmacist before use if you are • taking any other product containing acetaminophen, or any other pain reliever/fever reducer
- taking sedatives or tranquilizers
When using this product
- **do not use more than directed**
- marked drowsiness may occur
- alcohol, sedatives, and tranquilizers may increase drowsiness
- be careful when driving a motor vehicle or operating machinery
- excitability may occur, especially in children • avoid alcoholic drinks
Stop use and ask a doctor if
- you get nervous, dizzy, or sleepless
- pain, cough, or nasal congestion gets worse or lasts more than 5 days (children) or 7 days (adults)
- fever gets worse or lasts more than 3 days
- redness or swelling is present
- cough comes back or occurs with rash or headache that lasts. These could be signs of a serious condition.
- new symptoms occur

If pregnant or breast-feeding, ask a health professional before use.
Keep out of reach of children. In case of overdose, get medical help or contact a Poison Control Center right away. Prompt medical attention is critical for adults as well as for children, even if you do not notice any signs or symptoms.

Directions:
- do not take more than 4 doses in any 24-hour period
- do not exceed recommended dosage. Taking more than the recommended dose (overdose) may cause serious liver damage.
- adults and children 12 yrs and over: 4 tsp every 4 hours
- children 6 to under 12 yrs: 2 tsp every 4 hours
- children under 6 yrs: ask a doctor

Other Information:
- **each teaspoon contains:** sodium 4 mg
- store at 20–25°C (68–77°F)
- alcohol free

Inactive Ingredients: citric acid, D&C red no. 33, FD&C yellow no. 6, flavor, glycerin, high fructose corn syrup, polyethylene glycol, purified water, sodium benzoate, sodium citrate, sorbitol solution, sucralose

How Supplied: Bottles of 4 fl. oz.

ROBITUSSIN®
HONEY COUGH Drops
Honey-Lemon Tea, Honey Citrus, Natural Honey Center and Almond with Natural Honey Center

Active Ingredient (in each drop):
Natural Honey Center and *Honey Lemon Tea:*
Menthol, USP 5 mg
Honey Citrus and Almond with Natural Honey Center:
Menthol, USP 2.5 mg

Uses:
- temporarily relieves
  - occasional minor irritation, pain, sore mouth, and sore throat
  - cough associated with a cold or inhaled irritants

Warnings:
Sore throat warning: Severe or persistent sore throat or sore throat accompanied by high fever, headache, nausea, and vomiting may be serious. Consult a doctor right away. Do not use more than 2 days or give to children under 3 years of age unless directed by a doctor.
Ask a doctor before use if you have
- cough that occurs with too much phlegm (mucus)
- cough that lasts or is chronic such as occurs with smoking, asthma, or emphysema
Stop use and ask a doctor if cough lasts more than 7 days, comes back, or is accompanied by fever, rash, or persistent headache. These could be signs of a serious condition.
If pregnant or breast-feeding, ask a health professional before use.

Keep out of reach of children.

Directions:
- adults and children 4 years and over:
  - for cough or sore throat: *Honey Lemon Tea and Natural Honey Center*—allow 1 drop to dissolve slowly in mouth.
    May be repeated every 2 hours, as needed, or as directed by a doctor.
    Honey Citrus and Almond with Natural Honey Center—for cough or sore throat: allow 2 drops to dissolve slowly in mouth.
    May be repeated every 2 hours, as needed, or as directed by a doctor.
- children under 4 years: ask a doctor
Other Information: store at 20–25°C (68–77°F).

Inactive Ingredients:
Natural Honey Center: caramel, corn syrup, glycerin, high fructose corn syrup, honey, natural herbal flavor, sorbitol, sucrose
Honey Lemon Tea: caramel, citric acid, corn syrup, honey, natural flavor, sucrose, tea extract
Honey Citrus: citric acid, corn syrup, flavors, honey, sucrose
Almond with Natural Honey Center: caramel, corn syrup, glycerin, honey, natural almond flavor, natural anise flavor, natural coriander flavor, natural fennel flavor, natural honey flavor and other natural flavors, sorbitol, sucrose

How Supplied: Honey Lemon Tea and Honey Citrus in bags of 25 drops. Natural Honey Center and Almond with Natural Honey center in bags of 20 drops.

ROBITUSSIN® PM Cough & Cold
Nasal Decongestant, Cough Suppressant, Antihistamine

Active Ingredients: (in each 5 mL tsp):
Chlorpheniramine maleate, USP 1 mg
Dextromethorphan HBr, USP 7.5 mg
Pseudoephedrine HCl, USP 15 mg

Uses:
- temporarily relieves these symptoms occurring with a cold:
  - cough due to minor throat and bronchial irritation
  - nasal congestion
- temporarily relieves these symptoms due to hay fever or other upper respiratory allergies: • runny nose • sneezing • itchy, watery eyes • itching of the nose or throat

Warnings:
Do not use if you are now taking a prescription monoamine oxidase inhibitor (MAOI) (certain drugs for depression, psychiatric, or emotional conditions, or Parkinson's disease), or for 2 weeks after stopping the MAOI drug. If you do not know if your prescription drug contains an MAOI, ask a doctor or pharmacist before taking this product.
Ask a doctor before use if you have
- heart disease • high blood pressure
- thyroid disease • diabetes • trouble urinating due to an enlarged prostate gland • glaucoma • cough that occurs

with too much phlegm (mucus) • a breathing problem or chronic cough that lasts or as occurs with smoking, asthma, chronic bronchitis, or emphysema

Ask a doctor or pharmacist before use if you are taking sedatives or tranquilizers.

When using this product
• do not use more than directed
• marked drowsiness may occur
• avoid alcoholic drinks
• alcohol, sedatives, and tranquilizers may increase drowsiness
• be careful when driving a motor vehicle or operating machinery
• excitability may occur, especially in children

Stop use and ask a doctor if
• you get nervous, dizzy, or sleepless
• symptoms do not get better within 7 days or are accompanied by fever
• cough lasts more than 7 days, comes back, or is accompanied by fever, rash, or persistent headache. These could be signs of a serious condition.

If pregnant or breast-feeding, ask a health professional before use.

Keep out of reach of children. In case of overdose, get medical help or contact a Poison Control Center right away.

Directions:
• do not take more than 4 doses in any 24-hour period
• adults and children 12 years and older: 4 tsp every 6 hours
• children 6 to under 12 years: 2 tsp every 6 hours
• children under 6 years: ask a doctor

Other Information:
• **each teaspoon contains:** sodium 6 mg
• store at 20–25°C (68–77°F)
• not USP. Meets specifications when tested with a validated non-USP assay method
• dosage cup provided

Inactive Ingredients: citric acid, FD&C red no. 40, glycerin, high fructose corn syrup, natural and artificial flavors, propylene glycol, purified water, saccharin sodium, sodium benzoate, sodium chloride, sodium citrate

How Supplied:
Bottles of 4 fl. oz.

ROBITUSSIN® PE Syrup
Nasal Decongestant, Expectorant

Active Ingredients:
(in each 5 mL tsp):

Guaifenesin, USP 100 mg
Pseudoephedrine HCl, USP 30 mg

Uses: • temporarily relieves nasal congestion due to a cold • helps loosen phlegm (mucus) and thin bronchial secretions to make coughs more productive.

Warnings:
Do not use if you are now taking a prescription monoamine oxidase inhibitor (MAOI) (certain drugs for depression, psychiatric, or emotional conditions, or Parkinson's disease), or for 2 weeks after stopping the MAOI drug. If you do not

know if your prescription drug contains an MAOI, ask a doctor or pharmacist before taking this product.

Ask a doctor before use if you have
• heart disease • high blood pressure
• thyroid disease • diabetes
• trouble urinating due to an enlarged prostate gland
• cough that occurs with too much phlegm (mucus)
• cough that lasts or is chronic such as occurs with smoking, asthma, chronic bronchitis, or emphysema

When using this product do not use more than directed.

Stop use and ask a doctor if
• you get nervous, dizzy, or sleepless
• symptoms do not get better within 7 days or are accompanied by fever
• cough lasts more than 7 days, comes back, or is accompanied by fever, rash, or persistent headache. These could be signs of a serious condition.

If pregnant or breast-feeding, ask a health professional before use.

Keep out of reach of children. In case of overdose, get medical help or contact a Poison Control Center right away.

Directions:
• do not take more than 4 doses in any 24-hr period
• adults and children 12 yrs and over: 2 tsp every 4 hours
• children 6 to under 12 yrs: 1 tsp every 4 hours
• children 2 to under 6 yrs: ½ tsp every 4 hours
• children under 2 yrs: ask a doctor

Other Information:
• store at 20–25°C (68–77°F)
• alcohol-free
• dosage cup provided

Inactive Ingredients:
citric acid, FD&C red no. 40, flavors, glucose, glycerin, high fructose corn syrup, maltol, menthol, propylene glycol, saccharin sodium, sodium benzoate, water

How Supplied: Bottles of 4 fl oz, and 8 fl oz.

ROBITUSSIN® DM SYRUP
ROBITUSSIN® SUGAR FREE COUGH

ROBITUSSIN® DM INFANT DROPS
Cough Suppressant, Expectorant

Active Ingredients: (in each 5 mL tsp: Robitussin DM, Robitussin Sugar Free Cough)
Dextromethorphan HBr, USP 10 mg
Guaifenesin, USP 100 mg

Active Ingredients: (in each 2.5 mL Robitussin DM Infant Drops)
Dextromethorphan HBr, USP 5 mg
Guaifenesin, USP 100 mg

Uses:
• temporarily relieves cough due to minor throat and bronchial irritation as may occur with a cold
• helps loosen phlegm (mucus) and thin bronchial secretions to drain bronchial tubes

Warnings:
Do not use if you or your child are now taking a prescription monoamine oxidase inhibitor (MAOI) (certain drugs for depression, psychiatric, or emotional conditions, or Parkinson's disease), or for 2 weeks after stopping the MAOI drug. If you do not know if your child's or your prescription drug contains an MAOI, ask a doctor or pharmacist before taking this product or giving it to your child.

Ask a doctor before use if you or your child has
• cough that occurs with too much phlegm (mucus)
• cough that lasts or is chronic such as occurs with smoking, asthma, chronic bronchitis, or emphysema

Stop use and ask a doctor if cough lasts more than 7 days, comes back, or is accompanied by fever, rash, or persistent headache. These could be signs of a serious condition.

If pregnant or breast-feeding, ask a health professional before use.

Keep out of reach of children. In case of overdose, get medical help or contact a Poison Control Center right away.

Directions: (Robitussin DM, Robitussin Sugar Free Cough):
• do not take more than 6 doses in any 24-hour period
• adults and children 12 yrs and over: 2 tsp every 4 hours
• children 6 to under 12 yrs: 1 tsp every 4 hours
• children 2 to under 6 yrs: ½ tsp every 4 hours
• children under 2 yrs: ask a doctor

Directions: (Robitussin DM Infant Drops):
• repeat every 4 hrs
• do not use more than 6 doses in any 24-hr period
• choose by weight (if weight not known, choose by age)
• measure with the dosing device provided. Do not use with any other device.
• 24–47 lbs (2 to under 6 yrs): 2.5 mL
• under 24 lbs (under 2 yrs): ask a doctor

Inactive Ingredients: (Robitussin DM): citric acid, FD&C red no. 40, flavors, glucose, glycerin, high fructose corn syrup, menthol, saccharin sodium, sodium benzoate, water

Inactive Ingredients: (Robitussin Sugar Free Cough): acesulfame potassium, citric acid, flavors, glycerin, methylparaben, polyethylene glycol, povidone, propylene glycol, saccharin sodium, sodium benzoate, water

Inactive Ingredients: (Robitussin DM Infant Drops): citric acid, FD&C red no. 40, flavors, glycerin, high fructose corn syrup, maltitol, maltol, polyethylene glycol, povidone, propylene glycol, saccharin sodium, sodium benzoate, sodium chloride, sodium citrate, water

Other Information:
• store at 20–25°C (68–77°F)
• alcohol-free
• dosage cup or oral dosing device provided

Continued on next page

Robitussin DM/SF Cough—Cont.

How Supplied: Robitussin DM (cherry-colored) in bottles of 4, 8 and 12 fl oz, and single doses (premeasured doses 1/3 fl oz each)
Robitussin Sugar Free Cough in bottles of 4 fl oz
Robitussin DM Infant Drops in 1 fl oz bottles

ROBITUSSIN® SUGAR FREE Throat Drops (Natural Citrus and Tropical Fruit Flavors)

Active Ingredient (in each drop): Menthol, USP 2.5 mg

Uses:
• temporarily relieves
  • occasional minor irritation, pain, sore mouth, and sore throat
  • cough associated with a cold or inhaled irritants

Warnings:
Sore throat warning: Severe or persistent sore throat or sore throat accompanied by high fever, headache, nausea, and vomiting may be serious. Consult a doctor right away. Do not use more than 2 days or give to children under 3 years of age unless directed by a doctor.
Ask a doctor before use if you have
• cough that occurs with too much phlegm (mucus)
• cough that lasts or is chronic such as occurs with smoking, asthma, or emphysema
When using this product excessive use may have a laxative effect
Stop use and ask a doctor if cough lasts more than 7 days, comes back, or is accompanied by fever, rash, or persistent headache. These could be signs of a serious condition.
If pregnant or breast-feeding, ask a health professional before use.
Keep out of reach of children.

Directions:
• adults and children 4 years and over: allow 2 drops to dissolve slowly in the mouth
  • for sore throat: may be repeated every 2 hours, as needed, up to 9 drops per day, or as directed by a doctor
  • for cough: may be repeated every 2 hours, as needed, up to 9 drops per day, as or as directed by a doctor
• children under 4 years: ask a doctor

Other Information:
• **phenylketonurics:** contains phenylalanine 3.37 mg per drop
• store at 20–25°C (68–77°F)
• does not promote tooth decay
• product may be useful in a diabetic's diet on the advice of a doctor.
Exchange information*:
       3 Drops = FREE Exchange
       9 Drops = 1 Fruit
*The dietary exchanges are based on Exchange Lists for Meal Planning. Copyright 1995 by the American Diabetes Association Inc. and the American Dietetic Association.

Inactive Ingredients: aspartame, canola oil, citric acid, D&C yellow no. 10 aluminum lake (natural citrus only), FD&C blue no. 1 (natural citrus only), FD&C yellow no. 6 (tropical fruit only), isomalt, maltitol, natural flavor

How Supplied: Packages of 18 drops.

ROBITUSSIN® MAXIMUM STRENGTH COUGH
ROBITUSSIN® PEDIATRIC COUGH Formula
Cough Suppressant

Active Ingredients (in each 5 mL tsp Robitussin Maximum Strength Cough): Dextromethorphan HBr, USP 15 mg
(in each 5 mL tsp Robitussin Pediatric Cough Formula): Dextromethorphan HBr, USP 7.5 mg

Uses: temporarily relieves cough due to minor throat and bronchial irritation as may occur with a cold

Warnings:
Do not use if you are now taking a prescription monoamine oxidase inhibitor (MAOI) (certain drugs for depression, psychiatric, or emotional conditions, or Parkinson's disease), or for 2 weeks after stopping the MAOI drug. If you do not know if your prescription drug contains an MAOI, ask a doctor or pharmacist before taking this product.
Ask a doctor before use if you have
• cough that occurs with too much phlegm (mucus)
• cough that lasts or is chronic such as occurs with smoking, asthma, or emphysema
Stop use and ask a doctor if cough lasts more than 7 days, comes back, or is accompanied by fever, rash, or persistent headache. These could be signs of a serious condition.
If pregnant or breast-feeding, ask a health professional before use.
Keep out of reach of children. In case of overdose, get medical help or contact a Poison Control Center right away.

Directions:
• do not take more than 4 doses in any 24-hr period
Robitussin Maximum Strength Cough Suppressant
• adults and children 12 yrs and over: 2 tsp every 6 to 8 hours, as needed
• children under 12 yrs: ask a doctor
Robitussin Pediatric Cough Suppressant
• choose dosage by weight (if weight is not known, choose by age)
  • under 24 lbs (under 2 yrs): ask a doctor
  • 24–47 lbs (2 to under 6 yrs): 1 tsp every 6 to 8 hours
  • 48–95 lbs (6–under 12 yrs): 2 tsp every 6 to 8 hours
  • 96 lbs and over (12 yrs and older): 4 tsp every 6 to 8 hours

Other Information:
• store at 20–25°C (68–77°F)
• dosage cup provided

Inactive Ingredients (Robitussin Maximum Strength Cough): alcohol, citric acid, FD&C red no. 40, flavors, glucose, glycerin, high fructose corn syrup, menthol, saccharin sodium, sodium benzoate, water

(Robitussin Pediatric Cough Formula): citric acid, FD&C red no. 40, flavor, glycerin, high fructose corn syrup, saccharin sodium, sodium benzoate, sodium chloride, sodium citrate, water
• **each teaspoon contains:** sodium 5 mg

How Supplied: Robitussin Maximum Strength (dark red-colored) in bottles of 4 and 8 fl oz.
Robitussin Pediatric (cherry-colored) in bottles of 4 fl oz.

ROBITUSSIN® MAXIMUM STRENGTH COUGH& COLD
ROBITUSSIN® PEDIATRIC COUGH & COLD Formula
Cough Suppressant, Nasal Decongestant

Active Ingredients: (in each 5 mL tsp Robitussin Maximum Strength Cough & Cold) Dextromethorphan HBr, USP 15 mg
Pseudoephedrine HCl, USP 30 mg
(in each 5 mL tsp Robitussin Pediatric Cough & Cold Formula) Dextromethorphan HBr, USP 7.5 mg
Pseudoephedrine HCl, USP 15 mg

Uses:
• temporarily relieves these symptoms occurring with a cold:
  • nasal congestion • cough due to minor throat and bronchial irritation

Warnings:
Do not use if you are now taking a prescription monoamine oxidase inhibitor (MAOI) (certain drugs for depression, psychiatric, or emotional conditions, or Parkinson's disease), or for 2 weeks after stopping the MAOI drug. If you do not know if your prescription drug contains an MAOI, ask a doctor or pharmacist before taking this product.
Ask a doctor before use if you have
• heart disease • high blood pressure
• thyroid disease • diabetes
• trouble urinating due to an enlarged prostate gland
• cough that occurs with too much phlegm (mucus)
• cough that lasts or is chronic such as occurs with smoking, asthma, or emphysema
When using this product do not use more than directed.
Stop use and ask a doctor if
• you get nervous, dizzy, or sleepless
• symptoms do not get better within 7 days or are accompanied by fever
• cough lasts more than 7 days, comes back, or is accompanied by fever, rash, or persistent headache. These could be signs of a serious condition.
If pregnant or breast-feeding, ask a health professional before use.
Keep out of reach of children. In case of overdose, get medical help or contact a Poison Control Center right away.

Directions:
- repeat dose every 6 hrs, as needed
- do not take more than 4 doses in any 24-hr period

Robitussin Maximum Strength Cough & Cold. • adults and children 12 yrs and over: 2 tsp • children under 12 yrs: ask a doctor

Robitussin Pediatric Cough & Cold Formula • choose dosage by weight (if weight is not known, choose by age)
- under 24 lbs (under 2 yrs): ask a doctor
- 24–47 lbs (2 to under 6 yrs): 1 tsp
- 48–95 lbs (6 to under 12 yrs): 2 tsp
- 96 lbs and over (12 yrs and older): 4 tsp

Other Information: • store at 20–25°C (68–77°F)
- dosage cup provided

Inactive Ingredients (Robitussin Maximum Strength Cough & Cold): alcohol, citric acid, FD&C red no. 40, flavors, glucose, glycerin, high fructose corn syrup, menthol, saccharin sodium, sodium benzoate, water
(Robitussin Pediatric Cough & Cold Formula): citric acid, FD&C red no. 40, flavor, glycerin, high fructose corn syrup, saccharin sodium, sodium benzoate, sodium chloride, sodium citrate, water
- **each teaspoon contains:** sodium 5 mg

How Supplied:
Robitussin Maximum Strength Cough & Cold: Red syrup in bottles of 4 fl oz and 8 fl oz.
Robitussin Pediatric Cough & Cold Formula: (bright red) in bottles of 4 fl oz.

ROBITUSSIN®-CF Syrup
ROBITUSSIN® COUGH & COLD INFANT DROPS
Nasal Decongestant, Cough Suppressant, Expectorant

Active Ingredients: (in each 5 mL tsp Robitussin CF)

Dextromethorphan HBr, USP 10 mg
Guaifenesin, USP 100 mg
Pseudoephedrine HCl, USP 30 mg
(in each 2.5 mL Robitussin Cough & Cold Infant Drops)
Dextromethorphan HBr, USP 5 mg
Guaifenesin, USP 100 mg
Pseudoephedrine HCl, USP 15 mg

Uses:
- temporarily relieves these symptoms occurring with a cold:
  - nasal congestion
  - cough due to minor throat and bronchial irritation
- helps loosen phlegm (mucus) and thin bronchial secretions to make coughs more productive

Warnings:
Do not use if you or your child are taking a prescription monoamine oxidase inhibitor (MAOI) (certain drugs for depression, psychiatric, or emotional conditions, or Parkinson's disease), or for 2 weeks after stopping the MAOI drug. If you do not know if your child's or your prescription drug contains an MAOI, ask a doctor or pharmacist before taking this product or giving it to your child.
Ask a doctor before use if you or your child has
- heart disease • high blood pressure
- thyroid disease • diabetes
- trouble urinating due to an enlarged prostate gland
- cough that occurs with too much phlegm (mucus)
- cough that lasts or is chronic such as occurs with asthma

When using this product do not use more than directed.
Stop use and ask a doctor if
- you or your child gets nervous, dizzy, or sleepless
- symptoms do not get better within 7 days or are accompanied by fever
- cough lasts more than 7 days, comes back, or is accompanied by fever, rash, or persistent headache. These could be signs of a serious condition.

If pregnant or breast-feeding, ask a health professional before use.
Keep out of reach of children. In case of overdose, get medical help or contact a Poison Control Center right away.

Directions: (Robitussin CF Syrup):
- do not take more than 4 doses in any 24-hr period
- adults and children 12 yrs and over: 2 tsp every 4 hours
- children 6 to under 12 yrs: 1 tsp every 4 hours
- children 2 to under 6 yrs: ½ tsp or 2.5 mL
- children under 2 yrs: ask a doctor

Directions: (Robitussin Cough & Cold Infant Drops):
- do not use more than 4 doses in any 24-hour period
- repeat every 4 hours
- choose dosage by weight (if weight is not known, choose by age)
- measure with the dosing device provided. Do not use with any other device.
- 27–47 lbs (2 to under 6 yrs): 2.5 mL
- under 24 lbs (under 2 yrs): ask a doctor
Other Information:
- store at 20–25°C (68–77°F)
- alcohol-free
- dosage cup or oral dosing device provided

Inactive Ingredients: (Robitussin CF) citric acid, FD&C red no. 40, flavors, glycerin, propylene glycol, saccharin sodium, sodium benzoate, sorbitol, water
(Robitussin Cough & Cold Infant Drops) citric acid, FD&C red no. 40, flavors, glycerin, high fructose corn syrup, maltitol, maltol, polyethylene glycol, povidone, propylene glycol, saccharin sodium, sodium benzoate, sodium citrate, water

How Supplied: Robitussin CF (red-colored) in bottles of 4, 8, and 12 fl oz. Robitussin Cough & Cold Infant Drops in 1 fl oz bottles

DIETARY SUPPLEMENT INFORMATION

This section presents information on natural remedies and nutritional supplements marketed under the Dietary Supplement Health and Education Act of 1994. It is made possible through the courtesy of the manufacturers whose products appear on the following pages. The information concerning each product has been prepared, edited, and approved by the manufacturer's professional staff.

Products found in this section include vitamins, minerals, herbs and other botanicals, amino acids, other substances intended to supplement the diet, and concentrates, metabolites, constituents, extracts, and combinations of these ingredients. The descriptions of these products are designed to provide all information necessary for informed use, including, when applicable, active ingredients, inactive ingredients, actions, warnings, cautions, interactions, symptoms and treatment of oral overdosage, dosage and directions for use, and how supplied. Descriptions in this section must be in full compliance with the Dietary Supplement Health and Education Act, which permits claims regarding a product's effect on the structure or functioning of the body, but forbids claims regarding a product's ability to treat, diagnose, cure, or prevent any specific disease. Descriptions of products marketed under the act do not receive formal evaluation or approval from the Food and Drug Administration.

In compiling this section, the publisher has emphasized the necessity of describing products comprehensively. The descriptions seen here include all information made available by the manufacturer. The publisher does not warrant or guarantee any product described here, and does not perform any independent analysis of the information provided. Inclusion of a product in this book does not represent an endorsement, and the publisher does not necessarily advocate the use of any product listed.

A&Z Pharmaceutical Inc.
**180 OSER AVENUE, SUITE 300
HAUPPAUGE, NY 11788**

Direct Inquiries to:
(631) 952-3800

D-CAL™
**Calcium Supplement with Vitamin D
Chewable Caplets**

Ingredients: Calcium Carbonate, Vitamin D, Sorbitol, Flavor, D&C Red #27 Lake, Magnesium Stearate. No sugar, No salt, No lactose, No preservative.

Supplement Facts

Serving Size One Caplet

Each Caplet Contains		% Daily Value
Calcium (as		
calcium carbonate)	300 mg	30%
Vitamin D	100 IU	25%

Recommended Intake: Take two caplets daily for adult and one caplet for child, or as directed by your physician.

Warnings: KEEP OUT OF REACH OF CHILDREN. Do not accept if safety seal under cap is broken or missing.

Actions: D-Cal™ provides a concentrated form of calcium to help build healthy bones. It contains Vitamin D to help the body absorb calcium. D-Cal™ can also help prevent osteoporosis. It is helpful to pregnant and nursing women, children's growth, and calcium deficiency at all ages.

How Supplied: Bottles of 30 and 60 caplets

AkPharma Inc.
**P.O. BOX 111
PLEASANTVILLE, NJ 08232-0111**

Direct Inquiries To:
Elizabeth Klein: (609) 645-5100
FAX: (609) 645-0767

Medical Emergency Contact:
Alan E. Kligerman: (609) 645-5100

PRELIEF®

PRODUCT OVERVIEW
Key Facts: Prelief is AkPharma's brand name for calcium glycerophosphate which has a number of important uses. These fields include:
Urinary: As a palliative in interstitial cystitis, prostatitis, overactive bladder.

Intestinal: As a symptoms reducer in irritable bowel syndrome.
Prelief is taken in periodic dosages, regardless of meals or foods eaten. Clinical studies demonstrate that such use greatly reduces urinary pain and urgency in overactive bladder. Prelief is also used beneficially in terms of pain and urgency with interstitial cystitis and prostatitis. A pilot clinical study suggests beneficial use by persons with diarrhea-predominant irritable bowel syndrome (IBS) and a clinical study to confirm this is nearing completion. Clinical studies are also underway to confirm cellular effects in interstitial cystitis.
Safety Information: Prelief is made from an FDA Generally Recognized as Safe (GRAS)[1] mineral and is also listed in the Food Chemicals Codex (FCC).[2]

PRODUCT INFORMATION
Description:
Prelief Tablets: Each tablet contains 345 mg calcium glycerophosphate (65 mg of elemental calcium). The tablets also contain 0.25% magnesium stearate as a processing aid. Two tablets are equivalent to 690 mg calcium glycerophosphate (130mg of elemental calcium).
Prelief Powder: Each ¼ teaspoon usage of powder is comparable to two tablets. The powder dissolves rapidly in food or non-alcoholic beverages. Tablets are recommended for taking with alcoholic beverages.
Two tablets or about ¼ teaspoon of powder provides 15% (130 mg) of the FDA Recommended Daily Intake (RDI) for calcium and 10% (100 mg) of the FDA RDI for phosphorus. No sodium; no aluminum; no sugar; no potassium.
Reasons for Use: Prelief is used as an intervention in certain identifiable urinary and intestinal problems such as interstitial cystitis, prostatitis, overactive bladder and irritable bowel syndrome.
Action: Through a mechanism not fully elucidated, Prelief appears to reduce cellular inflammation in the urinary bladder. It also appears to non-irritatively encourage cellular reproduction. This is possibly a result of Prelief's uniquely free calcium ion and/or the glycerophosphate moiety, working singly or together. In addition, Prelief neutralizes the acid found in a large number of foods which many people find cause them discomfort.
Usage:
Tablets: 2–3 tablets, 2 times a day.
Powder: ¼ teaspoon of powder 2 times a day. More can be used when needed.
Kosher: Prelief is Kosher and Parve.

How Supplied:
Tablets: 60, 120 and 300-tablet bottles.
Powder: Portable 20-use (correspondent to 40 tablets) squeeze bottle and 150-serving shaker.
Use Limitations: None, except as may apply below.

Adverse Reactions: None known.
Toxicity: None known.

Interactions with Drugs: Calcium may interfere with the availability of some antibiotics. Check with drug publications.

Precautions: None, except for people who have been advised by their physician not to take calcium, phosphorus or glycerin/glycerol.

[1] 21 CFR §184.1201
[2] Food Chemicals Codex, 4th Edition, pp 60–61
For more information, please write or call toll-free 1-800-994-4711.
AkPharma Inc.
P.O. Box 111
Pleasantville, NJ 08232-0111
Shown in Product Identification Guide, page 503

Alpine Pharmaceuticals
**1940 FOURTH STREET
SAN RAFAEL, CA 94901**

Direct inquiries to:
phone (888) 746-3224
fax (415) 451-6981
www.alpinepharm.com

SINECCH
[sĭn' ĕk]
Homeopathic Arnica Montana

Active Ingredients: Homeopathic Arnica Montana 1M HPUS, Homeopathic Arnica Montana 12C HPUS.

Indications: Reduces pain, bruising, and swelling caused by trauma (major injuries from car accidents, falls, sports injuries, etc), or caused by plastic surgery or general surgery.

Inactive Ingredients: Sucrose, Lactose, Capsules contain gelatin, titanium dioxide, iron oxide, FD&C blue #1, D&C red #28, D&C green #3.

Directions: For adults and children over 6 years of age. Swallow the capsules with water, or twist open the capsules and pour the contents into your mouth. Let the pellets dissolve. If possible, do not eat or drink anything for 15 minutes before and after taking SinEcch.
For Surgery the three SinEcch 01 capsules of 500 mg Homeopathic Arnica Montana 1M are taken 1 pre-operatively, 1 post-operatively, and 1 at bedtime on the day of surgery. The nine SinEcch 02 capsules of 500 mg Homeopathic Arnica Montana 12C are taken one every morning, afternoon, and evening for the three days after surgery.
For Trauma the pre-op dose is taken as soon as possible, the post-op dose 4 hours after the first dose and the remainder of the capsules are taken in the same manner as the surgery dosage schedule. The

schedule is printed on the box and on the package of capsules.

Warnings: This product is safety sealed. The box is sealed and the capsules are individually blister sealed. Do not use if seals or blisters are broken. If you are pregnant or nursing consult your physician before taking SinEcch. Do not take together with the prescription pain medicine Talwin (pentazocine) or Talwin NX. Keep this and all medication out of the reach of children.

How Supplied: SinEcch is a programmed dosage regimen of two different strengths of Homeopathic Arnica Montana. Three SinEcch 01 capsules of 500 mg Homeopathic Arnica Montana 1M and nine SinEcch 02 capsules of 500 mg Homeopathic Arnica Montana 12C per blister card. Store at room temperature.

Shown in Product Identification Guide, page 503

American Longevity
**2400 BOSWELL ROAD
CHULA VISTA, CA 91914**

Direct Inquiries to:
Customer Service
800-982-3189
Fax:
619-934-3205
www.americanlongevity.net

Plant Derived Minerals

Description: Minerals which are so important to our health are not so readily available. Minerals never occured in a uniform blanket on the crust of the Earth. Therefore, unless you supplement with minerals, you can't guarantee that you will get all you need through the 4 food groups. Our Plant Derived Mineral products are liquid concentrates containing a natural assortment of up to 77 minerals from prehistoric plants in their unaltered colloidal form. A mineral deficiency can lead to disease or even death. Plant Derived Minerals can help you in your fight against deficiencies. Now, it even comes in a great tasting cherry flavor.

Supplement Facts:
Calories <5
Majestic Earth Plant   600mg *
  Derived Minerals
*daily value not established

Directions:
1) Store in cool environment after opening
2) Suggested as a dietary supplement. For adults, mix 1 or 2 ounces in a small glass of fruit or vegetable juice of your choice. Drink during or after meals, 1 to 3 times a day or as desired. For children reduce amount by two-thirds

Other Ingredients: Calcium, Chlorine, Magnesium, Phosphorus, Potassium, Sodium, Sulfur, Antimony, Arsenic, Aluminum Hydroxide, Barium, Beryllium, Bismuth, Boron, Bromine, Cadmium, Carbon, Cerium Cesium, Chromium, Cobalt, Copper, Dysprosium, Erbium, Europium, Fluorine, Gadolinium, Gallium, Germanium, Gold, Hafnium, Holmium Hydrogen, Indium, Iodine, Iridium, Iron, Lanthanum, Lead, Lithium, Lutetium, Manganese, Mercury, Molybdenum, Neodymium, Nickel, Niobium, Nitrogen, Osmium, Oxygen, Palladium, Platinum, Praseodymium, Rhenium, Rhodium, Rubidium, Ruthenium, Samarium, Scandium, Selenium, Silicon, Silver, Strontium, Tantalum, Tellurium, Terbium, Thallium, Thorium, Thulium, Tin, Titanium, Tungsten, Vanadium, Ytterbium, Yttrium, Zinc, Zirconium.

NONI PLUS PLUS
(morinda citrifolia)

Description:
*Noni Plus Plus, containing Noni and Aloe Vera Juice, promotes optimal health and well being. Noni (morinda citrifolia) is a fruit that is grown in the volcanic, mineral-rich soils of Hawaii and other tropical islands. It has been used for hundreds of years by the Polynesians, who believe in its health benefits. Aloe Vera has been regarded as a healing plant for over 2000 years. There are many benefits to using Noni Plus Plus, such as: immune support, joint support, digestive support, helps boost free radical absorption and supports collagen production for better looking skin.†

Supplement Facts:
Serving size: 1 Fluid Ounce (28.5 ml)
Servings per container: 34

	Amount per serving	% Daily Value
Calories:	9	<1%
Total Carbohydrates:	2.25 g	<2%
Sugars	2.25 g	**
Protein	0 g	0%
Vitamin A (as beta carotene)	1.1 IU	<2%
Vitamin C (as ascorbic acid)	7 mg	1%
Vitamin B 12 (as cyanocobalamin)	3.3 mcg	10%
Calcium (as calcium glycinate)	15.18 mg	<2%
Iron (from ferrous bis-glycinate)	1 mcg	<2%
Iodine (from potassium iodide)	0.2 mcg	<2%
Magnesium (from magnesium glycinate)	0.55 mg	<2%
Zinc (zinc glycinate)	2.5 mcg	<2%
Selenium (from selenium glycinate)	.5 mcg	<2%
Copper (copper glycinate)	.04 mcg	<2%
Manganese (manganese glycinate)	2.5 mcg	<2%
Chromium (chromium nicotinyl glycinate)	2.0 mcg	<2%
Molybdnum (molybdenum glycinate)	.15 mcg	<2%
Sodium (sodium iodide)	5.8 mg	<2%
Propriety Blend	6.6 g	**
Aloe Vera Gel, Noni (mo rinda cit rifolia) extract 5:**1PE, Grape Seed Extract		
Cobalt (cyanocobalamin)	3.5 mcg	**
Vanadium (vanadyl sulfate)	.2 mcg	**

Other Ingredients: Purified water, natural pineapple flavor, glycerine, citric acid, xanthan gum, sodium benzoate, and potassium sorbate as preservative.

Warning: as with any dietary supplement, if you are pregnant or nursing, seek the advice of your health care professional. **KEEP OUT OF THE REACH OF CHILDREN**

*Percent Daily Values are based on a 2,000 calorie diet
**Daily Value Not Established

Directions: Drink 1 oz per 100 lbs. daily, or as directed by your health care practitioner.

How Supplied: 32 fl. oz. bottle

Awareness Corporation/ dba AwarenessLife
**25 SOUTH ARIZONA PLACE, SUITE 500
CHANDLER, ARIZONA 85225**

Direct Inquiries to:
1-800-69AWARE
www.awarecorp.com
www.awarenesslife.com

AWARENESS CLEAR™

Description: May help with general digestion.*

Ingredients: Proprietary blend of Oregano Leaf, Clove Flowers, Black Walnut Seed Husk, Peppermint Leaf, Nigella, Grapefruit, Winter Melon Seed, Gentian, Hyssop Leaf, Crampbark, Thyme Leaf, Fennel.

Directions: Take 2 capsules each morning on an empty stomach, 1–2 hours before eating with 1 glass of water

Warnings: Do not use if Pregnant or Breastfeeding. Keep out of reach of children.

How Supplied: 90 Vegetarian Capsules per Bottle

*These statements have not been evaluated by the Food and Drug Administration. These products are not intended to diagnose, treat, cure, or prevent any disease.

Continued on next page

DAILY COMPLETE®

Description: Liquid Supplement. 100% vegetarian ingredients delivers 211 vitamins, minerals, antioxidants, enzymes, fruits and vegetables, amino acids and herbs, in one ounce liquid a day (great orange taste) Helps to Provide Energy & Reduce Stress Levels*.

Ingredients: Rich in Vitamins & Minerals, Ionic Plant Minerals, Botanical Antioxidants with Phenalgrin™, 32 Fruit & Vegetable Whole Juice Complex, Whole Superfood Green complex, 34 Herbal Ingredients, Essential Fatty Acid Complex, Special Ocean Vegetable Blend

Directions: Take 1 ounce (30 ml) per day, during or immediately after a meal

Warnings: Do not use if pregnant or breast-feeding. Keep out of reach of children.

How Supplied: 30 ounces per Bottle, Clinically Tested Ingredients.

EXPERIENCE®

Description: Promotes Regularity & Cleanses the Colon*

Ingredients: Proprietary Blend of Senna, Blonde Psyllium Seed Husk, Fennel Seed, Cornsilk, Solomon's seal, Rhubarb Root, Kelp

Directions: Take 1 to 2 Capsules before bedtime with a full glass of water.

Warnings: Do not use if pregnant or breast-feeding or if you have colitis. Keep out of reach of children

How Supplied: 90 Capsules per bottle, Clinically tested

PURE GARDENS CREAM®

Description: 100% natural may help to improve dry skin, fine lines and helps to tone the skin.

Ingredients: Apple oil, vitamin C, vitamin E, Aloe Vera Leaf, Almond Oil, Cold Press Virgin Olive Oil, Sesame Oil, Chamomile Flowers Oil, Calendula Officinalis Oil, Beeswax, Jojoba Oil, Linseed Oil.

Directions: Application for both face and body. External use only

How Supplied: 2 ounce jar, Clinically tested

PURETRIM™ WHOLEFOOD WELLNESS SHAKE

Description: Vegetarian Natural Wholefood High Protein Low Carb Energy Shake. No Dairy, No Soy

Ingredients: Vegetable Pea & Brown Rice Protein, Antioxidants, Prebiotics, Essential Fatty Acids & Enzyme Active Greens

Directions: Mix contents in 10 oz. of cold water.

Warnings: Not for use by pregnant or lactating women. Must be 18 years or older to use.

How Supplied: 10 Packets (Net Wt 500 g)

SYNERGYDEFENSE® CAPSULES

Description: Improves Digestion, Boosts the Immune System, & strengthens the body's natural defense*.

Ingredients: Proprietary Blend of Enzymes, Probiotics, Antioxidants, Prebiotics

Directions: Take 1 capsule with a glass of water during or before your largest meal of the day. Take once or twice a daily.

Warnings: Do not use if pregnant or lactating. If under 18, consult a physician before use.

How Supplied: 30 Vegetarian Capsules individually sealed

---

*These statements have not been evaluated by the Food and Drug Administration. These products are not intended to diagnose, treat, cure, or prevent any disease.

Bausch & Lomb

1400 NORTH GOODMAN STREET
ROCHESTER, NY 14609

Direct Inquiries to:
Main Office
(585) 338-6000
Consumer Affairs
1-800-553-5340

BAUSCH & LOMB PRESERVISION® AREDS

Eye Vitamin and Mineral Supplement
AREDS: The ONLY clinically proven effective formula.
New easy to swallow 2 per day Soft Gels

Description: Each Soft Gel contains:
[See first table at top of next page]

Other Ingredients: Gelatin, Glycerin, Soybean Oil, Unbleached Lecithin, Yellow Wax, Annatto Oil, Titanium Dioxide

- Age-related macular degeneration (AMD) is the leading cause of vision loss and blindness in people over 55. The landmark National Institutes of Health AREDS trial proved that a high potency antioxidant vitamin and mineral supplement was effective in helping to preserve the sight of certain people most at risk.**
- Now patented, Bausch & Lomb PreserVision® is the one and only eye vitamin and mineral supplement clinically proven effective in the 10 year National Institutes of Health (NIH) Age Related Eye Disease Study (AREDS).
- Bausch & Lomb PreserVision® is a high potency antioxidant and mineral supplement with the antioxidant vitamins A, C, E, and selected minerals in amounts above those in ordinary multivitamins and generally cannot be obtained through diet alone.
- **Recommended Intake:** Now instead of taking 4 tablets per day to get the high levels proven effective in the National Institutes of Health (NIH) Age Related Eye Disease Study (AREDS), you only need to take: 2 soft gels per day — 1 in the morning, 1 in the evening taken with meals.

Bausch & Lomb PreserVision® is the #1 recommended eye vitamin and mineral supplement among vitreoretinal eye doctors.*

For future savings and information along with a FREE 16 page brochure on age-related macular degeneration, call toll free 1-866-HOPE-AMD (1-866-467-3263) Reference 92.

CURRENT AND FORMER SMOKERS: Consult your eye doctor or eye care professional about the risks associated with smoking and Beta-Carotene.

---

* Date on file, Bausch & Lomb Incorporated.

** This statement has not been evaluated by the Food and Drug Administration. This product is not intended to diagnose, treat, cure or prevent any disease.

How Supplied: Available in bottles of 60 count and 120 count soft gels.
Orange, oval shaped soft gelatin capsule imprinted with BL-PV on one side.

BAUSCH & LOMB PRESERVISION® LUTEIN

Eye Vitamin and Mineral Supplement
Beta-carotene free formulation.
New easy to swallow 2 per day Soft Gels

Description: Each soft gel contains:
[See second table at top of next page]

Other Ingredients: Gelatin, Glycerin, Soybean Oil, Unbleached Lecithin, Yellow Wax, Annatto Oil, Titanium Dioxide

Contents	Source	Daily Dosage (2 Soft Gels) Amount	% of Daily Value
Vitamin A	(beta-carotene)	28,640 IU	573%
Vitamin C	(ascorbic acid)	452 mg	753%
Vitamin E	(dl-alpha tocopheryl acetate)	400 IU	1333%
Zinc	(zinc oxide)**	69.6 mg	464%
Copper	(cupric oxide)	1.6 mg	80%

** Zinc Oxide is the most concentrated form of zinc and contains more elemental zinc than any other zinc salt (zinc sulfate or zinc acetate).

Contents	Source	Daily Dosage (2 Soft Gels) Amount	% Daily Value
Vitamin C	(ascorbic acid)	452 mg	753%
Vitamin E	(dl-alpha tocopheryl acetate)	400 IU	1333%
Zinc	(zinc oxide)†	69.6 mg	464%
Copper	(cupric oxide)	1.6 mg	80%
Lutein		10 mg	††

† Zinc Oxide is the most concentrated form of zinc and contains more elemental zinc than any other zinc salt (zinc sulfate or zinc acetate).
†† Daily value not established

This product is Vitamin A (beta-carotene) Free.

STORE AT ROOM TEMPERATURE.

- The new Bausch & Lomb PreserVision® Lutein patented formula is based on the clinically proven Bausch & Lomb PreserVision® Age Related Eye Disease Study (AREDS) formula*, with the beta-carotene substituted with 10 mg of FloraGlo® Lutein.
- Lutein is a carotenoid found in dark leafy green vegetables such as spinach. Carotenoids are concentrated in the macula, the part of the eye responsible for central vision. Studies suggest that lutein plays an essential role in maintaining healthy central vision by protecting against free radical damage and filtering blue light.**
- Lutein levels in your eye are related to the amount in your diet. Bausch & Lomb PreserVision® Lutein contains 5 mg of lutein per soft gel, which gives you 10 mg of lutein per day. The leading multivitamin contains only a fraction of the amount of lutein used in clinical studies.

*Bausch & Lomb Ocuvite® Preser Vision® AREDS formula was the one and only antioxidant vitamin and mineral supplement proven effective in the 10-year National Institutes of Health (NIH) AREDS trial. AREDS was a 10-year, independent study conducted by the National Eye Institute (NEI) of the National Institutes of Health (NIH).

Age-related macular generation (AMD) is the leading cause of vision loss and blindness in people over 55. For future savings and information along with a FREE 16 page brochure on age-related macular degeneration, call toll free 1-866-HOPE-AMD (1-866-467-3263) Reference 93.

Recommended Intake: 2 soft gels per day – 1 in the morning, 1 in the evening taken with meals.

**This statement has not been evaluated by the Food and Drug Administration. This product is not intended to diagnose, treat, cure or prevent any disease.

FloraGLO® is a registered trademark of Kemin Industries, Inc.

How Supplied: Available in bottles of 50 count soft gels. Orange, oval shaped soft gelatin capsule, imprinted with BL-LPV on one side.

Beach Pharmaceuticals

Division of Beach Products, Inc.
5220 SOUTH MANHATTAN AVE.
TAMPA, FL 33611

Direct Inquiries to:
Richard Stephen Jenkins, Exec. V.P.:
(813) 839-6565

BEELITH Tablets
magnesium supplement with pyridoxine HCl

Description: Each tablet contains magnesium oxide 600 mg and pyridoxine hydrochloride (Vitamin B_6) 25 mg equivalent to Vitamin B_6 20 mg.

Supplement Facts
Serving Size: 1 Tablet

	Amount Per Tablet	% Daily Value
Vitamin B_6 (pyridoxine HCl)	20 mg	1000%
Magnesium (from magnesium oxide)	362 mg	90%

Inactive Ingredients: FD&C Yellow No. 6, hydroxypropyl methylcellulose, magnesium stearate, microcrystalline cellulose, polyethylene glycol, sodium starch glycolate, titanium dioxide. May also contain D&C Yellow No. 10, FD&C Yellow No. 5 (Tartrazine), hydroxypropyl cellulose, polydextrose, stearic acid and/or triacetin.

Indications: As a dietary supplement for patients with magnesium and/or Vitamin B_6 deficiencies resulting from malnutrition, alcoholism, magnesium depleting drugs, chemotherapy, and inadequate nutritional intake or absorption. Also, increases urinary magnesium levels.

Dosage: One tablet daily or as directed by a physician.

Warnings: Do not take this product if you are presently taking a prescription drug without consulting your physician or other health professional. If you have kidney disease, take only under the supervision of a physician. Excessive dosage may cause laxation. If pregnant or breast-feeding, ask a health professional before use. **KEEP OUT OF THE REACH OF CHILDREN.**

How Supplied: Golden yellow, film-coated tablet with the letters **BP** and the number **132** imprinted on each tablet. Packaged in bottles of 100 (Item No. 0486-1132-01) tablets.

Beutlich LP Pharmaceuticals

1541 SHIELDS DRIVE
WAUKEGAN, IL 60085-8304

Direct Inquiries to:
847-473-1100
800-238-8542 in US & Canada
FAX 847-473-1122
www.beutlich.com
e-mail beutlich@beutlich.com

PERIDIN-C®
Vitamin C Supplement

Dietary supplement helps alleviate hot flashes by improving capillary

Continued on next page

Peridin-C—Cont.

strength and maintaining vascular integrity, reducing the physiologic potential for flushing.

Suggested Use: As a Dietary Supplement - 1 tablet daily or as directed/For Hot Flashes - 2 tablets, 3 times per day after meals. Reduce servings gradually after one month until effective daily intake is determined.

Ingredients:
Ascorbic Acid (Vitamin C) 200 mg
Hesperidin Complex (Bioflavonoids) - 150 mg
Hesperidin Methyl Chalcone (Bioflavonoid) - 50 mg

Other Ingredients: hydroxypropyl methylcellulose, Microcrystalline cellulose, crospovidone, stearic acid, polydextrose, titanium dioxide, yellow 6 lake, polyethylene glycol, magnesium stearate, silicon dioxide, triacetin, carnauba wax and polysorbate 80.

How Supplied: In bottles of:
100 tablets NDC #0283-0597-01
500 tablets NDC #0283-0597-05

Dannmarie, LLC
2005 PALMER AVENUE #200
LARCHMONT, NY 10538

Direct Inquiries to:
phone: (877) 425-8767
www.premcal.com
info@premcal.com

PREMCAL

Description: PremCal is a combination calcium and vitamin D nutritional supplement that offers three different strengths of vitamin D3 per tablet-500 IU, 750 IU, and 1000 IU with 500 mg of elemental calcium as the carbonate. PremCal is indicated in those requiring higher than the currently recommended doses of vitamin D such as vitamin D deficiency, premenstrual syndrome, osteoporosis, osteomalacia or malabsorption.

Ingredients: PremCal tablets are supplied in 3 different strengths of vitamin D3 (Light- 500 IU; Regular- 750 IU; Extra strength -1000 IU) with a constant amount of calcium 500 mg as calcium carbonate and 15 mg of magnesium oxide. Each tablet also contains hypromellose, croscarmellose sodium, malto dextrin, povidone, stearic acid, magnesium stearate, triacetin, polyethylene glycol, silicon dioxide. Free of sugar, soy, wheat, gluten, corn, shellfish, and artificial colors.

Directions: One tablet two times a day with meals or as recommended by your physician.

Warnings: Do not take more than two tablets per day unless directed by your physician. Do not use with prolonged or intense exposure to sunlight unless directed by your physician. Do not use if you have a calcium disorder such as primary hyperparathyroidism, hypercalciuria, elevated calcium levels, kidney stones or kidney disease without consulting your physician.

How Supplied: PremCal Light, Regular and Extra strength are supplied in bottles of 180 tablets. UPC#8-80569-00014-3 (PremCal *Light); UPC#8-80569-00011-2 (PremCal -Regular); UPC#8-80569-00017-4 (PremCal -Extra strength).

Eminence Labs
LOS ANGELES, CA 90010

Direct Inquiries To:
Richard Shen
Phone: (626) 930-0254

Eminence Labs is dedicated to the cutting-edge biotechnologies to study cellular activities and protein molecules interaction, especially on the mechanism of pain, in order to elucidate the nuance of cellular, physical and chemical mechanisms. It is based on the super medical concepts to solve problems, to recreate cells and to help individuals reach normal and healthy body status, and moreover reach entire organ systems all over the whole body.*

201 GA Nano Bio-Chem Hair Protection: To employ the NanoTech and Transdermal Delivery to enforce nutrients into follicle cell with excellent clinical results. Used for treatment of Psilosis and Alopecia.

301 GA&B Nano Neuron Bio-Defense Liquid: To activate cells, adjust cellular action potentials and minor chemical elements. Used for complete relief of pain.

302 Nano joint Bio-Defense Liquid: To deliver into bone joint and joint cavities. Used for treatment of Gout and Osteoarthritis.

303 Nano Menes Bio-Defense Liquid: Aims at female menstrual pain and rebuild up healthy cells of propagation system.

305 Bio-Nano-Vital Refreshing Essence: To prevent and cure of buccal cells and inner membrane ulceration.

306 Bio-Nano-Nasal Rejuvenating Essence: To prevent and cure nasal tissue change and treat of allergic rhinitis.

606 Buccal Temper Essence: To assist with a cure for cure Periodontal disease and cariosity within a short period of time.

801 Bio-Nano Magic Gel: To rejuvenate and restore the tightness of female prolapsed vagina.

802 Bio-Nano Compact Gel: To cure pregnancy stretch marks, wrinkles and weakened muscle.

These statements have not been evaluated by the Food and Drug Administration. These products are not intended to diagnose, treat, cure, or prevent any disease.*

Eniva Corporation
MINNEAPOLIS, MN 55449

Direct Inquiries to:
www.eniva.com

VIBE™
Liquid Multi-Nutrient Supplement

Supplement Facts
Serving Size: 1 Fluid Ounce
Servings Per Container: 32

	Amount Per Serving	% Daily Value
Calories	24	
Total Carbohydrate	5 g	2%*
Sugars	3 g	†
Vitamin A	5,000 IU	100%
Vitamin C	120 mg	200%
Vitamin D	500 IU	125%
Vitamin E	30 IU	100%
Thiamin (B1)	1.5 mg	100%
Riboflavin (B2)	1.7 mg	100%
Niacin	20 mg	100%
Vitamin B6	2 mg	100%
Folic Acid	400 mcg	100%
Vitamin B12	6 mcg	100%
Biotin	300 mcg	100%
Pantothenic Acid	10 mg	100%
Calcium	100 mg	10%
Phosphorus	50 mg	5%
Iodine	150 mcg	100%
Magnesium	200 mg	50%
Zinc	4 mg	26%
Selenium	35 mcg	50%
Copper	.4 mg	20%
Manganese	1.5 mg	75%
Chromium	120 mcg	100%
Potassium	175 mg	5%
Boron	1 mg	†
Germanium	25 mcg	†
Strontium	500 mcg	†
Sulfur	35 mg	†
Vanadium	5 mcg	†
AntiOX²™ Proprietary Blend	6,000 mg	†

Natural Extracts: Cranberry, Raspberry, Blueberry, Blackberry, Strawberry, Cherry, Carrot, Elderberry, Hibiscus (flower), Lemon, Lime, Apple, Blackcurrant, Oregano, Chokeberry, Grape, Pumpkin, Tomato, Pomegranate, Katemfe, Wolfberry, Stevia (leaf), Citrus Bioflavonoids, Grape Seed

HeartMAX   280 mg   †
Proprietary Blend
  D-Ribose, CoQ10, L-Carnitine, Malic
  Acid, Lecithin

CollaMAX™   3,300 mg   †
Proprietary Blend
  Green Tea Leaf Extract, L-Lysine,
  L-Proline, Aloe Vera Gel, Glucosamine
  HCl (vegetable), Glycine, Alanine,
  Valine, Isoleucine, Leucine

---

* Percent Daily Values are based on a
  2,000 calorie diet.
† Daily Value not established.

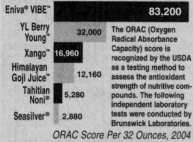

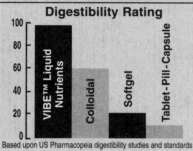

*Shown in Product Identification
Guide, page 503*

4Life Research

9850 S 300 W
SANDY, UT 84070

Direct Inquiries to:
Ph: (801) 562-3600
Fax: (801) 562-3699
Email: productsupport@4life.com
Website: www.4life.com

4LIFE® TRANSFER FACTOR
PLUS® ADVANCED FORMULA

Description: Transfer factors are
small peptides of approximately 44
amino acids that "transfer" or have the
ability to express cell-mediated immunity from immune donors to non-immune
recipients. 4Life® Transfer Factor™
products are derived from egg yolk and
cow colostrum extracts containing anti-
gen information, providing the broadest
spectrum transfer factor available. The
extraction of 4Life Transfer Factor is
protected by US patents 6,468,534;
4,816,563; with other patents pending.
Transfer factors educate the immune
system to recognize self from non-self,
thus support healthy immune system
function. Because it instructs the immune system to act appropriately, transfer factors are effective in supporting
normal inflammatory response in the
body, a key to healthy body system function.
4Life Transfer Factor Plus Advanced
Formula combines Transfer Factor E-
XF™ with a proprietary formulation of
innate and adaptive immune system en-
hancers such as Inositol Hexaphosphate,
Cordyceps, Beta Glucans, Maitake and
Shiitake Mushrooms. These ingredients
work together to trigger and enhance the
various immune protective mechanisms
of the body. Clinical studies show that
4Life Transfer Factor Plus Advanced
Formula can increase Natural Killer cell
activity up to 437 percent above baseline.*

---

*Blind Independent study conducted by
Dr. Anatoli Vorobiev, Head of Immunol-
ogy, at the Russian Academy of Medical
Science.
Summary of Research: In 1949
transfer factors were discovered by Dr.
H. Sherwood Lawrence. Since that time
hundreds of studies have been completed
involving transfer factors' effect on various diseases. Due to new studies conducted in Russia, the Russian Health
Ministry has approved 4Life Transfer
Factor and 4Life Transfer Factor Plus to
be the first supplements used by doctors
and hospitals in Russia. Recent studies
on transfer factor include:
**Rak, AV et al. Effectiveness of Transfer
Factor (TF) in the Treatment of Osteo-
myelitis Patients.** *International Symposium* in Moscow 2002, Nov 5–7, 62–63.
**Granitov, VM et al. Usage of Transfer
Factor Plus in Treatment of HIV – Infected Patients.** *Russian Journal of HIV,
AIDS and Related Problems* 2002, 1, 79–
80.
**Karbysheva, NV et al. Enhanced Trans-
fer Factor in the Complex Treatment of
Patients with Opisthorchiasis.** *Interna-
tional Symposium in* Moscow 2002,
May, 104–105.
**Luikova, SG et al. Transfer Factor in
Dermatovenerology.** *Syberian Journal
of Dermatology and Venerology* 2002,
3, 34–35.

Directions for Use: 4Life Transfer
Factor Plus – Take two (2) capsules daily
with 8 oz. of fluid.

How Supplied: 60ct/bottle
**4Life Transfer Factor™ Products
Include:**
  4Life Transfer Factor Advanced
  Formula
  4Life Transfer Factor Plus Advanced
  Formula

4Life® Transfer Factor RioVida™
4Life® Transfer Factor Cardio™
4Life® Transfer Factor ReCall®
4Life® Transfer Factor MalePro™
4Life® Transfer Factor GluCoach™
4Life® Transfer Factor™ Chewable
4Life® Transfer Factor™ Immune
Spray
4Life® Transfer Factor™ RenewAll
4Life® Transfer Factor™ Kids
4Life® Transfer Factor™ Toothpaste
4Life® Transfer Factor Age-Defying
Effects™
*See www.transferfactorinstitute.com for
more information on transfer factor*

GlaxoSmithKline
Consumer Healthcare,
L.P.

P.O. BOX 1467
PITTSBURGH, PA 15230

Direct Inquiries to:
Consumer Affairs
1-800-245-1040

For Medical Emergencies Contact:
Consumer Affairs
1-800-245-1040

ALLUNA™ SLEEP
Herbal Supplement Tablet

Use: Alluna Sleep is an herbal supplement that can relieve occasional
sleeplessness.* It works by helping you
relax, so you can drift off to sleep naturally.*
Alluna Sleep has been clinically tested
and shown to be effective in actually promoting your body's own natural sleep
pattern – safely and gently.* This is a
natural process. Depending upon your
particular circumstances, benefits are
typically seen within a few nights with
more consistent results within two
weeks.
Alluna Sleep is not habit forming and is
safe to take over time. You can expect to
wake up refreshed, with no groggy side
effects, because you experience a natural, healthy sleep through the night.*

Supplement Facts:
Serving Size: 2 Tablets

	Amount Per 2 Tablets	% Daily Value
Calories	5	
Valerian Root Extract	500 mg	†
Hops Extract	120 mg	†

†Daily Value Not Established

Continued on next page

Alluna—Cont.

Other Ingredients: microcrystalline cellulose, soy polysaccharide, hydrogenated castor oil, hypromellose. Contains less than 2% of titanium dioxide, propylene glycol, magnesium stearate, silica, polyethylene glycol (400, 6,000 and 20,000), blue 2 lake, artificial flavoring.

Directions: Take **two** (2) tablets one hour before bedtime with a glass of water.

Warning: As with all dietary supplements, contact your doctor before use if you are pregnant or lactating. Keep this and all dietary supplements out of the reach of children. Driving or operating machinery while using this product is not recommended. Chronic insomniacs should consult their doctor before using this product.

Please Note: The herbs in this product have a distinct natural aroma.

Store in a cool, dry place. Avoid temperatures above 86°F.

How Supplied: Packets of 28 and 56 Tablets

BEANO®
[*bēan ō*]
Food Enzyme Dietary Supplement

PRODUCT INFORMATION

Description:
Beano drops: each 5 drop dosage follows Food Chemical Codex (FCC) standards for activity and contains 150 GalU (galactosidase units) of alpha-D-galactosidase derived from *Aspergillus niger* mold. The enzyme is in a liquid carrier of water and xylitol. Add about 5 drops on the first bite of problem food serving, but remember a normal meal has 2-3 servings of the problem foods.

Beano tablets: each tablet follows Food Chemical Codex (FCC) standards for activity and contains 150 GalU (galactosidase units) of alpha-D-galactosidase derived from *Aspergillus niger* mold. The enzyme is in a carrier of cellulose gel, mannitol, invertase, potato starch, magnesium stearate, gelatin (fish), colloidal silica. 3 tablets swallowed, chewed, or crumbled onto food should be enough for a normal meal of 3 servings of problem foods (1 tablet per ½ cup serving). Beano® will hydrolyze complex sugars, raffinose, stachyose and verbascose, into the simple sugars - glucose, galactose and fructose, and the easily digestible disaccharide, sucrose. (Sucrose hydrolysis happens simultaneously with normal digestion.) In some cases, more enzyme than 5 drops or 3 tablets will be required, and this is a function of the quantity of food eaten, the levels of alpha-linked sugars in the food, and the gas-producing propensity of the person.

Use: Helps prevent flatulence and/or bloat from a variety of grains, cereals, nuts, seeds, and vegetables containing the sugars raffinose, stachyose and/or verbascose. This includes all or most legumes and all or most cruciferous vegetables. Examples of such foods are oats, wheat, beans of all kinds, chickpeas, peas, lentils, peanuts, soy-content foods, broccoli, brussel sprouts, cabbage, carrots, corn, leeks, onions, parsnips, squash. Note: Most vegetables and beans also contain fiber, which is gas productive in some people, but usually far less so than the alpha-linked sugars. Beano® has no effect on fiber.

Usage: About 5 drops per food serving or 3 tablets per meal (1 tablet per ½ cup serving) of 3 servings of problem foods; higher levels depending on symptoms.

Precautions: If you are pregnant or nursing, ask your doctor before product use. Beano is made from a safe, food-grade mold. However, if a rare sensitivity occurs, discontinue use. Galactosemics should not use without physician's advice, since one of the breakdown sugars is galactose.

How Supplied: Beano® is supplied in both a liquid form (30 and 75 serving sizes, at 5 drops per serving), and a tablet form (30, 60, and 100 tablet sizes as well as 24 tablets in packets of 3). These statements have not been evaluated by the Food and Drug Administration. This product is not intended to diagnose, treat, cure or prevent any disease.
For more information and free samples, please write or call toll-free 1-800-257-8650 or visit www.beano.net.

FEOSOL® Caplets
Hematinic
Iron Supplement

Description: FEOSOL Caplets contain pure iron micro particles called carbonyl iron. Replacing FEOSOL Capsules, this advanced formula is specially designed to be well absorbed, gentle on the stomach and offers enhanced safety in the event of an accidental overdose. Each FEOSOL carbonyl iron caplet delivers 45 mg of pure elemental iron, the same amount of elemental iron contained in the 225 mg ferrous sulfate capsule. At equivalent doses, carbonyl iron and ferrous sulfate were shown to be equally efficacious in correcting hemoglobin, hematocrit and serum iron levels in iron-deficient patients[1].

Safety: According to the American Association of Poison Control Centers, iron containing supplements are the leading cause of pediatric poisoning deaths for children under six in the United States[2]. Widely used as a food additive, carbonyl iron must be gastrically solubilized before it can be absorbed, giving it lower toxicity and enhancing its safety versus any of the ferrous salts[3]. As a result, carbonyl iron presents less chance of harm from accidental overdose. In addition, at equivalent doses, carbonyl iron side effects are no greater than those experienced with ferrous sulfate[4].

Warnings: Do not exceed recommended dosage. The treatment of any anemic condition should be under the advice and supervision of a physician. Since oral iron products interfere with absorption of oral tetracycline antibiotics, these products should not be taken within two hours of each other. Occasional gastrointestinal discomfort (such as nausea) may be minimized by taking with meals. Iron containing medication may occasionally cause constipation or diarrhea. If you are pregnant or nursing a baby, seek the advice of a health professional before using this product.

WARNING: Accidental overdose of iron-containing products is a leading cause of fatal poisoning in children under 6. Keep this product out of reach of children. In case of accidental overdose, call a doctor or poison control center immediately.

SUPPLEMENT FACTS
Serving Size: 1 Caplet

Amount per Caplet	% Daily Value
Iron 45 mg	250%

Ingredients: Lactose, Sorbitol, Carbonyl Iron, Hypromellose. Contains 1% or less of the following ingredients: Carnauba Wax, Crospovidone, FD&C Blue #2 Al Lake, FD&C Red #40 Al Lake, FD&C Yellow #6 Al Lake, Magnesium Stearate, Polydextrose, Polyethylene Glycol, Polyethylene Glycol 8000 (Powder), Stearic Acid, Titanium Dioxide, Triacetin.

Directions: Adults—one caplet daily or as directed by a physician. Children under 12 years: Consult a physician.

Tamper-Evident Feature: Each caplet is encased in a plastic cell with a foil back; do not use if cell or foil is broken.

References: [1]Devasthali SD, Gordeuk VR, Brittenham GM, et al, "Bioavailability of Carbonyl Iron: A randomized, double-blind study." Eur J Haematology, 1991; 46:272–278.
[2]FDA Consumer; March 1996:7
[3]Heubers, JA, Brittenham GM, Csiba E and Finch CA. "Absorption of carbonyl iron." J Lab Clin Med 1986; 108:473–78.
[4]Devasthali SD, Gordeuk VR, Brittenham GM, et al, "Bioavailability of a Carbonyl Iron: A randomized, double-blind study." Eur J Haematology, 1991; 46:272–278.

Store at room temperature, avoid excessive heat (greater than 100°F) or humidity.

How Supplied: Boxes of 30 and 60 caplets in blisters. Also available in single unit packages of 100 caplets intended for institutional use
Also available: Feosol Tablets.

Comments or Questions? Call Toll-Free 1-800-245-1040 Weekdays. GlaxoSmithKline Consumer Healthcare, L.P.
Moon Township, PA 15108
Made in USA
Shown in Product Identification Guide, page 504

FEOSOL® TABLETS
Hematinic
Iron Supplement

Description: Feosol tablets provide the body with ferrous sulfate—an iron supplement for iron deficiency and iron deficiency anemia when the need for such therapy has been determined by a physician.

SUPPLEMENT FACTS
Serving Size: 1 Tablet

Amount per Tablet	% Daily Value
Iron 65 mg	360%

Ingredients: Dried ferrous sulfate 200 mg (65 mg of elemental iron) equivalent to 325 mg of ferrous sulfate per tablet. Lactose, Sorbitol, Crospovidone, Magnesium Stearate, Carnauba Wax. Contains 2% or less of the following ingredients: FD&C Blue #1, FD&C Yellow #6, Hypromellose, Polydextrose, Polyethylene Glycol, Titanium Dioxide, Triacetin.

Directions: Adults and children 12 years and over—One tablet daily or as directed by a physician. Children under 12 years—Consult a physician.

Tamper-Evident Feature: Each tablet is encased in a plastic cell with a foil back; do not use if cell or foil is broken.

Warnings: Do not exceed recommended dosage. The treatment of any anemic condition should be under the advice and supervision of a physician. Since oral iron products interfere with absorption of oral tetracycline antibiotics, these products should not be taken within two hours of each other. Occasional gastrointestinal discomfort (such as nausea) may be minimized by taking with meals. Iron containing medication may occassionally cause constipation or diarrhea.

If you are pregnant or nursing a baby, seek the advice of a health professional before using this product.

WARNING: Accidental overdose of iron-contraining products is a leading cause of fatal poisoning in children under 6. Keep this product out of reach of children. In case of accidental overdose, call a doctor, or poison control center immediately.

Store at room temperature (59–86°F). Not USP for dissolution.

How Supplied: Cartons of 100 tablets in child-resistant blisters. Previously packaged in bottles. Also available: Feosol caplets.

Supplement Facts
Serving Size 1 Tablet

Amount Per Serving	% Daily Value for Pregnant or Lactating Women	% Daily Value for Adults and Children 4 or more years of age
Calories 5		
Calcium 500 mg	38%	50%

Amount Per Tablet	% Daily Value for Pregnant or Lactating Women	% Daily Value for Adults and Children 4 or More Years of Age
Vitamin D 125 IU	31%	31%
Calcium 250 mg	19%	25%

Comments or Questions? Call toll-free 1-800-245-1040 weekdays. GlaxoSmithKline Consumer Healthcare, L.P.
Moon Township, PA 15108
Made in USA
Shown in Product Identification Guide, page 504

OS-CAL® CHEWABLE
Calcium Supplement

Description: Calcium supplement to help reduce the risk of osteoporosis. Osteoporosis affects middle-aged and older persons, especially Caucasian and Asian women, and those whose families tend to have fragile bones in later years. A lifetime of regular exercise and eating a healthful diet that includes enough calcium, especially during teen and early adult years, builds and maintains good bone health and may reduce the risk of osteoporosis in later life.

Adequate calcium intake is important, but daily intakes above 2000 mg are not likely to provide any additional benefit. [See first table above]

Ingredients: Calcium carbonate, dextrose monohydrate, maltodextrin, microcrystalline cellulose, magnesium stearate, artificial flavors, sodium chloride. Each tablet provides 500 mg of elemental calcium

Directions: One tablet two to three times a day with meals, or as recommended by your physician.

How Supplied: Bottle of 60 tablets
Store at room temperature.
Keep out of reach of children.

OS-CAL® 250 + D
Calcium with Vitamin D Supplement

Description: Calcium supplement to help reduce the risk of osteoporosis (see below*). Also contains Vitamin D.

Supplement Facts
Serving Size 1 Tablet
[See second table above]

Ingredients: Oyster shell powder, corn syrup solids, talc, corn starch, hypromellose. Contains less than 1% of calcium stearate, polysorbate 80, titanium dioxide, polyethylene glycol, Vitamin D, propylparaben and methylparaben (preservative), simethicone, yellow 5 lake, blue 1 lake, carnauba wax, edetate sodium.

Directions: One tablet three times a day with meals, or as recommended by your physician.

How Supplied: Bottle of 100 and 240 tablets
Store at room temperature.
Keep out of reach of children.

*Osteoporosis affects middle-aged and older persons, especially Caucasian and Asian women, and those whose families tend to have fragile bones in later years. A lifetime of regular exercise and eating a healthful diet that includes enough calcium, especially during teen and early adult years, builds and maintains good bone health and may reduce the risk of osteoporosis in later life.

Adequate calcium intake is important, but daily intakes above 2000 mg are not likely to provide any additional benefit.

Shown in Product Identification Guide, page 505

OS-CAL® 500
Calcium Supplement

Description: Calcium supplement to help reduce the risk of osteoporosis. Osteoporosis affects middle-aged and older persons, especially Caucasian and Asian women, and those whose families tend to have fragile bones in later years. A lifetime of regular exercise and eating a healthful diet that includes enough calcium, especially during teen and early adult years, builds and maintains good bone health and may reduce the risk of osteoporosis in later life.

Adequate calcium intake is important, but daily intakes above 2000 mg are not likely to provide any additional benefit.

Continued on next page

Os-Cal 500—Cont.

Supplement Facts
Serving Size 1 Tablet
[See first table at right]

Ingredients: Oyster shell powder, corn syrup solids, talc, corn starch. Contains less than 1% of sodium starch glycolate, calcium stearate, polysorbate 80, hypromellose, polydextrose, titanium dioxide, propylparaben and methylparaben (preservative), triacetin, yellow 5 lake, blue 1 lake, polyethylene glycol, carnauba wax.

Directions: One tablet two to three times a day with meals, or as recommended by your physician.

How Supplied: Bottles of 75 and 160 tablets
Store at room temperature.
Keep out of reach of children.

Shown in Product Identification Guide, page 505

OS-CAL® 500 + D
Calcium with Vitamin D Supplement

Description: Calcium supplement to help reduce the risk of osteoporosis (see below*). Also contains Vitamin D.
[See second table above]

Ingredients: Oyster shell powder, corn syrup solids, talc, corn starch. Contains less than 1% of sodium starch glycolate, calcium stearate, polysorbate 80, hypromellose, polydextrose, titanium dioxide, Vitamin D, propylparaben and methylparaben (preservative), triacetin, yellow 5 lake, blue 1 lake, polyethylene glycol, carnauba wax.

Directions: One tablet two to three times a day with meals, or as recommended by your physician.

How Supplied: Bottle of 75 and 160 tablets
Store at room temperature.
Keep out of reach of children.
*Osteoporosis affects middle-aged and older persons, especially Caucasian and Asian women, and those whose families tend to have fragile bones in later years. A lifetime of regular exercise and eating a healthful diet that includes enough calcium, especially during teen and early adult years, builds and maintains good bone health and may reduce the risk of osteoporosis in later life.
Adequate calcium intake is important, but daily intakes above 2000 mg are not likely to provide any additional benefit.

Shown in Product Identification Guide, page 505

REMIFEMIN Menopause
Drug Free
Herbal Supplement
A safe, natural, effective way to help ease the physical and emotional symptoms of menopause*

Remifemin Menopause is a unique, natural formula. For over 40 years in Europe, it has helped reduce the unpleasant physical and emotional symptoms associated with menopause, such as hot flashes, night sweats and mood swings. Clinically shown to be safe and effective. Not a drug.
Remifemin Menopause helps you approach menopause with confidence – naturally.*

Supplement Facts Serving Size 1 tablet		
Ingredients:	Amount Per Tablet:	% Daily Value:
Black Cohosh Extract (Root and Rhizome) Equivalent to	20 mg	†

†Daily Value Not Established.

Other Ingredients: Lactose, Cellulose, Potato Starch, Magnesium Stearate, and Natural Peppermint Flavor.
Standardized to be equivalent to 20 mg Black Cohosh (*Cimicifuga racemosa*) root and rhizome.
Contains no salt, yeast, wheat, gluten, corn, soy, coloring, or preservatives.

Directions: Take one tablet in the morning and one tablet in the evening, with water. You can expect to notice improvements within a few weeks with full benefits after using Remifemin twice a day for 4 to 12 weeks. This product is intended for use by women who are experiencing menopausal symptoms. Does not contain estrogen. Remifemin is not meant to replace any drug therapy.

Warnings: This product should not be used by women who are pregnant or considering becoming pregnant or are nursing. As with any dietary supplement, always keep out of reach of children. For a few consumers, gastric discomfort may occur but should not be persistent. If gastric discomfort persists, discontinue use and see your health care practitioner. As part of an overall good health care program, we encourage you to see your health care practitioner on a regular basis.

Making Sense Out of Menopause with Remifemin Menopause
Today, women are leading very dynamic and diverse lifestyles. Despite this diversity, there is one constant. They are all experiencing physiological changes.

They will all experience menopause. The time when you have menopausal symptoms is a multiphasic period. Technically, the change or transitional process of menopause is known as the *"Climacteric"*. There are different phases of the climacteric that a woman experiences:

1. *Perimenopause* is the transitional phase when hormone levels begin to drop. This phase lasts typically 3 to 5 years but can last up to 10 years. This gradual decline in estrogen levels causes the troublesome effects of menopause.

2. *Menopause* is the permanent cessation of menstruation. The average age at menopause is 51, but there is considerable variation in this timing among women. Menopause is medically defined as one year without menstruation.

3. *Postmenopause* is the phase following menopause. During this phase, your body gets used to the loss of estrogen and eventually the symptoms such as hot flashes go away.

Some Commonly Asked Questions Regarding Remifemin Menopause
1. What is Remifemin Menopause?
Remifemin Menopause is a uniquely formulated natural herbal supplement derived from the black cohosh plant. It is formulated to work with your body to promote physical and emotional balance during menopause. Over 40 years of clinical research has shown Remifemin Menopause helps reduce hot flashes, night sweats, related occasional sleeplessness, irritability and mood swings. In a recent clinical study, on average, women experienced the following overall improvements:

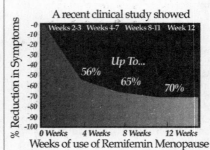

A recent clinical study showed
Weeks 2-3 Weeks 4-7 Weeks 8-11 Week 12
Up To...
56% 65% 70%
% Reduction in Symptoms
0 Weeks 4 Weeks 8 Weeks 12 Weeks
Weeks of use of Remifemin Menopause

2. What makes Remifemin Menopause so special? Remifemin Menopause contains an *exclusive* extract of black cohosh. Unlike many other black cohosh products, it is developed with specific modern analytical techniques which pro-

---

Amount Per Tablet	% Daily Value for Pregnant or Lactating Women	% Daily Value for Adults and children 4 or more years of age
Calcium 500 mg	38%	50%

Supplement Facts Serving Size 1 Tablet		
Amount Per Tablet	% Daily Value for Pregnant or Lactating Women	% Daily Value for Adults and Children 4 or more years of age
Vitamin D 200 IU	50%	50%
Calcium 500 mg	38%	50%

duce a standardized extract of the black cohosh root and rhizome. In addition, Remifemin is estrogen free and does not influence hormone levels, unlike estrogens and phytoestrogens such as soy.

3. With so many products out there claiming to be "natural," how can I be sure that this product is safe and effective? Remifemin Menopause's formulation is supported by over 40 years of clinical research, and millions of women in Europe have safely used it. Remifemin Menopause is drug free and estrogen free. And it is brought to you from a world-renowned health care company.

4. How does Remifemin Menopause work? Remifemin Menopause contains a proprietary standardized extract taken from the rootstock of the black cohosh plant. Studies have shown that the compounds found within this standardized herbal extract seem to interact with certain hormone receptors – without influencing hormone levels.*

5. How long does it take for Remifemin Menopause to work? Remifemin Menopause is a natural herbal supplement, not a drug. It will take time for your body's cycles to respond to its gentle onset. Personally, you may notice improvements within a few weeks. But for some women, it may take 4 to 12 weeks to benefit fully from Remifemin Menopause. Since the effects of Remifemin Menopause increase after extended twice daily use, we recommend that you take Remifemin Menopause for at least 12 weeks. If you do not find any difference in your well being after 12 weeks, please consult your physician to discuss other options.

6. Can I take it over a long period of time, since the menopausal period lasts for years? Every woman's menopause symptoms are different. Depending on your particular circumstances, you should expect that over time your body will be adjusted to its lower level of estrogen and you may find that you no longer need to take Remifemin. You should listen to your body. We recommend that you take Remifemin Menopause twice daily for up to 6 months continuously. If, after discontinuing use your symptoms return, you may start taking Remifemin Menopause again. Keep in mind that Remifemin Menopause is a natural herbal supplement that supports a natural change that may take you years to go through. As part of an overall good healthcare program, we encourage you to see your health care practitioner on a regular basis.

7. Are there any known side effects? When used properly following the package directions, Remifemin Menopause has few side effects, if any. In clinical research, there was a small percentage of gastric discomfort complaints. If you have been taking Remifemin Menopause and find that this or any other condition develops and persists, please discontinue use and see your physician.

8. Is there a certain time of the day when I should take this product? Do I need to take it with food? You can take Remifemin Menopause with or without food any time of the day. We recommend that you take one tablet in the morning with your breakfast and one tablet in the evening with water.

9. Can I take my herbal tea, vitamins, or other dietary supplements with

Remifemin Menopause? Typically, dietary supplements can be taken with other dietary supplements. Always follow package directions. If you should notice any undesirable effects, discontinue taking them together.

Expiration and Storage Information
The expiration date of this package is printed on the side panel flap of the outer carton as well as on the blister packs. Do not use this product after this date.
Store this product in a cool, dry place. Keep out of the reach of children. Avoid storing at temperatures above 86°F.

---

*These statements have not been evaluated by the Food and Drug Administration. This product is not intended to diagnose, treat, cure, or prevent any disease.

Questions or Comments? Call toll-free 1-800-965-8804 weekdays, or visit www.remifemin.com anytime.

Remifemin ® is a trademark of Schaper & Brümmer GmbH & Co. KG, licensed to GlaxoSmithKline.

Greek Island Labs.

**7620 E. MCKELLIPS RD.
SUITE 4 PMB 86
SCOTTSDALE, AZ 85257 USA**

Direct Inquires To:
www.GreekIslandLabs.com
1-888-841-7363

ATHENA HAIR SYSTEM
Shampoo

Description: Women's Shampoo

Ingredients: Proprietary Greek Blend: Water, Cocamidopropyl Betaine, Sodium Methyl Cocoyl Taurate, Cocamide MEA, Sodium Chloride, Alcohol, Panthenol, Lecithin, Tocopherol Acetate, Caffeine, Biotin, Borage Oil, Azelaic Acid, Phytosterols, Zinc Sulfate Monohydrate, Saw Palmetto Extract

Directions: Use Daily Apply to wet hair then rinse

Warnings: Keep out of eyes

How Supplied: 8 fl. oz Per Bottle

ATHENA HAIR SYSTEM
Supplement

Description: Women's Supplement for Promoting Healthy Hair Growth*

Ingredients: Proprietary Greek Blend of: Rosemary (aerial parts), Ashwagandha Root, Atlantic Kelp, Olive Leaf, artichoke Leaf, Black cumin Seed,

Eleuthero Root, Grape Leaf Extract, and Pomegranate Fruit Extract Fruit & Veggie Blend, Raspberry, Strawberry, Watermelon, Radish, Cantaloupe, Cherry, Leek, Onion, Papaya, Peach, Pear, Collagen, MSM, Vitamin A, Vitamin C, Vitamin E Thiamin, Riboflavin, Niacin, Vitamin B6, Folate, Vitamin B12 Alfalfa Leaf, Asparagus Spear, Broccoli Floret, Brussels Sprout Leaf, Cabbage Leaf, Cauliflower Floret, Garlic Bulb, Kale Leaf, Mustard Greens, and Spinach Leaf

Directions: 2 Capsules daily with food

Warnings: Consult your doctor prior to using this product if you are taking any prescription medication

How Supplied: 60 Capsules (Vegetarian) Per Bottle

*The statements have not been reviewed or approved by the Food & Drug Administration. This product is not intended to diagnose, treat, cure or prevent any disease.

SPARTAN HAIR SYSTEM
Shampoo

Description: Men's Shampoo

Ingredients: Proprietary Greek Blend: Water, Cocamidopropyl Betaine, Sodium Methyl Cocoyl Taurate, Cocamide MEA, Sodium Chloride, Alcohol, Panthenol, Lecithin, Tocopherol Acetate, Caffeine, Biotin, Borage Oil, Azelaic Acid, Phytosterols, Zinc Sulfate Monohydrate, Saw Palmetto Extract

Directions: Use Daily Apply to wet hair and rinse

Warnings: Keep out of eyes

How Supplied: 8 fl. oz Per Bottle

SPARTAN HAIR SYSTEM
Supplement

Description: Men's Supplement for Promoting Healthy Hair Growth*

Ingredients: Proprietary Greek Blend of: Rosemary (aerial parts), Ashwagandha Root, Atlantic kelp, Olive Leaf, artichoke Leaf, Black cumin Seed, Eleuthero Root, Grape Leaf Extract, and Pomegranate Fruit Extract Fruit & Veggie Blend, Raspberry, Strawberry, Watermelon, Radish, Cantaloupe, Cherry, Leek, Onion, Papaya, Peach, Pear, Collagen, MSM, Vitamin A, Vitamin C, Vitamin E Thiamin, Riboflavin, Niacin, Vitamin B6, Folate, Vitamin B12 Alfalfa Leaf, Asparagus Spear, Broccoli Floret, Brussels Sprout Leaf, Cabbage Leaf, Cauliflower Floret, Garlic Bulb, Kale Leaf, Mustard Greens, and Spinach Leaf

Directions: 2 Capsules daily with food

Continued on next page

Spartan Hair System—Cont.

Warnings: Consult your doctor prior to using this product if you are taking any prescription medication

How Supplied: 60 Capsules (Vegetarian) Per Bottle

*The statements have not been reviewed or approved by the Food & Drug Administration. This product is not intended to diagnose, treat, cure or prevent any disease.

Legacy for Life, LLC
P.O. BOX 410376
MELBOURNE, FL 32941-0376

Direct Inquiries to:
(800) 557-8477
(321) 951-8815
www.legacyforlife.net

IMMUNE[26®]

Description: immune[26®] ("hyperimmune" egg) is derived from both the white, and the yolk, of eggs of hens stimulated with over 26 inactivated pathogens. The polyvalent preparation is primarily of enteric human origin.

Clinical Background: Upon oral administration, a wide range of molecular weight immune components, of both a specific, and non-specific nature, are passively transferred to the recipient. immune[26®] supports immune function, modulates autoimmune responses, supports and balances cardiovascular function, helps maintain healthy cholesterol levels, a vital circulatory system, a fully functional digestive tract, flexible and healthy joints, and energy levels. immune[26®] appears to help the body "balance" immune function, rather than "boost" immune function. It may be used concomitantly with prescription medications.

How Supplied: One serving (4.5g) of immune[26®] is available as: pure hyperimmune egg powder, capsules (9/serving), and as chewable tablets (3/serving). immune[26®] COMPLETE Support, with 4.5g of hyperimmune egg, is enriched with protein, minerals, and 100% of the daily value of more than 13 essential vitamins. immune[26®], at 4.5g, is also the essential ingredient in the high protein, low carbohydrate Legacy BALANCE Shake, utilized for weight management and athletic performance.

Precautions: Those with known allergies to eggs should consult with a health practitioner before consuming this product.

Note: immune[26®] is not intended to diagnose, treat, cure, or prevent any disease. These statements have not been evaluated by the Food and Drug Administration.

Mannatech, Inc.
600 S. ROYAL LANE
SUITE 200
COPPELL, TX 75019

For Medical Professional Inquiries Contact:
Stephen Boyd, MD, PhD
(972) 471-7400
sboyd@mannatech.com

Direct Inquiries to:
Customer Service
(972) 471-8111

Product Information:
www.mannatech.com

Ingredient Information:
www.glycoscience.com

AMBROTOSE®
A Glyconutritional Dietary Supplement

Supplement Facts:
Ambrotose® powder:
Serving Size 0.44 g (approx. ¼ teaspoon)
Powder canister: 100g or 50g

Amount Per Serving	% Daily Value
0.44g	*

* Daily Values not established.

Ambrotose® capsules:
Serving Size: one capsule (2 times daily)
Capsules per container: 60

Amount Per Serving	% Daily Value
1 capsule	*

* Daily Values not established.

Ambrotose® with Lecithin capsules:
Ambrotose® with Lecithin Supplement Facts:
Serving Size: one capsule (2 times daily)
Capsules per container: 60

Amount Per Serving	% Daily Value
1 capsule	*

* Daily Values not established.

Ingredients:
Ambrotose® Powder
Ambrotose® complex
(patent pending)

Arabinogalactan (Larix decidua) (gum), rice starch, Manapol® aloe vera gel extract (inner leaf gel), gum ghatti, Glucosamine HCl, and gum tragacanth.
Ambrotose® capsules
Ambrotose® complex
(patent pending)
Arabinogalactan (Larix decidua) (gum), Manapol® aloe vera gel extract (inner leaf gel), gum ghatti and gum tragacanth.
Other ingredients: Brown rice flour, silicon dioxide, magnesium stearate, gelatine.
Ambrotose® with Lecithin capsules
Ambrotose® complex
(patent pending)
Arabinogalactan (Larix decidua) (gum), Manapol® aloe vera gel extract (inner leaf gel), gum ghatti and gum tragacanth.
Lecithin powder.
Other ingredients: Calcium carbonate, dibasic calcium phosphate, gelatin, brown rice flour, cellulose, silicon dioxide, magnesium stearate.
For additional information on ingredients, visit www.glycoscience.com

Use: Ambrotose® complex is a proprietary formula designed to help provide saccharides used in glycoconjugate synthesis to promote cellular communication and immune support.** Consumers who are healthy may notice improved concentration, more energy, better sleep, improved athletic performance, and a greater sense of well-being.

Directions: The recommended intake of Ambrotose® powder is ¼ teaspoon two times a day; the recommended intake of Ambrotose® capsules or Ambrotose® with Lecithin is one capsule two times daily. If desired, you may begin by taking less than the recommended intake. If well tolerated, you may gradually increase to the recommended intake. As a blend of plant saccharides, Ambrotose complex is safe in amounts well in excess of the label recommendations. Children between the ages of 12 and 48 months with growth/nutritional problems (failure to thrive) have been given 1 tablespoon a day of Ambrotose powder for 3 months with no adverse effects. Individuals have reported taking as much as 10 tablespoons of Ambrotose powder (approx. 50 grams) each day for several months with no adverse effects. The amount needed by each individual may vary with time, age, genetic makeup, metabolic rate, and activities, stress level, current dietary intake, and health challenges of the moment. A health care professional experienced with use of Ambrotose complex may be helpful.

Warning: Anyone who is taking medication may wish to advise his/her physician. One teaspoon of Ambrotose® powder (equivalent to approximately 12 Ambrotose® capsules) contains the amount of glucose equivalent to 1/25 teaspoon of sucrose (table sugar)
KEEP BOTTLE TIGHTLY CLOSED.

STORE IN A COOL, DRY PLACE.

How Supplied: Bottle of 3.50 oz (100g) powder. Bottle of 1.75 oz (50g) powder. Bottle of 60 (150mg) capsules.

** This statement has not been evaluated by the Food and Drug Administration. This product is not intended to diagnose, treat, cure or prevent any disease.

Mannatech Inc.
600 S. Royal Lane, Suite 200
Coppell, Texas 75019
www.mannatech.com
Shown in Product Identification Guide, page 506

AMBROTOSE AO™
[ăm-brō-tōs]
Glyco-Antioxidant Supplement

[See table below]
For additional information on ingredients, Visit www.glycoscience.com

Use: Ambrotose AO™ capsules helps protect both water and fat soluble portions of cells from free radical attacks while supporting your immune system.** Defend your health by supporting overall immune function through the natural glyconutrients in Ambrotose® complex.** Protect against the daily onslaught of toxins, poor food, stress and the environment, all of which contribute to an increase in free radicals, accelerating the aging process. ** Help restore cellular damage and the overall balance your body may have lost due to the harmful effect of free radical damage that results from pollutants in the air we breathe, the water we drink and the lives we live.**

** This statement has not been evaluated by the Food and Drug Administration. This product is not intended to diagnose, treat, cure or prevent any disease.

Directions: The recommended intake of Ambrotose AO™ capsules is one capsule two times daily.

Oxygen Radical Absorption Capacity (ORAC) can be used to assess the antioxidant status of human blood and serum. One recent study reported that increasing fruit and vegetable consumption from the usual five to an experimental ten servings per day over two weeks can increase serum ORAC values by roughly 13%.[1] In an open-label pilot study of 12 healthy human volunteers, the antioxidant effects of increasing amounts of supplementation with Ambrotose AO™ were evaluated. A battery of tests was selected in order to assess both oxidative damage and protection. Independent companies were contracted to conduct blood and urine chemistry tests and statistical data analyses. An increase in $ORAC_{\beta\text{-PE}}$, a measure of oxidative protection, was found at all three doses: 19.1% at 500 mg per day, 37.4% at 1.0 g per day, and 14.3% at 1.5 g per day. A trend of decreased urinary lipid hydroperoxides/creatinine, a marker of oxidative damage, was observed as well. No significant trends were found in regard to urinary alkenal or 8-OHdG levels.[2] Thus, over the same time period, 1.0 g per day of Ambrotose AO™ provided over twice the antioxidant protection (37.4%) provided by 5 servings of fruits and vegetables (13%).

1. Cao G;Booth SL;Sadowski JA;Prior RL;. Increases in human plasma antioxidant capacity after consumption of controlled diets high in fruit and vegetables. *Am J Clin Nutr.* 1998 Nov; 68: 1081-1087.

2. Boyd S, Gary K, Koepke CM, et al. An open-label pilot study of the antioxidant activity in humans of Ambrotose AO™: Results. *GlycoScience & Nutrition (Official Publication of GlycoScience com: The Nutrition Science Site).* 2003;4(6).
   Shown in Product Identification Guide, page 506

PLUS with AMBROTOSE® Complex
Dietary Supplement Caplets

Supplement Facts:
Serving Size - 1 Caplet (3 times daily)

	Amount Per Serving	% Daily Value
Iron	1mg	5
Wild Yam (root)	200mg	*
Standardized for 25mg Phytosterols		
L-Glutamic acid	200mg	*
L-Glycine	200mg	*
L-Lysine	200mg	*
L-Arginine	100mg	*
Beta Sitosterol	25mg	*
Ambrotose® Complex (patent pending)	2.5mg	*

Arabinogalactan (Larix decidua) (gum), Manapol® aloe vera gel extract (inner leaf gel), gum ghatti and gum tragacanth.

Other Ingredients: Microcrystalline cellulose, stearic acid, croscarmellose sodium, silicon dioxide, magnesium stearate, titanium dioxide coating.

*Daily value not established.

For additional information on ingredients, visit www.glycoscience.com

Use: PLUS caplets provide nutrients to help support the endocrine system's production and balance of hormones.** A well-functioning endocrine system works in harmony with the body's immune system, helps support the efficient metabolism of fat, and supports natural recovery from physical or emotional stress.** The functional components of PLUS caplets are wild yam extract, amino acids, and beta sitosterol. PLUS caplets contain no hormones.

Directions: The recommended intake of PLUS caplets is one caplet three times daily.

Warning: After an extensive review of the literature, no documented evidence was found linking the ingredients in PLUS caplets with any form of human cancer or with any problems associated with pregnancy. However, as with all supplements, you should consult your health care professional if you are pregnant.

Supplement Facts:
Serving Size - 1 Capsule

	Amount Per Serving	% Daily Value
Vitamin E (as mixed d-alpha-, d-beta, d-delta and d-gamma tocopherols)	18 IU	60%
Mtech AO Blend™	113mg	
Quercetin dihydrate		*
Grape pomace extract (fruit)		*
Green tea extract (leaves)		*
Australian Bush Plum (Terminalia ferdinandiana) (fruit)		*
Ambrotose® Phyto Formula	333mg	
Gum Arabic		*
Xanthan Gum		*
Gum Tragacanth		*
Gum Ghatti		*
Aloe vera gel extract (inner leaf gel)- Manapol® powder		*
Phyt • Aloe complex (broccoli, Brussels sprout, cabbage, carrot, Cauliflower, garlic, kale, onion, Tomato, turnip, papaya, pineapple)		*

Other Ingredients: Vegetable-based cellulose capsules

*Daily value not established.

Continued on next page

PLUS with Ambrotose—Cont.

KEEP BOTTLE TIGHTLY CLOSED. STORE IN A COOL, DRY PLACE.

How Supplied: Bottle of 90 caplets.

** This statement has not been evaluated by the Food and Drug Administration. This product is not intended to diagnose, treat, cure or prevent any disease.

Shown in Product Identification Guide, page 506

McNeil Consumer & Specialty Pharmaceuticals

Division of McNeil-PPC, Inc.
FORT WASHINGTON, PA 19034

Direct Inquiries to:
Consumer Relationship Center
Fort Washington, PA 19034
(800) 962-5357

LACTAID® ORIGINAL STRENGTH CAPLETS
(lactase enzyme)

LACTAID® EXTRA STRENGTH CAPLETS
(lactase enzyme)

LACTAID® ULTRA CAPLETS AND CHEWABLE TABLETS
(lactase enzyme)

LACTAID® FAST ACT CAPLETS AND CHEWABLE TABLETS
(lactase enzyme)

Description: Each serving size (3 caplets) of *LACTAID® Original Strength* contains 9000 FCC (Food Chemical Codex) units of lactase enzyme (derived from *Aspergillus oryzae*).
Each serving size (2 caplets) of *LACTAID® Extra Strength* contains 9000 FCC units of lactase enzyme (derived from *Aspergillus oryzae*).
Each serving size (1 caplet) of *LACTAID® Ultra Caplet* contains 9000 FCC units of lactase enzyme (derived from *Aspergillus oryzae*).
Each serving size (1 tablet) of *LACTAID® Ultra Chewable Tablet* contains 9000 FCC units of lactase enzyme (derived from *Aspergillus oryzae*).
Each serving size (1 caplet) of *LACTAID® Fast Act Caplet* contains 9000 FCC units of lactase enzyme (derived from *Aspergillus oryzae*).
Each serving size (1 tablet) of *LACTAID® Fast Act Chewable Tablet* contains 9000 FCC units of lactase enzyme (derived from *Aspergillus oryzae*).

LACTAID® is the original lactase dietary supplement that makes milk and dairy foods more digestible for individuals with lactose intolerance. *LACTAID®* lactase enzyme hydrolyzes lactose into two digestible simple sugars: glucose and galactose. *LACTAID® Caplets/Chewable Tablets* are taken orally for *in vivo* hydrolysis of lactose.

Actions: *LACTAID® Caplets/Chewable Tablets* work by providing the enzyme that hydrolyzes the milk sugar lactose (disaccharide) into the two monosaccharides, glucose and galactose.

Uses: LACTAID® Supplements help prevent the gas, bloating, or diarrhea that many people may experience after eating foods containing dairy.*

---

*This statement has not been evaluated by the Food and Drug Administration. This product is not intended to diagnose, treat, cure, or prevent any disease.

Directions: Original Strength: Swallow 3 caplets with your first bite of dairy foods to help prevent symptoms. **Extra Strength:** Swallow 2 caplets with your first bite of dairy foods to help prevent symptoms. **Ultra Caplets:** Take 1 caplet with your first bite of dairy foods to help prevent symptoms. You may have to take more than 1 caplet, but no more than 2 at a time. **Ultra Chewables:** Chew 1 chewable tablet with your first bite of dairy foods to help prevent symptoms. You may have to take more than 1 chewable tablet but no more than 2 at a time. **Fast Act Caplets:** Swallow 1 caplet with your first bite of dairy foods. If necessary, you may swallow 2 caplets at one time. If you continue to eat foods containing dairy after 30–45 minutes, we recommend taking another caplet. **Fast Act Chewable Tablets:** Chew 1 tablet with your first bite of dairy foods. If necessary, you may take 2 chewable tablets at one time. If you continue to eat foods containing dairy after 30–45 minutes, we recommend taking another chewable tablet.

Warnings: *Consult your doctor if* your symptoms continue after using the product or if your symptoms are unusual and seem unrelated to eating dairy. Keep out of reach of children. **Do not use if carton is open or if printed plastic neckwrap is broken or if single serve packet is open.**

LACTAID® Ultra Chewable Tablets: **Phenylketonurics Contains: Phenylalanine.**

Ingredients: *LACTAID® Original Strength Caplets:* Lactase Enzyme (9000 FCC Lactase units/3 caplets), Mannitol, Cellulose, Sodium Citrate, Magnesium Stearate.
LACTAID® Extra Strength Caplets: Lactase Enzyme (9000 FCC Lactase units/2 caplets), Mannitol, Cellulose, Sodium Citrate, Magnesium Stearate.

LACTAID® Ultra Caplets: Lactase Enzyme (9000 FCC Lactase units/Caplet), Cellulose, Sodium Citrate, Magnesium Stearate, Colloidal Silicon Dioxide.
LACTAID® Ultra Chewable Tablets: Lactase Enzyme (9000 FCC Lactase units/tablet), Mannitol, Cellulose, Sodium Citrate, Magnesium Stearate, Natural and Artificial Flavor, Citric Acid, Acesulfame K, Aspartame.
LACTAID® Fast Act Chewable Tablets: Lactase Enzyme (9000 FCC Lactase units/tablet), Mannitol, Microcrystalline Cellulose, Croscarmellose Sodium, Crospovidone, Magnesium Stearate, Natural and Artificial Flavor, Citric Acid, Sucralose.
LACTAID® Fast Act Caplets: Lactase Enzyme (9000 FCC Lactase units/caplet), Microcrystalline Cellulose, Croscarmellose Sodium, Crospovidone, Magnesium Stearate, Colloidal Silicon Dioxide.

How Supplied: *LACTAID® Original Strength Caplets* are available in bottles of 120 count. Store at or below room temperature (below 77°F) but do not refrigerate. Keep away from heat. *LACTAID® Extra Strength Caplets* are available in bottles of 50 count. Store at or below room temperature (below 77°F) but do not refrigerate. Keep away from heat. *LACTAID® Ultra Caplets* are available in single serve packets in 12, 32, 60 and 90 count packages. Store at or below 86°F. Keep away from heat. *LACTAID® Ultra Chewable Tablets* are available in single serve packets of 32 and 60 counts. Store at or below room temperature (below 77°F), but do not refrigerate. Keep away from heat and moisture.
LACTAID® Caplets and *LACTAID® Ultra Chewable Tablets* are certified kosher from the Orthodox Union.
Also available: 100% lactose-free Lactaid Milk.

Shown in Product Identification Guide, page 507

Memory Secret
1221 BRICKELL AVENUE
SUITE 1000
MIAMI, FL 33131 USA

For Direct Inquiries Contact:
(866) 673 2738
fax 1-305-675-2279
e-mail intelectol@memorysecret.net

INTELECTOL® MEMORY ENHANCER
VINPOCETINE TABLETS MEMORY SECRET

Description: INTELECTOL® is the purest form of Vinpocetine available. Vinpocetine is a derivative of Vincamine, which is extracted from the Periwinkle plant (*Vinca Minor, Vinca Pervinca*). Research suggests that Vinpocetine helps to maintain healthy blood circulation in the brain and supports certain neurotransmitters in the memory process.* Vinpocetine supports and protects brain blood vessel health and aids mental function.*

Directions: As a dietary supplement, take 2 tablets twice daily with meals. Vinpocetine should be taken as part of an on-going regimen with exercise, a healthy diet and keeping active the mind. Do not use if tamper-evident seal is broken.

Cautions: Take product with food to avoid stomach upset. Not recommended for use by pregnant women, nursing mothers or anyone under 18 years old. Consult a doctor or health care professional before use if you have any medical condition or if taking any medication. Not recommended for use by anyone with hemophilia, heart problems or low blood pressure. **Keep out of reach of children.**

Store in a cool, dry place.

Supplement Facts
Serving Size 2 tablets
Servings Per Container: 25

	Amount Per Serving	% DV
Vinpocetine	10 mg	*
(from Periwinkle seed extract)		

*Daily Value not established.
Other Ingredients: Lactose, hydroxypropylcellulose, magnesium stearate and talc.

> ***These statements have not been evaluated by the Food & Drug Administration. This product is not intended to diagnose, treat, cure, or prevent any disease.**

Distributed by: The Memory Secret, Inc.
1221 Brickell Ave., Suite 1000, Miami, FL 33131/USA
memorysecret™
www.memorysecret.net
Shown in Product Identification Guide, page 512

UNKNOWN DRUG?
Consult the
Product Identification Guide
(Gray Pages)
for full-color photos of
leading over-the-counter
medications

Mission Pharmacal Company
10999 IH 10 WEST
SUITE 1000
SAN ANTONIO, TX 78230-1355

Direct Inquiries to:
PO Box 786099
San Antonio, TX 78278-6099
TOLL FREE: (800) 292-7364
(210) 696-8400
FAX: (210) 696-6010
For Medical Information Contact:
In Emergencies:
Mary Ann Walter

CITRACAL® ⓤ
[sĭ' trə-kăl]
Ultradense® calcium citrate dietary supplement

Ingredients: Calcium (as Ultradense® calcium citrate) 200 mg, polyethylene glycol, croscarmellose sodium, polyvinyl alcohol-part hydrolyzed, color added, magnesium silicate, magnesium stearate.

Sensitive Patients: CITRACAL® contains no wheat, barley, yeast or rye; is sugar, dairy and gluten free.
One Tablet Provides:
200 mg. calcium (elemental), equaling 20% of the U.S. recommended Daily Value for adults and children 4 or more years of age.

Directions: Take 1 to 2 tablets two times daily or as recommended by a physician, pharmacist or health professional. Store at room temperature.

How Supplied: Supplied as white, barrel shaped, coated tablets in bottles of 100 (UPC 0178-0800-01), and bottles of 200 (UPC 0178-0800-20).
ⓤ=Kosher Parvae approved by Orthodox Union.

CITRACAL® 250 MG + D
[sĭ'trə-kăl]
Ultradense® calcium citrate-Vitamin D dietary supplement

Ingredients: Calcium (as Ultradense® calcium citrate) 250 mg., polyethylene glycol, croscarmellose sodium, polyvinyl alcohol-part hydrolyzed, color added, magnesium silicate, magnesium stearate, vitamin D_3 (200 IU).

How Supplied: Supplied as white, modified rectangle shaped, coated tablets in bottles of 150 (UPC 0178-0837-15).

CITRACAL® Caplets + D
[sĭ ' trə-kăl]
Ultradense® calcium citrate-Vitamin D dietary supplement

Ingredients: Calcium (as Ultradense® calcium citrate) 315 mg., polyethylene glycol, croscarmellose sodium, polyvinyl alcohol-part hydrolyzed, color added, magnesium silicate, magnesium stearate, vitamin D_3 (200 IU).

How Supplied: Supplied as white, arc rectangle shaped, coated tablets in bottles of 60 (UPC 0178-0815-60), and bottles of 120 (UPC 0178-0815-12), and bottles of 180 (UPC 0178-0815-18).

CITRACAL® PLUS
[sĭ'trə-kăl]
Ultradense® calcium citrate-Vitamin D-multimineral dietary supplement

Ingredients: Calcium (as Ultradense® calcium citrate) 250 mg., polyethylene glycol, magnesium oxide, croscarmellose sodium, polyvinyl alcohol-part hydrolyzed, color added, magnesium silicate, pyridoxine hydrochloride, zinc oxide, sodium borate, manganese gluconate, copper gluconate, magnesium stearate, vitamin D_3 (125 IU).

How Supplied: Supplied as white, arc rectangle shaped, coated tablets in bottles of 150 (UPC 0178-0825-15).

Novartis Consumer Health, Inc.
200 KIMBALL DRIVE
PARSIPPANY, NJ 07054-0622

Direct Product Inquiries to:
Consumer & Professional Affairs
(800) 452-0051
Fax: (800) 635-2801

Or write to above address.

BENEFIBER® Fiber Supplement
Non-Thickening Powder

Description: Benefiber® is a 100% natural fiber, that can be mixed with almost anything. It's taste free, grit-free, and will never thicken. So it won't alter the taste or texture of foods or non-carbonated beverages. It can be used in coffee, pudding, soup, or whatever is desired.[††]

Supplement Facts:
Serving Size: 1 tbsp (4g)
(makes 4 fl oz prepared)

Amount Per Serving	%DV
Calories 20	
Total Carbohydrate 4g	1%*
Dietary Fiber 3g	12%*
Soluble Fiber 3g	†
Sodium 20mg	1%

*Percent Daily Values (DV) are based on a 2,000 calorie diet.
†Daily Value not established.

Continued on next page

Information on Novartis Consumer Health, Inc. products appearing on these pages is effective as of November 2004.

Benefiber—Cont.

Ingredients: Partially Hydrolyzed Guar Gum (A 100% natural fiber).

Guar Gum is derived from the seed of the cluster bean.

ⓤ 100% Natural Fiber–Sugar Free

Directions for use: Stir 1 tablespoon (tbsp) of Benefiber into at least 4 oz. of any beverage or soft food (hot or cold). Use 8 oz. if using 2 tbsp. Stir until dissolved.††

Age	Dosage
12 yrs. to adult	1–2 tbsp up to 3 times daily*
7 to 11 yrs.	1/2–1 tbsp up to 3 times daily**
Under 6 yrs.	Ask your doctor

tbsp=tablespoon

* Not to exceed 5 tbsp per day.

**Not to exceed 2.5 tbsp per day.

†† Not recommended for carbonated beverages.

Store at controlled room temperature 20–25°C (68–77°F). Protect from moisture.

Use within 6 months of opening.

Keep out of reach of children.

If you are pregnant or nursing a baby, ask a health professional before use.

Tamper Evident Feature: Do not use if printed bottle inner seal is broken or missing or if sealed packet is broken or torn.

How Supplied:
- 12 serving cannister = 1.7 oz/48 g
- 24 serving cannister = 3.4 oz/96 g
- 42 serving cannister = 6 oz/168 g
- 60 serving cannister = 6 oz/240 g
- 80 serving cannister = 11.3 oz/320 g

Packaged by weight, not volume. Contents may settle during shipping and handling.

Benefiber® guarantees your satisfaction or your money back.

Questions? Call **1-800-452-0051** 24 hours a day, 7 days a week or visit us at **www.benefiber.com** for recipe ideas and additional information.

Shown in Product Identification Guide, page 512

BENEFIBER® CAPLETS
Fiber Supplement

Supplement Facts
Serving Size: 6 Caplets
Servings Per Container: about 16

Amount Per Serving	%DV*
Calories 25	
Total Carbohydrate 6g	2%*
Dietary Fiber 3g	12%*
Soluble Fiber 3g	†
Sodium 5mg	<1%

*Percent Daily Values (DV) are based on a 2,000 calorie diet.
†Daily Value not established.

Directions for use:

Adults: Take 2–6 caplets up to 3 times daily to supplement the fiber content of your diet. Swallow with liquid.

Do not exceed 18 caplets per day.

Tamper Evident Feature: Notice! Protective printed inner seal "sealed for your protection" beneath cap. If missing or damaged, do not use contents.

Keep out of reach of children.

If you are pregnant or nursing a baby, ask a health professional before use.

Ingredients: partially hydrolyzed guar gum, microcrystalline cellulose, confectioner's sugar, maltodextrin, hypromellose, titanium dioxide, magnesium stearate, polydextrose, colloidal silicon dioxide, triacetin, polyethylene glycol 8000, methylparaben

Store at controlled room temperature 20–25°C (68–77°F).

Protect from excessive heat and moisture.

Benefiber® guarantees your satisfaction or your money back.

Questions? call **1-800-452-0051** 24 hours a day, 7 days a week.

How Supplied: 100 ct, 160 ct caplets www.benefiber.com for additional information.

Shown in Product Identification Guide, page 512

BENEFIBER®
Fiber Supplement
Chewable Tablets Orange Creme Flavor

Benefiber Chewable Tablets are an easy way to add fiber to your diet. These great tasting tablets provide as much fiber per dose as the leading bulk fiber powder, but because there's no need for water or mixing, you can take them virtually anywhere, anytime.

Supplement Facts:
Serving Size: 3 Tablets
Servings Per Container: Varies

Amount Per Serving	%DV*
Calories 35	
Total Carbohydrate 8g	3%*
Dietary Fiber 3g	12%*
Soluble Fiber 3g	†
Sugars 3g	
Sodium 10mg	<1%

*Percent Daily Values (DV) are based on a 2,000 calorie diet.
†Daily Value (DV) not established.

Ingredients: partially hydrolyzed guar gum, sorbitol, maltodextrin, confectioner's sugar, dextrates, citric acid, magnesium stearate, sucralose, sucrose, natural and artificial flavors, modified food starch, acacia, FD&C yellow 6 aluminum lake, silicon dioxide, lecithin, tocopherols, soybean oil

Directions for use: Adults: Chew 1 to 3 tablets up to 5 times daily to supplement the fiber content of your diet. Do not take more than 15 tablets in a 24 hour period.

Age	Dosage
12 yrs. to adult	1–3 tablets up to 5 times daily*
7 to 11 yrs.	1/2–1 1/2 tablets up to 5 times daily**
Under 6 yrs.	ask your doctor

* Not to exceed 15 tablets per day.
**Not to exceed 7 1/2 tablets per day.

Other Information: Store at controlled room temperature 20–25°C (68–77°F). Protect from excessive heat and moisture.

Keep out of reach of children.

If you are pregnant or nursing a baby, ask a health professional before use.

Tamper Evident Feature: Notice! Protective printed inner seal beneath cap. If missing or damaged, do not use contents.

Product may contain dark specks due to the processing of natural ingredients.

Questions? call **1-800-452-0051** 24 hours a day, 7 days a week.
www.benefiber.com
for additional information.
Benefiber guarantees your satisfaction or your money back.

How Supplied: Available in bottles of 36 ct. and 100 ct. tablets.

Shown in Product Identification Guide, page 512

SLOW FE®
Slow Release Iron Tablets

Drug Facts:
Active Ingredient
(in each tablet): **Purpose:**
160 mg dried ferrous sulfate, USP (equivalent to 50 mg elemental iron) .... Iron deficiency

Uses: For use in the prevention of iron deficiency when the need for such therapy has been determined by a doctor.

Warnings:
- The treatment of any anemic condition should be under the advice and supervision of a doctor.
- As oral iron products interfere with absorption of oral tetracycline antibiotics, these products should not be taken within two hours of each other.
- **If pregnant or breast-feeding,** ask a health professional before use.

> **Warning:** Accidental overdose of iron-containing products is a leading cause of fatal poisoning in children under 6. Keep this product out of reach of children. In case of accidental overdose, call a doctor or poison control center immediately.

Directions:
- Tablets must be swallowed whole.
- ADULTS: One or two tablets daily or as recommended by a doctor. A maximum of four tablets daily may be taken.
- CHILDREN UNDER 12: consult a doctor

Other Information:
- store at controlled room temperature 20–25°C (68–77°F)
- protect from moisture

Inactive Ingredients: cetosteryl alcohol, FD&C blue #2 aluminum lake, hypromellose, lactose, magnesium stearate, polysorbate 80, talc, titanium dioxide, yellow iron oxide
Questions? call **1-800-452-0051** 24 hours a day, 7 days a week.

How Supplied: Child-resistant blister packages of 30 ct., 60 ct. and 90 ct. NDC 0067-0125-47.
Child Resistant
Blister packaged for your protection. Do not use if individual seals are broken. Tablets non-USP (disintegration, content uniformity)
Tablets made in Great Britain
Shown in Product Identification Guide, page 513

SLOW FE® WITH FOLIC ACID
(Slow Release Iron, Folic Acid)
Dietary Supplement

Description: Slow Fe with Folic Acid delivers 47.5 mg elemental iron as ferrous sulfate plus 350 mcg folic acid using the unique wax matrix delivery system described above (for SLOW FE® Slow Release Iron Tablets).
Provides women of childbearing potential with folic acid to help reduce the risk of neural tube birth defects. These birth defects are rare, but serious, and occur within 28 days of conception, often before a woman knows she's pregnant.

Formula: Each tablet contains: 47.5 mg elemental iron as ferrous sulfate and 350 mcg folic acid.

Other Ingredients: lactose, hypromellose, talc, magnesium stearate, cetostearyl alcohol, polysorbate 80, titanium dioxide, yellow iron oxide.

Dosage: ADULTS—One or two tablets once a day or as recommended by a physician. A maximum of two tablets daily may be taken. CHILDREN UNDER 12—Consult a physician. Tablets must be swallowed whole.

Warning: The treatment of any anemic condition should be under the advice and supervision of a physician. As oral iron products interfere with absorption of oral tetracycline antibiotics, these products should not be taken within two hours of each other. Intake of folic acid from all sources should be limited to 1000 mcg per day to prevent the masking of Vitamin B_{12} deficiencies. Should you become pregnant while using this product, consult a physician as soon as possible about good prenatal care and the continued use of this product. If you are already pregnant or nursing a baby, seek the advice of a health care professional before using this product.

> **Warning:** Accidental overdose of iron-containing products is a leading cause of fatal poisoning in children under 6. Keep this product out of reach of children. In case of accidental overdose, call a doctor or poison control center immediately.

How Supplied: Blister packages of 20 supplied in Child-Resistant packaging. Store at controlled room temperature 20–25°C (68°–77°F). Protect from moisture.
Tablets made in Great Britain
Novartis Consumer Health, Inc.
Parsippany, NJ 07054-0622 © 2003
Shown in Product Identification Guide, page 513

Pharmics, Inc.
PO BOX 27554
SALT LAKE CITY, UT 84127

Direct Inquiries to:
Customer Service: 800-456-4138
FAX: 801-966-4177
service@pharmics.net
www.pharmics.com

FERRETTS
[fĕ-rĕts]
Ferrous Fumarate
Iron Supplement

Description: Ferrets tablets are for use as a dietary iron supplement.
Each tablet contains:
Iron (from 325 mg ferrous fumarate) 106 mg

Other Ingredients: Microcrystalline cellulose, sodium starch glycolate, magnesium stearate, Opadry II clear, Opadry II Red 40L15175.

Suggested Use: One tablet daily or as directed by a physician.

> **Warning:** Accidental overdose of iron containing products is a leading cause of fatal poisoning in children under 6. Keep this product out of the reach of children. In case of accidental overdose, call a doctor or poison control center immediately.

Caution: As with any drug, if you are pregnant or nursing a baby, seek the advise of a health care professional before using this product.

How Supplied: Ferretts are supplied in tamper evident, child resistant unit dose packages of 60 tablets (NDC 00813-0012-06). Do not use if blister or seal is broken. Ferretts are a scored red film coated caplet shape tablet, embossed "P-Fe".

FERRETTS IPS LIQUID
[fĕ-rĕts]
Iron Protein Succinylate
Iron Supplement

Description: Iron Protein Succinylate is a proprietary stabilized iron compound. The iron is wrapped in a casein protective layer, which allows the iron to pass through the stomach to the intestinal tract for immediate safe and efficacious absorption.
Ferretts IPS liquid is for use as a dietary supplement.

Each 1 ml contain:	2.67 mg iron*
Each 5 ml contains:	13.33 mg iron*
Each 7.5 ml contain:	20 mg iron*
Each 10 ml contains:	26.67 mg iron*
Each 15 ml contain:	40 mg iron*

*elemental iron

Suggested Use: 15 ml daily or as directed by a health care professional.
Supplement Facts

Serving Size:	15 ml	
Amount per 15 ml		% Daily Value
Iron	40 mg	222%*
(from Iron Protein Succinylate)		

*Based on 18 mg Daily Value

Other Ingredients: Purified water, sorbitol solution, propylene glycol, casein (milk protein) strawberry flavor, sodium hydroxide, methylparaben sodium, propylparaben sodium, saccharin sodium.

> **Warning:** Accidental overdose of iron containing products is a leading cause of fatal poisoning in children under 6. Keep this product out of the reach of children. In case of accidental overdose, call a doctor or poison control center immediately.

Continued on next page

Ferretts IPS—Cont.

Caution: As with any drug, if you are pregnant or nursing a baby, seek the advise of a health care professional before using this product.

How Supplied: 8 fl. oz bottles with tamper evident seal and child resistant cap. Strawberry flavor. Do not use if tamper evident seal is broken.
Store at controlled room temperature 15°–30° C (59°–86°F).

The Procter & Gamble Company

P. O. BOX 599
CINCINNATI, OH 45201

Direct Inquiries to:
Consumer Relations
(800) 832–3064

METAMUCIL®
DIETARY FIBER SUPPLEMENT

[met uh-mū sil]
(psyllium husk)
*Also see **Metamucil Fiber Laxative** in Nonprescription Drugs section*

Description: Metamucil contains psyllium husk (from the plant *Plantago ovata*), a concentrated source of soluble fiber which can be used to increase one's dietary fiber intake. When used as part of a diet low in saturated fat and cholesterol, 7g per day of soluble fiber from psyllium husk (the amount in 3 doses of Metamucil) may reduce the risk of heart disease by lowering cholesterol. Each dose of Metamucil powder and Metamucil Fiber Wafers contains approximately 3.4 grams of psyllium husk (or 2.4 grams of soluble fiber). A listing of ingredients and nutrition information is available in the listing of Metamucil Fiber Laxative in the Nonprescription Drug section. Metamucil Smooth Texture Sugar-Free Regular Flavor and Metamucil capsules contains no sugar and no artificial sweeteners. Metamucil Smooth Texture Sugar-Free Orange Flavor contains aspartame (phenylalanine content of 25 mg per dose). Metamucil powdered products are gluten-free.

Uses: Metamucil Dietary Fiber Supplement can be used as a concentrated source of soluble fiber to increase the dietary intake of fiber. Diets low in saturated fat and cholesterol that include 7 grams of soluble fiber per day from psyllium husk, as in Metamucil, may reduce the risk of heart disease by lowering cholesterol. One adult dose of Metamucil has 2.4 grams of this soluble fiber. Consult a doctor if you are considering use of this product as part of a cholesterol-lowering program.

Warnings: Read entire Drug Facts section in listing for Metamucil Fiber Laxative in the Nonprescription Drug section.

Directions: Adults 12 yrs. & older: 1 dose in 8 oz of liquid *3 times daily*. Capsules: 2–6 capsules for increasing daily fiber intake; 6 capsules for cholesterol lowering use. Up to three times daily. Under 12 yrs.: Consult a doctor. See mixing directions in Drug Facts in listing for Metamucil Fiber Laxative in the Nonprescription Drug section.
NOTICE: Mix this product with at least 8 oz (a full glass) of liquid. Taking without enough liquid may cause choking. Do not take if you have difficulty swallowing.
For listing of ingredients and nutritional information for Metamucil Dietary Fiber Supplement, and for laxative indications and directions for use, see Metamucil Fiber Laxative in the Nonprescription Drug section.
Notice to Health Care Professionals: To minimize the potential for allergic reaction, health care professionals who frequently dispense powdered psyllium products should avoid inhaling airborne dust while dispensing these products. Handling and Dispensing: To minimize generating airborne dust, spoon product from the canister into a glass according to label directions.

How Supplied: Powder: canisters and cartons of single-dose packets. Capsules: 100 and 160 count bottles. For complete ingredients and sizes for each version, see Metamucil Table 1, page 718, Nonprescription Drug section.
Questions? 1-800-983-4237

Purdue Products L.P.

ONE STAMFORD FORUM
STAMFORD, CT 06901-3431

For Medical Information Contact:
(888) 726-7535
Adverse Drug Experiences:
(888) 726-7535
Customer Service:
(800) 877-5666
FAX: (800) 877-3210

SENOKOT™ Brand Wheat Bran

[sĕn'-ō-kaht]
Natural Fiber Supplement
• Orange Flavor
• Orange Flavor, Sugar-Free
• Flavor-Free, Sugar-Free

Description: Senokot™ Brand Wheat Bran, made with 100% natural bran, provides 4.6 grams of wheat bran per serving. Wheat bran is one of nature's best sources of fiber. This natural fiber supplement mixes easily with liquids and is smooth and grit free.

Actions/Uses: Senokot™ Brand Wheat Bran helps maintain regularity. A natural dietary supplement, it is gentle enough to use every day.

Ingredients:

Orange Flavor: Fructose, wheat bran, sucrose, gum arabic, citric acid, locust bean gum, natural orange flavor, beta-carotene, xanthan gum.

Supplement Facts
Serving Size: 1 scoop (17.56 g)
Servings Per Container: 66

Amount Per Serving	%DV*
Calories 70	
Sodium 5 mg	<1%
Total Carbohydrates 16 g	5%
Dietary Fiber 3 g	12%
Soluble Fiber 1 g	†
Insoluble Fiber 2 g	†
Sugars 12 g	†
Iron 0.6 mg	4%

* Percent Daily Values (DV) are based on a 2000 calorie diet
† Daily Value not established

Orange Flavor, Sugar-Free: Wheat bran, maltodextrin, gum arabic, citric acid, natural and artificial orange flavors, locust bean gum, beta-carotene, xanthan gum, aspartame.

Phenylketonurics: Contains phenylalanine 30.02 mg per scoop of Orange Flavor, Sugar-Free only.

Supplement Facts
Serving Size: 1 scoop (10.28 g)
Servings Per Container: 72

Amount Per Serving	%DV*
Calories 40	
Sodium 5 mg	<1%
Total Carbohydrates 9 g	3%
Dietary Fiber 3 g	12%
Soluble Fiber 1 g	†
Insoluble Fiber 2 g	†
Sugars 0 g	†
Iron 0.6 mg	4%

* Percent Daily Values (DV) are based on a 2000 calorie diet
† Daily Value not established

Flavor-Free, Sugar-Free: Wheat bran, maltodextrin, gum arabic, locust bean gum, xanthan gum.

Supplement Facts
Serving Size: 1 scoop (9.3 g)
Servings Per Container: 76

Amount Per Serving	%DV*
Calories 40	
Sodium 5 mg	<1%
Total Carbohydrates 8 g	3%
Dietary Fiber 3 g	12%
Soluble Fiber 1 g	†
Insoluble Fiber 2 g	†
Sugars 0 g	†
Iron 0.6 mg	4%

* Percent Daily Values (DV) are based on a 2000 calorie diet
† Daily Value not established

Directions: Fill glass with 8 oz. of water or other beverage. Add one scoop of Senokot Brand Wheat Bran. Stir until completely mixed.

Warnings:
- To prevent trouble swallowing or choking, mix each dose in at least 8 oz. of water or other beverage.
- Do not use if you have a bowel obstruction or abdominal symptoms such as nausea, vomiting, abdominal pain, or a sudden change in bowel habits that lasts over two weeks.
- Do not use if you have Celiac Disease or an allergy to wheat.

Introducing quantities of bran into the diet may temporarily cause minor gas or bloating in some people. If this occurs, reduce the amount of Senokot™ Brand Wheat Bran and then slowly increase the dose over several days as tolerable.

Bulk-forming products may affect how medications work. Take Senokot™ Brand Wheat Bran two or more hours before or after taking medications.

Keep out of reach of children.

Other Information: Does not contain senna. Store at room temperature tightly closed to protect from humidity.

How Supplied:
Orange Flavor: Plastic bottles of 2 lb. 8.8 oz. net weight (1159 g) containing 66 servings and bottles of 1 lb. 1.3 oz. (492 g) containing 28 servings.

Orange Flavor, Sugar-Free: Plastic bottles of 1 lb. 10.1 oz. net weight (740 g) containing 72 servings and bottles of 10.8 oz. (308 g) containing 30 servings.

Flavor-Free, Sugar-Free: Plastic bottles of 1 lb. 8.9 oz. net weight (707 g) containing 76 servings and bottles of 10.4 oz. (298 g) containing 32 servings.

© 2004, Purdue Products L.P., Stamford, CT 06901-3431

Shown in Product Identification Guide, page 515

SLOW-MAG® Tablets
[slō'-măg]
magnesium chloride

Description: Each enteric-coated tablet contains 64 mg elemental magnesium and 106 mg elemental calcium. Magnesium is an essential mineral of a healthy diet. SLOW-MAG® Tablets are a dietary supplement that provides a magnesium chloride formulation that is enteric-coated to help prevent the stomach upset commonly associated with oral magnesium supplements. SLOW-MAG Tablets provide magnesium chloride for increased absorption versus magnesium oxide.

Actions/Uses: SLOW-MAG is a dietary supplement. Magnesium may help to maintain the function of the heart, muscles, and nervous system. Magnesium is necessary for normal protein syntheses, carbohydrate metabolism, and proper muscle function. It is necessary for the role it plays in helping the body utilize calcium and potassium properly. Proper magnesium levels help maintain normal heart rhythms.

Ingredients: Magnesium chloride hexahydrate, calcium carbonate, cellulose acetate phthalate, pregelatinized starch, povidone, diethyl phthalate, talc, titanium dioxide, magnesium stearate, carnauba wax, FD&C Blue No. 2 Lake.

Directions for Use: As a dietary supplement, take 2 tablets daily or as directed by a physician. Two 64 mg tablets (128 mg) contain 32% of the recommended daily allowance for magnesium and 212 mg of calcium.

Other: Store in a cool dry place 59°–77°F (15°–25°C). Store tablets in original container with desiccant. Do not repackage.

Warnings: Keep out of reach of children.

How Supplied: Plastic bottles of 60 tablets.

Supplement Facts
Serving Size 2 Tablets
Servings Per Container 30

Amount Per Serving	% Daily Value
Calcium 212 mg	21%
Magnesium 128 mg	32%
Chloride 373 mg	11%

Dist. Purdue Products L.P., Stamford, CT 06901-3431

Shown in Product Identification Guide, page 515

Sunny Health Co., Ltd.
YAESU CENTER BLDG.
1-6-6 YAESU, CHUO-KU,
TOKYO 103-0028, JAPAN

Direct Inquiries to:
Consumer Service
Tel: 81-33-276-5589
Fax:81-33-276-5333
URL: http://www.sunnyhealth.com

MICRODIET DIETARY SUPPLEMENT
Specially formulated to control body weight

Description: Microdiet (MD)™ dietary supplement is a low calorie diet formulated with proteins, fat, carbohydrates, food fibers, and a complete multivitamins. The products are formulated as either drinks (shakes) with all natural flavors of coca, coffee, milk tea, green tea, berry mix, banana, strawberry or soups with flavors of corn, potato, pumpkin, and curry. Each pack contains 50 grams and the details of the content is described below.
[See table at top of next page]
Microdiet (MD)™ was developed as a low calorie dietary supplement by Sunny Health in 1989, and has marketed for the past 16 years to help reduce weight for obesity. Since its inception, 70 million packets of Microdiet (MD)™ has been consumed by 1.1 million consumers to help reduce their body weights and has shown to be clinically safe and effective.‡
Scientific Support: A very low calorie diet (VLCD) was originally developed as a very low calorie diet (VLCD) for weight control by Dr. J. Stordy, University of Surrey, England in 1983 and subsequently, this low calorie diet was marketed in 40 different countries. Since 1989, Sunny Health in Japan, introduced Microdiet (MD)™ dietary supplement to control body weight and obesity. Since 1993 to date, 9 clinical studies were carried out with Microdiet (MD)™ and its effectiveness of weight control against moderate to severe obesity of adult males, adult females either with or without combination of physical exercise with modified diet, older adults with age-related disease, and stress-induced obesity were clinically evaluated (Kagoshima et al, New Food 35(12): 1–8, 1993; Hirao, J., Diagnosis and New Drugs 32(3): 259–266, 1995; Terashita et al, Therapeutics Res. 16(10): 451–461, 1995: Yano et al, Therapeutic Res. 17(4): 365–371, 1996; Dota, T., Therapeutics Res. 17(11): 245–251, 1996; Dota, T., Diagnosis and New Drugs, 34 (8): 43–49, 1997; Tanaka et al, Body Composition, Monograph (Nov. issue) 26–30, 1997; Nakanishi et al, Clin. Sports Med. 15 (9):1047–1053, 1998; Yonei et al, Diagnosis and Therapy 92(4):

Continued on next page

Microdiet—Cont.

704–709, 2004).‡ The study results demonstrated that when one or two normal meals are replaced with one or two packets of Microdiet (MD)™, body weights were significantly reduced without any severe side effects based on a variety of clinical parameters that were monitored simultaneously during the studies. Furthermore. Effectiveness of Microdiet (MD)™ in weight control in older age groups with age-related disease was aslo observed without compromising their respective therapy. No cases of severe side effects were observed in older age groups with age-related disease undergoing therapy. So far Microdiet (MD)™ has been used in more than 400 hospitals and clinical centers to control body weights and/or as a nutritional supplement in Japan.

Ingredients:

Drink-formulation ingredients include Milk Protein, Soy Protein, Soy Peptide, Dextrose, Water Soluble Fibers, Skim Milk Powder, 6 different Natural Flavors of Cocoa Powder, Coffee, Milk Tea, Green Tea, Berry Mix, Banana, Strawberry as listed in Description), Vegetable Oil, Magnesium Carbonate, Calcium Carbonate, Yeast Powder, Malt Dextrin, Sodium Chloride, Sodium Caseinate, Tripostassium Citrate, Artificial flavor, Aspartame (Sweetener)†, Sodium L-Ascorbate, Vitamin E, Ferric Pyrophosphate, Vitamin A, Nicotinamide, Calcium Pantothenic Acid, Cyanocobalamin, Pyridoxine Hydrochloride, Thiamin Mononitrate, Riboflavin, Vitamin D, and Folic Acid.

Soup-formulation ingredients include Soy Protein, Milk Protein, Cane Sugar, Natural Flavor of Sweet Corn, Potato, Pumpkin, and Curry as listed in Description), Dextrin, Water Soluble Fibers, Skim Milk Powder, Vegetable Oil, Magnesium Carbonate, Calcium Carbonate Yeast Powder, Sodium Chloride, Onion, Butter Powder, Seasoning, Artificial Flavor, Sodium Caseinate, Tripostassium Citrate, Non-cooked Egg Shell Calcium, Gardenia Natural, Gelatinizing Agent, Sodium L-Ascorbate, Vitamin E, Ferric Pyrophosphate, Vitamin K2, Vitamin A, Nicotinamide, Calcium Pantothenic Acid, Cyanocobalamin, Pyridoxine Hydrochloride, Thiamin Mononitrate, Riboflavin, Vitamin D, and Folic Acid.

†**Phenylketonurics: contains phenylalanine**

Directions for Use: As a dietary supplement, take either 1 or 2 packets of drink-formulation or soup formulations of choice to substitute one or two meals per day. In case of drink type, 350 ml of portable water is poured into a shaker followed by adding 1 packet (50g pack) of Microdiet™ of choice and shake well before drink. In case of soup formulation, 1 packet of soup (49~52g) is placed into bowel, and followed by adding 250 ml (more or less) of hot water and stir until complete mixing. When taking this product, drink plenty of waters (1.5~2.0 liters) daily to promote normal bowel movement.

Safety: Since 1989, Microdiet (MD)™ has been marketed as a low calorie diet to control body weight and has sold 170 million packets to approximately 1.1 million consumers and no cases of severe side effects have been reported by consumers since Microdiet (MD)™ was placed for consumers in Japan. Microdiet (MD)™ has been used in more than 400 hospitals and clinical centers to control body weights and as nutritional supplement. Furthermore, 19 clinical studies have been completed and no cases of severe side effects have been reported by either physicians or dieticians.

Warning: Microdiet™ products should not be used more than recommended daily amount unless directed by a physician. In addition, consumers, who are allergic to any of the ingredients listed in the product description should be avoided or consult a physician. These products have not been evaluated in pregnant, breast feeding mothers or children under 17 years of age, or over 70 years age, patients of heart, kidney, liver, disease, or diabetes should consult a physician prior to use. Also consult a physician prior to use if taking a prescription medication. **Keep this product out of the reach of children. Do not use if you are pregnant, can become pregnant or breast feeding.**

How Supplied: Drink formulation is supplied with 2 packets of each (50g) of 7 flavors, Cocoa, Coffee, Milk Tea, Green Tea, Berry Mix, Banana, and Strawberry and total of per 14 packets per box. or 14 packets of any of the 7 flavors of choice per box.. **Soup formulation** is supplied with 4 packets of each (49–52g) of corn, and potatoes flavors and 3 packets of pumpkin, and curry flavors per box. or 14 packets of any single flavor of choice per box. All products should be kept at room temperature and avoid direct heat or any sunlight.

‡**These statements have not been evaluated by the Food and Drug Administration. These products are not intended to diagnose, treat, cure or prevent any disease.**

Sunpower Nutraceutical Inc.

**8850 RESEARCH DRIVE
IRVINE, CA 92618**

Direct Inquiries to:
Richard Lynn
Tel: (949) 553-8899
Fax: (949) 553-9084

PRODUCT LISTING

Descriptions: Sunpower Nutraceutical System combined vitamins, minerals, special formulated herbs, Pycnogenol® and proprietary Traditional Chinese Medicines (TCM) from S.P. Pharmaceutical Inc. (S.P.) which manufactured at GMP facility and under FDA Act and U.S. Pharmacopeia quality, purity and potency standards.*

Time-released, Double-layered tablets are made by advanced manufacturing techniques which allows nutrients to be

Supplement Facts: Serving Size: 1 Packet (g)	Drink Formulation*	% Daily Value*	Soup Formulation	% Daily Value*
	50		49~52	
Total calories (Cal)	173		172	
Total Protein (g)	21	35	20.6	34
Total fat (g)	2.5	4.2	3.3	5.5
Total Carbohydrate (g)	16.7	5.6	14.3	4.8
Dietary fibers	5.0	2.0	5.0	2.0
Sodium (mg)	347	14.4	752	31.3
Vitamin A (ug)	350	23.3	350	23.3
Vitamin B1 (mg)	0.9	60	1.0	66.6
Vitamin B2 (mg)	0.9	52.9	0.9	52.9
Niacin (mg)	6.0	30	6.0	20
Pantothenic acid (mg)	3.3	33	3.3	33
Vitamin B6 (mg)	1.3	65	1.3	65
Vitamin B12 (mcg)	2.2	36.7	2.2	36.7
Folic Acid (mcg)	163	40.8	163	40.8
Vitamin C (mg)	43.3	72.2	56.3	93.8
Vitamin D (mcg)	4.2	42	4.2	42
Vitamin E (mg)	4.4	22	4.4	22
Iron (mg)	6.7	44.7	6.7	44.7
Calcium (mg)	380	38	380	38
Magnesium (mg)	116	33.1	116	33.1
Potassium (mg)	700	23.3	700	23.3
Phosphorus (mg)	268	33.5	204	25.5

*% daily values as based on a 2,000 Calories diet.

released slowly for better absorption during digestion.*

Sunpower Product Overview:

Sun Liver™: contains vitamins, minerals, Pycnogenol® and S.P. Pro-Liver Formula to help to fight free radical damage, and provide nutrients essential for healthy liver function.

Sun Cardio™: contains CoQ10, OPC, Ginkgo Biloba, Red Wine Extract and S.P. Pro-Cardio Formula to help maintain normal cardiovascular system.

Power Circulation™: contains Ginkgo Biloba, Barley Grass, Lecithin and S.P. Pro-Circulation Formula to help maintain a healthy blood circulatory system.

Sun Joint™: contains Glucosamine, Chondroitin, Collagen Type II, Chitosan Oligo and S.P. Pro-Connection Formula to provide essential nutrients for bone, joint, ligament and cartilage function.

Power Lasting™: contains Yohimbe, Damiana, Saw Palmetto, Pumpkin Seed, Sarsaparilla Root, and S.P. Pro-Long Formula to help maintain normal kidney and sexual function and enhance endurance.

Sun Beauty™ 1: Formulated for women ages 14–28 contains Alfalfa, St. John's Wort, Cranberry, Royal Jelly, and S.P. Beauty I Formula to help establish healthy hormonal rhythms and basic immunity.

Sun Beauty™ 2: Formulated for women ages 29–42 contains Alfalfa, Selenium, Green Tea, Uva Ursi Leaves, Cranberry, and S.P. Beauty II Formula to support and balance a woman's vitality and healthy immunity during the menstrual cycle.

Sun Beauty™ 3: Formulated for women ages over 43 contains chromium, Burdock Root, Fo-Ti, Black Cohoshe, Red Clover, Chaste Tree Berries, and S.P. Beauty III Formula to support general well-being during menopause and post-menopause.

Power Refresh™: Contains Cordyceps Sinensis, American Ginseng, Grape Seeds Extract, Bee Pollen and Licorice.

Sun Decan: Contains Agaricus Blazei Murill, Reishi Extract, Hedyotis Diffusa Extract, and Lonicera Japonica Extract to provide essential nutrients for healthy immune system.

BioMarine Protein: This patented product contains Pure Biomarine Amino Peptide Powder, Oat Bran Extract, Dicalcium, and Microcrystalline Cellulose Fiber that can help induce death of weak or shrinking bad cells.

*The statements have not been reviewed or approved by the Food & Drug Administration. This product is not intended to diagnose, treat, cure or prevent any disease.

Shown in Product Identification Guide, page 516

Tahitian Noni International
333 WEST RIVER PARK DRIVE PROVO, UT 84604 USA

Direct Inquiries to:
Ph: (801) 234-1000
Website: www.tahitiannoni.com

TAHITIAN NONI® LIQUID DIETARY SUPPLEMENT

Description: TAHITIAN NONI® Juice has a heritage, a pedigree that distinguishes it from every other product on the market. This pedigree extends back 2,000 years to the people who used the noni fruit for its benefits. The countless benefits of this unique fruit can only be enjoyed if the fruit is revealed in its most pure form. Our proprietary formulation captures this precisely. It's no wonder that TAHITIAN NONI Juice touches the lives of millions worldwide. You'll find 2,000 years of goodness in every bottle of TAHITIAN NONI Juice! Always look for the TAHITIAN NONI Juice Footprint: Your only assurance of quality, purity, and authenticity.

Supplement Facts
Serving Size: 1 fluid ounce (30 ml)
Servings Per Container 33

Amount Per Serving	% Daily Value*
Calories 13	
Total Carbohydrate 3g	1%
Sugars 2g	†

*Percent Daily Values are based on a 2,000 calorie diet.
†Daily Value not established.

Ingredients: Reconstituted *Morinda citrifolia* fruit juice from pure juice puree from French Polynesia, natural grape juice concentrate, natural blueberry juice concentrate, and natural flavors. Not made from dried or powdered *Morinda citrifolia*.

How Supplied: 1 FL. OZ./30 mL daily. Preferably before meals
Shake well before using and refrigerate after opening
Do not use if seal around cap is broken
Packaged by Tahitian Noni International, a subsidiary of Morinda, Inc. Provo, UT 84604. USA.

References:
Mugglestone C, Davies S, et al., A single centre, double-blind, three dose level, parallel group, and placebo controlled safety study with TAHITIAN NONI® Juice in Healthy subjects. BI-BRA International LtD, Clinical Studies Department. Woodmansterne Road, Carshalton UK. 2003
TAHITIAN NONI® Juice (TNJ) liquid dietary supplement was used in a human clinical trial investigating the effects of different dosage on 96.

Wang MY et al., Morinda citrifolia (Noni): A Literature Review and Recent Advances in Noni Research. Acta Pharmacol Sin. 2002 Dec; 23 (12): 1127–41.
Morinda citrifolia L. fruit juice has been used in folk remedies by Polynesians for over 2000 years, and is reported to have a broad range of therapeutic effects, including antibacterial, antiviral, antifungal, antitumor, anthelmintic, analgesic, hypotensive, anti-inflammatory, and immune enhancing effects.
Furusawa E, Hirazumi A, Story SP, Jensen CJ Antitumor Potential of a Polysaccharide-rich Substance from the Fruit Juice of *Morinda citrifolia* (Noni) on Sarcoma 180 Ascites Tumor in Mice. 2003 Phytother Res. 17(1158–1164)
The fruit juice of *Morinda citrifolia* L.(Noni) from Hawaii and from the Brand TAHITIAN NONI® Juice contain a polysaccharide-rich substance (noni-ppt) with significant antitumor activity on Sarcoma 180 Ascites Tumor in mice. The therapeutic administration of noni-ppt produced a cure rate of 25%–45% in allogeneic mice. Noni-ppt also showed synergistic or additive benefits when combined with a broad spectrum of chemotherapeutic drugs.
Gerson, S. Green, L. Preliminary Evaluation of the Antimicrobial Activity of Extracts of *Morinda citrifolia* L. 2002 General Meeting of American Society for Microbiology.
Morinda citrifolia was shown to have antimicrobial and antifungal properties against *A. niger, C. albicans, E. coli, S. aureus* and *T. mentagrophytes*.
Opinion of the Scientific Committee on Foods on Tahitian Noni® Juice, European Commission. SCF/CS/NF/DOS/18 ADD 2 Final. 11, December 2002.
Sub-chronic and acute oral toxicity studies of TAHITIAN NONI® Juice measured clinical signs, food consumption, weight gain, hematology, clinical chemistry, selective organ weights, and tissue samples of 55 organs (for histology). The No-Observable-Adverse-Effect-Level (NOAEL) was >80 ml/kg which is more than 8% of the animals' body weight. Genotoxicity and allergenicity tests revealed no effects.
B. A. Mueller, et al. Am J. Kidney Dis. 2000 Feb; 35(2): 330–2.
They reported that "The potassium concentration in noni juice samples was determined and found to be 56.3 mEq/L, similar to that in orange juice and tomato juice... [and]...may be surreptitious source of potassium in patients with renal disease." Tahitian Noni® Juice is not a significant source of potassium. B.A. Mueller in USA Today, March 28, 2000 clarified his previous conclusion, stating that his analysis was made on a different noni product and not on Tahitian Noni® Juice and the amount of potassium in the brand of noni juice he analyzed in his study was "only 65 milligrams of potassium per 1 ounce serving, as much as you'd get in 2 inches of a banana."

Continued on next page

Tahitian Noni—Cont.

Tolson CB, Vest RG, West BJ. Quantitative ICP Mineral Analysis of TAHITIAN NONI® Juice. Tahitian Noni International Research Center. American Fork, Utah. USA 84003. Internal Data.
Potassium content of TAHITIAN NONI® Juice is 40 mg per 1 ounce serving. Compared to Grape juice* 42 mg per 1 ounce serving, Banana* 102 mg per 1 ounce serving and Yogurt* 66 mg per 1 ounce.

———

* Source: USDA Nutrient Database for Standard Reference
Carr ME, Koltz J. Bergeron M. Coumadin Resistance and the Vitamin Supplement "Noni." 2004 Am J. Hematology 77:103–104.
Carr et al reported a case of a 41-year-old female developing a coumadin resistance after drinking "Noni Juice 4 Everything" brand that "...has vitamin K and vitamin K was listed as a separate component, indicating that the juice might be fortified with vitamin K." They concluded that "...if you are on warfarin or coumadin, NO "NONI JUICE" for YOU!" This conclusion does not apply to the Brand TAHITIAN NONI® Juice as no vitamin K is added nor detected in TAHITIAN NONI® Juice.
Su Chen. HPLC Analysis of Vitamins in TAHITIAN NONI® Juice. Tahitian Noni International Research Center. American Fork, Utah. USA 84003. Internal Data.
Vitamin K is not present or is below detection limits in HPLC analysis of TAHITIAN NONI® Juice. AOAC Method was followed.

---

*This statement has not been evaluated by the Food and Drug Administration. This product is not intended to diagnose, treat, cure or prevent any disease

---

Shown in Product Identification Guide, page 516

Vemma™ Nutrition Company
8322 E. HARTFORD DR.
SCOTTSDALE, AZ 85255

For Direct Inquiries Contact:
Tel: 1-800-577-0777
Email:
productknowledge@govemma.com

VEMMA NUTRITION PROGRAM™

Description: The Vemma Nutrition Program provides two powerful liquid formulas that make it easy to get the vitamins, minerals and antioxidants you need to form a solid nutritional foundation. The first half of the program is Mangosteen Plus™, a powerful multivitamin formulation that contains 12 full-spectrum vitamins in a base of antioxidant-rich mangosteen fruit and mangosteen pericarp (rind) extract, whole leaf aloe vera and decaffeinated green tea. This amazing formula provides these powerful benefits:

Mangosteen Powered Antioxidants. Mangosteen provides powerful plant-based antioxidant protection and features a full array of phytonutrients including naturally-occurring xanthones.* Xanthones are effective antioxidants and provide the body with important nutritional benefits.*

Vitamin Powered Antioxidants. Contains critical antioxidant vitamins A (as beta carotene), C and E to help fight free radical damage and prevent oxidative stress to the body.* Some scientific evidence suggests that consumption of antioxidant vitamins may reduce the risk of certain forms of cancer. However, the FDA has determined that this evidence is limited and not conclusive.

Whole Leaf Aloe Vera. This wonderful leaf succulent contains an impressive selection of minerals, amino acids and nu-

Mangosteen Plus™
Supplement Facts
Serving Size 2 Tbsp (30 mL/1 fl oz)
Servings Per Container 32

	Amount Per Serving	% Daily Value
Calories	20	
Total Carbohydrate	5 g	2%*
Sugars	5 g	†
Vitamin A (100% as beta carotene)	5000 IU	100%
Vitamin C (as ascorbic acid)	300 mg	500%
Vitamin D (as cholecalciferol)	400 IU	100%
Vitamin E (as d-alpha tocopheryl acetate)	60 IU	200%
Thiamin (as thiamine hydrochloride)	1.5 mg	100%
Riboflavin (as riboflavin U.S.P.)	1.7 mg	100%
Niacin (as niacinamide)	20 mg	100%
Vitamin B6 (as pyridoxine hydrochloride)	5 mg	250%
Folate (as folic acid)	800 mcg	200%
Vitamin B12 (as cyanocobalamin)	15 mcg	250%
Biotin (as d-Biotin)	300 mcg	100%
Pantothenic Acid (as calcium d-pantothenate)	10 mg	100%
Selenium (as amino acid chelate)	140 mcg	200%
Proprietary Mangosteen, Whole Leaf Aloe Vera and Green Tea Blend	25.2 g	†

Reconstituted Mangosteen (*Garcinia mangostana L.*) (fruit), Aloe Vera Leaf (*Aloe barbadensis Miller*), Green Tea (*Camellia sinensis*) (leaf) (decaffeinated), Mangosteen Extract (pericarp) (standardized for 10% xanthones).
* Percent Daily Values are based on a 2,000 calorie diet.
† Daily Value not established.
Other ingredients: fructose, natural flavors, potassium sorbate, sodium benzoate, malic acid and xanthan gum.

Essential Minerals®
Supplement Facts
Serving Size 2 Tbsp (1 fl oz)
Servings Per Container 32

	Amount Per Serving	% Daily Value
Calories	15	
Total Carbohydrate	3 g	1%*
Sugars	3 g	†
Proprietary Mineral Blend	956 mg	†

Carbon (Organic), Calcium, Sodium, Sulfur, Magnesium, Chloride, Bromide, Fluoride, Iodine, Potassium, Niobium, Aluminum, Iron, Phosphorus, Silica, Manganese, Boron, Strontium, Titanium, Tungsten, Copper, Zinc, Tin, Zirconium, Molybdenum, Vanadium, Chromium, Selenium, Nickel, Cobalt, Lithium, Gallium, Barium, Yttrium, Neodymium, Hafnium, Cadmium, Thorium, Antimony, Cerium, Tellurium, Beryllium, Samarium, Dysprosium, Erbium, Bismuth, Gadolinium, Cesium, Lanthanum, Praseodymium, Europium, Lutetium, Terbium, Ytterbium, Holmium, Thallium, Thulium, Tantalum, Germanium, Gold, Platinum, Rhodium, Rubidium, Ruthenium, Scandium, Silver, Indium.
* Percent Daily Values are based on a 2,000 calorie diet.
† Daily Value not established.
Other ingredients: purified water, fructose, plant mineral extract, natural kiwi flavor, natural strawberry flavor, citric acid, xanthan gum and carmine color.

PRODUCT INFORMATION

tritional sugars such as polysaccharides, enzymes, lignins, saponins and anthraquinones that are known to provide the body with many beneficial effects for health and wellness.*

Beneficial Levels of Selenium. Some scientific evidence suggests that consumption of selenium may produce anticarcinogenic effects in the body. However, the FDA has determined that this evidence is limited and not conclusive.

Powerful B Vitamins. Supplies additional B vitamins at heart-healthy levels for added energy and provides a good source of folate.* Healthful diets with adequate folate may reduce a woman's risk of having a child with a brain and spinal cord defect.

Green Tea. Well-studied and documented for its traditional use and for its healing properties, it is also a powerful antioxidant.

The second half of the program is Essential Minerals®. Minerals support the health of organs, bones and the immune system.* The body does not inherently produce the minerals it needs, this is why supplementation and diet are important. In fact, our physical well-being is more directly dependent upon the minerals we take into our bodies than almost any other factor.* Vemma's Essential Minerals is a completely balanced, 100% natural mineral supplement that contains a combination of 65 major, trace and ultra-trace minerals. Essential Minerals is offered in a bioavailable (body-ready) liquid form that consists of pristine plant-sourced minerals totally dissolved in an ionic state.

The Vemma Nutrition Program's bioavailable (body-ready) formulas are easy to take and easy for the body to use. They are ideal supplements for patients who have trouble swallowing pills or tablets.

---

*These statements have not been approved by the Food and Drug Administration. This product is not intended to diagnose, treat, or prevent any disease.

Supplement Facts:
[See first table at top of previous page]
[See second table at top of previous page]

Directions: Shake well and serve cold. Take one fluid ounce (2 tablespoons) of Mangosteen Plus and one fluid ounce (2 tablespoons) of Essential Minerals daily. For best results, take both products together. For children ages two to twelve, take ½ dosages daily. Children under two, seek the advice of a healthcare professional.

Warnings: Keep out of reach of children. As with any nutritional supplement, always consult your healthcare professional if you are pregnant, lactat-

ing or if you have any other health condition. Discontinue if allergic reaction occurs.

Note: Store in a cool, dry place. Refrigerate after opening. Avoid exposure to direct sunlight.

How Supplied: 32 oz. bottle of Mangosteen Plus and 32 oz. bottle of Essential Minerals.

Shown in Product Identification Guide, page 516

Wyeth Consumer Healthcare Wyeth
FIVE GIRALDA FARMS
MADISON, NJ 07940

Direct Inquiries to:
Wyeth Consumer Healthcare Product Information 800-322-3129

CALTRATE® 600 + D

SUPPLEMENT FACTS
Serving Size 1 Tablet

Amount Per Serving	% DV
Vitamin D 200 IU	50%
Calcium 600 mg	60%

Ingredients: Calcium Carbonate, Starch. Contains less than 2% of the following: cholecalciferol, Croscarmellose Sodium, dl-Alpha Tocopherol, FD&C Yellow No. 6 Aluminum Lake, Gelatin, Magnesium Stearate, Partially Hydrogenated Soybean Oil, Sucrose, Titanium Dioxide. May contain less than 2% of the following: Glycerin, Hypromellose, Polydextrose, Polyethylene Glycol, Polyvinyl Alcohol, Talc.
As with any supplement, if you are pregnant or nursing a baby, contact your healthcare professional. **Keep out of reach of children.**

Suggested Use: Take one tablet twice daily with food or as directed by your physician. Not formulated for use in children.
Bottle sealed with printed foil under cap. Do not use if foil is torn.
Storage: Store at Room temperature. Keep bottle tightly closed.

How Supplied:
Bottles of 60, 120 tablets

CALTRATE® 600 PLUS™ Tablets
CALTRATE® 600 PLUS™ Chewables
Calcium Carbonate

Calcium Supplement With Vitamin D & Minerals

Supplement Facts
Serving Size 1 Tablet

Amount Per Serving	% DV
Vitamin D 200 IU	50%
Calcium 600 mg	60%
Magnesium 45 mg	11%
Zinc 7.5 mg	50%
Copper 1 mg	50%
Manganese 1.8 mg	90%
Boron 250 mcg	*

* Daily Value (% DV) not established.

Ingredients: Calcium Carbonate, Starch, Microcrystalline Cellulose, Magnesium oxide.

Contains <2% of: Cholecalciferol (Vit. D), Croscarmellose Sodium, Cupric Sulfate, dl-Alpha Tocopherol (Vit. E), FD&C Blue #1 Aluminum Lake, FD&C Red #40 Aluminum Lake, FD&C Yellow #6 Aluminum Lake, Gelatin, Hypromellose, Magnesium Stearate, Manganese Sulfate, Partially Hydrogenated Soybean Oil, Polysorbate 80, Sodium Borate, Sucrose, Titanium Dioxide, Triacetin, Zinc Oxide.

Chewables

Supplement Facts
Serving Size 1 Tablet

Amount Per Serving	% DV
Calories 10	
Total Carbohydrate 2 g	<1%+
Sugars 2 g	*
Vitamin D 200 IU	50%
Calcium 600 mg	60%
Magnesium 40 mg	10%
Zinc 7.5 mg	50%
Copper 1 mg	50%
Manganese 1.8 mg	90%
Boron 250 mcg	*

* Daily Value (%DV) not established.
+ Percent Daily Value based on a 2,000 calorie diet

Ingredients: Dextrose, Calcium Carbonate, Maltodextrin, Magnesium Stearate, Magnesium Oxide, Adipic Acid, Natural and Artificial Flavors, Mineral Oil, Cellulose, Zinc Oxide, Manganese Sulfate, Sodium Borate, FD&C Red #40 Aluminum Lake, Cupric Oxide, Gelatin, Sucrose, FD&C Yellow #6 Aluminum Lake, FD&C Blue #2 Aluminum Lake, Corn Starch, Canola Oil, Crospovidone, Cholecalciferol (Vit. D), Hydroxypropyl Methylcellulose, Stearic Acid, dl-Alpha Tocopherol.

Suggested Use: Take one tablet twice daily with food or as directed by your physician. Not formulated for use in children.

As with any supplement, if you are pregnant or nursing a baby, contact your healthcare professional.

Continued on next page

Caltrate 600 Plus—Cont.

Keep out of reach of children.
Bottle sealed with printed foil under cap.
Do not use if foil is torn.
Store at room temperature. Keep bottle tightly closed.
© 1999

How Supplied: Tablets; Bottles of 60 & 120
Chewables, Bottles of 60.
(Orange, cherry and fruit flavors)

CENTRUM®
High Potency Multivitamin-Multimineral Supplement, Advanced Formula From A to Zinc®

Supplement Facts:
Serving Size 1 Tablet

Each Tablet Contains	% DV
Vitamin A 3500 IU (29% as Beta Carotene)	70%
Vitamin C 60 mg	100%
Vitamin D 400 IU	100%
Vitamin E 30 IU	100%
Vitamin K 25 mcg	31%
Thiamin 1.5 mg	100%
Riboflavin 1.7 mg	100%
Niacin 20 mg	100%
Vitamin B_6 2 mg	100%
Folic Acid 400 mcg	100%
Vitamin B_{12} 6 mcg	100%
Biotin 30 mcg	10%
Pantothenic Acid 10 mg	100%
Calcium 162 mg	16%
Iron 18 mg	100%
Phosphorus 109 mg	11%
Iodine 150 mcg	100%
Magnesium 100 mg	25%
Zinc 15 mg	100%
Selenium 20 mcg	29%
Copper 2 mg	100%
Manganese 2 mg	100%
Chromium 120 mcg	100%
Molybdenum 75 mcg	100%
Chloride 72 mg	2%
Potassium 80 mg	2%
Boron 150 mcg	*
Nickel 5 mcg	*
Silicon 2 mg	*
Tin 10 mcg	*
Vanadium 10 mcg	*
Lutein 250 mcg	*
Lycopene 300 mcg	*

*Daily Value (%DV) not established.

Ingredients: Dibasic Calcium Phosphate, Magnesium Oxide, Potassium Chloride, Microcrystalline Cellulose, Ascorbic Acid (Vit. C), Ferrous Fumarate, Calcium Carbonate, Gelatin, dl-Alpha Tocopheryl Acetate (Vit. E). Contains less than 2% of the following: Acacia Senegal Gum, Ascorbyl Palmitate, Beta Carotene, Biotin, Boron, Butylated Hydroxytoluene, Calcium Pantothenate, Chromic Chloride, Citric Acid, Colloidal Silicon Dioxide, Crospovidone, Cupric Acid, Cyanocobalamin (Vit. B_{12}), Ergocalciferol (Vit. D), FD&C Yellow No. 6 Aluminum Lake, Folic Acid, Hypromellose, Lutein, Lycopene, Magnesium Stearate, Manganese Sulfate, Niacinamide, Nickelous Sulfate, Phytonadione (Vit. K), Polysorbate 80, Potassium Iodide, Potassium Sorbate, Pregelatinized Starch, Purified Water, Pyridoxine Hydrochloride (Vit. B_6), Riboflavin (Vit. B_2), Silicon Dioxide, Sodium Ascorbate, Sodium Benzoate, Sodium Citrate, Sodium Metavanadate, Sodium Molybdate, Sodium Selenate, Sodium Silicoaluminate, Sorbic Acid, Stannous Chloride, Starch, Sucrose, Thiamine Mononitrate (Vit. B_1), Titanium Dioxide, Tocopherol, Tribasic Calcium Phosphate, Triethyl Citrate, Vitamin A Acetate (Vit. A), Zinc Oxide. May also contain: Calcium Stearate, Glucose, Lactose Monohydrate.

Suggested Use:
One tablet daily with food. Not formulated for use in children.

Warning: Accidental overdose of iron-containing products is a leading cause of fatal poisoning in children under 6. Keep this product out of reach of children. In case of accidental overdose, call a doctor or poison control center immediately.

As with any supplement, if you are pregnant or nursing a baby, contact your healthcare professional.

IMPORTANT INFORMATION: Long-term intake of high levels of vitamin A (excluding that sourced from beta-carotene) may increase the risk of osteoporosis in postmenopausal women. Do not take this product if taking other vitamin A supplements.

How Supplied: Light peach, engraved CENTRUM C1.
Bottles of 15, 50, 130, 180, 250 tablets
Storage: Store at room temperature. Keep bottle tightly closed.
Bottle sealed with printed foil under cap.
Do not use if foil is torn.

CENTRUM KIDS COMPLETE
Rugrats®
Chewable Multivitamin Supplement (Orange, Cherry, Fruit Punch)

Supplement Facts:
[See table below]

Ingredients: Sucrose, Dibasic Calcium Phosphate, Mannitol, Calcium Carbonate, Stearic Acid, Magnesium Oxide, Ascorbic Acid (Vit. C), Pregelatinized Starch, Microcrystalline Cellulose, dl-Alpha Tocopheryl Acetate (Vit. E). Contains less than 2% of the following: Acacia, Aspartame**, Beta Carotene, Biotin, Butylated Hydroxytoluene (BHT), Calcium Pantothenate, Carbonyl Iron, Carrageenan, Chromic Chloride, Citric Acid, Cupric Oxide, Cyanocobalamin (Vit. B_{12}), Dextrose, Ergocalciferol (Vit. D), FD&C Blue 2 Aluminum Lake, FD&C Red 40 Aluminum Lake, FD&C Yellow 6 Aluminum Lake, Folic Acid, Gelatin, Glucose, Guar Gum, Lactose, Magnesium Stearate, Malic Acid, Manganese Sulfate, Mono and Diglycerides, Natural and Artificial Flavors, Niacinamide, Phytonadione (Vit. K), Potassium Iodide, Potassium Sorbate, Purified Water, Pyri-

Serving Size:	½ Tablet	1 Tablet
Amount Per Serving:	% DV for Children 2 and 3 Years (1/2 Tablet)	% DV for Adults and Children 4 Years and Older (1 Tablet)
Total Carbohydrate <1g	*	<1%+
Vitamin A 3500 IU (29% as Beta Carotene)	70%	70%
Vitamin C 60 mg	75%	100%
Vitamin D 400 IU	50%	100%
Vitamin E 30 IU	150%	100%
Vitamin K 10 mcg	*	13%
Thiamin 1.5 mg	107%	100%
Riboflavin 1.7 mg	106%	100%
Niacin 20 mg	111%	100%
Vitamin B_6 2 mg	143%	100%
Folic Acid 400 mcg	100%	100%
Vitamin B_{12} 6 mcg	100%	100%
Biotin 45 mcg	15%	15%
Pantothenic Acid 10 mg	100%	100%
Calcium 108 mg	7%	11%
Iron 18 mg	90%	100%
Phosphorus 50 mg	3%	5%
Iodine 150 mcg	107%	100%
Magnesium 40 mg	10%	10%
Zinc 15 mg	94%	100%
Copper 2 mg	100%	100%
Manganese 1 mg	*	50%
Chromium 20 mcg	*	17%
Molybdenum 20 mcg	*	27%

*Daily Value (%DV) not established.
+Percent Daily Values based on a 2,000 calorie diet.

doxine Hydrochloride (Vit. B_6), Riboflavin (Vit. B_2), Silicon Dioxide, Sodium Ascorbate, Sodium Benzoate, Sodium Citrate, Sodium Molybdate, Sodium Silicoaluminate, Sorbic Acid, Starch, Thiamine Mononitrate (Vit. B_1), Tocopherol, Tribasic Calcium Phosphate, Vanillin, Vitamin A Acetate (Vit. A), Zinc Oxide. May also contain: Fructose, Maltodextrin.

Suggested Use: Children 2 and 3 years of age, chew approximately ½ tablet daily with food. Adults and children 4 years of age and older, chew 1 tablet daily with food. Not formulated for use in children less than 2 years of age.

Warning: Accidental overdose of iron-containing products is a leading cause of fatal poisoning in children under 6. Keep this product out of reach of children. In case of accidental overdose, call a doctor or poison control center immediately. **CONTAINS ASPARTAME. ** PHENYLKETONURICS: CONTAINS PHENYLALANINE.**

Storage: Store at room temperature. Keep bottle tightly closed. Bottle sealed with printed foil under cap. Do not use if foil is torn.

How Supplied: Assorted Flavors—Uncoated Tablet—Bottles of 60, 100 tablets
Also available as: Centrum® Kids™ + Extra C (250 mg); and as: **Centrum® Kids™ + Extra Calcium** (200 mg).
Marketed by: Wyeth Consumer Healthcare, Madison, NJ 07940

CENTRUM® PERFORMANCE COMPLETE MULTIVITAMIN SUPPLEMENT Tablets

Supplement Facts
Serving Size 1 Tablet

Each Tablet Contains	% DV
Vitamin A 3500 IU	70%
(29% as Beta Carotene)	
Vitamin C 120 mg	200%
Vitamin D 400 IU	100%
Vitamin E 60 IU	200%
Vitamin K 25 mcg	31%
Thiamin 4.5 mg	300%
Riboflavin 5.1 mg	300%
Niacin 40 mg	200%
Vitamin B_6 6 mg	300%
Folic Acid 400 mcg	100%
Vitamin B_{12} 18 mcg	300%
Biotin 40 mcg	13%
Pantothenic Acid 10 mg	100%
Calcium 100 mg	10%
Iron 18 mg	100%
Phosphorus 48 mg	5%
Iodine 150 mcg	100%
Magnesium 40 mg	10%
Zinc 15 mg	100%
Selenium 70 mcg	100%
Copper 2 mg	100%
Manganese 4 mg	200%
Chromium 120 mcg	100%
Molybdenum 75 mcg	100%
Chloride 72 mg	2%
Potassium 80 mg	2%
Ginseng Root (*Panax ginseng*) Standardized Extract 50 mg	*
Ginkgo Biloba Leaf (*Ginkgo biloba*) Standardized Extract 60 mg	*
Boron 60 mcg	*
Nickel 5 mcg	*
Silicon 4 mg	*
Tin 10 mcg	*
Vanadium 10 mcg	*

*Daily Value (%DV) not established.

Ingredients: Dibasic Calcium Phosphate, Potassium Chloride, Ascorbic Acid (Vit. C), Microcrystalline Cellulose, Calcium Carbonate, dl-Alpha Tocopheryl Acetate (Vit. E), Magnesium Oxide, Ginkgo Biloba Leaf (*Ginkgo biloba*) Standardized Extract, Gelatin, Ginseng Root (*Panax ginseng*) Standardized Extract, Ferrous Fumarate, Niacinamide, Crospovidone, Starch. Contains less than 2% of the following: Acacia Senegal Gum, Beta Carotene, Biotin, Butylated Hydroxytoluene, Calcium Pantothenate, Chromic Chloride, Citric Acid, Cupric Oxide, Cyanocobalamin (Vit. B_{12}), Ergocalciferol (Vit. D), FD&C Red No. 40 Aluminum Lake, FD&C Yellow No. 6 Aluminum Lake, Folic Acid, Glucose, Hypromellose, Lactose Monohydrate, Magnesium Borate, Magnesium Stearate, Manganese Sulfate, Nickelous Sulfate, Phytonadione (Vit.K), Polyethylene Glycol, Polysorbate 80, Potassium Iodide, Potassium Sorbate, Purified Water, Pyridoxine Hydrochloride (Vit. B_6), Riboflavin (Vit. B_2), Silicon Dioxide, Sodium Ascorbate, Sodium Benzoate, Sodium Borate, Sodium Citrate, Sodium Metavanadate, Sodium Molybdate, Sodium Selenate, Sodium Silicoaluminate, Sorbic Acid, Stannous Chloride, Sucrose, Thiamin Mononitrate (Vit. B_1), Titanium Dioxide, Tocopherol, Tribasic Calcium Phosphate, Vitamin A Acetate (Vit. A), Zinc Oxide. May also contain: Maltodextrin.

Suggested Use: Adults—One tablet daily with food. Not formulated for use in children.

Warning: Accidental overdose of iron-containing products is a leading cause of fatal poisoning in children under 6. Keep this product out of reach of children. In case of accidental overdose, call a doctor or poison control center immediately.

Precaution: As with any supplement, if you are taking a prescription medication, or if you are pregnant or nursing a baby, contact your physician before using this product.

Important Information: Long-term intake of high levels of vitamin A (excluding that sourced from beta-carotene) may increase the risk of osteoporosis in postmenopausal women. Do not take this product if taking other vitamin A supplements.

Store at room temperature. Keep bottle tightly closed. Bottle sealed with printed foil under cap. Do not use if foil is torn.

How Supplied: Bottles of 45, 75 and 120 Tablets.

CENTRUM® SILVER®
Multivitamin/Multimineral Dietary Supplement for Adults 50+ From A to Zinc®

Supplement Facts
Serving Size 1 Tablet

Each Tablet Contains	% DV
Vitamin A 3500 IU	70%
(29% as Beta Carotene)	
Vitamin C 60 mg	100%
Vitamin D 400 IU	100%
Vitamin E 45 IU	150%
Vitamin K 10 mcg	13%
Thiamin 1.5 mg	100%
Riboflavin 1.7 mg	100%
Niacin 20 mg	100%
Vitamin B_6 3 mg	150%
Folic Acid 400 mcg	100%
Vitamin B_{12} 25 mcg	417%
Biotin 30 mcg	10%
Pantothenic Acid 10 mg	100%
Calcium 200 mg	20%
Phosphorus 48 mg	5%
Iodine 150 mcg	100%
Magnesium 100 mg	25%
Zinc 15 mg	100%
Selenium 20 mcg	29%
Copper 2 mg	100%
Manganese 2 mg	100%
Chromium 150 mcg	125%
Molybdenum 75 mcg	100%
Chloride 72 mg	2%
Potassium 80 mg	2%
Boron 150 mcg	*
Nickel 5 mcg	*
Silicon 2 mg	*
Vanadium 10 mcg	*
Lutein 250 mcg	*
Lycopene 300 mcg	*

*Daily Value (%DV) not established.

Ingredients: Calcium Carbonate, Dibasic Calcium Phosphate, Magnesium Oxide, Potassium Chloride, Microcrystalline Cellulose, Ascorbic Acid (Vit. C), dl-Alpha Tocopheryl Acetate (Vit. E), Gelatin, Pregelatinized Starch, Crospovidone. Contains less than 2% of the following: Acacia Senegal Gum, Ascorbyl Palmitate, Beta Carotene, Biotin, Boron, Butylated Hydroxytoluene, Calcium Panto-

Continued on next page

Centrum Silver—Cont.

thenate, Chromic Chloride, Citric Acid, Colloidal Silicon Dioxide, Cupric Oxide, Cyanocobalamin (Vit. B_{12}), Ergocalciferol (Vit. D), FD&C Blue No. 2 Aluminum Lake, FD&C Red No. 40 Aluminum Lake, FD&C Yellow No. 6 Aluminum Lake, Folic Acid, Hypromellose, Lutein, Lycopene, Magnesium Stearate, Manganese Sulfate, Niacinamide, Nickelous Sulfate, Phytonadione (Vit. K), Polysorbate 80, Potassium Iodide, Potassium Sorbate, Purified Water, Pyridoxine Hydrochloride (Vit. B_6), Riboflavin (Vit. B_2), Silicon Dioxide, Sodium Ascorbate, Sodium Benzoate, Sodium Citrate, Sodium Metavanadate, Sodium Molybdate, Sodium Selenate, Sodium Silicoaluminate, Sorbic Acid, Starch, Sucrose, Thiamine Mononitrate (Vit. B_1), Titanium Dioxide, Tocopherol, Tribasic Calcium Phosphate, Triethyl Citrate, Vitamin A Acetate (Vit. A), Zinc Oxide. May also contain: Calcium Stearate, Glucose, Lactose Monohydrate.

Recommended Intake:

Adults, 1 tablet daily with food. Not formulated for use in children.

Warnings: Keep out of the reach of children. As with any supplement, if you are pregnant or nursing a baby, contact your healthcare professional.

Important Information: Long-term intake of high levels of vitamin A (excluding that sourced from beta-carotene) may increase the risk of osteoporosis in postmenopausal women. Do not take this product if taking other vitamin A supplements.

How Supplied: Bottles of 60, 100, 150, and 220 tablets

Storage: Store at Room Temperature. Keep bottle tightly closed. Bottle is sealed with printed foil under cap. Do not use if foil is torn.

PROFILES OF COMMON DIETARY SUPPLEMENTS

This section features clinical information on frequently used supplements, including vitamins, minerals, glucosamine, coenzyme Q10, and other products. Organized alphabetically by common name, each profile includes the following: description, actions and pharmacology, clinical trials, indications and usage, contraindications, precautions and adverse reactions, overdosage (when available), dosage, and literature citations.

Calcium

DESCRIPTION

Calcium is an essential mineral. Average adult weight is made up of about 2% calcium, most of which is stored in the skeleton and teeth. A small amount of calcium circulates in the blood, muscles, and fluid between cells to help transmit nerve impulses. Along with keeping teeth and bones strong, calcium also promotes blood coagulation and plays an essential role in enabling muscles, including the heart, to relax and contract. Food sources of calcium include dairy products (milk, yogurt, cheese), sea vegetables, sardines, almonds, hazelnuts, legumes, collards, kale, parsley, and tofu (Pitchford 1993).

The scope of this discussion will be limited to the oral salt formulations, including carbonate, citrate, glubionate, gluconate, lactate, phosphate, and other calcium salts. (Calcium acetate, calcium chloride, calcium gluceptate, and calcium gluconate may be administered intravenously.) Because calcium salts are bound with other molecules such as oxygen and carbon, supplements often list the percentage of elemental calcium in each tablet along with the total salt weight, usually in milligrams. The table below lists common examples.

Type of oral calcium salt	Elemental calcium per 1,000 mg (percentage and weight)
Carbonate	40% (400 mg)
Citrate	21% (210 mg)
Lactate	13% (130 mg)
Gluconate	9% (90 mg)

Other Names: Ca, calcium carbonate, calcium chloride, calcium citrate, calcium gluceptate, calcium gluconate, calcium malate

ACTIONS AND PHARMACOLOGY

EFFECTS

Calcium has anti-osteoporotic, antihypertensive, antihyperlipidemic, and possible anticarcinogenic properties. It is an electrolyte, a nutrient, and a mineral. Calcium functions as a regulator in the release and storage of neurotransmitters and hormones, in the uptake and binding of amino acids, and in vitamin B12 absorption and gastrin secretion. Calcium is required to maintain the function of the nervous, muscular, and skeletal systems and cell membrane and capillary permeability. It is an activator in many enzyme reactions and is essential in the transmission of nerve impulses; contraction of cardiac, smooth, and skeletal muscles; respiration; blood coagulation; and renal function (Product Info: Calcium gluconate 1992; AHFS 1979).

Antiproliferative Effects: Calcium precipitates soluble colonic luminal surfactants (bile acids and free fatty acids) resulting in reduced cytolytic activity of these substances and, consequently, reduced epithelial damage and colonic proliferation. This antiproliferative effect was found for calcium provided as milk, calcium carbonate, and calcium phosphate and may explain the inverse association between calcium intake and colorectal neoplasia reported in some studies (Govers et al 1994).

CLINICAL TRIALS

Complications of Pregnancy

A meta-analysis of studies evaluating the effect of calcium supplementation on pregnancy-related hypertension and pre-eclampsia has raised controversy. The meta-analysis (n=2,260 subjects) reports a significant and substantial 62% reduction in risk of pre-eclampsia as well as decreases in both systolic (-5.4 mm Hg) and diastolic (-3.4 mm Hg) blood pressure with calcium supplementation (typically, 1 to 2 g per day). Many of these studies were conducted in countries where there is low dietary calcium intake. The authors acknowledge that there is insufficient data to determine whether calcium supplementation affects the meaningful outcomes of maternal and fetal morbidity and mortality. Nevertheless, they suggest a policy of offering calcium supplementation to all pregnant women in whom there is a concern about the development of pre-eclampsia (Bucher et al 1996). Numerous criticisms of the authors' methods of analysis, of their conclusions, and of their advice have been offered (Cher 1997; Cappuccio 1996; Roberts et al 1996; Levine et al 1996).

Fluorosis

A combination of calcium, ascorbic acid, and vitamin D3 reversed dental, clinical, and early skeletal fluorosis in children in a double-blind, placebo-controlled study. Twenty-five children (aged 6 to 12 years), living in an area where the drinking water contained fluorides at a concentration of 4.5 mg/liter (mg/L), were administered either placebo (n=10) or ascorbic acid 250 mg and calcium compound (125 mg elemental calcium) twice a day and vitamin D3 60,000 IU once a week (n=15) for 180 days. Intake of fluoride-rich water continued as usual. At the end of the treatment period, there was significant improvement in dental, clinical, and skeletal grades of fluorosis in the treated children (p=0.05) but not in the placebo group. There were significantly reduced fluoride levels in the blood and serum and increased urinary fluoride levels in the treated group (p=0.05 for all three parameters) but not in the placebo group, indicating increased removal of fluoride from the body. The results of this small study indicate that calcium, ascorbic acid, and vitamin D3 supplementation can reverse fluorosis in children (Gupta et al 1996).

Osteoporosis

A review of studies in which postmenopausal women were treated with antiresorptive drugs (estrogen or calcitonin) or with antiresorptive drugs plus calcium showed greater increases in bone mass when treatment included supplemental calcium. Calcitonin alone stopped bone loss in the spine, but calcitonin plus calcium increased bone mass of the spine (Nieves et al 1998).

Intermittent fluoride treatment plus calcium increased bone mineral density and was associated with a lower fracture rate than calcium supplementation alone in men with idiopathic osteoporosis. Fifty men with osteoporosis but no history of vertebral fractures were given either calcium 1,000 mg/day, or intermittent monofluorophosphate (MFP, 114 mg=15 mg fluoride ions daily, 3 months on, 1 month off) plus calcium 950 to 1,000 mg/day for 36 months. There was a progressive decrease in back pain in the MFP group over the three years, whereas there was no significant change in the calcium-only group. The fracture rate (new fractures per 100 patient-years) at the end of 3 years was 4.9 for the MFP group and 20.5 for the calcium-only group (Ringe et al 1998).

Concurrent administration of oral vitamin D3 and calcium reduced the incidence of nonvertebral fractures and hip fractures and increased bone density of the total proximal femoral region in elderly women (mean age 84 years). Compared with the placebo group (n=888), the treated women (n=877) had 32% fewer nonvertebral fractures and 43% fewer hip fractures. Eighteen months of treatment resulted in an increase of 2.7% in bone density of the total proximal femoral region compared with a decrease of 4.6% in the placebo group (p<0.001). The dosage of vitamin D3 was 20 mcg (800 IU)/day and elemental calcium was 1.2 g/day (Chapuy et al 1992). In a smaller 3-year study (n=318) in women and men over the age of 65 and living at home, calcium 500 mg/day (as calcium citrate malate) plus 700 IU of cholecalciferol/day, in comparison to placebo, reduced the rate of bone loss of both men and women and significantly reduced the incidence of nonvertebral fractures. Rates of loss of bone mass were lower for femoral neck, spine, and total body in treatment groups after 1 year. However, significant differences between treatment groups in years 2 and 3 were maintained only for total-body bone mineral density (Dawson-Hughes et al 1997).

Premenstrual Pain

Calcium supplementation was effective in reducing premenstrual pain, but not menstrual pain, in a prospective, randomized, double-blind, placebo-controlled, parallel-group, multicenter clinical trial of premenstrual syndrome. Subjects (n=497) were given calcium 1,200 mg daily or placebo for three menstrual cycles. Outcome measures included a daily subjective rating scale with 17 core symptoms, of which three were pain-related, and four symptom factors, of which one was pain-related. Significantly lower scores occurred for all pain measures in the treatment group during the luteal phase of the third menstrual cycle (p=0.001) while scores did not change significantly in controls. Pain scores did not decrease significantly during the menstrual phase of the third menstrual cycle for both calcium and placebo groups (Thys-Jacobs et al 1998).

INDICATIONS AND USAGE
Approved by the FDA:

- Prophylaxis of calcium deficiency and treatment of osteoporosis
- Calcium acetate: Treatment of hyperphosphatemia related to renal failure and hemodialysis
- Calcium carbonate: Used alone or in combination products as an antacid to relieve symptoms of heartburn, acid indigestion, and stomach upset

Unproven Uses: Calcium supplementation may reduce premenstrual pain, total and LDL cholesterol, hypertension, and the occurrence of colorectal polyps. Studies show it may also reverse fluorosis in children (when combined with vitamins C and D), control age-related increases in parathyroid hormone, and reduce plasma bilirubin in patients with Crigler-Najjar syndrome (calcium phosphate only).

Weaker evidence shows calcium supplementation may be helpful for leg cramps, pre-eclampsia, and prophylaxis of urinary crystallization of calcium oxalate in patients with nephrolithiasis (calcium citrate only).

CONTRAINDICATIONS
Calcium supplements are contraindicated in patients with hypercalcemia (Gilman et al 2001).

PRECAUTIONS AND ADVERSE REACTIONS
Calcium enhances the effect of cardiac glycosides on the heart and may precipitate arrhythmias (Dukes 1980).

Oral calcium supplementation can cause constipation. Additionally, oral calcium—including antacids containing calcium carbonate or other absorbable calcium salts—can cause hypercalcemia (especially in patients with hypothyroidism) and milk-alkali syndrome with doses higher than 4 g daily. Hypercalcemia may result in nephrolithiasis, anorexia, nausea, vomiting, and ocular toxicity. Symptoms of milk-alkali syndrome include hypercalcemia, uremia, calcinosis, nausea, vomiting, headache, weakness, azotemia, and alterations in taste.

High intake of calcium, whether from food alone or including supplements, was associated in an epidemiological study with an increased incidence of prostate cancer, possibly due to calcium's inhibitory effect on vitamin D conversion (Giovannucci et al 1998).

Pregnancy: FDA-rated as Pregnancy Category C. Calcium is safe in normal dietary amounts.

Breastfeeding: Calcium is safe in normal dietary amounts.

Drug Interactions

Aspirin: Concurrent use may result in decreased effectiveness of aspirin due to increased urinary pH and subsequent increased renal elimination of salicylates. *Clinical Management:* Monitor for reduced aspirin effectiveness upon initiation of calcium-containing products or for possible aspirin toxicity upon withdrawal of calcium-containing products. Adjust the dose accordingly. Using buffered aspirin may limit the degree to which the urine is alkalinized.

Atenolol: Concomitant use may decreased bioavailability of atenolol. *Clinical Management:* Instruct patients to avoid taking atenolol and calcium-containing products at the same time. Atenolol should be administered 2 hours before or 6 hours after calcium-containing products.

Bismuth Subcitrate: Concomitant use may result in decreased effectiveness of bismuth subcitrate. *Clinical Management:* Bismuth subcitrate and calcium-containing products should be administered at least 30 minutes apart.

Bisphosphonates: Concurrent use may interfere with the absorption of bisphosphonates such as alendronate, etidronate, and risedronate. *Clinical Management:* Administer bisphosphonates 2 hours before and 3 to 4 hours after a dose of calcium.

Calcium channel blockers: Concomitant use can result in decreased effectiveness of calcium channel blockers. *Clinical Management:* Monitor the patient and adjust dose accordingly.

Cefpodoxime: Concomitant use may result in decreased effectiveness of cefpodoxime. *Clinical Management:* Concurrent administration of cefpodoxime and calcium-containing products is not recommended. If concurrent use cannot be avoided, cefpodoxime should be taken at least 2 to 3 hours before the administration of calcium. Because staggered administration may not be completely reliable, aggressively monitor patients for continued antibiotic efficacy. Alternative antibiotic therapy (eg, another third-generation cephalosporin or a second-generation cephalosporin with similar activity) may need to be considered.

Digitoxin: Coadministration of digitoxin and parenteral calcium is contraindicated (Product Info: Crystodigin 1995). Early case reports describe cardiovascular collapse after administration of intravenous calcium in patients receiving digitalis. *Clinical Management:* Administration of parenteral calcium to digitoxin-treated patients is contraindicated.

Digoxin: Most textbooks and reviews state that a contraindication exists in giving calcium intravenously in the presence of digitalis glycosides, though this is based on relatively few reports. The similar actions of digitalis glycosides and calcium are documented, and deaths have occurred during simultaneous administration. *Clinical Management:* If calcium is needed in a digitalized patient, it should be infused over several hours or given orally.

Diuretics: Thiazide and thiazide-like diuretics may cause hypercalcemia by decreasing renal calcium excretion. Concomitant ingestion of calcium salts and thiazide diuretics may predispose patients to developing the milk-alkali syndrome. *Clinical Manage-*

ment: Instruct patients to avoid excessive ingestion of calcium in any form (eg, antacids, dairy products) during thiazide diuretic therapy. Consider monitoring the patient's serum calcium level and/or parathyroid function if calcium replacement therapy is clinically necessary.

Fluoroquinolones: Concomitant use may result in decreased effectiveness of fluoroquinolones such as ciprofloxacin and enoxacin. *Clinical Management:* Concurrent administration of fluoroquinolones with calcium—including calcium-fortified foods and drinks such as orange juice—should be avoided. Fluoroquinolones may be taken 2 hours before or 6 hours after taking calcium-containing products.

Gentamicin: A retrospective study conducted on 267 patients who had undergone elective coronary artery bypass graft (CABG) surgery showed an increased incidence of renal failure in patients who had received gentamicin and bypass prime solutions containing high amounts of calcium (Schneider et al 1996). *Clinical Management:* Avoid concurrent use of gentamicin and solutions containing a high amount of calcium during CABG surgery.

Hyoscyamine: Concomitant use may result in decreased absorption of hyoscyamine. *Clinical Management:* Hyoscyamine should be taken prior to meals and calcium-containing products should be taken after meals.

Itraconazole: Concomitant use may result in decreased effectiveness of itraconazole. *Clinical Management:* Calcium-containing products should be taken at least 1 hour before or 2 hours after itraconzaole.

Ketoconazole: Concomitant use may result in decreased effectiveness of ketoconazole. *Clinical Management:* Concurrent administration of ketoconazole and calcium-containing products is not recommended. If concurrent use cannot be avoided, ketoconazole should be taken at least 2 hours before calcium-containing products. Because staggered administration may not be completely reliable, aggressively monitor patients for continued antifungal efficacy.

Levothyroxine: Concurrent use with calcium carbonate may result in decreased absorption of levothyroxine. *Clinical Management:* Separate the administration of levothyroxine and calcium carbonate by at least 4 hours.

Methscopolamine: Concomitant use may result in decreased absorption of methscopolamine, although the effect is minor. *Clinical Management:* Monitor the patient for drug effectiveness.

Polystyrene Sulfonate: Concomitant administration of calcium-containing antacids and sodium polystyrene sulfonate resin therapy has resulted in the elevation of serum carbon dioxide content levels, associated with varying degrees of metabolic alkalosis. *Clinical Management:* Separate the oral administration of sodium polystyrene sulfonate and calcium-containing products by as much time as possible. Another alternative is to administer the sodium polystyrene sulfonate rectally. If concurrent oral administration cannot be avoided, monitor the patient for evidence of alkalosis.

Ranitidine bismuth citrate: Concurrent use may result in decreased plasma concentrations of ranitidine; however, the effect is clinically insignificant.

Sucralfate: Concurrent use may result in decreased effectiveness of sucralfate. *Clinical Management:* Calcium-containing products should not be taken 30 minutes before or after sucralfate administration.

Sulfasalazine: Concomitant sulfasalazine and calcium gluconate therapy has been reported to result in delayed absorption of sulfasalazine.

Tetracyclines: Concurrent use may result in decreased effectiveness of tetracyclines. *Clinical Management:* Concurrent administration of any of the tetracyclines and calcium-containing products is not recommended. If concurrent use cannot be avoided, tetracyclines should be taken at least 1 to 3 hours before calcium-containing products. Because staggered administration may not be completely reliable, aggressively monitor patients for continued antibiotic efficacy.

Ticlopidine: Concurrent use may result in decreased effectiveness of ticlopidine. *Clinical Management:* Concurrent administration of ticlopidine and calcium-containing products is not recommended. If concurrent use cannot be avoided, ticlopidine should be taken at least 1 to 2 hours before the administration of calcium.

Zicaltibine: Concurrent use may result in decreased effectiveness of zicaltibine. *Clinical Management:* Separate the administration of zalcitabine and calcium-containing products as far apart as possible.

Food and Supplement Interactions

Dairy foods: Phosphorus, found in dairy products, may inhibit calcium absorption by forming insoluble compounds with calcium ions. This binds the mineral into a form that is poorly absorbed through the intestinal wall. *Clinical Management:* Calcium products should not be taken within 2 hours of a dairy product or other foods high in phosphorous.

Foods containing oxalic acid or phytic acid: Oxalic acid (found in foods such as spinach, parsley, rhubarb, and beans) and phytic acid (found in bran and whole cereals) may inhibit calcium absorption by forming insoluble compounds with calcium ions. This binds the mineral into a form that is poorly absorbed through the intestinal wall. *Clinical Management:* Calcium products should not be taken within 2 hours of eating foods high in oxalic acid or phytic acid.

Iron: Concurrent use may result in reduced absorption of iron, although the effect is usually not clinically significant.

Zinc: Concurrent use may result in reduced absorption of zinc, although the effect is usually not clinically significant.

OVERDOSAGE

Active treatment is required when serum calcium levels reach 12 mg/dL, and intensive treatment is necessary for levels greater than 15 mg/dL (AMA 1980).

DOSAGE

Mode of Administration: Oral

How Supplied: Capsule, liquid, tablet

Daily Dosage: The National Institute of Medicine recommends the following Adequate Intakes (AIs) for males and females: *0 to 6 months* — 210 mg/day; *7 to 12 months* — 270 mg/day; *1 to 3 years* — 500 mg/day; *4 to 8 years* — 800 mg/day; *9 to 18 years* — 1,300 mg/day; *19 to 50 years* — 1,000 mg/day; *51+ years* — 1,200 mg/day. The same AIs apply to pregnant or lactating women.

ADULTS

Colorectal cancer prevention: 1,200 to 2,000 mg/d (Hofstad et al 1998; Duris et al 1996; Lipkin & Newmark 1993; Zimmerman 1993).

Crigler-Najjar Syndrome: 4,000 mg/d (Van der Veere et al 1997).

Dysmenorrhea: 1,000 to 1,300 mg/d (Penland et al 1993; Thys-Jacobs et al 1989).

Hypercholesterolemia: 250 to 400 mg/d with meals (Denke et al 1993; Bell et al 1992; Karanja et al 1994).

Hyperphosphatemia: 1,334 mg of calcium acetate with each meal initially. Most patients will require 2,001 to 2,668 mg with each meal. The dosage may be increased as necessary to obtain serum phosphate levels below 6 mg/dL as long as hypercalcemia does not occur (Product Info: PhosLo 1996); or alternatively, 1 to 17 grams of calcium carbonate daily in divided doses (Malberti et al 1988; Slatopolsky et al 1986).

Hyperphosphatemia of renal failure and hemodialysis: 4,000 to 8,000 mg/d of calcium acetate (Product Info: PhosLo 1996) or 2,500 to 8,500 mg/d of calcium carbonate (Malberti et al 1988; Slatopolsky et al 1986).

Hypertension, idiopathic: 1,000 to 2,000 mg/d (Bucher et al 1996; Takagi et al 1991; Lyle et al 1987; Tabuchi et al 1986).

Hypertension, pregnancy-related: 1,000 to 2,000 mg/d (Bucher et al 1996).

Hypocalcemia: calcium carbonate, 1 to 2 grams 3 times a day with meals (AMA 1986); calcium citrate, 950 mg to 1.9 g given 3 or 4 times a day after meals (AMA 1986); calcium gluconate, 15 g daily in divided doses (AMA 1986); calcium lactate, 7.7 grams daily in divided doses with meals (USPDI 2004; AMA 1980); calcium glubionate, 15 grams/d in divided doses (AMA 1986); dibasic calcium phosphate, 4.4 g daily in divided doses with or after meals (USPDI 2004; AMA 1980); tribasic calcium phosphate, 1.6 grams twice daily with or after meals (USPDI 2004).

Nephrolithiasis, prevention: 200 to 300 mg with meals or as the citrate salt between meals (Liebman et al 1997; Levine et al 1994; Barilla et al 1978).

Osteoporosis, glucocorticoid-induced, prevention of bone loss:1,000 mg/d (Buckley et al 1996).

Osteoporosis, idiopathic, prevention of bone loss and fractures: 500 to 2,400 mg/d including a bedtime dose (Nieves et al 1998; Dawson-Hughes et al 1997; Fujita et al 1997; McKane et al 1996; Blumsohn et al 1994; Reid et al 1993; Chapuy et al 1992).

Pre-eclampsia, prevention: 1,000 to 2,000 mg/d (Bucher et al 1996).

Premenstrual syndrome: 1,000 to 1,200 mg/d (Thys-Jacobs et al 1998; Penland et al 1993; Thys-Jacobs et al 1989).

PEDIATRICS

Bone mass accretion (adolescents): 500 mg/d (Lloyd et al 1993).

Fluorosis: 250 mg/d (Gupta et al 1996).

Hypertension, prevention: 600 mg/d (Gillman et al 1995).

Hypocalcemia: calcium chloride, 200 mg/kg/d in divided doses every 4 to 6 hours (Benitz et al 1988); calcium glubionate: infants up to 1 year old should receive 1.8 grams of calcium glubionate 5 times a day before meals, and children 1 to 4 years old should receive 3.6 grams 3 times a day before meals. Children over age 4 should receive adult and adolescent doses (USPDI 2004); calcium gluconate, 200 to 800 mg/kg/d in divided doses (USPDI 2004; Benitz et al 1988); calcium lactate, 500 mg/kg/24 hours given orally in divided doses (USPDI 2004; Benitz et al 1981; Shirkey 1980; AMA 1980; Pagliaro et al 1979); calcium levulinate: 500 mg/kg/24 hours (12 g/square meter/24 hours) given orally in divided doses (Shirkey 1980); dibasic calcium phosphate: 200 to 280 mg/kg of body weight a day, in divided doses with or after meals (USPDI 2004).

LITERATURE

American Society of Health-System Pharmacists (AHFS): *American Hospital Formulary Service Drug Information*. ASHP, Bethesda, MD; 1997.

AMA Department of Drugs: *AMA Drug Evaluations*, 4th ed. American Medical Association, Chicago, IL, USA; 1980.

Bell L, Halstenson CE, Halstenson CJ et al: Cholesterol-lowering effects of calcium carbonate in patients with mild to moderate hypercholesterolemia. *Arch Intern Med*; 152(12):2441-2444. 1992

Benitz WE, Tatro DS: *The Pediatric Drug Handbook*, 2nd ed. Year Book Medical Publishers, Chicago, IL, USA; 1988.

Blumsohn A, Herrington K, Hannon RA et al: The effect of calcium supplementation on the circadian rhythm of bone resorption. *J Clin Endocrinol Metab*; 79(3):730-735. 1994

Bucher HC, Cook RJ, Guyatt GH et al: Effects of dietary calcium supplementation on blood pressure - a meta-analysis of randomized controlled trials. *JAMA*; 275(13):1016-1022. 1996

Bucher HC, Guyatt GH, Cook RJ et al: Effect of calcium supplementation on pregnancy-induced hypertension and preeclampsia. *JAMA*; 275(14):1113-1117. 1996

Buckley LM, Leib ES, Cartularo KS et al: Calcium and vitamin D3 supplementation prevents bone loss in the spine secondary to low dose corticosteroids in patients with rheumatoid arthritis: a randomized, double-blind placebo-controlled trial. *Ann Intern Med*; 125(12):961-968. 1996

Cappuccio FP, Markandu ND, Singer DRJ et al: Does oral calcium supplementation lower high blood pressure? A double blind study. *J Hypertens*; 5(1):67-71. 1987

Chapuy MC, Arlot ME, Duboeuf F et al: Vitamin D3 and calcium to prevent hip fractures in elderly women. *N Engl J Med*; 327(23):1637-1642. 1992

Cher DJ: Dietary calcium and blood pressure (letter). *JAMA*; 126(6):492. 1997

Dawson-Hughes B, Harris SS, Krall EA et al: Effect of calcium and vitamin D supplementation on bone density in men and women 65 years of age or older. *N Engl J Med*; 337(10):670-676. 1997

Denke MA, Fox MM, Schulte MC: Short-term dietary calcium fortification increases fecal saturated fat content and reduces serum lipids in men. *J Nutr*; 123(6):1047-1053. 1993

Deroisy R, Zartarian M, Meurmans L et al: Acute changes in serum calcium and parathyroid hormone circulating levels induced by the oral intake of five currently available calcium salts in healthy male volunteers. *Clin Rheumatol*; 16(3):249-253. 1997

Dukes MNG: *Meyler's Side Effects of Drugs*, vol 9. Excerpta Medica, New York, NY; 1980.

Duris I, Hruby D, Pekarkova B et al: Calcium chemoprevention in colorectal cancer. *Hepatogastroenterology*; 43(7):152-154. 1996

Fujita T, Ohgitani S, Fujii Y: Overnight suppression of parathyroid hormone and bone resorption markers by active absorbable algae calcium: a double-blind crossover study. *Calcif Tissue Int*; 60(6):506-512. 1997

Gilman AG, Hardman JG, Limbird LE (eds): *Goodman & Gilman's The Pharmacological Basis of Therapeutics*, 10th ed. McGraw-Hill, New York, NY; 2001.

Giovannucci E, Rimm EB, Wolk A et al: Calcium and fructose intake in relation to risk of prostate cancer. *Cancer Res*; 58(3):442-447. 1998

Govers MJAP, Termont DSML, Van der Meer R: Mechanism of the antiproliferative effect of milk mineral and other calcium supplements on colonic epithelium. *Cancer Res*; 54(1):95-100. 1994

Gupta SK, Gupta RC, Seth AK et al: Reversal of fluorosis in children. *Acta Paediatr Jpn*; 38(5):513-519. 1996

Harvey JA, Kenny P, Poindexter J et al: Superior calcium absorption from calcium citrate than calcium carbonate using external forearm counting. *J Am Coll Nutr*; 9(6):583-587. 1990

Heaney RP, Smith KT, Recker RR et al: Meal effects on calcium absorption. *Am J Clin Nutr*; 49(2):372-376. 1989

Hofstad B, Almendingen K, Vatn M et al: Growth and recurrence of colorectal polyps: a double-blind 3-year intervention with calcium and antioxidants. *Digestion*; 59(2):148-156. 1998

Ivanovich P, Fellows H, Rich C: The absorption of calcium carbonate. *Ann Intern Med*; 66(5):917-923. 1967

Karanja N, Morris CD, Rufolo P et al: Impact of increasing calcium in the diet on nutrient consumption, plasma lipids, and lipoproteins in humans. *Am J Clin Nutr*; *59(4):900-907*. 1994

Levine BS, Rodman JS, Wienerman S et al: Effect of calcium citrate supplementation on urinary calcium oxalate saturation in female stone formers: implications for prevention of osteoporosis. *Am J Clin Nutr*; 60(4):592-596. 1994

Levine R, DerSimonian R: Effects of calcium supplementation on pregnancy-induced hypertension (letter). *JAMA*; 276(17):1387. 1996

Liebman M, Chai W: Effect of dietary calcium on urinary oxalate excretion after oxalate loads. *Am J Clin Nutr*; 65(5):1453-1459. 1997

Lipkin M, Newmark H: Calcium and colon cancer (letter). *Nutr Rev*; 51(7):213-214. 1993

Lloyd T, Andon MB, Rollings N et al: Calcium supplementation and bone mineral density in adolescent girls. *JAMA*; 270(7):841-844. 1993

Lopez-Jaramillo P, Delgado F, Jacome P et al: Calcium supplementation and the risk of preeclampsia in Ecuadorian pregnant teenagers. *Obstet Gynecol*; 90(2):162-167. 1997

Lyle RM, Melby CL, Hyner GC et al: Blood pressure and metabolic effects of calcium supplementation on normotensive white and black men. *JAMA*; 257(13):1772-1776. 1987

Malberti F, Surian M, Poggio F et al: Efficacy and safety of long-term treatment with calcium carbonate as a phosphate binder. *Am J Kidney Dis*; 12(6):487-491. 1988

McKane WR, Khosla S, Egan KS et al: Role of calcium intake in modulating age-related increases in parathyroid function and bone resorption. *J Clin Endocrinol Metab*; 81(5):1699-1703. 1996

Newmark K, Nugent P: Milk-alkali syndrome: a consequence of chronic antacid abuse. *Postgrad Med*; 93(6):149-150, 156. 1993

Nieves JW, Komar L, Cosman F et al: Calcium potentiates the effect of estrogen and calcitonin on bone mass: review and analysis. *Am J Clin Nutr*; 67(1):18-24. 1998

Penland JG, Johnson PE: Dietary calcium and manganese effects on menstrual cycle symptoms. *Am J Obstet Gynecol*; 168(5):1417-1423. 1993

Parfitt K (ed): *Martindale: The Complete Drug Reference*. London: Pharmaceutical Press (electronic version). Thomson Micromedex, Greenwood Village, CO, 2000.

Pitchford P: *Healing with Whole Foods*. North Atlantic Books, Berkeley, CA; 1993.

Product Information: Calcium gluconate. LyphoMed, Deerfield, IL; 1992.

Product Information: Crystodigin (digitoxin). Eli Lilly and Company, Indianapolis, IN; 1995.

Product Information: PhosLo (calcium acetate). Braintree Laboratories, Braintree, MA; 1996.

Recker RR: Calcium absorption and achlorhydria. *N Engl J Med*; 313(2):70-73. 1985

Reid IR, Ames RW, Evans MC et al: Effect of calcium supplementation on bone loss in postmenopausal women. *N Engl J Med*; 328(7):460-464. 1993

Riley BB: Incompatibilities in intravenous solutions. *J Hosp Pharm*; 28:228-240. 1970

Ringe JD, Dorst A, Kipshoven C et al: Avoidance of vertebral fractures in men with idiopathic osteoporosis by a three year therapy with calcium and low-dose intermittent monofluorophosphate. *Osteoporos Int*; 8(1):47-52. 1998

Roberts JM, D'Abarno J: Effects of calcium supplementation on pregnancy-induced hypertension (letter). *JAMA*; 276(17):1386-1387. 1996

Schneider M, Valentine S, Clarke G et al: Acute renal failure in cardiac surgical patients, potentiated by gentamicin and calcium. *Anaesth Intensive Care*; 24:647-650. 1996

Shirkey HC: *Pediatric Dosage Handbook*. American Pharmaceutical Association, Washington, DC, USA; 1980.

Slatopolsky E, Weerts C, Lopez-Hilker S et al: Calcium carbonate as a phosphate binder in patients with chronic renal failure undergoing dialysis. *N Engl J Med*; 315(3):157-161. 1986

Tabuchi Y, Ogihara T, Hashizume K et al: Hypotensive effect of long-term oral calcium supplementation in elderly patients with essential hypertension. *J Clin Hypertens*; 2:254-262. 1986

Takagi Y, Fukase M, Takata S et al: Calcium treatment of essential hypertension in elderly patients evaluated by 24 h monitoring. *Am J Hypertens*; 4(10 pt 1):836-839. 1991

Thys-Jacobs S, Ceccarelli S, Bierman A et al: Calcium supplementation in premenstrual syndrome: a randomized crossover trial. *J Gen Intern Med*; 4(3):183-189. 1989

Thys-Jacobs S, Starkey P, Bernstein D et al: Calcium carbonate and the premenstrual syndrome: effects on premenstrual and menstrual symptoms (Premenstrual Syndrome Study Group). Am J Obstet Gynecol; 179(2):444-452. 1998

United States Pharmacopeial Convention, Inc.: *USP DI: Drug Information for the Health Care Professional*, 24th ed. Thomson Micromedex, Greenwood Village CO; 2004.

Van der Veere CN, Jansen PL, Sinaasappel M et al: Oral calcium phosphate: a new therapy for Crigler-Najjar disease? *Gastroenterology*; 112(2):455-462. 1997

Wabner CL, Pak CYC: Modification by food of the calcium absorbability and physicochemical effects of calcium citrate. *J Am Coll Nutr*; 11(5):548-552. 1992

Young LY, Koda-Kimble MA: *Applied Therapeutics: The Clinical Use of Drugs*, 6th ed. Applied Therapeutics, Inc, Vancouver, WA, USA; 1995.

Zimmerman J: Does dietary calcium supplementation reduce the risk of colon cancer (letter)? *Nutr Rev*; 51(4):109-112. 1993

Chondroitin Sulfate

DESCRIPTION

Chondroitin sulfate is a mucopolysaccharide found in most mammalian cartilaginous tissues. It has a molecular configuration similar to sodium hyaluronate, although chondroitin has a considerably shorter chain length (Liesegang 1990). In clinical settings, chondroitin is commonly used as a viscoelastic agent during ophthalmic procedures. Its major use as a supplement is for relieving symptoms of osteoarthritis and rheumatic diseases. It has also been used to treat heart disease, nephrolithiasis, and hypercholesterolemia. The chondroprotective properties of chondroitin have led to speculative use in the prevention and/or treatment of disorders of other connective tissue structures such as the aorta, vascular tissues, and soft tissues involved in musculoskeletal trauma. Chondroitin has demonstrated some efficacy in small clinical trials for treating dry eyes, interstitial cystitis, and temporomandibular joint (TMJ) disorder.

Other Names: CDS, chondroitin sulfate A, chondroitin sulfate C, chondroitin-4-sulfate, chondroitin-6-sulfate, CSA, CSC, and galactosaminoglucuronoglycan sulfate

ACTIONS AND PHARMACOLOGY
EFFECTS
Chondroitin sulfate has protective effects on cartilage as well as viscoelastic effects. Preliminary evidence suggests it may also have antilipidemic, anticoagulant, and antithrombogenic properties.

Cardiovascular Effects: Chondroitin sulfate administered orally or parentally has been reported to produce beneficial effects on serum lipids and "lipid clearing." (Morrison 1971; Morrison 1969). In a 22-week evaluation, phospholipid levels were significantly reduced after 14 weeks of treatment with chondroitin sulfate. However, this benefit was not sustained through trial completion (Izuka et al 1968).

Chondroprotective Effects: Chondroitin sulfate is a galactosaminoglucuronoglycan sulfate (GAG) that has demonstrated some efficacy in the treatment of osteoarthritis. Exogenously administered GAGs concentrate in cartilage where they can be used in the synthesis of new cartilaginous matrix. The chondroprotective action of chondroitin sulfate has been demonstrated in vitro. Chondroitin sulfate inhibits the effect of leukocyte elastase, which can alter fundamental components of the cartilaginous matrix (proteoglycans and collagen fibers). Leukocyte elastase is found in high concentrations in the blood and synovial fluid of patients with rheumatic diseases (Shankland 1998; Morreale et al 1996; Pipitone 1991).

Viscoelastic Effects: Similar to sodium hyaluronate, chondroitin sulfate is used primarily as a viscoelastic agent for ophthalmic surgical procedures. Viscoelastic agents possess rheologic properties (e.g., viscosity, pseudoplasticity, and coatability) that make them amenable to ocular surgical procedures. Specifically, these agents are used to protect cells and tissues from mechanical trauma (coating actions), to allow space for surgical manipulation, to separate tissues and break adhesions, and to provide lubrication to manipulate tissue (Liesegang 1990; Barron et al 1985). Viscoelastic agents are also postoperatively employed to maintain space, diminish localized bleeding, and lubricate and separate tissues to prevent adhesions; they are also used as tissue substitutes (e.g., vitreous) (Liesegang 1990).

CLINICAL TRIALS
Interstitial Cystitis
Some benefit was noted for patients with interstitial cystitis after treatment with chondroitin sulfate. Eighteen patients with the disorder who tested positive to the potassium stimulation test received 40 mL chondroitin sulfate 0.2% intravesically once weekly for 4 weeks and then once monthly for 1 year in an open-label study. Of the 13 patients followed for the entire 13-month study, six showed good response, four had partial response, two had fair response, and one patient had no response. Patients with epithelial permeability as demonstrated by the positive potassium challenge test may be more likely to respond to treatment with glucosaminoglycans (Steinhoff et al 2002).

Osteoarthritis
A meta-analysis of 15 randomized, placebo-controlled trials evaluated the structural and symptomatic efficacy of oral glucosamine or chondroitin in knee osteoarthritis. Glucosamine improved scores on all outcomes measures, including joint space narrowing. Chondroitin demonstrated improvement on two outcome measures: the Lequesne Index (e.g., distance walked, duration of morning stiffness, and discomfort) and a visual analogue scale for pain and mobility. Safety was excellent for both compounds (Richy et al 2003).

Another meta-analysis of 16 studies on the use of chondroitin in osteoarthritis recognized a general positive trend, with supplementation demonstrating improvement in functional capacity, reduction of pain, reduction of nonsteroidal anti-inflammatory drugs (NSAIDs) or analgesic consumption, and tolerability. In each study, an analgesic or NSAID was concurrently used with chondroitin. However, nine of the trials in this analysis suffered from a variety of methodological problems and did not meet evaluation criteria. The authors concluded that larger long-term, randomized clinical trials are needed to define chondroitin's specific place in therapy (Leeb et al 2000).

Treatment with naproxen and chondroitin helped to decrease the number of joints affected by erosive osteoarthritis over a 2-year radiological investigation (n=24). However, chondroitin sulfate did not modify disease progression, and the authors concluded there was no overall clinical significance in this trial. Patient assessment of pain and adverse effects were not evaluated (Rovetta et al 2002).

Combination therapy with glucosamine, chondroitin, and manganese ascorbate improved symptoms of knee arthritis but had equivocal effects on low-back arthritis in a 16-week, randomized, double-blind, placebo-controlled, cross-over pilot study involving 34 men from the United States Navy. Subjects were randomized to receive either oral Cosamin (consisting of glucosamine hydrochloride 500 mg, chondroitin sulfate 400 mg, and manganese ascorbate 76 mg) or placebo three times daily for 8 weeks. Improvement under treatment was statistically significant by patient assessment of results (p=0.02) and the visual analog scale for pain, both recorded in examinations (p=0.02) or patient diaries (p=0.02). Running times and knee range of motion were unaffected by treatment, and trends in acetaminophen use, Lequesne scores, and patient and examiner assessment of severity did not reach significance (Leffler et al 1999).

TMJ

Decreased temporomandibular joint (TMJ) tenderness, fewer TMJ sounds, and fewer over-the-counter analgesics resulted with supplementation of glucosamine and chondroitin. In a 12-week, double-blind, placebo-controlled study, patients received 750 mg of glucosamine HCl and 600 mg of chondroitin sulfate twice daily (n=23) or placebo (n=22). Statistically significant improvements were demonstrated in one scale of the McGill Pain Questionnaire in the treatment group (evaluative pain rating index) and four scales in the placebo group (sensory, evaluative, number of words, and miscellaneous pain rating indices). There was also a significant decrease in the visual analog scale in the placebo group. TMJ noises significantly decreased in the treatment group with no change in patients in the control group. The mean number of over-the-counter medications (mainly acetaminophen) was significantly fewer in the treatment group (Nguyen et al 2001).

Administration of 1,600 mg of glucosamine HCl, 1,000 mg of calcium ascorbate, and a 1,200-mg mixture of chondroitin sulfate-4 and -6, all taken twice daily, produced beneficial effects in TMJ arthritis. Of the 50 participants in the uncontrolled, preliminary study, 80% reported a decrease in joint noises; 2% reported a worsening in symptoms of pain and/or swelling; 10% failed to comply with conditions of the study, and 8% reported no change. Responses were noted an average of 14 to 21 days after starting treatment; however, patients were allowed to take aspirin and ibuprofen when TMJ pain interfered with daily activities (Shankland 1998).

INDICATIONS AND USAGE
Approved by the FDA:

- For protection during cataract extraction with intraocular lens implantation
- For use as a corneal preservation medium

Unproven Uses: People with osteoarthritis and rheumatic diseases take chondroitin sulfate to reduce pain, improve functional capacity, and reduce the use of painkillers. Chondroitin therapy is sometimes used to treat the following: TMJ disorder, coronary heart disease, hypercholesterolemia, nephrolithiasis, interstitial cystitis (intravesical), dry eye syndrome (ophthalmic), snoring (intranasal), and to prevent or treat disorders of connective tissue structures such as the aorta, vascular tissues, and soft tissues involved in musculoskeletal trauma.

PRECAUTIONS AND ADVERSE REACTIONS

Intraocular pressure changes may occur when chondroitin is used in the eye. Patients with asthma may be at risk for symptom exacerbation when taking a combination of glucosamine and chondroitin (Tallia et al 2002).

Drug Interactions:

Antiplatelet and Anticoagulant Agents: Theoretically, concurrent use with chondroitin may increase the risk of bleeding.

DOSAGE
Mode of Administration: Intramuscular, intravenous, oral

How Supplied: Capsule, tablet, sterile solution derived from bovine tracheal cartilage or shark cartilage

Daily Dosage:

Cataract extraction/lens implantation (ophthalmic solution): 0.2 to 0.5 mL using standard sterile technique into the anterior chamber with the provided needle/cannula prior to capsulotomy.

Osteoarthritis: 800 to 1200 mg orally in single or divided doses

LITERATURE
Alpar JJ, Alpar AJ, Baca J et al: Comparison of Healon® and Viscoat® in cataract extraction and intraocular lens implantation. *Ophthalmic Surg*; 19(9):636-642. 1988

Bourne WM: Endothelial cell survival on transplanted human corneas preserved at 4 degrees C in 2.5% chondroitin sulfate for one to 13 days. *Am J Ophthalmol*; 102(3):382-386. 1986

Cohen M, Wolfe R, Mai T et al: A randomized, double blind, placebo controlled trial of a topical cream containing glucosamine sulfate, chondroitin sulfate, and camphor for osteoarthritis of the knee. *J Rheumatol*; 30(3):523-528. 2003

Conte A, de Bernardi M, Palmieri L et al: Metabolic fate of exogenous chondroitin sulfate in man. *Arzneimittelforschung*; 41(7):768-772. 1991

Leeb BF, Schweitzer H, Montag K et al: A meta-analysis of chondroitin sulfate in the treatment of osteoarthritis. *J Rheumatol*; 27(1):205-211. 2000

Leffler CT, Philippi AF, Leffler SG et al: Glucosamine, chondroitin, and manganese ascorbate for degenerative joint disease of the knee or low back: a randomized, double-blind, placebo-controlled pilot study. *Mil Med*; 164(2):85-91. 1999

Liesegang TJ: Viscoelastic substances in ophthalmology. *Surv Ophthalmol*; 34(4):268-293. 1990

Mazieres B, Combe B, Phan Van A et al: Chondroitin sulfate in osteoarthritis of the knee: a prospective, double blind, placebo controlled multicenter clinical study. *J Rheumatol*; 28(1):173-178. 2001

Morreale P, Manopulo R, Galati M et al: Comparison of the antiinflammatory efficacy of chondroitin sulfate and diclofenac sodium in patients with knee osteoarthritis. *J Rheumatol*; 23(8):1385-1391. 1996

Nguyen P, Mohamed SE, Gardiner D et al: A randomized, double-blind clinical trial of the effect of chondroitin sulfate and glucosamine hydrochloride on temporomandibular joint disorder: a pilot study. *J Craniomandibular Pract*; 19(2):130-139. 2001

Product Information: DuoVisc® Ophthalmic Viscosurgical Device; Alcon Labs, Fort Worth, TX, 2001.

Richy F, Bruyere O, Ethgen O et al: Structural and symptomatic efficacy of glucosamine and chondroitin in knee osteoarthritis. *Arch Intern Med*; 163(13):1514-1522. 2003

Rovetta G: Galactosaminoglycuronoglycan sulfate (matrix) in therapy of tibiofibular osteoarthritis of the knee. *Drugs Exp Clin Res*; 17(1):53-57. 1991

Rovetta G, Monteforte P, Molfetta G et al: Chondroitin sulfate in erosive osteoarthritis of the hands. *Int J Tissue React*; 24(1):29-32. 2002

Shankland WE: The effects of glucosamine and chondroitin sulfate on osteoarthritis of the TMJ: a preliminary report of 50 patients. *J Craniomandibular Pract*; 16(4):230-235. 1998

Steinhoff G, Ittah B, and Rowan S: The efficacy of chondroitin sulfate 0.2% in treating interstitial cystitis. *Can J Urol*; 9(1): 1454-1458. 2002

Tallia A, Cardone D: Asthma exacerbation associated with glucosamine- chondroitin supplement. *J Am Board Fam Pract*; 15(6):841-848. 2002

Verbruggen G, Goemaere S, Veys E: Chondroitin sulfate: S/MOAD (structure/disease modifying anti-osteoarthritis drug) in the treatment of finger joint OA. *Osteoarthritis Cartilage*; 6(suppl A): 37-38. 1998[TAB]

Coenzyme Q10

DESCRIPTION

Coenzyme Q10 is a fat-soluble quinone that is synthesized intracellularly and participates in a variety of important cellular processes. It has vitamin-like characteristics and is structurally similar to vitamin K. Coenzyme Q10 is a vital component of the inner mitochondrial membrane, with the highest concentrations found in the heart, liver, kidneys, and pancreas. The total body content ranges from 0.5 to 1.5 grams (Lampertico et al 1993; Mortensen 1993; Beyer 1992; Greenberg et al 1990; Langsjoen et al 1988; Farah et al 1984). Its most common clinical use is for treating heart disease, hypertension, and immunodepression. Although coenzyme Q10 is necessary for energy production and function, further studies are needed to warrant its use for performance enhancement.

An endogenous deficiency of coenzyme Q10 has been suggested in a variety of disorders, including cancer, congestive heart failure, hypertension, chronic hemodialysis, mitochondrial disease, and periodontal disease (Lockwood et al 1994; Triolo et al 1994; Matthews et al 1993; Greenberg et al, 1990; Ogasahara et al 1986).

Other Names: Coenzyme Q, CoQ, CoQ10, ubidecarenone, ubiquinone, ubiquinone-Q10

ACTIONS AND PHARMACOLOGY
EFFECTS

Coenzyme Q10 is an antioxidant and cardiotonic. Some evidence suggests it may also have cytoprotective and neuroprotective qualities.

Cardiovascular Effects: The most extensive studies of coenzyme Q10 have been in cardiovascular disease, most specifically for its purported benefit in preventing cellular damage during myocardial ischemia and reperfusion (Mortensen 1993; Rengo et al 1993; Greenberg et al 1990). Numerous potential therapeutic mechanisms have been considered. The most notable of these are: (1) correction of coenzyme Q10 deficiency, (2) direct free-radical scavenging activity via semiquinone species, (3) direct membrane-stabilizing properties due to phospholipid protein interactions, (4) and correction of a mitochondrial "leak" of electrons during oxidative respiration (Ma et al 1996; Mortensen 1993; Rengo et al 1993; Greenberg et al 1990; Greenberg et al 1988). Other potential mechanisms include effects on prostaglandin metabolism, inhibition of intracellular phospholipases, and stabilization of the integrity of calcium-dependent slow channels (Greenberg et al 1990).

Migraine Prophylaxis: Because some migraine sufferers show dysfunction in mitochondrial energy metabolism, researchers speculate that coenzyme Q10 reduces migraine frequency by improving mitochondrial oxidative phosphorylation (Rozen et al 2002).

Mitochondrial Electron Transfer Effects: Coenzyme Q10 has a significant role in mitochondrial electron transfer and the synthesis of adenosine triphosphate (ATP). The oxidation-reduction cycling of coenzyme Q10 during electron transport has been directly observed. Coenzyme Q10 may also have direct membrane-stabilizing properties as well as free-radical scavenging abilities, especially against lipid peroxidation (Lampertico et al 1993; Matthews et al 1993; Beyer 1992; Permanetter et al 1992; Greenberg et al 1990).

CLINICAL TRIALS
Heart Failure

Numerous open studies of patients with congestive heart failure, some involving more than 1,000 participants, have reported clinical benefits with oral coenzyme Q10 added to conventional therapy such as digitalis, diuretics, and ACE inhibitors. Trials were both short-term (1 to 4 weeks) and long-term (3 months to 6 years), with typical doses ranging from 50 to 100 mg (Baggio et al 1993; Lampertico et al 1993; Mortensen 1993; Greenberg et al 1990; Langsjoen et al 1990; Langsjoen et al 1988; Mortensen et al 1985; Ishiyama et al 1976). Most placebo-controlled studies support these findings, demonstrating a significant improvement in left-ventricular ejection fraction, stroke volume, clinical symptoms, and functional status during coenzyme Q10 add-on therapy (100 to 150 mg daily for up to 1 year) in chronic heart failure patients (Morisco et al 1993; Mortensen 1993; Rengo et al 1993; Greenberg et al 1990).

Controlled studies have reported an improvement in quality of life and a significant reduction in hospitalizations for patients with worsening heart failure who took coenzyme Q10 (Morisco et al 1993; Mortensen 1993). Beneficial effects were attributed to enhanced myocardial contractility, with the most benefit appearing in patients with severe heart failure (NYHA class III or IV) and in those with dilated cardiomyopathy and the lowest plasma or tissue levels of coenzyme Q10. A meta-analysis of eight of these clinical trials concluded that addition of coenzyme Q10 to standard CHF regimens was associated with significant improvements in ejection fraction, stroke volume, and cardiac output (Soja et al 1997).

Migraine prophylaxis

Coenzyme Q10 reduced migraine frequency in 29 of 31 patients with episodic migraine (with or without aura) in an open-label study. Subjects took 150 mg of coenzyme Q10 daily with breakfast for 3 months after a 1-month baseline period. Average headache frequency was reduced from 7.34 days during the 30-day baseline to 2.95 days during the last 60 days of treatment (p<0.002). However, headache intensity was not affected. No side effects were observed (Rozen et al 2002).

INDICATIONS AND USAGE
Approved by the FDA:

■ For use as an orphan product in the treatment of Huntington's disease and mitochondrial cytopathies

Unproven Uses: Coenzyme Q10 is used mainly for the treatment of congestive heart failure and cardiomyopathy. Studies have shown it may benefit patients having cardiovascular surgery such as cardiac valve replacement, coronary artery bypass grafting, and repair of abdominal aortic aneurysms. Coenzyme Q10 has also been used for asthenozoospermia, central nervous system problems, and muscle disorders. Athletes sometimes take it to improve performance, but current evidence does not justify this use.

PRECAUTIONS AND ADVERSE REACTIONS

Hepatic failure is a precaution for use, since the primary site of metabolism is the liver. However, coenzyme Q10 has a very low toxicity profile, and higher plasma levels seem to be well-tolerated. There have been no reports of overt hepatotoxicity with coenzyme Q10.

Gastrointestinal problems are the most common adverse effects (less than 1% in large studies), including nausea, epigastric discomfort, diarrhea, heartburn, and appetite suppression. Rare side effects may include skin rash, pruritus, photophobia, irritability, agitation, headache, and dizziness.

Transient minor abnormalities of urinary sediment (protein, granular, and hyaline casts) were reported in patients with Parkinson's disease given doses of 400 to 800 mg of coenzyme Q10 daily for 1 month. Problems resolved following discontinuation of therapy (Shults et al 1998).

Fatigue and increased involuntary movements were reported in patients with Huntington's chorea taking high doses (Feigin et al 1996).

Drug Interactions:

HMG-CoA Reductase Inhibitors (e.g., lovastatin, simvastatin): Use of these drugs may inhibit the natural synthesis of coenzyme Q10. Reduced levels of coenzyme Q10 may place patients at risk for side effects of HMG-CoA reductase inhibitors, particularly myopathy (Mortensen et al 1997; Bargossi et al 1994; Watts et al 1993; Folkers et al 1990).

Oral Hypoglycemic Agents and Insulin: Dosage adjustment may be necessary, since coenzyme Q10 could reduce insulin requirements.

Warfarin: Concurrent use could reduce anticoagulant effectiveness; monitor the INR as necessary.

DOSAGE

Mode of Administration: Intravenous, oral, topical

How Supplied: Capsule, gelcap, solution

Daily Dosage:

Note: For best absorption, coenzyme Q10 should be taken with food.

ADULTS

Angina (stable): 150 to 600 mg orally in divided doses; 1.5 mg/kg IV once daily for 7 days.

Cardiac Surgery: 100 mg daily for 14 days before surgery, followed by 100 mg daily for 30 days postoperatively.

Congestive Heart Failure: 50 to 150 mg daily in two or three divided doses; 50 to 100 mg IV daily for 3 to 35 days.

Migraine Prevention: 150 mg daily.

Neurological Disease: (associated with mitochondrial ATP-producing deficiency): 150 mg or more daily.

Parkinson's Disease/Huntington's Disease: 800 to 1,200 mg daily.

Periodontal Disease: 25 mg twice daily; or topical solution consisting of 85 mg/mL in soybean oil applied twice daily.

PEDIATRIC

General Use: 2.4 to 3.8 mg/kg daily.

Pediatric Mitochondrial Encephalomyopathy: 30 mg daily.

Storage: Store at room temperature away from heat, moisture, and direct light.

LITERATURE

Baggio E, Gandini R, Plancher AC et al: Italian multicenter study on the safety and efficacy of coenzyme Q10 as adjunctive therapy in heart failure (interim analysis). *Clin Invest*; 71:145-149. 1993

Baggio E, Gandini R, Plancher AC et al: Italian multicenter study on the safety and efficacy of coenzyme Q10 as adjunctive therapy in heart failure. *Mol Aspects Med*; 15(suppl):S287-S294. 1994

Beyer RE: An analysis of the role of coenzyme Q in free radical generation and as an antioxidant. *Biochem Cell Biol*; 70:390-403. 1992

Farah AE, Alousi AA, Schwarz RP: Positive inotropic agents. *Ann Rev Pharmacol Toxicol*; 24:275-328. 1984

Feigin A, Kieburtz K, Como P et al: Assessment of coenzyme Q10 tolerability in Huntington's disease. *Movement Disord*; 11:321-323. 1996

Folkers K, Langsjoen P, Willis P et al: Lovastatin decreases coenzyme Q levels in humans. *Proc Natl Acad Sci USA*; 87:8931-8934. 1990

Greenberg S, Frishman WH: Co-enzyme Q10: a new drug for cardiovascular disease. *J Clin Pharmacol*; 30:596-608. 1990

Ishiyama T, Morita Y, Toyama S et al: A clinical study of the effect of coenzyme Q on congestive heart failure. *Jpn Heart J*; 17:32-42. 1976

Kamikawa T, Kobayashi A, Tamashita T et al: Effects of coenzyme Q10 on exercise tolerance in chronic stable angina pectoris. *Am J Cardiol*; 56:247-251. 1985

Lampertico M, Comis S: Italian multicenter study on the efficacy and safety of coenzyme Q10 as adjuvant therapy in heart failure. *Clin Invest*; 71:129-133. 1993

Langsjoen H, Langsjoen P, Langsjoen P et al: Usefulness of coenzyme Q10 in clinical cardiology: a long-term study. *Mol Aspects Med* 1994; 15(suppl):S165-S175.

Langsjoen PH, Folkers K, Lyson K et al: Effective and safe therapy with coenzyme Q10 for cardiomyopathy. *Klin Wochenschr*; 66:583-590. 1988

Langsjoen PH, Langsjoen A, Willis R et al: Treatment of hypertrophic cardiomyopathy with coenzyme Q10. *Mol Aspects Med*; 18(suppl):S145-S151. 1997

Langsjoen PH, Langsjoen PH, Folkers K: Isolated diastolic dysfunction of the myocardium and its response to CoQ10 treatment. *Clin Invest*; 71(suppl):S140-S144. 1993

Langsjoen PH, Langsjoen PH, Folkers K: Long-term efficacy and safety of coenzyme Q10 therapy for idiopathic dilated cardiomyopathy. *Am J Cardiol*; 65:521-523. 1990

Lockwood K, Moesgaard S, Folkers K: Partial and complete regression of breast cancer in patients in relation to dosage of coenzyme Q10. *Biochem Biophys Res Commun*; 199:1504-1508. 1994

Lockwood K, Moesgaard S, Hanioka T et al: Apparent partial remission of breast cancer in high risk patients supplemented with nutritional antioxidants, essential fatty acids and coenzyme Q10. *Mol Aspects Med*; 10(suppl):S231-S240. 1994

Ma A, Zhang W, Liu Z: Effect of protection and repair of mitochondrial membrane-phospholipid on prognosis in patients with dilated cardiomyopathy. *Blood Press*; 5:53-55. 1996

Matthews PM, Ford B, Dandurand RJ et al: Coenzyme Q10 with multiple vitamins is generally ineffective in treatment of mitochondrial disease. *Neurology*; 43:884-890. 1993

Mortensen SA, Leth A, Agner E et al: Dose-related decrease of serum coenzyme Q10 during treatment with HMG-CoA reductase inhibitors. *Mol Aspects Med*; 18(Suppl):137-144. 1997

Mortensen SA: Perspectives on therapy of cardiovascular diseases with coenzyme Q10 (Ubiquinone). *Clin Invest*; 71:116-123. 1993

Ogasahara S, Nishikawa Y, Yorifuji S et al: Treatment of Kearns-Sayre syndrome with coenzyme Q10. *Neurology*; 36:45-53. 1986

Permanetter B, Rossy W, Klein G et al: Ubiquinone (coenzyme Q10) in the long-term treatment of idiopathic dilated cardiomyopathy. *Eur Heart J*; 13:1528-1533. 1992

Rengo F, Abete P, Landino P et al: Role of metabolic therapy in cardiovascular disease. *Clin Invest*; 71:124-128. 1993

Rozen TD, Oshinsky ML, Gebeline CA et al: Open label trial of coenzyme Q10 as a migraine preventive. *Cephalalgia*; 22:137-141. 2002

Shults CW, Beal MF, Fontaine D et al: Absorption, tolerability, and effects on mitochondrial activity of oral coenzyme Q10 in parkinsonian patients. *Neurology*; 50:793-795. 1998

Soja AM, Mortensen SA: Treatment of congestive heart failure with coenzyme Q10 illuminated by meta-analyses of clinical trials. *Mol Aspects Med*; 18(suppl):S159-S168. 1997

Triolo L, Lippa S, Oradei A et al: Serum coenzyme Q10 in uremic patients on chronic hemodialysis. *Nephron*; 66:153-156. 1994

Watts GF, Castelluccio C, Rice-Evans C et al: Plasma coenzyme Q (Ubiquinone) concentrations in patients treated with simvastatin. *J Clin Pathol*; 46:1055-1057. 1993

Zimmerman JJ: Therapeutic application of oxygen radical scavengers. *Chest*; 100:189-192. 1991

Folic Acid

DESCRIPTION

Folic acid is a water-soluble B vitamin found in a variety of foods, especially green leafy vegetables. Folium, the Latin word for leaf, is the source of the term folic acid. This vitamin is required for DNA synthesis and a variety of other key reactions in normal metabolism.

Folic acid has emerged as an important preventive nutrient, most notably for neural tube defects in pregnancy and atherosclerotic disease due to elevated homocysteine. Sexually active women of child-bearing potential should be encouraged to use folic acid supplements if dietary intake is not sufficient. Individuals with vascular disease risks should be tested for hyperhomocysteinemia or given prophylactic supplementation. Cancer prevention is inadequately supported, yet intriguing relationships exist at several sites, including the cervix, colon, and lung.

As a therapeutic intervention, the treatment of megaloblastic anemia has been the primary application of folic acid supplementation for some time in both traditional and alternative medicine, though a concerted attempt to rule out vitamin B_{12} deficiency is required before initiating monotherapy with folic acid. Deficiencies secondary to pharmaceutical therapy with anticonvulsants and oral contraceptives increase the need for folic acid supplementation. Topical folic acid solutions for use in periodontal disease are available but remain underutilized.

Other Names: folate, folinic acid, pteroylglutamic acid, vitamin B9

ACTIONS AND PHARMACOLOGY

EFFECTS

Folic acid has the following effects: antidepressant, antiproliferative, antiteratogenic, antihomocysteinemic, and anti-inflammatory (gingival). The coenzymes formed from folic acid are instrumental in the following intracellular metabolisms: conversion of homocysteine to methionine, conversion of serine to glycine, synthesis of thymidylate, histidine metabolism, synthesis of purines, and utilization or generation of formate (Gilman et al 2001).

CLINICAL TRIALS

Cardiovascular Disease

While no prospective intervention trials using folic acid supplements have been conducted, low folic acid status has been associated with cardiovascular disease (Omenn et al 1998), and folic acid supplementation is associated with reduced risk of coronary heart disease in epidemiological studies (Rimm et al 1998). The plan to fortify cereal-grain products with 140 mcg of folate per 100 grams is projected to reduce the U.S. population risk of coronary artery disease by 5% (Tucker et al 1996), presumably by lowering blood homocysteine levels (Boers 1998).

Folic acid supplementation can reduce elevated plasma homocysteine levels and may reduce atherosclerosis progression and risk of cardiovascular events. Folic acid has been combined with vitamin B_6 and vitamin B_{12} with greater effect on homocysteine levels A meta-analysis of 12 trials examining the effects of supplemental folic acid on blood homocysteine levels showed that supplements of 0.5 to 5 mg of folic acid could be expected to reduce blood homocysteine by a quarter to a third. Addition of vitamin B_{12} reduced blood homocysteine by another 7%. Vitamin B_6 did not lower homocysteine any further (Anon 1998).

Contraceptive-Induced Folic Acid Deficiency

Using oral contraceptives may result in folic acid deficiency that may occasionally manifest as megaloblastic anemia and thrombocytopenia. Administration of folic acid can correct the folic acid deficiency and thereby promptly reverse any abnormalities associated with the deficiency (Lewis 1974; Luhby et al 1971). The FDA-approved minimum optimal dose of oral folic acid is 2 milligrams/day for oral contraceptive-induced folate deficiency.

Depression

Folic acid deficiency may cause psychiatric disturbances such as depression. Low folate status is more common in depressed patients and has been linked with poor response to antidepressant therapy. Two controlled studies have suggested that supplementation of folate or its derivatives may improve clinical outcomes in the treatment of depression (Alpert et al 1997; Bottiglieri 1996).

Lung Cancer

Low folate status may increase lung cancer risk, and large doses may reduce precancerous changes in bronchial tissues. Epidemiological studies have suggested a relationship between low folate status and cancer of the lung (Glynn et al 1994). One study found that folic acid (10 mg) with vitamin B_{12} (500 mcg) reduced evidence of atypical bronchial squamous metaplasia in smokers.

However, the authors cautioned that the spontaneous variation in sputum cytology results along with other limitations of this study temper the significance of these findings (Heimberger et al 1988).

Methotrexate Toxicity

A meta-analysis of all published double-blind, randomized, controlled trials (n=7) testing the influence of folate supplementation on rheumatoid arthritis patients treated with methotrexate (MTX) showed an 80% reduction of side effects (mainly gastrointestinal) with folic acid supplementation and no compromise of MTX efficacy. However, high-dose folinic acid was associated with an increase in tender and swollen joints (Ortiz et al 1998).

Prevention of Neural Tube Defects

Folic acid should be administered at least 1 month before and during the first 3 months of pregnancy. The Centers for Disease Control and Prevention and various other committees recommend that all women of childbearing age who are capable of becoming pregnant receive 400 mcg/day. The reduction in neural tube defects in patients receiving folic acid therapy has been 60% to 70% (NHMRC 1994). Patients with previous history of neural tube defects during pregnancy should receive 4 milligrams/day starting 1 month before pregnancy and throughout the first 3 months of pregnancy (NHMRC 1991 and 1994; AAP 1993; Mulinare 1993).

Neural tube defects were decreased by approximately 60% in 3,051 pregnant mothers treated with 0.4 milligram of folic acid during the periconceptional period (28 days before the last menstrual period through 28 days after the last menstrual period) (Werler et al 1993).

A significant reduction in risk for first-time occurrence of neural tube defects was observed in 18,508 pregnant women consuming folic acid-containing multivitamins compared to no folic acid consumption (Milunsky et al 1989). Similar results were reported in another study (Czeizel et al 1992).

Ulcerative Colitis and Colonic Adenomas

Folate supplementation can reduce cell abnormalities in the rectal mucosa of patients with ulcerative colitis. Folic acid 15 mg/day (as calcium folate) or a placebo was taken (double-blind) for 3 months by 24 patients with UC of more than 7 years' duration. Patients had been in remission (no acute inflammation) for more than 1 month. In the placebo group, there was no difference in proliferative index between baseline and 3-month measures. In the folate group, proliferation was significantly reduced at 3 months compared to baseline (Biasco et al 1997).

Epidemiological studies have suggested a relationship between low folate status and colorectal cancer (Glynn et al, 1994). Folic acid supplementation had a nonsignificant but dose-response effect on protecting ulcerative colitis patients against colonic neoplasia. Use of higher doses (1,000 mcg daily) of folic acid was associated with greater risk reduction (46%, nonsignificant) (Lashner et al 1997).

INDICATIONS AND USAGE
Approved by the FDA

- Prevention of neural tube defects in pregnancy
- Treatment of megaloblastic anemias caused by folic acid deficiency
- Treatment of folic acid deficiency caused by oral contraceptive or anticonvulsant therapy

Unproven Uses: Strong evidence shows that folic acid therapy can reduce high levels of homocysteine, which has been linked to coronary heart disease. Other studies have suggested that folic acid supplementation may be helpful for atherosclerosis, colon cancer prevention, coronary heart disease, depression, gingival hyperplasia, hyperhomocysteinemia, iron-deficiency or sickle-cell anemia, lung cancer prevention, methotrexate toxicity, prevention of restenosis following coronary angiography, ulcerative colitis, and vitiligo. Weaker evidence suggests that folic acid may be of some benefit for cervical cancer prevention (some studies were inconclusive), aphthous ulcers, geriatric memory deficit, and prevention of fragile X syndrome in children.

CONTRAINDICATIONS

Pernicious anemia and megaloblastic anemia caused by vitamin B_{12} deficiency (Prod Info: Folic acid tablets 1995).

PRECAUTIONS AND ADVERSE REACTIONS

Folic acid doses above 0.1 mg/day may obscure pernicious anemia. Side effects of folic acid therapy include erythema, pruritus, urticaria, irritability, excitability, nausea, bloating, and flatulence.

A variety of central nervous system effects have been reported following 5 mg of folic acid three times a day, including altered sleep patterns, vivid dreaming, irritability, excitability, and overactivity (Hunter et al 1970). Discontinuation of the drug usually results in rapid improvement but in some cases may require 3 weeks before complete restoration.

Gastrointestinal disturbances following oral doses of 5 mg three times daily have been reported and include nausea, abdominal distention, discomfort, flatulence, and a constant bad or bitter taste in the mouth (Prod Info: Folic acid tablets 1995).

High-dose folic acid has been associated with zinc depletion. (Kakar et al 1985). Evidence suggests that up to 5 to 15 milligrams daily of folic acid does not have significant adverse effects on zinc status in healthy, nonpregnant individuals (Butterworth et al 1989).

Pregnancy: FDA-rated as Pregnancy Category A (relatively safe) at doses below 0.8 mg/day; doses higher than this are rated as Pregnancy Category C (effects unknown).

Drug Interactions:

Pancreatic enzymes: Concurrent use may interfere with the absorption of folic acid. Clinical Management: Patients taking pancreatin may require folic acid supplementation.

Phenytoin and fosphenytoin: Concurrent use may decrease phenytoin or fosphenytoin levels and increase seizure frequency. Clinical Management: If folic acid is added to phenytoin therapy, monitor patients for decreased seizure control.

Pyrimethamine: Concurrent use may reduce the effectiveness of pyrimethamine. Clinical Management: Folic acid should not be used as a folate supplement during pyrimethamine therapy as it is ineffective in preventing megaloblastic anemia. Leucovorin (folinic acid) may be added to pyrimethamine therapy to prevent hematologic toxicity without affecting pyrimethamine efficacy. However, the use of leucovorin may worsen leukemia.

Sulfasalazine: Concurrent use may decrease the absorption of folic acid. Clinical Management: Monitor patient for signs of deficiency.

Triamterine: Concurrent use may cause decreased utilization of dietary folate. Clinical Management: Monitor patient for signs of deficiency.

DOSAGE

Mode of Administration: Intramuscular, intravenous, oral, subcutaneous

How Supplied: Capsule, tablet, sterile solution for injection

Daily Dosage: All doses are for oral administration unless otherwise noted.

ADULTS

Recommended dietary allowance (RDA): *adults and adolescents ≥14 years* — 400 mcg/day; *pregnancy* — 600 mcg/day; *lactation* — 500 mcg/day.

Anticonvulsant-induced folate deficiency: 15 mg daily.

Aphthous ulcers (canker sores): treat folic acid deficiency.

Hyperhomocysteinemia: 500 to 5,000 mcg daily.

Methotrexate toxicity: 5 mg orally per week.

Oral contraceptive-induced folate deficiency: 2 mg daily.

Periodontal disease: 2 mg twice daily, or 5 mL of 0.1% topical mouth rinse twice daily.

Prevention of birth defects: 400 to 4,000 mcg orally daily beginning 1 month before conception.

Prevention of cerebrovascular disease: treat folic acid deficiency or hyperhomocysteinemia.

Prevention of cervical cancer: 800 to 10,000 mcg daily.

Prevention of colorectal cancer: 1 to 5 mg daily.

Prevention of lung cancer: 10 mg daily.

Prevention of neural tube defects (first occurrence prevention): 0.4 mg of folic acid daily. Doses from 0.5 to 1 mg daily are often administered during pregnancy.

Prevention of neural tube defects (prevention of recurrence): Patients with a previous history of neural tube defects during pregnancy should receive 4 mg daily starting 1 month before pregnancy and throughout the first 3 months of pregnancy.

Prevention of restenosis following coronary angiography: 1 mg in combination with 400 mcg vitamin B_{12} and 10 mg vitamin B_6 daily.

Sickle cell anemia: 1 mg daily.

Treatment of folic acid deficiency (intramuscular, intravenous, or oral): Up to 1 mg daily until clinical symptoms of deficiency have resolved and blood levels have returned to normal.

Ulcerative colitis: 15 mg daily.

Vitiligo: 2,000 to 10,000 mcg daily.

PEDIATRICS

Recommended dietary allowance (RDA): *Infants and children: 0 to 6 months* — 65 mcg/day; *7 to 12 months* — 80 mcg/day; *1 to 3 years* — 150 mcg/day; *4 to 8 years* — 200 mcg/day; *9 to 13 years* — 300 mcg/day.

Anticonvulsant-induced folate deficiency: 5 mg daily.

Folic acid deficiency (intramuscular, intravenous, subcutaneous, or oral): Up to 1 mg daily until clinical symptoms of deficiency have resolved and blood levels have returned to normal.

Folic acid deficiency in preterm neonates (intramuscular): 100 mcg daily from day 7 until discharge from hospital.

Gingival hyperplasia: 5 mg daily (Backman et al 1989).

Hyperhomocysteinemia: 500 to 5,000 mcg daily.

Storage: Store oral and parenteral folic acid at room temperature.

LITERATURE

Alpert JE, Fava M: Nutrition and depression: the role of folate. *Nutr Rev*; 55(5):145-149. 1997

American Academy of Pediatrics (AAP): AAP Committee on Genetics: folic acid for the prevention of neural tube defects. *Pediatrics*; 92(3):493-494. 1993

Anon: Lowering blood homocysteine with folic acid based supplements: meta-analysis of randomized trials. Homocysteine Lowering Trialists' Collaboration. *BMJ*; 316(7135):894-898. 1998

Anon: Use of folic acid for prevention of spina bifida and other neural tube defects: 1983-1991. *MMWR*; 40(30):513-516. 1991

Anon: Vitamin supplements. *Med Lett Drugs Ther*; 27(693):66-68. 1985

Backman N, Holm A-K, Hanstrom L et al: Folate treatment of diphenylhydantoin-induced gingival hyperplasia. *Scand J Dent Res*; 97(3):222-232. 1989

Bailey LB: Evaluation of a new recommended dietary allowance for folate. *J Am Diet Assoc*; 92(4):463-468, 471. 1992

Berg MJ, Rivey MP, Vern BA et al: Phenytoin and folic acid: individualized drug-drug interaction. *Ther Drug Monit*; 5(4):395-399. 1983

Biasco G, Zannoni U, Paganelli GM et al: Folic acid supplementation and cell kinetics of rectal mucosa in patients with ulcerative colitis. *Cancer Epidemiol Biomarkers Prev*; 6(6):469-471. 1997

Boers G: Moderate hyperhomocysteinemia and vascular disease: evidence, relevance and the effect of treatment (review). *Eur J Pediatr*; 157(suppl 2):S127-S130. 1998

Bottiglieri T: Folate, vitamin B_{12}, and neuropsychiatric disorders. *Nutr Rev*; 54(12):382-390. 1996

Butterworth CE Jr: Folate status, women's health, pregnancy outcome, and cancer. *J Am Coll Nutr*; 12(4):438-441. 1993

Butterworth CE Jr, Hatch KD, Gore H et al: Improvement in cervical dysplasia associated with folic acid therapy in users of oral contraceptives. *Am J Clin Nutr*; 35(1):73-82. 1982

Czeizel AE, Dudas I: Prevention of the first occurrence of neural-tube defects by periconceptional vitamin supplementation. *N Engl J Med*; 327(26):1832-1835. 1992

Dickinson CJ: Does folic acid harm people with vitamin B_{12} deficiency (review)? *QJM*; 88(5):357-364. 1995

Gilman AG, Hardman JG, Limbird LE (eds): *Goodman & Gilman's The Pharmacological Basis of Therapeutics*, 10th ed. McGraw-Hill, New York, NY; 2001.

Glynn SA, Albanes D: Folate and cancer: a review of the literature. *Nutr Cancer*; 22:101-119. 1994

Guidolin L, Vignoli A, Canger R: Worsening in seizure frequency and severity in relation to folic acid administration. *Eur J Neurol*; 5(3):301-303. 1998

Heimburger DC, Alexander CB, Birch R et al: Improvement in bronchial squamous metaplasia in smokers treated with folate and vitamin B_{12}: report of a preliminary randomized double-blind intervention trial. *JAMA*; 259(10):1525-1530. 1988

Hunter R, Barnes J, Oakeley HF et al: Toxicity of folic acid given in pharmacological doses to healthy volunteers. *Lancet*; 1(7637):61-63. 1970

Kakar F, Henderson MM: Potential toxic side effects of folic acid (letter). *J Natl Cancer Inst*; 74(1):263. 1985

Lashner BA, Heidenreich PA, Su GL et al: The effect of folate supplementation on the incidence of dysplasia and cancer in chronic ulcerative colitis: a case-control study. *Gastroenterology*; 97(2):255-59. 1989

Lashner BA, Provencher KS, Seidner DL et al: The effect of folic acid supplementation on the risk for cancer or dysplasia in ulcerative colitis. *Gastroenterology*; 112(1):29-32. 1997

Leung CF, Lao TT, Chang AMZ: Effect of folate supplement on pregnant women with beta-thalassaemia minor. *Eur J Obstet Gynecol Reprod Biol*; 33(3):209-213. 1989

Melikian V, Paton A, Leeming RJ et al: Site of reduction and methylation of folic acid in man. *Lancet*; 2(7731):955-957. 1971

Milunsky A, Jick H, Jick SS et al: Multivitamin/folic acid supplementation in early pregnancy reduces the prevalence of neural tube defects. *JAMA*; 262(20):2847-2852. 1989

Morita H, Tagushi J, Kurihara H et al: Genetic polymorphism of 5, 10-methylenetetrahydrofolate reductase (MTHFR) as a risk factor for coronary artery disease. *Circulation*; 95(8):2032-2036. 1997

Mulinaire J: Epidemiologic associations of multivitamin supplementation and occurrence of neural tube defects. *Ann N Y Acad Sci*; 678:130-136. Mar 15, 1993

National Health and Medical Research Council (NHMRC): Prevention of neural tube defects: results of the Medical Research Council Vitamin Study, MRC Vitamin Study Research Group. *Lancet*; 338(8760):131-137. 1991

National Health and Medical Research Council (NHMRC): Revised statement on the relationship between dietary folic acid and neural tube defects such as spina bifida. *J Paediatr Child Health*; 30:476-477. 1994

Nguyen TT, Dyer DL Dunning DD et al: Human intestinal folate transport: cloning, expression, and distribution of complementary RNA. *Gastroenterology*; 112(3):783-791. 1997

Omenn GS, Beresford SAA, Motulsky AG: Preventing coronary heart disease: B vitamins and homocysteine. *Circulation*; 97(5):421-424. 1998

Pack ARC: Folate mouthwash: effects on established gingivitis in periodontal patients. *J Clin Periodontol*; 11(9):619-628. 1984

Pack AR, Thomson ME: Effects of topical and systemic folic acid supplementation on gingivitis in pregnancy. *J Clin Periodontol*; 7(5):402-414. 1980

Prakash R, Petrie WM: Psychiatric changes associated with an excess of folic acid. *Am J Psychiatry*; 139(9):1192-1193. 1982

Product Information: Folic acid tablets, USP. Halsey Drug Co, Inc, Brooklyn, NY; 1995.

Product Information: Folvite® (folic acid). Lederle Labs, Pearl River, NY; 1990.

Rieder MJ: Prevention of neural tube defects with periconceptual folic acid. *Clin Perinatol*; 21(3):483-503. 1994

Rimm EB, Willett WC, Hu FB: Folate and vitamin B6 from diet and supplements in relation to risk of coronary heart disease among women. *JAMA*; 279(5):359-364. 1998

Russell RM, Dutta SK, Oaks EV et al: Impairment of folic acid absorption by oral pancreatic extracts. *Dig Dis Sci*; 25(5):369-373. 1980

Skoutakis VA, Acchiardo SR, Meyer MC et al: Folic acid dosage for chronic hemodialysis patients. *Clin Pharmacol Ther*; 18(2):200-204. 1975

Thomson ME, Pack ARC: Effects of extended systemic and topical folate supplementation on gingivitis of pregnancy. *J Clin Periodontol*; 9(3):275-280. 1982

Tucker KL, Mahnken B, Wilson PWF et al: Folic acid fortification of the food supply: potential benefits and risks for the elderly population. *JAMA*; 276(23):1879-1885. 1996

Werler MM, Shapiro S, Mitchell AA: Periconceptional folic acid exposure and risk of occurrent neural tube defects. *JAMA*; 269(10):1257-1261. 1993

Glucosamine

DESCRIPTION
Glucosamine is an endogenous aminomonosaccharide synthesized from glucose and utilized for biosynthesis of two larger compounds, glycoproteins and glycosaminoglycans. These compounds are necessary for the construction and maintenance of virtually all connective tissues and lubricating fluids in the body (Reichelt et al 1994; Reuser 1994; Setnikar et al 1993). The sulfate salt of glucosamine forms half of the disaccharide subunit of keratan sulfate, which is decreased in osteoarthritis, and of hyaluronic acid, which is found in both articular cartilage and synovial fluid (Leffler et al 1999).

Supplemental glucosamine is generally used to reduce pain and immobility associated with osteoarthritis, especially in the knee joint. The supplements are usually derived from crab shells, although a corn source is also available. Most studies of osteoarthritis have used the sulfate form of glucosamine (D'Ambrosio et al 1981; Pujalte et al 1980). Other forms include glucosamine hydrochloride and N-acetyl glucosamine.

Other Names: 2-amino-2-deoxy-beta-D-glucopyranose, chitosamine, glucosamine hydrochloride, glucosamine sulfate, N-acetyl glucosamine (NAG)

ACTIONS AND PHARMACOLOGY
EFFECTS
Anti-arthritic Effects:

Preclinical studies with glucosamine have suggested tropism for cartilage and bone. Glucosamine seems to enhance cartilage proteoglycan synthesis, thereby inhibiting deterioration of cartilage brought about by osteoarthritis and helping to maintain equilibrium between cartilage catabolic and anabolic processes (Setnikar et al 1993; D'Ambrosio et al 1981; Vidal y Plana et al 1980, 1978). Exogenous administration of glucosamine in animals has been reported to retard cartilage degradation and rebuild experimentally damaged cartilage tissue (D'Ambrosio et al 1981; Pujalte et al 1980; Crolle et al 1980). Protection against metabolic impairment of cartilage induced by nonsteroidal anti-inflammatory drugs and corticosteroids has been described. An anti-inflammatory action of glucosamine has also been proposed, unrelated to cyclo-oxygenase inhibition (Reichelt et al 1994).

Glucose Metabolism Effects: It has been hypothesized that glucosamine may impair insulin secretion through competitive inhibition of glucokinase in pancreatic beta cells and/or alteration of peripheral glucose uptake (Monauni et al 2000; Balkan et al 1994).

Wound Healing Effects: Hyaluronic acid (HA), which is synthesized by fibroblasts, promotes proliferation of epithelial cells. Oral glucosamine may enhance HA synthesis, thus accelerating healing and minimizing scarring in fresh wounds (McCarty 1996).

CLINICAL TRIALS
Knee Pain

In a randomized, placebo-controlled study, patients reported improvement in unspecified knee pain and function after glucosamine supplementation. Glucosamine hydrochloride 2,000 mg (n=24) or placebo (n=22) was given once daily in the morning for 3 months. Between the groups, there was no difference in joint line palpation, duck walk, or stair-climb results. There were significant improvements in the glucosamine group on the knee pain scale at week 8 of evaluation (p=0.004) and on the knee injury and osteoarthritis outcome score (KOOS) on weeks 8 and 12 (p=0.038). Self-reported improvements in perceived pain began to occur between weeks 4 and 8 and at week 12. Eighty-eight percent of patients who were receiving glucosamine reported some level of pain relief, compared to 17% in the placebo group. Side effects were reported as mild and short-lived, with gastrointestinal effects and headache cited most frequently and occurring equally in both groups (Braham et al 2003).

A topical preparation of glucosamine, chondroitin, and shark cartilage reduced pain associated with osteoarthritis of the knee. Sixty-three patients were randomized to receive a water-soluble cream (30 mg/g of glucosamine sulfate; 50 mg/g of chondroitin sulfate, 140 mg/g of shark cartilage, 32 mg/g of camphor, and 9 mg/g of peppermint oil) or placebo for 8 weeks. Both groups reported improvement on the visual analog scale pain scores, with the treatment group improving a further 1.2 points (p=0.03) at 4 weeks and 1.8 points (p=0.002) at 8 weeks compared to the placebo group. Patients were instructed to apply cream generously to painful joints, gently massage until cream disappears, and repeat as necessary (Cohen et al 2003).

Two randomized, double-blind, parallel trials of glucosamine reported no improvement in osteoarthritis of the knee. In the first, patients were randomized to receive 500 mg of glucosamine three times daily (n=49) or a placebo (n=49) for 2 months. No statistical difference was noted between the groups in mean scores for resting and walking after 30 and 60 days (Rindone et al 2000). In the second study, glucosamine was no better than placebo as an analgesic for knee pain due to osteoarthritis. In the 6-month evaluation, patients with varying degrees of pain were randomized to receive 500 mg of glucosamine sulfate three times daily (n=38) or placebo (n=37). There were no differences between the groups in any assessment marker at any time during the trial. The authors suggested that their results differ from previous glucosamine studies because the patients in this trial were more symptomatic and had more structural damage than patients in trials with positive glucosamine results. In addition, this trial had a high placebo response of 33%, perhaps an indication of selection bias to those who have an affinity for complementary therapies (Hughes et al 2002).

Osteoarthritis

A meta-analysis of 15 randomized, placebo-controlled trials evaluating the structural and symptomatic efficacy of oral glucosamine and chondroitin in knee osteoarthritis demonstrated efficacy for glucosamine on joint space narrowing (JSN) and Western Ontario MacMaster University Osteoarthritis Index (WOMAC). Similar efficacies were demonstrated for chondroitin and glucosamine on the Lequesne Index (LI) and visual analogue scale (VAS) for pain and mobility. Joint cartilage degeneration was slowed by the long-term daily administration of oral glucosamine at the minimal dose of 1,500 mg during a minimal period of 3 years (Richy et al 2003).

Oral glucosamine was effective for osteoarthritis of the spine in a multicenter, randomized, double-blind, placebo-controlled trial. Subjects (n=160) with symptomatic cervical and/or lumbar spine osteoarthritis of at least 6 months' duration received 1,500 mg of glucosamine sulfate daily or placebo for 6 weeks. Outcome measures included visual analogue scales and/or clinical measurements for pain, morning stiffness, tenderness, and mobility. Analysis of variance found significant improvement compared to placebo at both locations for pain at rest and at night, tenderness and lateral flexion, and at the lumbar level for pain on active movement, flexion, rotation, and morning stiffness. Improvement persisted 4 weeks after discontinuation of treatment (Giacovelli et al 1993).

Temporomandibular Joint (TMJ) Disorder

In a 12-week, double-blind, placebo-controlled study, patients received 750 mg of glucosamine hydrochloride and 600 mg of chondroitin sulfate twice daily (n=23) or placebo (n=22). Statistically significant improvements were seen in measures of joint tenderness and jawbone noises (e.g., cracking). In addition, the mean number of over-the-counter analgesics (mainly acetaminophen) used was significantly lower in the treatment group (p=0.03). Adverse effects were mainly gastrointestinal, which were reported as transient and resolved spontaneously (Nguyen et al 2001).

INDICATIONS AND USAGE

Unproven Uses: Glucosamine, especially the sulfate form, is a popular treatment for pain and immobility associated with osteoarthritis. Glucosamine is classified by the European League Against Rheumatism (EULAR) as a Symptomatic Slow-Acting Drug in Osteoarthritis. This drug group is characterized by slow-onset improvement in osteoarthritis with persistent benefits after discontinuation (Jordan et al 2003). Whether long-term use of glucosamine can reverse the course of osteoarthritis is a theory that has yet to be investigated. Supplemental glucosamine has also been used for articular injury repair, TMJ, and cutaneous aging (wrinkles).

PRECAUTIONS AND ADVERSE REACTIONS

Glucosamine should be used with caution in patients with an allergy to shellfish and shellfish products. Asthma patients may be at risk for symptom exacerbation when taking the combination of glucosamine and chondroitin. Patients with diabetes should also be cautious, since glucosamine may affect insulin sensitivity or glucose tolerance.

The most commonly reported adverse effects are gastrointestinal disturbances, including nausea, dyspepsia, heartburn, vomiting, constipation, diarrhea, anorexia, and epigastric pain. Less than 1% of patients have reported edema, tachycardia, drowsiness, insomnia, headache, erythema, and pruritus.

Drug Interactions

Antidiabetic Drugs: Glucosamine may reduce their effectiveness. *Clinical Management:* Glucosamine is likely safe for patients with diabetes that is well-controlled with diet only or with one or two oral antidiabetic agents (HbA1c less than 6.5%). In patients with higher HbA1c concentrations or for those requiring insulin, closely monitor blood glucose concentrations.

Doxorubicin, Etoposide, and Teniposide: Glucosamine may reduce their effectiveness. *Clinical Management:* Avoid concomitant use.

OVERDOSAGE

In mice, the LD50 for glucosamine hydrochloride is 15 g/kg oral, 1,100 mg/kg intravenous, and 6,200 mg/kg subcutaneous (RTECS 2001). No mortality in mice or rats resulted from glucosamine sulfate at doses of 5,000 mg/kg oral, 3,000 mg/kg intramuscular, and 1,500 mg/kg intravenous (Kelly 1998).

DOSAGE

Mode of Administration: Intra-articular, intramuscular, intravenous, oral, topical

How Supplied: Cream, liquid, tablet, solution

Daily Dosage: Osteoarthritis

Oral: 1,500 mg in single or three divided doses daily. Results were seen after a minimum of 4 weeks and up to 3 years later (Pavelka et al 2002; Reginster et al 2001; Noack et al 1994).

Intramuscular: 400 mg of glucosamine sulfate once daily (Reichelt et al 1994; D'Ambrosio et al 1981; Crolle et al 1980). A regimen of 400 mg twice weekly for 6 weeks has also been given (Reichelt et al 1994).

LITERATURE

Balkan B, Dunning BE: Glucosamine inhibits glucokinase in vitro and produces a glucose-specific impairment of in vivo insulin secretion in rats. *Diabetes*; 43(10):1173-1179. 1994

Braham R, Dawson B, Goodman C et al: The effect of glucosamine supplementation on people experiencing knee pain. *Br J Sports Med*; 37(1):45-49. 2003

Cohen M, Wolfe R, Mal T et al: A randomized, double blind, placebo controlled trial of a topical cream containing glucosamine sulfate, chondroitin sulfate, and camphor for osteoarthritis of the knee. *J Rheumatol*; 30(3):523-528. 2003

Crolle G, D'Este E: Glucosamine sulphate for the management of arthrosis: a controlled clinical investigation. *Curr Med Res Opin*; 7(2):104-109. 1980

D'Ambrosio E, Casa B, Bompani R et al: Glucosamine sulphate: a controlled clinical investigation in arthrosis. *Pharmatherapeutica* 1981; 2(8):504-508.

Giacovelli G, Rovati LC: Clinical efficacy of glucosamine sulfate in osteoarthritis of the spine (abstract). *Rev Esp Rheumatol*; 20(suppl 1):325. 1993

Higgins G: Optimistic look for disease modifiers in osteoarthritis. *Inpharma*; 896:3-4. 1993

Jordan KM, Arden NK, Doherty M et al: EULAR Recommendations 2003: an evidence based approach to the management of knee osteoarthritis: Report of a Task Force of the Standing Committee for International Clinical Studies Including Therapeutic Trials (ESCISIT). *Ann Rheumatic Dis*; 62:1145-1155. 2003

Kelly G: The role of glucosamine sulfate and chondroitin sulfates in the treatment of degenerative joint disease. *Alt Med Review*; 3(1):27-39. 1998

Leffler CT, Philippi AF, Leffler SG et al: Glucosamine, chondroitin, and manganese ascorbate for degenerative joint disease of the knee or low back: a randomized, double-blind, placebo-controlled pilot study. *Mil Med*; 164(2):85-91. 1999

McCarty MF: Glucosamine for wound healing. *Med Hypotheses*; 47:273-275. 1996

Monauni T, Zenti MG, Cretti A et al: Effects of glucosamine infusion on insulin secretion and insulin action in humans. *Diabetes*; 49(6): 926-935. 2000

Nguyen P, Mohamed SE, Gardiner D et al: A randomized, double-blind clinical trial of the effect of chondroitin sulfate and glucosamine hydrochloride on temporomandibular joint disorder: a pilot study. *J Craniomandibular Pract*; 19(2):130-139. 2001

Noack W, Fischer M, Foerster KK et al: Glucosamine sulfate in osteoarthritis of the knee. *Osteoarthritis Cartilage*; 2:51-59. 1994

Pavelka K, Gatterova J, Olejarova M et al: Glucosamine sulfate use and delay of progression of knee osteoarthritis: a 3-year, randomized, placebo-controlled, double-blind study. *Arch Intern Med*;162(18):2113-2123. 2002

Pujalte JM, Llavore EP, Ylescupidez FR: Double-blind clinical evaluation of oral glucosamine sulphate in the basic treatment of osteoarthrosis. *Curr Med Res Opin*; 7(2):110-114. 1980

Reginster JY, Deroisy R, Rovati LC et al: Long-term effects of glucosamine sulfate on osteoarthritis progression: a randomized, placebo-controlled clinical trial. *Lancet*; 357(9252):251-256. 2001

Reichelt A, Forster KK, Fischer M et al: Efficacy and safety of intramuscular glucosamine sulfate in osteoarthritis of the knee: a randomised, placebo-controlled, double-blind study. *Arzneimittelforschung*; 44(1):75-80. 1994

Reuser AJJ, Wisselaar HA: An evaluation of the potential side-effects of alpha-glucosidase inhibitors used for the management of diabetes mellitus. *Eur J Clin Invest*; 24(suppl 3):19-24. 1994

Richy F, Bruyere O, Ethgen O et al: Structural and symptomatic efficacy of glucosamine and chondroitin in knee osteoarthritis. *Arch Intern Med*; 163(13):1514-1522. 2003

RTECS: Registry of Toxic Effects of Chemical Substances. National Institute for Occupational Safety and Health, Cincinnati, OH (internet version), Thomson Micromedex, Greenwood Village, CO; 2001.

Setnikar I, Palumbo R, Canali S et al: Pharmacokinetics of glucosamine in man. *Arzneimittelforschung*; 43(10):1109-1113. 1993

Vidal y Plana RR, Karzel K: Glukosamin. Seine Bedeutung fuer den Knorpelstoffwechsel der Gelenke. 2. Gelenkknorpel-Untersuchungen. *Fortschr Med*; 21:801-806. 1980

Iron

DESCRIPTION

Iron is an essential trace mineral involved in the entire process of respiration, including oxygen and electron transport. The function and synthesis of hemoglobin, which carries most of the oxygen in the blood, is dependent on iron. Iron is also involved in the production of cytochrome oxidase, myoglobin, L-carnitine, and aconitase, all of which are involved in energy production in the body. In addition to its fundamental roles in energy production, iron is involved in DNA synthesis and may also play roles in normal brain development and immune function. Iron is also involved in the synthesis of collagen and the neurotransmitters serotonin, dopamine, and norepinephrine.

Iron-deficiency anemia is the most common nutritional disorder in the world. Although about 25% of the world's population is iron deficient, it should be noted that anemia is not always associated with iron deficiency. Low iron levels can occur from insufficient dietary intake, impairment of iron absorption, or loss of iron through bleeding. It is important to determine the cause before treating. Whether to treat iron deficiency (ferritin <20 mcg/L) in the absence of anemia (hemoglobin 11 g/dL or greater) is controversial. Preliminary data from NHANES III demonstrate that the prevalence of iron-deficiency anemia in the United States is very low. There is no known benefit of high iron storage status, and some evidence exists that a moderate increase in iron stores is a possible risk factor for ischemic heart disease and cancer. The safe upper range of iron intake is difficult to specify due to the complexity of the Western diet and iron physiology (Lynch et al 1996).

The best dietary sources of iron are green vegetables, legumes, and meat. Much of the iron ingested in the American diet in the form of enriched breads and cereals is not well absorbed. The average dietary intake of iron in the United States ranges from 10 to 20 mg daily. Some individuals, including adolescents and pregnant and lactating women, may be at risk for iron deficiency.

ACTIONS AND PHARMACOLOGY
EFFECTS
Iron has putative immune-enhancing, anticarcinogenic, and cognition-enhancing activities.

Antibacterial Effects: The role of iron in resistance to infection is complex. Iron deficiency is known to impair response of T lymphocytes to mitogens and to decrease the bactericidal activity of neutrophils. On the other hand, bacteria require iron for growth, and bacterial virulence is enhanced by increased iron availability. Also, the presence of infection or inflammation changes the cytokine-mediated metabolism of iron, which complicates attempts to define the relative benefits and hazards of iron therapy for prophylaxis of infectious disease (Walter et al 1997). Some studies have shown that iron supplementation given to infants reduces the incidence of respiratory infections. Other studies have found no difference in groups of infants given either iron or a placebo. Adult studies cited in this review found no benefit of iron use for reducing infection rates, and suggested that more illness may occur with supplementation (Oppenheimer 2001).

Cardiac Effects: Breath-holding spells in children have been overcome by iron supplementation. Along with improved iron status in these children, autonomic cardiovascular control during sleep was improved (i.e., increased heart rate variability, reduced ratio of low-frequency/high-frequency powers) (Orii et al 2002).

Oxidative Effects: Researchers have theorized that excess iron could play a role in the etiology of cancer and coronary heart disease. Iron is able to catalyze reactions that produce free radical metabolites, which may damage cell membranes, cause chromosomal mutations, or oxidize low-density lipoproteins (LDL) into more atherogenic particles (Sempos et al 1996; Minotti 1993; Imlay et al 1988). Animal studies have confirmed that atherosclerotic plaques contain a high concentration of iron, and rats given large amounts of iron have increased LDL lipid peroxidation. In human studies, atherosclerosis has been associated with increased iron levels (Meyers 2000).

CLINICAL TRIALS
Cognitive Function in Adolescents

Iron supplementation improved hematological status and some measures of cognitive functioning in a double-blind, placebo-controlled study of 81 iron-deficient, nonanemic adolescent girls. Participants were randomly assigned to receive oral ferrous sulfate 650 mg twice daily or placebo for 8 weeks. Four tests of attention and memory were administered before and after the intervention. The supplemented group had significantly higher serum ferritin levels and performed significantly better than controls on a test of verbal learning and memory. Other measures of attention and learning were unchanged (Bruner et al 1996).

Positive results were also found in a randomized, double-blind, placebo-controlled study of 59 primarily nonanemic girls aged 16 or 17 years who took 105 mg daily of elemental iron as a liquid syrup or placebo. After 2 months, iron supplementation significantly improved subjective reports of lassitude, ability to concentrate in school, and mood. The majority of subjects reporting improvement had been hypoferremic prior to treatment. Physical fitness scores and subjective measures of appetite and sleep quality were unaffected by iron therapy (Ballin et al 1992).

Fatigue
Iron supplementation may reduce unexplained fatigue in nonanemic women. In a randomized, double-blind, placebo-controlled trial, 144 nonanemic women (aged 18 to 55 years, hemoglobin above 11.7 g/dL) with fatigue as a primary complaint were given placebo or long-acting ferrous sulfate providing 80 mg of elemental iron per day for 4 weeks. On a 10-point visual analog scale, fatigue scores at 1 month, relative to baseline, were reduced significantly more in the iron group than in the placebo group (p=0.004). After adjustments for age, depression and anxiety, and serum ferritin concentration, iron supplementation was the variable most associated with decrease in fatigue. Younger age was associated with a greater decrease in intensity of fatigue (Verdon et al 2003).

Iron-Deficiency Anemia

In adult and pediatric trials, both oral and intravenous iron supplementation was shown to overcome documented iron-deficiency anemia (Komolafe et al 2003; Shobha et al 2003; Kianfar et al 2000; Fridge et al 1998; Singh et al 1998). However, one study found that intravenous iron sucrose therapy was more effective, convenient, and safe than oral ferrous sulfate in the treatment of severe anemia in pregnant women (Al-Momen et al 1996).

Pediatric Studies

The frequency of breath-holding spells (BHS) diminished significantly in children with this disorder (n=33) given iron 5 mg/kg/day for 16 weeks compared with controls (n=34). Some 88% of those given iron had complete or partial responses compared with 6% in the placebo group (Daoud et al 1997). In another study, children receiving iron supplements showed improved autonomic cardiovascular control during sleep (e.g., increased heart rate variability and reduced ratio of low-frequency/high-frequency powers) (Orii et al 2002).

INDICATIONS AND USAGE
Approved by the FDA:

■ Iron-deficiency anemia (prophylaxis and treatment)

Unproven Uses: Limited research suggests that supplemental iron could be helpful for reducing the frequency of breath-holding spells in children. It may also enhance cognition in children and adolescents who have a documented iron deficiency. Likewise, iron may have some favorable effects on immunity and exercise performance—but again, these benefits are most likely limited to those with acute or borderline iron deficiency. Iron supplementation has also been used for the following: Plummer-Vinson syndrome, malaria, herpes simplex outbreaks, pediatric diarrhea, intestinal helminth infection, microcephaly prophylaxis, and decreased thyroid function during very-low-calorie diets.

CONTRAINDICATIONS

Iron supplements are contraindicated in patients with hemochromatosis and hemosiderosis. They are also contraindicated for treating anemias not caused by iron deficiency, such as hemolytic anemia or thalassemia, due to the risk of excess iron storage.

Parenteral preparations are not for subcutaneous administration. Sustained-release dosage forms should be avoided in patients who have conditions associated with intestinal strictures.

PRECAUTIONS

Treatment of iron-deficiency anemia must only be done under medical supervision. Iron supplements should be used with extreme caution in those with chronic liver failure, alcoholic cirrhosis, chronic alcoholism, and pancreatic insufficiency. Iron should also be used cautiously in those with a history of gastritis, peptic ulcer disease, and gastrointestinal bleeding. Patients with elevated serum ferritin levels should generally avoid iron supplements, as should those with an active or suspected infection.

In addition, patients should be aware that a moderate increase in iron stores has been associated with an increased risk of ischemic heart disease and cancer (Lynch et al 1996).

The most common side effects of iron supplements are gastrointestinal problems, including nausea, vomiting, bloating, abdominal discomfort, black stools, diarrhea, constipation, and anorexia. Enteric-coated iron preparations may prevent some of the gastrointestinal complaints associated with iron therapy. Temporary staining of teeth may occur from iron-containing liquids. Adverse effects from intramuscular iron injections include cutaneous pigmentation with iron deposits, sarcoma, nausea, vomiting, fever, chills, backache, headache, myalgia, malaise, and dizziness.

Pregnancy: FDA-rated as Pregnancy Category C. Pregnant women should not use supplemental doses of iron higher than RDA amounts (27 mg daily) unless their physician recommends it.

Breastfeeding: Nursing mothers should not use supplemental doses of iron higher than RDA amounts (9 or 10 mg daily, depending on age) unless their physician recommends it.

Pediatrics: Iron supplements can be highly toxic or lethal to small children. Those who take iron supplements should use childproof bottles and store them away from children.

Drug Interactions

Proton Pump Inhibitors (lansoprazole, omeprazole, pantoprazole, rabeprazole): Concomitant use may suppress the absorption of carbonyl iron.

Antacids: Concomitant use of aluminum- or magnesium-containing antacids may decrease the absorption of iron.

Bisphosphonates (alendronate, etidronate, risedronate): Concomitant use with ferrous (II) iron supplements may decrease the absorption of bisphosphonates.

H_2 Blockers (cimetidine, famotidine, nizatidine, ranitidine): Concomitant use may suppress the absorption of carbonyl iron.

Levodopa: Concomitant use with iron may reduce the absorption of levodopa.

Levothyroxine: Concomitant use with iron may decrease the absorption of levothyroxine.

Penicillamine: Concomitant use with iron may decrease the absorption of penicillamine.

Quinolones (ciprofloxacin, gatifloxacin, levofloxacin, lomefloxacin, moxifloxacin, norfloxacin, ofloxacin, sparfloxacin, trovafloxacin): Concomitant use may decrease the absorption of both the quinolone and iron supplement.

Tetracyclines (doxycycline, minocycline, tetracycline): Concomitant use may decrease the absorption of both the tetracycline and iron supplement.

Supplement Interactions

Beta-Carotene: Concomitant use may enhance the absorption of iron.

Calcium Carbonate: Concomitant use may decrease the absorption of iron.

Copper: Concomitant use with iron supplements may decrease the copper status of tissues.

Inositol Hexaphosphate: Concomitant use may decrease the absorption of iron.

L-Cysteine: Concomitant use may increase the absorption of iron.

Magnesium: Concomitant use may decrease the absorption of iron.

N-Acetyl-L-Cysteine: Concomitant use may increase the absorption of iron.

Tocotrienols: Concomitant use of tocotrienols-which are typically used in their nonesterified forms-and iron may cause oxidation of tocotrienols.

Vanadium: Concomitant use may decrease the absorption of iron.

Vitamin C: Concomitant use may enhance the absorption of iron.

Vitamin E (alpha-tocopherol, gamma-tocopherol, mixed tocopherols): Concomitant use of nonesterified tocopherols and iron may cause oxidation of the tocopherols.

Zinc: Concomitant use may decrease the absorption of iron.

Food Interactions

Caffeine (e.g., coffee): Concomitant use may decrease the absorption of iron.

Cysteine-Containing Proteins (e.g., meat): Concomitant use may increase the absorption of iron.

Dairy Foods and Eggs: Concomitant use may decrease the absorption of iron.

Oxalic Acid (e.g., spinach, sweet potatoes, rhubarb, beans): Concomitant use may decrease the absorption of iron.

Phytic Acid (e.g., unleavened bread, raw beans, seeds, nuts and grains, soy isolates): Concomitant use may decrease the absorption of iron.

Teas and Other Tannin-Containing Herbs: Concomitant use may cause decrease the absorption of iron.

OVERDOSAGE

Acute iron overdose can be divided into four stages. In the first, which occurs up to 6 hours after ingestion, the principal symptoms are vomiting and diarrhea. Other symptoms include hypotension, tachycardia, and CNS depression ranging from lethargy to coma. The second phase may occur at 6 to 24 hours after ingestion and is characterized by a temporary remission. In the third phase, gastrointestinal symptoms recur accompanied by shock, metabolic acidosis, coma, hepatic necrosis and jaundice, hypoglycemia, renal failure, and pulmonary edema. The fourth phase may occur several weeks after ingestion and is characterized by gastrointestinal obstruction and liver damage.

In a young child, 75 mg/kg is considered extremely dangerous. A dose of 30 mg/kg can lead to symptoms of toxicity. The lethal dosage range is estimated at ≥180 mg/kg. A peak serum iron concentration of 5 mcg/mL or more is associated with moderate to severe poisoning.

DOSAGE

Mode of Administration: Intramuscular, oral

How Supplied: Capsule, elixir, suspension, tablet

Ferrous fumarate is available in the following forms and strengths:

Chewable tablets — 100 mg

Suspension — 100 mg/5 mL

Tablets — 200 mg, 300 mg, 325 mg, 350 mg

Ferrous gluconate is available in the following forms and strengths:

Enteric-coated tablets — 325 mg

Tablets — 300 mg, 320 mg, 324 mg, 325 mg

Ferrous sulfate is available in the following forms and strengths:

Capsules, extended-release — 250 mg

Enteric-coated tablets — 324 mg, 325 mg

Elixir — 220 mg/5 mL

Liquid — 75 mg/0.6 mL

Tablets — 195 mg, 300 mg, 324 mg, 325 mg

Exsiccated ferrous sulfate is available in the following forms and strengths:

Capsules — 150 mg, 159 mg

Enteric-coated tablets — 200 mg

Tablets — 200 mg

Tablet, extended-release — 160 mg

The following lists the elemental iron content of various forms:

Iron Salt	% Iron
Ferrous fumarate	33
Ferrous gluconate	11.6
Ferrous sulfate	20
Ferrous sulfate, anhydrous	30

Daily Dosage: All doses are for oral administration unless otherwise note. Iron supplementation should be done only under a physician's supervision.

The following lists the Recommended Dietary Allowance (RDA) for iron:

Males and females — Infants to 6 months: 0.27 mg/d; *7 to 12 months:* 11 mg/d; *1 to 3 years:* 7 mg/d; *4 to 8 years:* 10 mg/d; *9 to 13 years:* 8 mg/d.

Males — 14 to 18 years: 11 mg/d; *≥19 years:* 8 mg/d

Females — 14 to 18 years: 15 mg/d; *19 to 50 years:* 18 mg/d; *≥51 years:* 8 mg/d

Pregnancy — all ages: 27 mg/d

Lactation — 14 to 18 years: 10 mg/d; *19 to 50 years:* 9 mg/d

ADULTS

Decreased Thyroid Function During Very-Low-Calorie Diets: 9 mg/d or more to bring total iron intake to 1.5 times the RDA.

Impaired Athletic Performance: Treat only confirmed iron deficiency.

Inflammatory Bowel Disease: Treat only confirmed iron deficiency.

Iron-Deficiency Anemia (intramuscular injection): The total parenteral dose required for restoration of hemoglobin and body stores of iron can be approximated using the following formula: Adults and children over 15 kg: dose (mL) = 0.0442(desired hemoglobin – observed hemoglobin) x lean body weight in kg + (0.26 x lean body weight in kg).

Iron Deficiency In Pregnancy: 60 to 100 mg/d.

Iron Insufficiency Therapy: immediate-release dosage forms: 2 to 3 mg/kg daily in 3 divided doses; sustained-release dosage forms: 50 to 100 mg daily.

Plummer-Vinson Syndrome: 2 to 3 mg/kg/d.

Prevention of Iron Deficiency in Pregnancy: 400 to 1,000 mg daily.

PEDIATRICS

Adolescent Girls With Low Ferritin: 105 to 260 mg daily.

Breath-Holding Syndrome (ferrous sulfate solution): 5 mg/kg daily.

Cognitive Function: 105 to 260 mg daily.

Iron Deficiency: 6 mg/kg/d for 2 to 3 months; absorption of iron is increased if given with a source of vitamin C.

Iron-Deficiency Anemia: *premature infants*, 2 to 4 mg/kg/d in 2 to 4 divided doses, up to a maximum of 15 mg/d; *children*, 3 to 6 mg/kg/d in 1 to 3 divided doses. *Intramuscular injection:* The total parenteral dose required for restoration of hemoglobin and body stores of iron can be approximated using the following formula: Children 5 to 15 kg: dose (mL) = 0.0442(desired hemoglobin – observed hemoglobin) x weight in kg + (0.26 x weight in kg).

LITERATURE

Abdel-Salam G, Czeizel AE: A case-control etiologic study of microcephaly. *Epidemiology*; 11(5):571-575. 2000

Al-Momen A, Al-Meshari A, Al-Nuaim L et al: Intravenous iron sucrose complex in the treatment of iron deficiency anemia during pregnancy. *Eur J Obstet Gynecol*; 69:121-124. 1996

Anderson BD, Turchen SG, Manoguerra AS et al: Retrospective analysis of ingestions of iron containing products in the United States: are there differences between chewable vitamins and adult preparations? *J Emerg Med*; 19(3):255-258. 2000

Anon: NKF-DOQI clinical practice guidelines for the treatment of anemia of chronic renal failure. *Am J Kidney Dis*; 30:S137-S192. 1997

Anon: Routine iron supplementation during pregnancy: policy statement: US Preventive Task Force. *JAMA*; 270(23):2846-2848. 1993

Baker WF: Iron deficiency in pregnancy, obstetrics, and gynecology. *Hematol Oncol Clin North Am*; 14(5):1061-1077. 2000

Ballin A, Berar M, Rubinstein U et al: Iron state in female adolescents. *Am J Dis Child*; 146(7):803-805. 1992

Beard J, Borel M & Peterson FJ: Changes in iron status during weight loss with very-low-energy diets. *Am J Clin Nutr*; 66(1):104-110. 1997

Beard JL: Iron deficiency anemia: reexamining the nature and magnitude of the public health problem. *J Nutr*; 131:568S-580S. 2001

Brolin RE, Gorman JH, Gorman RC et al: Prophylactic iron supplementation after Roux-en-Y gastric bypass: a prospective, double-blind, randomized study. *Arch Surg*; 133:740-744. 1998

Bruner AB, Joffe A, Duffan AK: Randomized study of cognitive effects of iron supplementation in non-anemic iron-deficient adolescent girls. *Lancet*; 348(9033):992-996. 1996

Campbell NRC, Hasinoff BB: Iron supplements: a common cause of drug interactions. *Br J Clin Pharmacol*; 31(3):251-255. 1991

Cogswell ME, Parvanta I, Ickes L et al: Iron supplementation during pregnancy, anemia, and birth weight: a randomized controlled trial. *Am J Clin Nutr*; 78:773-781. 2003

Dantas RO & Villanova MG: Esophageal motility impairment in Plummer-Vinson syndrome: correction by iron treatment. *Dig Dis Sci*; 38(5):968-971. 1993

Daoud AS, Batieha A, Al-Sheyyab M et al: Effectiveness of iron therapy on breath-holding spells. *J Pediatr*; 130(4):547-550. 1997

Herrinton LJ, Friedman GD, Baer D et al: Transferrin saturation and risk of cancer. *Am J Epidemiol*; 142(7):692-698. 1995

Hoffman RM, Jaffe PE: Plummer-Vinson syndrome: a case report and literature review. *Arch Intern Med*; 155(18):2008-2011. 1995

Horl WH, Cavill I, Macdougall IC et al: How to diagnose and correct iron deficiency during r-huEPO therapy — a consensus report. *Nephrol Dial Transplant*; 11(2):246-250. 1996

Hurrell RF: Bioavailability of iron. *Eur J Clin Nutr*; 51(suppl 1):S4-S8. 1997

Kianfar H, Kimiagar M & Ghaffarpour M: Effect of daily and intermittent iron supplementation on iron status of high school girls. *Int J Vitam Nutr Res*; 70(4):172-177. 2000

Knekt P, Reunanen A, Takkunen H et al: Body iron stores and risk of cancer. *Int J Cancer*; 56(3):379-382. 1994

LaManca JJ & Haymes EM: Effects of iron repletion on VO2max, endurance, and blood lactate in women. *Med Sci Sports Exerc*; 25(12):1386-1392. 1993

Looker AC, Dallman PR, Carroll MD et al: Prevalence of iron deficiency in the United States. *JAMA*; 277(12):973-976. 1997

Lynch SR & Baynes RD: Deliberations and evaluations of the approaches, endpoints and paradigms for iron dietary recommendations. *J Nutr*; 126(9 suppl):2404S-2409S. 1996

Lynch SR: Interactions of iron with other nutrients. *Nutr Rev*; 55(4):102-110. 1997

Lynch SR: The effect of calcium on iron absorption. *Nutr Res Rev*; 13(2):141-158. 2000

Makrides M, Crowther CA, Gibson RA et al: Efficacy and tolerability of low-dose iron supplements during pregnancy: a randomized controlled trial. *Am J Clin Nutr*; 78:145-153. 2003

Makrides M, Leeson R, Gibson RA et al: A randomized controlled clinical trial of increased dietary iron in breast-fed infants. *J Pediatr*; 133:559-562. 1998

Meyers DG: The iron hypothesis: does iron play a role in atherosclerosis? *Transfusion*; 40(8):1023-1029. 2000

Milman N, Bergholt T, Byg KE et al: Iron status and iron balance during pregnancy. A critical reappraisal of iron supplementation. *Acta Obstet Gynecol Scand*; 78(9):749-757. 1999

Nelson RL: Iron and colorectal cancer risk: human studies. *Nutr Rev*; 59(5):140-148. 2001

Nishiyama S, Inomoto T, Nakamura T et al: Zinc status relates to hematological deficits in women endurance runners. *J Am Coll Nutr*; 15(4):359-363. 1996

Oppenheimer SJ: Iron and its relation to immunity and infectious disease. *J Nutr*; 131(2s-2):616S-635S. 2001

Orii KE, Kato Z, Osamu F et al: Changes of autonomic nervous system function in patients with breath-holding spells treated with iron. *J Child Neurol*; 17:337-340. 2002

Salonen JT, Nyyssonen K, Korpela H et al: High stored iron levels are associated with excess risk of myocardial infarction in eastern Finnish men. *Circulation*; 86(3):803-811. 1992

Sempos CT, Looker AC, Gillum RF: Iron and heart disease: the epidemiologic data. *Nutr Rev*; 54(3):73-84. 1996

Shobha S & Sharada D: Efficacy of twice weekly iron supplementation in anemic adolescent girls. *Indian Pediatr*; 40:1186-1190. 2003

Stellon AJ & Kenwright SE: Iron deficiency anaemia in general practice: presentations and investigations. *Br J Clin Pract*; 51(2):78-80. 1997

Stevens RG, Graubard BI, Micozzi MS et al: Moderate elevation of body iron level and increased risk of cancer occurrence and death. *Int J Cancer*; 56(3):364-369. 1994

Tam DA, Rash FC: Breath-holding spells in a patient with transient erythroblastopenia of childhood. *J Pediatr*; 130(4):651-653. 1997

Tseng M, Sandler RS, Greenberg ER et al: Dietary iron and recurrence of colorectal adenomas. *Cancer Epidemiol Biomarkers Prev*; 6(12):1029-1032. 1997

Tzonou A, Lagiou P, Trichopoulou A et al: Dietary iron and coronary heart disease risk: a study from Greece. *Am J Epidemiol*; 147(2):161-166. 1998

Ullen H, Augustsson K, Gustavsson C et al: Supplementary iron intake and risk of cancer: reversed causality? *Cancer Lett*; 114(1-2):215-216. 1997

van Asperen IA, Feskens EJ, Bowles CH et al: Body iron stores and mortality due to cancer and ischaemic heart disease: a 17-year follow-up study of elderly men and women. *Int J Epidemiol*; 24(4):665-670. 1995

Verdon F, Burnand B, Fallab Stubi CL et al: Iron supplementation for unexplained fatigue in non-anaemic women: double blind randomised placebo controlled trial. *BMJ*; 326:1124-1126. 2003

Walter T, Olivares M, Pizarro F et al: Iron, anemia, infection. *Nutr Rev*; 55(4):111-124. 1997

Young YE, Koda-Kimble M: *Applied Therapeutics: The Clinical Use of Drugs*, 6th ed. Applied Therapeutics, Inc, Vancouver, WA; 1995.

Zhu YI, Haas JD: Iron depletion without anemia and physical performance in young women. *Am J Clin Nutr*; 66(2):334-341. 1997

Magnesium

DESCRIPTION

Magnesium is an essential mineral. Average daily intakes of dietary magnesium have declined in recent years due to processing of food. The average daily intake has been estimated to be approximately 300 to 360 mg. Some experts suggest an increased daily intake of 440 to 490 mg, especially if the patient is pregnant, taking potent loop diuretics, or rarely eating a well-balanced meal containing green leafy vegetables, legumes, nuts, or animal protein (Whang et al, 1994).

Magnesium sulfate is used for replacement therapy for hypomagnesemia; in total parenteral nutrition to correct or prevent deficiencies; to control or prevent seizures in preeclampsia; and in the oral form as a cathartic. Magnesium may also be effective in treating certain cardiac arrhythmias, in asthma when unresponsive to other treatments, during alcohol withdrawal, and for ischemic heart disease.

Patients with congestive heart failure often take medications that may deplete magnesium to the extent that arrhythmias occur or are worsened. Magnesium therapy has inconsistent effects on hypertension, but should be considered in those at risk of deficiency, including women and patients taking magnesium-depleting medications.

The scope of this discussion will be limited to the oral formulations.

ACTIONS AND PHARMACOLOGY
EFFECTS

Magnesium is said to exhibit antiosteoporotic activity; anti-arrhythmic, antihypertensive, glucose regulatory, bronchodilator. It is an electrolyte, a nutrient, and a mineral.

Magnesium is important as a cofactor in many enzymatic reactions in the body (Gilman et al, 1990; Havel et al,1989). There are at least 300 enzymes that are dependent upon magnesium for normal functioning. Actions on lipoprotein lipase have been found to be important in reducing serum cholesterol (Davis et al, 1984). Magnesium is necessary for maintaining serum potassium and calcium levels due to its effect on the renal tubule (Rasmussen et al, 1988).

In the heart magnesium acts as a calcium channel blocker. It also activates sodium-potassium ATPase in the cell membrane to promote resting polarization and reduce arrhythmias (Shattock et al, 1987).

CLINICAL TRIALS
Osteoporosis

A cross-sectional analysis was conducted to assess dietary components in bone mineral density (BMD). Cohorts in a heart study were analyzed for changes in BMD and dietary intake. Baseline BMDs were obtained in individuals (n=628) and dietary intake was assessed by questionnaires. Changes in a 4-year period were analyzed in BMD. Greater magnesium intake was associated with a lesser decline in BMD (Tucker et al, 1999).

Patients with gluten-sensitive enteropathy (sprue) and associated osteoporosis showed increases in BMD after 2 years of magnesium therapy. Five patients took Mg 504 to 576 mg daily, as either Mg chloride or Mg lactate, for 2 years. Erythrocyte Mg rose from 137 mcmol at baseline to 193 mcmol at 2 years (p<0.02) (normal 202+/-6 mcmol). Serum parathyroid hormone rose from 37 to 63 pg/mL at the 3-month point (p<0.04) (normal 10 to 55 pg/mL). BMD increased at all sites measured—significantly so at both the femoral neck and proximal femur (p<0.04). Increases in BMD correlated well (r=0.95) with the rise in erythrocyte Mg, which had been significantly below normal at the start of study (Rude & Olerich, 1996).

Diabetes

High doses of magnesium significantly reduced plasma fructosamine in type 2 diabetics, but did not affect fasting glucose or hemoglobin A1 (HbA1); half of that dose was without effect on any of those parameters. In a randomized, double-blind trial, 128 type 2 diabetics with poor glycemic control while being treated by diet or diet plus hypoglycemic drugs were given placebo, Mg (as MgO) 20.7 mmol/day, or Mg 41.4 mmol/day for 30 days. Before supplementation, 31% of subjects had low intramononuclear Mg levels, compared to a control group of blood donors. In the 29 patients with peripheral neuropathy, intracellular Mg was significantly lower (p<0.05) than in those without it. After 30 days, no change in plasma or intracellular Mg or improvement in glycemic control was evident in the placebo group or the lower dose Mg group. In the higher dose Mg group, fructosamine fell from 4.1 to 3.8 mmol (p<0.05) and urinary Mg increased. There were no significant changes in plasma or intracellular Mg, HbA1, or fasting glucose (Lima et al, 1998).

Three months of magnesium supplementation 15 mmol/day did not improve glycemic control in insulin-requiring type 2 diabetics. Fifty patients who were not necessarily hypomagnesemic but had used insulin for at least 6 months were randomized to receive Mg as Mg-asparate-HCl or placebo. Plasma Mg concentration and urinary Mg excretion were significantly higher in the Mg group than in the placebo group after 3 months' treatment (p<0.05 and p=0.004, respectively), but there were no differences between the groups in plasma glucose, glycosylated hemoglobin (HbA1c), plasma cholesterol, or plasma triglycerides (de Valk et al, 1998).

A randomized, double-blind, cross-over study was conducted to assess effects of magnesium in noninsulin diabetes. Patients with type 2 diabetes (n=9) treated by diet only received either 15.8 mmol Mg daily or a placebo for 4 weeks. Serum levels were measured after each treatment period. Increased plasma Mg levels, total body glucose disposal (p<0.005) and glucose oxidation (p<0.01) were observed with Mg supplementation (Paolisso et al, 1994).

A randomized, double-blind, placebo-controlled study was done to assess effects of magnesium treatment in type 2 diabetes. Patients with type 2 diabetes (n=40) were given 30 mmol Mg daily or a placebo for 3 months. Serum and urine measurements were done at the beginning, and at 2 and 3 months. Plasma Mg levels increased after the 3-month treatment but declined to pretreatment levels after 6 months (Eibl et al, 1995).

Hypertension

A meta-analysis of randomized studies investigating the effects of magnesium supplementation on blood pressure (BP) showed a dose-dependent effect. Twenty trials (total n=1,220), including 14 trials with hypertensive subjects, met inclusion criteria of randomization, a control group, Mg as the sole treatment, and sufficient data to calculate the difference in blood pressure change between the active and control treatments. The dose of magnesium varied from 10 to 40 mmol/day. For every 10-mmol increase in daily Mg intake, there was a reduction in systolic BP of 4.3 mm Hg (p<0.001) and in diastolic BP 2.3 mmHg (p=0.09). This result needs to be tested in adequately powered trials. Uncertainty remains as to the clinical utility of Mg supplements for controlling BP (Jee et al, 2002).

Migraine

Oral magnesium was effective in reducing the frequency of migraine headaches in a 12-week, multicenter, placebo-controlled, double-blind study. Of 81 patients, 43 were administered magnesium 600 mg (24 mmol) (trimagnesium dicitrate) every day for 12 weeks and 38 were given placebo. After 9 weeks of therapy, the average frequency of attacks was reduced in the Mg-treated group compared with the placebo-treated group (41.6% vs 15.8%, p=0.03) and compared with baseline (p=0.04). The number of days with migraine was also reduced in the Mg group (52.3%) compared with placebo (19.5%) (p=0.03). The average duration of attack, pain intensity, and amount of acute medication required per person were also reduced in the treatment group compared with placebo; these differences were not statistically significant. The major adverse events reported consisted of diarrhea and gastric irritation (Peikert et al, 1996).

A similarly designed study showed no difference between magnesium and placebo treatment in prevention of migraine. Sixty-nine patients with confirmed history of migraine without aura were randomly assigned to a 12-week treatment of either 20 mmol Mg-L-aspartate-hydrochloride twice daily (n=35) or an identical-appearing placebo (n=34). Responders were identified as those with a 50% reduction in the duration of migraine in hours or in the intensity of migraine at the end of the third month of treatment in comparison to baseline values. There were 10 responders in each group. There was no difference between groups in the absolute number of migraine days or the number of migraine attacks during the study. Although physicians' assessments of efficacy were nearly the same for the two treatments, 33% of the patients of the magnesium group and only 11% of the placebo group regarded the study medication to be superior to previously used migraine prophylactics. The authors mentioned that some patients started using sumatriptan to treat migraine attacks; this may have biased outcomes. They recommended that future studies provide a standardized scheme for treatment of attacks during the study (Pfaffenrath et al, 1996).

INDICATIONS AND USAGE
Approved by the FDA:

- Magnesium sulfate (Epsom salt) is approved as a laxative for the temporary relief of constipation.

Unproven Uses: Magnesium is used for migraine, bone resorption, diabetes, hypertension, arrhythmias, PMS, nephrolithiasis, spasms, and leg cramps during pregnancy.

CONTRAINDICATIONS
Magnesium is not to be used in the presence of heart block, severe renal disease, or toxemia in the 2 hours preceding delivery.

PRECAUTIONS AND ADVERSE REACTIONS
Side effects include blurred vision, photophobia, diarrhea, hypermagnesemia, hypotension, increased bleeding times, neuromuscular blockade (in higher doses), and vasodilation.

Administration of magnesium, especially in renally impaired patients, may lead to loss of deep tendon reflexes, hypotension, confusion, respiratory paralysis, cardiac arrhythmias, or cardiac arrest. Increased bleeding time has been reported. Monitor to avoid magnesium toxicity.

Pregnancy: Rickets in the newborn may result from prolonged magnesium sulfate administration in the second trimester of pregnancy.

Drug Interactions

Aminoglycosides: Concomitant use with magnesium may precipitate neuromuscular weakness and possibly paralysis. *Clinical Management:* Monitor patients for respiratory dysfunction and apnea. If neuromuscular blockade occurs, discontinue the aminoglycoside and change antibiotic therapy. Patients receiving large cumulative doses of aminoglycosides should have serum calcium, magnesium, potassium, and creatinine monitored.

Calcium channel blockers: Concomitant use with magnesium may enhance hypotensive effects. *Clinical Management:* Monitor blood pressure closely when adding or deleting calcium channel blockers in patients receiving magnesium

Fluoroquinolones: Concomitant use with magnesium may decrease absorption and effectiveness. *Clinical Management:* Fluoroquinolones should be administered at least 4 hours before magnesium or any product containing magnesium.

Labetalol: Concomitant use with magnesium may cause bradycardia and reduced cardiac output. *Clinical Management:* Myocardial function should be monitored when using concomitant magnesium sulfate and labetalol.

Levomethadyl: Concomitant use with magnesium may precipitate QT prolongation *Clinical Management:* Caution should be used when prescribing concomitant drugs known to induce hypokalemia or hypomagnesemia, such as laxatives, as they may precipitate QT prolongation and interact with levomethadyl.

Neuromuscular blockers: Concomitant use with magnesium may enhance neuromuscular blocking effects. *Clinical Management:* The dose of neuromuscular blocker may need to be adjusted downward in patients receiving large doses of magnesium salts administered for toxemia of pregnancy.

OVERDOSAGE
Hypermagnesemia from magnesium administration is most commonly seen in patients with renal insufficiency. Hypermagnesemia presents as muscle weakness, electrocardiogram changes, sedation, hypotension, and confusion. These symptoms will progress to absent deep-tendon reflexes, respiratory paralysis, and heart block (Gilman et al, 1990).

Respiratory paralysis occurs at 12 to 15 mEq/L, while concentrations greater than 15 mEq/L result in cardiac conduction abnormalities and cardiac arrest (Gilman et al, 1990).

DOSAGE
Mode of Administration: Intramuscular, intravenous, oral, topical

How Supplied: Capsule, cream, solution, tablet

Daily Dosage: The following chart lists the Recommended Dietary Allowance (RDA) for magnesium:

Age	Males	Females	Pregnancy	Lactation
0 to 6 months	30 mg/day	30 mg/day		
7 to 12 months	75 mg/day	75 mg/day		
1 to 3 years	80 mg/day	80 mg/day		
4 to 8 years	130 mg/day	130 mg/day		
9 to 13 years	240 mg/day	240 mg/day	400 mg/day	400 mg/day
14 to 18 years	410 mg/day	360 mg/day	400 mg/day	360 mg/day

Age	Males	Females	Pregnancy	Lactation
19 to 30 years	400 mg/day	310 mg/day	350 mg/day	310 mg/day
31+ years	420 mg/day	320 mg/day	360 mg/day	320 mg/day

ADULTS

Abdominal and Perineal Incision Wound Healing (magnesium hydroxide ointment, topical): apply twice daily along with zinc chloride spray for 7 days.

Congestive Heart Failure (enteric-coated magnesium chloride): 3,204 mg/d in divided doses (equal to 15.8 mmol elemental Mg).

Dentine Hypersensitivity: 4% Magnesium sulfate solution applied by iontophoresis.

Detrusor Instability (magnesium hydroxide): 350 mg for 4 weeks; double after 2 weeks if there is an unsatisfactory response.

Diabetes Mellitus Type 2: 15.8 to 41.4 mmol/d.

Dietary Supplement: 54 to 483 mg daily in divided doses.

Dyslipidemia (enteric-coated magnesium chloride): a mean dose of 17.92 mmol for a mean duration of 118 days; OR magnesium oxide, 15 mmol/d for 3 months.

Hypertension: 360 to 600 mg/d.

Migraine Prophylaxis: 360 to 600 mg/d.

Mitral Valve Prolapse (magnesium carbonate capsules): During the first week of treatment, 21 mmol/d is used; then 14 mmol/d is used during the second to fifth weeks.

Nephrolithiasis Prophylaxis (magnesium hydroxide): 400 to 500 mg/d.

Osteoporosis: 250 mg taken at bedtime on an empty stomach, increased to 250 mg three times daily for 6 months, followed by 250 mg daily for 18 months.

Premenstrual Syndrome: 200 to 360 mg/d.

PEDIATRICS

Deficiency: The oral dose of magnesium sulfate to treat hypomagnesemia in children is 100 to 200 mg/kg four times daily.

Dietary Supplement: 3 to 6 mg/kg body weight per day in divided doses 3 to 4 times daily, up to a maximum of 400 mg daily.

Laxative: The recommended dose of magnesium citrate for children 2 to 5 years of age is 2.7 to 6.25 g daily as a single or divided dose. For children 6 to 11 years of age, the dose is 5.5 to 12.5 g daily in single or divided doses.

LITERATURE

Abraham GE. Nutritional factors in the etiology of the premenstrual tension syndromes. *J Reprod Med*; 28(7):446-464. 1983

de Valk HW, Verkaaik R, van Rijn HJM et al. Oral magnesium supplementation in insulin-requiring type 2 diabetic patients. *Diabet Med*; 15:503-507. 1998

Davis WH, Leary WP, Reyes AJ et al. Monotherapy with magnesium increases abnormally low high density lipoprotein cholesterol: a clinical assay. *Curr Ther Res*; 36:341-346. 1984

Eibl NL, Kopp HP, Nowak HR et al. Hypomagnesemia in type II diabetes: Effect of a 3-month replacement therapy. *Diabetes Care*; 18(2):188-192. 1995

Gilman AG, Rall TW, Nies AS et al (eds). Goodman and Gilman's The Pharmacological Basis of Therapeutics, 8th ed. Pergamon Press, New York, NY, 1990.

Havel RJ, Calloway DH, Gussow JD et al. Recommended Dietary Allowances, 10th ed. National Academy Press, Washington, DC, 1989.

Lima M, Cruz T, Pousada JC et al. The effect of magnesium supplementation in increasing doses on the control of type 2 diabetes. *Diabetes Care*; 21:682-686. 1998

Jee SH, Miller ER III, Guallar E et al. The effect of magnesium supplementation on blood pressure: a meta-analysis of randomized clinical trials. *Am J Hypertens*; 15(8):691-696. 2002

Paolisso G, Scheen A, Cozzolino D et al. Changes in glucose turnover parameters and improvement of glucose oxidation after 4-week magnesium administration in elderly noninsulin-dependent (type II) diabetic patients. *J Clin Endocrinol Metab*; 78:1510-514. 1994

Peikert A, Wilimzig C & Kohne-Volland R. Prophylaxis of migraine with oral magnesium: results from a prospective, multi-center, placebo-controlled and double-blind randomized study. *Cephalagia*; 16:257-263. 1996

Pfaffenrath V, Wessely P, Meyer C et al. Magnesium in the prophylaxis of migraine—a double-blind, placebo-controlled study. *Cephalagia*; 16:436-440. 1996

Rasmussen HS, Aurup P, Goldstein K et al. Influence of magnesium substitution therapy on blood lipid composition in patients with ischemic heart disease. *Arch Intern Med*; 149:1050-1053. 1989

Rasmussen HS, Cintin C, Aurup P et al. The effect of intravenous magnesium therapy on serum and urine levels of potassium, calcium, and sodium in patients with ischemic heart disease, with and without acute myocardial infarction. *Arch Intern Med*;148:1801-1805. 1988

Rude RK & Olerich M. Magnesium deficiency: possible role in osteoporosis associated with gluten-sensitive enteropathy. *Osteoporos Int*; 6(6):453-461. 1996

Rude RK. Physiology of magnesium metabolism and the important role of magnesium in potassium deficiency. *Am J Cardiol*; 63(14):31G-34G. 1989

Shattock MJ, Hearse DJ & Fry CH. The ionic basis of the anti-ischemic and anti-arrhythmic properties of magnesium in the heart. *J Am Coll Nutr*; 6:27-33. 1987

Stendig-Lindberg G, Tepper R & Leichter. Trabecular bone density in a two-year controlled trial of peroral magnesium in osteoporosis. *Mag Res*; 6(2):155-163. 1993

Stuart A, Smellie A, O'Reilly J et al. Magnesium replacement and glucose tolerance in elderly subjects. *Am J Clin Nutr*; 57(4):594-595. 1993

Tucker AK, Hannan MT, Chen H et al. Potassium, magnesium, and fruit and vegetable intakes are associated with greater bone mineral density in elderly men and women. *Am J Clin Nutr*; 69:727-736. 1999

Whang R, Hampton EM & Whang DD. Magnesium homeostasis and clinical disorders of magnesium deficiency. *Ann Pharmacother*; 28:220-226. 1994

Melatonin

DESCRIPTION

Melatonin (N-acetyl-5-methoxytryptamine) is a neurohormone produced by pinealocytes in the pineal gland during the dark hours of the day-night cycle. Serum levels of melatonin are very low during most of the day, and it has been labeled the "hormone of darkness." Melatonin is involved in the induction of sleep, may play a role in the internal synchronization of the mammalian circadian system, and may serve as a marker of the "biologic clock" (Haimov & Lavie, 1995; Garfinkel et al, 1995; Dollins et al, 1994; Tzischinsky & Lavie, 1994; Jan et al, 1994; Cavallo, 1993; Short, 1993).

Other Names: N-acetyl-5-methoxytryptamine

ACTIONS AND PHARMACOLOGY

EFFECTS

Melatonin is thought to have antioxidant, immunomodulator, and hypnotic effects.

In general, the pineal gland (projecting from diencephalon into third ventricle) is a neuroendocrine transducer, related to its secretion of melatonin. The hormone serves as a messenger to the neuroendocrine system regarding environmental conditions (especially the photoperiod). Putative functions of endogenous melatonin in this regard include regulation of sleep cycles, hormonal rhythms, and body temperature (Deacon et al, 1994; Dollins et al, 1993; Cavallo, 1993). Melatonin may also have a role in influencing the maturation and function of the hypothalamic-pituitary-gonadal axis and in determining the onset of puberty (Cavallo, 1993).

Production of melatonin is regulated by postsynaptic receptors originating in the superior cervical ganglion, which innervate the pineal gland. The suprachiasmatic nucleus of the hypothalamus (entrained by the light-dark cycle and considered the anatomic site for the biologic clock) receives stimuli from the retina (retinohypothalamic tract), and during dark hours the suprachiasmatic nuclei forward a stimulus to the superior cervical ganglion and pineal gland, resulting in melatonin secretion (Haimov & Lavie, 1995; Cavallo, 1993). This stimulatory activity is suppressed by light, especially bright light (Thalen et al, 1995; Cavallo, 1993; Strassman et al, 1987). Melatonin synthesis in the pinealocyte is dependent upon noradrenergic stimulation (Cavallo, 1993). The normal endogenous production rate is 28 to 30 mcg/d (Short, 1993; Lane & Moss, 1985). Production of the hormone is reduced in cirrhotic patients (12 mcg/day) (Lane & Moss, 1985) and in the elderly (Garfinkel et al, 1995).

Antioxidant Effects: Melatonin possesses free-radical scavenging properties, protecting cells against many oxidative agents. The mechanism of free-radical scavenging action is not well elucidated. Melatonin reacts with nitric oxide in the presence of doublet oxygen, producing N-nitrosomelatonin. Since nitric oxide can cause some cellular destruction, melatonin may protect the cell against such oxidative damage (Turjanski et al, 2000). Melatonin also inhibits the production of nitric oxide by inhibiting nitric oxide synthase. Nitric oxide's damaging effects are mediated through its reaction with superoxide to form peroxynitrite. Peroxynitrite stimulates lipid peroxidation, inactivates various enzymes, and depletes glutathione (Cuzzocrea et al, 2000).

Antitumor Effects: In vitro and animal studies have reported that melatonin is capable of inducing direct cytostatic actions on some human cancer cell lines, stimulating host immune responses, and inhibiting release of somatomedin-C (Lissoni et al, 1995; Lissoni et al, 1991). Melatonin has been used alone and in combination with interleukin-2 as an immunotherapeutic regimen in the treatment of cancer (Lissoni et al, 1995; Lissoni et al, 1994).

Sleep-Regulating Effects: Prolonged administration of oral melatonin has reportedly induced phase-setting effects on circadian rhythms, such as the sleep-wake cycle and rest-activity. The hormone has been reported to produce re-entrainment of circadian rhythms after time-zone shifts, and entrainment of previously free-running rhythms in the blind (Dollins et al, 1993; Cavallo, 1993; Dahlitz et al, 1991; Arendt et al, 1988; Arendt et al, 1986).

CLINICAL TRIALS
Cancer

Tumor regression rate and 5-year survival results were significantly increased in metastatic non-small cell lung cancer subjects who were concomitantly treated with chemotherapy and melatonin. One hundred subjects were randomized to receive chemotherapy only or chemotherapy and melatonin. Chemotherapy subjects received cisplatin 20 mg/m^2 per day intravenously and etoposide 100 mg/m^2 per day intravenously for 3 consecutive days. Four chemotherapy cycles were planned at 21-day intervals. Melatonin 20 mg orally was given 7 days every evening before chemotherapy and was continued after chemotherapy. Toxicity and clinical response were evaluated according to criteria of the World Health Organization. A complete response (CR) was achieved in 2 of 49 (4%) subjects treated with chemotherapy and melatonin. No patient achieved a CR with only chemotherapy. Fifteen of 49 (31%) subjects treated with chemotherapy and melatonin achieved a partial response (PR) compared to 9 of 51 (18%) chemotherapy-only subjects. Disease progression occurred in 20 of 51 chemotherapy-only subjects while 6 of 49 chemotherapy-melatonin subjects had progression (p<0.01). At 5 years, chemotherapy plus melatonin compared to chemotherapy alone improved survival (3 vs 0, p<0.001). Chemotherapy treatment was also better tolerated in subjects treated concomitantly with melatonin (Lissoni et al, 2003).

Sixteen patients with glioblastoma who were treated with melatonin 20 mg/d and radiotherapy (RT) experienced prolonged overall survival time compared to 14 patients given RT alone. Both groups were given steroids and anticonvulsants. The melatonin-treated group had a higher rate of survival at 1 year than did the RT-only group (p<0.02). Patients with RT alone experienced a significantly higher number of infections compared to melatonin plus RT group (p<0.025) (Lissoni et al, 1996a).

Tamoxifen and melatonin administered to 25 patients with metastatic solid tumors showed beneficial effects in terms of controlling cancer-cell proliferation or improving performance status. Patients included those diagnosed with melanoma, uterine cervix carcinoma, pancreatic cancer, heptocarcinoma, ovarian cancer, small cell cancer, or unknown primary tumor. Tamoxifen 20 mg and melatonin 20 mg were given daily. In 3 patients (12%) a partial response was seen. Stable disease was observed in 13 patients (52%) with the remaining 9 patients demonstrating progressive disease. No toxicity was seen (Lissoni et al, 1996b).

Other studies have reported significantly prolonged survival and greater improvement in performance status with oral melatonin plus supportive care compared to supportive care alone in patients with non-small cell lung cancer (n=63) (Lissoni et al, 1992a) and brain metastases of solid tumors (n=50) (Lissoni et al, 1994a). In the non-small cell lung cancer patients, a dose of 10 mg daily for 21 of 28 days was administered. No complete or partial responses were observed, although stable disease was achieved in significantly more patients treated with melatonin (32% versus 9%). A dose of 20 mg daily until progression was given to patients with brain metastases; the free-from-progression period was greater and the frequency of steroid-induced metabolic and infective complications was significantly lower with melatonin therapy relative to supportive care alone in this study. In both studies, patients had failed or progressed on prior chemotherapy, although details of previous therapy or criteria for failure were not provided. Methods of randomization and pretreatment clinical status of patients (such as underlying conditions) in each group, which could affect outcome, were also not specified, and the numbers of patients may have been too small for adequate statistical analysis. The same group of investigators conducted all studies.

The combination of subcutaneous recombinant interleukin-2 (aldesleukin) given 5 or 6 days/week for 4 weeks, plus oral melatonin 10 to 50 mg daily produced complete or partial tumor responses in 23% of pretreated patients with various digestive tract tumors (ie, colorectal, gastric, hepatic, or pancreatic carcinoma) (Lissoni et al, 1993a), 21% with solely metastatic gastric carcinoma and low performance status (Lissoni et al, 1993), and 20% of patients with non-small cell lung cancer (first-line therapy) (Lissoni et al, 1992) in small uncontrolled studies. A partial response rate was also observed with this combination in 3 of 12 previously treated or untreated patients (25%) with locally unresectable or metastatic endocrine tumors; responses occurred in carcinoid tumor, neuroendocrine lung tumor, and pancreatic islet cell tumor (Lissoni et al, 1995).

Chemotherapy-Induced Toxicity

Evening administration of melatonin throughout chemotherapy treatment and every day thereafter resulted in significant reductions in manifestations of chemotherapy-induced toxicity. Eighty patients were given melatonin 20 mg/d concomitantly with chemotherapy or chemotherapy only. Supportive care was the same in both groups of patients. Thrombocytopenia was significantly less (p<0.006) in the group receiving melatonin. Leukopenia and anemia were also less frequent. Asthenia and malaise were significantly less frequent (p<0.006) in the melatonin group. Stomatitis, neuropathy, and cardiac complications also occurred less frequently in the group receiving concomitant melatonin than in the group receiving chemotherapy alone. There was no difference between groups in the frequency of alopecia, nausea and vomiting, or diarrhea. The antitumor activity of cytotoxic drugs was not negatively influenced by concomitant administration of melatonin (Lissoni et al, 1997b).

Delayed Sleep Phase Syndrome

Melatonin advanced sleep onset in subjects with delayed sleep phase syndrome. Five mg melatonin given 5 hours before endogenous melatonin secretion advanced sleep onset and improved quality of life for 16 patients with delayed sleep phase syndrome (Smits & Nagtegaal, 2000).

Daily nighttime melatonin decreased sleep systolic and diastolic blood pressure in subjects with untreated mild to moderate essential hypertension in a randomized, double-blind, placebo-controlled, crossover trial. Sixteen men (aged 36 to 68 years) were orally supplemented with melatonin 2.5 mg or placebo 1 hour before bedtime one time only (acute); this dosage was then repeated daily for 3 weeks. Twenty-four hour ambulatory blood pressure and sleep quality were evaluated for both the acute and repeated treatment period. A significant decrease in sleep systolic (6 mm Hg) and diastolic (4 mm Hg) blood pressure was demonstrated during the 3 weeks of melatonin compared to placebo (p=0.046 and p=0.020). The 1-day only treatment had no effect on systolic and diastolic blood pressures while asleep (p=0.89 and p=0.86, respectively). No significant improvement in awake systolic and diastolic blood pressure was demonstrated during the 3 weeks of melatonin compared to placebo. Repeatedly used melatonin significantly increased sleep efficiency (p=0.017) and sleep time (p=0.013) (Scheer et al, 2004).

Headache

Melatonin reduced the number of daily attacks of cluster headache and the consumption of analgesics in acute sufferers. In a double-blind study of 20 sufferers of cluster headaches, subjects were given either melatonin 10 mg in a single evening dose or placebo for 2 weeks, during a cluster period. Fifty percent of melatonin-treated patients responded. Improvement began 3 days after the onset of treatment, and responders were free of headaches after 5 days. There was no improvement in the placebo group. Discontinuation of treatment by responders was followed by gradual recurrence of cluster attacks, obliging re-institution of treatment (Leone & Bussone, 1998; Leone et al, 1996).

Melatonin eliminated the occurrence of headaches of various kinds (migraine, cluster, tension headache) in 5 patients with delayed sleep phase syndrome. Each patient received either melatonin 5 mg or a placebo nightly for 14 days, followed by the other treatment for 14 days. Thereafter, each patient took melatonin nightly for at least 3 months. Melatonin was given 5 hours before the time when endogenous melatonin reached 10 picograms/mL. The endogenous nocturnal melatonin level of all subjects was normal and did not differ from those of patients who had delayed sleep phase syndrome without headache, suggesting that the headaches were not caused by melatonin deficiency. Rather, relief from headaches may have been a result of increased sleep and synchronicity of the biological clock to lifestyle (Nagtegaal et al, 1998).

Jet Lag

Melatonin has not been statistically superior to placebo in some jet lag studies (Claustrat et al, 1992; Petrie et al, 1989). In particular, mood, sleep quality, and morning sleepiness were not altered significantly in one study (Claustrat et al, 1992). Effective doses of melatonin have been either 5 mg daily (at various times) for 3 days prior to the flight, then the same dose for 4 additional days, or an 8 mg dose on the day of the flight and for 3 further days. The former regimen appears more effective.

Sedation and Anxiolysis

In a randomized, double-blind, dose-ranging study, melatonin (MLN) was as efficacious as midazolam (MZ) and more efficacious than placebo in provoking sedation and anxiolysis in preoperative surgical patients. Adult women scheduled for laparoscopic surgery were assigned to receive 1 of the following 7 sublingual premedication regimens (n=12 each group): MZ 0.05, 0.1, or 0.2 mg/kg; MLN 0.05, 0.1, or 0.2 mg/kg; or placebo. All patients were premedicated 2 hours prior to surgery; in each case, the patient was instructed to avoid swallowing the sublingual preparation of their respective study drug for 3 minutes after dosing, after which they were allowed to swallow. Sedation and anxiety were measured by a 4-point sedation scale and a visual analogue scale, respectively. Both MZ and MLN induced significantly greater reductions in preoperative anxiety when compared with placebo (p<0.05), and sedation was attained at 60 and 90 minutes after dosing by significantly more patients receiving MZ and MLN than placebo (p<0.02). With the exception of patients receiving MZ 0.2 mg/kg, there were no differences between groups with regard to the level of postoperative sedation; patients receiving MZ 0.2 mg/kg experienced an increased depth of sedation compared with patients receiving MLN 0.05 and 0.1 mg/kg. Postoperative pain scores were not different between groups at any time during postanesthesia recovery (Naguib & Samarkandi, 2000).

Sleep Disorders

Nine patients with periodic limb movement disorder showed improvements when given melatonin for 6 weeks in an open trial. Patients were given melatonin 3 mg taken 30 minutes before bedtime, between 10 and 11 p.m. for 6 weeks. Polysomnography was performed at baseline and during the last week of treatment. A wrist actigraph was worn during 2 weeks prior to treatment and during the last 14 days of supplementation in order to measure motor activity during sleep. Seven patients subjectively reported feelings of improved daytime symptoms of fatigue and excessive sleepiness within 7 days of treatment. Polysomnographic recordings reported significant decreases in parameters of periodic limb movements (p<0.05), which were confirmed through actigraphy. The investigators hypothesized that a resynchronization of circadian rhythms enhanced REM sleep and produced the observed effects (Kunz & Bes, 2001).

Improved sleep parameters were seen when melatonin was given to schizophrenic patients with insomnia in a randomized, double-blind, placebo-controlled, crossover study. Nineteen subjects were given either controlled-release melatonin 2 mg or placebo 2 hours before bedtime for 3 weeks, with a 1 week washout between the treatments. Wrist actigraphs were used to assess sleep quality for 3 nights during the last week of each treatment period. Sleep efficiency was significantly improved in the melatonin group compared to placebo (p=0.038). There was an insignificant decrease in sleep latency and increased total sleep time with melatonin versus placebo. Twenty-seven patients entered the study, but only 19 were assessed due to lack of compliance (n=4) and technical problems with the actigraphs (n=4) (Shamir et al, 2000).

Melatonin was effective in improving the sleep of patients with major depressive disorder. This double-blind, placebo-controlled study treated 24 outpatients with fluoxetine 20 mg and either slow-release melatonin 2.5 to 10 mg or placebo nightly for 4 weeks. No other medications were used. Patients treated with melatonin showed significant improvement in sleep variables compared with controls (p=0.01). No effect of melatonin on depression symptoms was found (Dolberg et al, 1998).

Limited data suggest benefits of oral melatonin in blind adults with free-running sleep-wake rhythms (Haimov & Lavie, 1995; Cavallo, 1993; Arendt et al, 1988). Sleep problems in these patients were considered related to an inability to remain synchronized to the normal 24-hour day, due at least in part to lack of light-dark perception. Therapy with melatonin resulted in normal sleep (without early awakening and day sleeps), attributed to resynchronization of the sleep-wake activity cycle. Effective doses have been 5 mg nightly at normal bedtime.

Ten children with neurologic and developmental disorders were given 3 mg melatonin 1 to 2 hours before bedtime and monitored for a mean of 7.5 months. In eight (80%) of the children, the average number of hours of sleep, average number of nighttime awakenings, average number of nights with early morning arousal, and average number of nights with delayed sleep onset greatly improved after treatment. Use of melatonin also improved day-time activities and behaviors (Jan, 2000). Another study examining 5 severely psychomotor retarded children showed improved sleep patterns after 4 weeks of treatment with 3 mg melatonin given every day at 6:30 p.m. (Pillar et al, 2000).

In a study of 100 pediatric patients (ages 3 months to 21 years) with chronic sleep disorders, 54% were visually impaired and 85% had multiple neurodevelopmental disabilities (including visual loss, deafness, blindness, mental retardation, cerebral palsy, epilepsy, chromosomal abnormalities, head injuries, degenerative central nervous system disorders, autism, and brain tumors). Of the 15 patients not having the above conditions, diagnoses were attention deficit hyperactive disorder, anxiety, bowel disorders, and nocturnal seizures. Treatment with oral melatonin doses of 2.5 to 10 mg resulted in improved sleep in 82% of these patients. Factors involved in non-response were recurrent pain, malfunction or absence of the suprachiasmatic nucleus, noisy sleep environments, psychological reasons for delayed sleep onset, multiple medications, and organically driven behavior. In 2 children with pineal glands destroyed by brain tumor or trauma, oral melatonin doses of 25 mg were required to produce a beneficial improvement in sleep quality. A secondary benefit was that improved patient sleep allowed caretakers to also have improved sleep (Jan & O'Donnell, 1996).

Tinnitus

Patients reported more subjective improvement in tinnitus with melatonin than with placebo in a randomized, crossover study. Twenty-three subjects were given melatonin 3 mg or placebo, to be taken 1 to 2 hours before retiring, for 30 days. After a 7-day washout, patients took the alternate treatment for 30 days. Average improvements in Tinnitus Handicap Inventory (THI) scores were significant and were the same with melatonin and placebo. However, on a follow-up questionnaire, 39% of patients reported an overall improvement with melatonin, whereas only 17% reported improvement with placebo. Among those reporting difficulty sleeping due to their tinnitus, 46.7% had overall improvement with melatonin and 20% with placebo (p=0.04). Eight of 16 patients with bilateral tinnitus reported improvement with melatonin and only 3 of the 16 had improvement with placebo. Overall, 35% of subjects had a decrease in loudness of their tinnitus with melatonin, compared with 13% with placebo. The only side effect reported in the study was bad dreams, which was equally distributed between the melatonin and placebo trials (Rosenberg et al, 1998).

INDICATIONS AND USAGE

Melatonin is used as a sleep aid, in the treatment of a variety of solid tumors (in combination with interleukin-2), and can be used to improve thrombocytopenia and other toxicities induced by cancer chemotherapy and from other conditions. Melatonin is also used for cluster headaches and tinnitus.

PRECAUTIONS AND ADVERSE REACTIONS

Adverse effects of exogenous melatonin have generally been minimal. Drowsiness, fatigue, headache, confusion, gastrointestinal complaints, and reduced body temperature have been reported. Melatonin has exacerbated dysphoria in depressed patients and has caused mood swings. It has caused depressive symptoms and fever when used with interleukin-2 in cancer therapy. Rarely, tachycardia, seizures, acute psychotic reactions, autoimmune hepatitis, and pruritus have been reported.

Drug Interactions:

Fluvoxamine: Increased central nervous system depression with concomitant use. *Clinical Management:* Monitor patients taking fluvoxamine with melatonin supplementation for changes in sleep patterns and signs of excessive central nervous system depression. Downward titration of melatonin dosages may be required during concomitant administration with fluvoxamine.

Nifedipine: Increased blood pressure with concomitant use. *Clinical Management:* Close monitoring of blood pressure is advised with appropriate dose adjustment of nifedipine or withdrawal of melatonin.

Warfarin: Increased risk of bleeding with concomitant use. *Clinical Management:* Avoid concomitant use of melatonin and warfarin. If both agents are taken together, monitor prothrombin time, INR, and signs and symptoms of excessive bleeding frequently. Only adjust the warfarin dose if the patient takes a consistent dosage of melatonin with a consistent and standardized brand.

DOSAGE

Mode of Administration: intramuscular, intravenous, oral, oral transmucosal, transdermal

How Supplied: tablet, tincture

Daily Dosage:

Cancer as combination therapy: 40 or 50 mg oral tablets given once daily at night, initiated 7 days prior to interleukin-2 and continued throughout the cycle

Cancer as single agent therapy: Melatonin 20 mg intramuscularly daily for 2 months (induction phase), followed by oral doses of 10 mg daily until progression, has been given for the treatment of solid tumors

Chronic insomnia: 1 to 10 mg orally daily

Delayed sleep phase syndrome: 5 mg orally daily

Jet lag: 5 mg orally daily for 3 days prior to departure, then 5 mg for 4 additional days

Normalization of nocturnal levels: constant intravenous daytime infusion of melatonin 4 mcg/hour for 5 hours (0.1 and 0.3 mg oral tablets have also been used)

Sleep disorders: 5 mg at the usual bedtime

Pediatric Dosage:

Congenital sleep disorder: 2.5 mg oral tablet

Neurological disability: 0.5 to 10 mg oral tablet at bedtime

Sleep-wake cycle disorder (controlled release tablets, oral: An average of 5.7 mg was used in children ages 4 to 21 years

LITERATURE

Arendt J, Aldhous J & Marks V. Alleviation of jet lag by melatonin: preliminary results of controlled double blind trial. *BMJ*; 292(6529):1170. 1986

Arendt J, Aldhous M & Wright J. Synchronisation of a disturbed sleep-wake cycle in a blind man by melatonin treatment (letter). *Lancet*; 1(8588):772-773. 1988

Cavallo A. The pineal gland in human beings: relevance to pediatrics. *J Pediatr*; 123(6):843-851. 1993

Claustrat B, Brun J, David M et al. Melatonin and jet lag: confirmatory result using a simplified protocol. *Biol Psychiatry*; 32(8):705-711. 1992

Cuzzocrea S, Constantino G, Gitto E et al. Protective effects of melatonin in ischemic brain injury. *J Pineal Res*; 29(4):217-227. 2000

Dahlitz M, Alvarez B, Vignau J et al. Delayed sleep phase syndrome response to melatonin. *Lancet*; 337(8750):1121-1124. 1991

Deacon S, English J & Arendt J. Acute phase-shifting effects of melatonin associated with suppression of core body temperature in humans. *Neuroscience*; 178(1):32-34. 1994

Dolberg OT, Hirschmann S & Grunhaus L. Melatonin for the treatment of sleep disturbances in major depressive disorder. *Am J Psychiatry*; 155(8): 1119-1121. 1998

Dollins AB, Lynch HJ, Wurtman RJ et al. Effect of pharmacological daytime doses of melatonin on human mood and performance. *Psychopharmacology* (Berl); 112(4):490-496. 1993

Dollins AB, Zhdanova IV, Wurtman RJ et al. Effect of inducing nocturnal serum melatonin concentrations in daytime on sleep, mood, body temperature, and performance. *Proc Natl Acad Sci USA*; 91(5):1824-1828. 1994

Dollins AB, Zhdanova IV, Wurtman RJ et al. Effect of inducing nocturnal serum melatonin concentrations in daytime on sleep, mood, body temperature, and performance. *Proc Natl Acad Sci USA*; 91(5):1824-1828. 1994

Garfinkel D, Laudon M, Nof D et al. Improvement of sleep quality in elderly people by controlled-release melatonin. *Lancet*; 346(8974):541-544. 1995

Haimov I & Lavie P. Potential of melatonin replacement therapy in older patients with sleep disorders. *Drugs Aging*; 7(2):75-78. 1995

James SP, Mendelson WB, Sack DA et al: The effect of melatonin on normal sleep. *Neuropsychopharmacology*; 1(1):41-44. 1988

Jan JE & O'Donnell ME. Use of melatonin in the treatment of paediatric sleep disorders. *J Pineal Res*; 21(4):193-199. 1996

Jan JE, Espezel H & Appleton RE. The treatment of sleep disorders with melatonin. *Dev Med Child Neurol*; 36(2):97-107. 1994

Kunz D & Bes F. Exogenous melatonin in periodic limb movement disorder: an open clinical trial and a hypothesis. *Sleep*; 24(2):183-187. 2001

Lane EA & Moss HB. Pharmacokinetics of melatonin in man: first pass hepatic metabolism. *J Clin Endocrinol Metab*; 61(6):1214-1216. 1985

Lissoni P, Barni S, Ardizzoia A et al. A randomized study with the pineal hormone melatonin versus supportive care alone in patients with brain metastases due to solid neoplasms. *Cancer* 1994a; 73(3):699-701.

Lissoni P, Barni S, Ardizzoia A et al. Randomized study with the pineal hormone melatonin versus supportive care alone in advanced nonsmall cell lung cancer resistant to a first-line chemotherapy containing cisplatin. *Oncology*; 49(5):336-339. 1992a

Lissoni P, Barni S, Cattaneo G et al. Clinical results with the pineal hormone melatonin in advanced cancer resistant to standard antitumor therapies. *Oncology*; 48(6):448-450. 1991

Lissoni P, Chilelli M, Villa S et al. Five years survival in metastatic non-small cell lung cancer patients treated with chemotherapy alone or chemotherapy and melatonin: a randomized trial. *J Pineal Res*; 35(1):12-15. 2003

Lissoni P, Meregalli S, Nosetto L et al. Increased survival time in brain glioblastomas by a radioneuroendocrine strategy with radiotherapy plus melatonin compared to radiotherapy alone. *Oncology*; 53(1):43-46. 1996a

Lissoni P, Paolorossi F, Tancini G et al. A phase II study of tamoxifen plus melatonin in metastatic solid tumor patients. *Br J Cancer*; 74(9):1466-1468. 1996b

Lissoni P, Tancini G, Barni S et al. Treatment of cancer chemotherapy-induced toxicity with the pineal hormone melatonin. *Support Care Cancer*; 5(2):126-129. 1997b

Lissoni P, Barni S, Tancini G et al. A randomised study with subcutaneous low-dose interleukin 2 alone vs interleukin 2 plus the pineal neurohormone melatonin in advanced solid neoplasms other than renal cancer and melanoma. *Br J Cancer*; 69(1):196-199. 1994

Mallo C, Zaidan R, Galy G et al. Pharmacokinetics of melatonin in man after intravenous infusion and bolus injection. *Eur J Clin Pharmacol*; 38(3):297-301. 1990

MacFarlane JG, Cleghorn JM, Brown GM et al. The effects of exogenous melatonin on the total sleep time and daytime alertness of chronic insomniacs: a preliminary study. *Biol Psychiatry*; 30(4):371-376. 1991

Naguib M & Samarkandi AH. The comparative dose-response effects of melatonin and midazolam for premedication of adult patients: a double-blinded, placebo-controlled study. *Anesth Analg*; 91:473-479. 2000

Nagtegaal JE, Smits MG, Swart ACW et al. Melatonin-responsive headache in delayed sleep phase syndrome: preliminary observations. *Headache*; 38(4):303-307. 1998

Rosenberg SE, Silverstein H, Rowan PT et al. Effect of melatonin on tinnitus. *Laryngoscope*; 108(3):305-310. 1998

Petrie K, Conaglen JV, Thompson L et al: Effect of melatonin on jet lag after long haul flights. *BMJ*; 298(6675):705-707. 1989

Pillar G, Shahar E, Peled N et al. Melatonin improves sleep-wake patterns in psychomotor retarded children. *Pediatr Neurol*; 23(3):225-228. 2000

Scheer F, Van Montfrans G, van Someren E et al. Daily nighttime melatonin reduces blood pressure in male patients with essential hypertension. *Hypertension*; 43(2):192-197. 2004

Shamir E, Barak Y, Shalman I et al. Melatonin treatment for tardive dyskinesia. *Arch Gen Psychiatry*; 58(11):1049-1052. 2001

Strassman RJ, Peake GT, Qualls CR et al. A model for the study of the acute effects of melatonin in man. *J Clin Endocrinol Metab*; 65(5):847-852. 1987

Thalen BE, Kjellman BF, Morkrid L et al. Melatonin in light treatment of patients with seasonal and nonseasonal depression. *Acta Psychiatr Scand*; 92(4):274-284. 1995

Tzischinsky O & Lavie P. Melatonin possesses time-dependent hypnotic effects. *Sleep*; 17(7):638-645. 1994

Waldhauser F, Waldhauser M, Lieberman HR et al. Bioavailability of oral melatonin in humans. *Neuroendocrinology*; 39(4):307-313. 1984

Vitamin C

DESCRIPTION
Vitamin C is an important biological antioxidant and has been a popular nutritional supplement for decades. Vitamin C is often used to prevent or ameliorate a wide variety of infections and to enhance the effectiveness of the immune system. It is popular as a promoter of connective-tissue health in conditions such as minor trauma and capillary fragility.

Other Names: ascorbic acid, calcium ascorbate

ACTIONS AND PHARMACOLOGY
EFFECTS
Vitamin C has antioxidant, atherogenic, anticarcinogenic, antihypertensive, antiviral, antihistamine, immunomodulatory, ophthalmoprotective, airway-protective, and heavy-metal detoxifying properties.

Antioxidant effects have been demonstrated as increased resistance of red blood cells to free radical attack in elderly persons and reduced activated oxygen species in patients receiving chemotherapy and radiation. Antioxidant mechanisms have been shown in the reduction of LDL oxidation as well, though studies on the prevention of heart disease and stroke are conflicting.

CLINICAL TRIALS
Alzheimer's disease
Vitamin C and vitamin E supplements in combination were associated with reduced prevalence and incidence of Alzheimer's disease (AD) in a cross-sectional, prospective study. A population of 4,740 adults 65 years of age and older were assessed for cognitive status, and their use of vitamin supplements was determined. Vitamin C users were those who took at least 500 mg of ascorbic acid, either as a single supplement or as part of a multivitamin preparation. Vitamin E users were defined as those who took a multivitamin preparation or an individual vitamin E supplement providing more than 400 IU per day. Multiple vitamin users were those whose preparation provided lower amounts of vitamin E and vitamin C. There were 200 prevalent cases of AD in the starting population. At the end of follow-up (up to 5 years), there were 104 incident cases of AD and 3,123 subjects who were free of dementia. The group of 1,429 people lost to follow-up comprised individuals who were older, less educated, and had performed less well on their cognitive screen than those who completed the protocol. Hence, AD incidence during the follow-up period may have been underestimated. After adjustment for age, sex, education, and apolipoprotein E genotype, prevalence analysis showed a significant inverse relation between prevalence of AD and vitamin E and multivitamin use. Vitamin E alone, vitamin C alone, or vitamin C in combination with multivitamins were not associated with AD prevalence. The strongest association was with the combination of vitamin E and vitamin C, with or without multivitamins (multivariate adjusted odds ratio, 0.22; 95% confidence interval (CI), 0.05 to 0.6). The combination of vitamin E and vitamin C also apparently reduced incidence (adjusted hazard ratio, 0.36; 95% CI, 0.09 to 0.99). For incidence, associations were not significant for vitamin E alone, vitamin C alone, multivitamin use alone or in combination (Zandi et al, 2004).

Antioxidant Defense Status
Supplementation with antioxidant vitamins, including vitamin C, improved antioxidant defense status in elderly subjects. Eighty-one subjects were stratified by sex and age and randomized to receive daily either placebo, a mineral combination (20 mg zinc,

100 mcg selenium), a vitamin combination (120 mg vitamin C, 6 mg beta-carotene, 15 mg vitamin E) or both combinations for a period of 2 years. Antioxidant defense, measured by in vitro challenge of red blood cells with free radicals, was improved in the vitamin group only (Girodon et al, 1997).

Supplementation with antioxidant vitamins, including vitamin C, prior to conditioning therapy (chemotherapy and radiation) for bone-marrow transplantation resulted in less of a rise in plasma lipid hydroperoxides than did conditioning therapy without pres-supplementation. Sixteen patients with leukemia were supplement-ed with alpha-tocopherol 825 mg, beta-carotene 45 mg, and ascorbic acid 450 mg for 3 weeks before beginning conditioning therapy. Ten other patients received conditioning therapy without supplementation with antioxidant vitamins. The rise in plasma lipid hydroperoxide level between the start of conditioning therapy and the completion of transplantation was from 20.1 to 36.2 mmol/liter in the supplemented group and from 23.3 to 83.5 mmol/liter in the unsupplemented group. The increase was significant (p<0.05) only in the unsupplemented group. Condition-ing therapy causes delayed toxic effects in several tissues, which is thought to be caused by free-radical damage. The authors speculated that reducing lipid peroxide formation may reduce the toxicity of conditioning therapy (Clemens et al, 1997).

Vitamin C Deficiency

Ascorbic acid deficiency in the institutionalized elderly may be corrected by daily vitamin C supplements. In a double-blind, placebo-controlled trial of 94 elderly inpatients with low levels of plasma and leukocyte vitamin C, patients received placebo or vitamin C 1 g for 60 days. Plasma and leukocyte vitamin C levels rose significantly during therapy. Treated patients showed signifi-cant increases in the mean values of body weight (0.41 kg), plasma albumin (0.46 g/liter), and prealbumin (25.4 mg/liter), and untreat-ed patients showed decreases of these values, 0.6 kg, 0.53 g/liter, and 7 mg/liter, respectively. Reductions in purpura and petechial hemorrhages were also noted in the vitamin C group; however, no change in mood or mobility was observed (Schorah et al, 1981).

Cardiovascular Disease Protection

In a Finnish prospective population study (n=1605), subjects with low plasma vitamin C (less than 11.4 mmol/liter, or 2 mg/liter) had a relative risk of acute myocardial infarction of 2.5 compared with those who were not deficient, after adjustments of the model for the strongest risk factors of myocardial infarction. The authors suggest that supplementation of vitamin C may be beneficial in individuals with low plasma levels but not in those whose plasma levels are above 2 mg/liter (Nyyssonen et al, 1997).

Cold Symptoms

Most controlled trials have found no significant effect of ascorbic acid on the incidence of colds, except for individuals under heavy acute physical stress. However, the effect of ascorbic acid supplementation on severity and duration of cold symptoms has been repeatedly, though not consistently, shown to be measurable and statistically significant, with a median decrease of 22% compared to placebo (Hemila, 1997a). Some authorities have called these effects minor at best (AMA, 1986). Significant reductions in incidence of pneumonia with ascorbic acid supple-mentation have been reported in 3 studies, including a random-ized, double-blind, placebo-controlled trial (Hemila, 1997b).

Fluorosis

A combination of calcium, ascorbic acid, and vitamin D_3 reversed dental, clinical, and early skeletal fluorosis in children in a double-

blind, placebo-controlled study. Twenty-five children (aged 6 to 12 years) living in an area where the drinking water contained 4.5 mg fluoride/liter were administered either placebo (n=10) or ascorbic acid 250 mg and calcium compound (125 mg elemental calcium) twice a day and vitamin D_3 60,000 IU once a week (n=15) for 180 days. Intake of fluoride-rich water continued as usual. At the end of the treatment period, there was significant improvement in dental, clinical, and skeletal grades of fluorosis in the treated children (p<0.05) but not in the placebo group. There were significantly reduced fluoride levels in the blood and serum and increased urinary fluoride levels in the treated group (p<0.05 for all 3 parameters) but not in the placebo group, indicating increased removal of fluoride from the body. The results of this small study indicate that calcium, ascorbic acid, and vitamin D_3 supplementation can reverse fluorosis in children (Gupta et al, 1996).

Hypertension

Oral ascorbic acid reduced blood pressure and arterial stiffness in patients with type 2 diabetes. In a randomized, double-blind, placebo-controlled trial, 30 patients (aged 45 to 70 years) with type 2 diabetes that was controlled with diet or hypoglycemic agents received either placebo or oral ascorbic acid 500 mg daily. After 4 weeks of treatment, mean brachial systolic pressure was reduced from 142 to 132 mm Hg in the ascorbic acid group (p=0.001 in comparison to baseline), and brachial diastolic pres-sure was reduced from 83.9 to 79.5 (p=0.003 in comparison to baseline). In the placebo group, blood pressure was not changed. The difference between treatments was statistically significant (p<0.001). The aortic augmentation index and the time to wave reflection, both indicators of aortic stiffness, showed improve-ment in the ascorbic acid group but not in the placebo group. Differences between treatments were significant (p=0.026 and p<0.01, respectively) (Mullan et al, 2002).

Vitamin C reduced daytime ambulatory but not nighttime blood pressure in older persons with hypertension; blood pressure of normotensive older persons was unaffected. In a double-blind, randomized, placebo-controlled crossover study (1 week washout between treatments), 40 nonsmokers between the ages of 60 and 80 years took ascorbic acid 250 mg twice daily or placebo, each for 3 months. Within the group of 17 participants who were hyperten-sive (systolic blood pressure 140 mm Hg or greater), SBP decreased significantly, by 3.7 mm Hg (95% confidence interval 1.5 to 5.9 mm Hg), with ascorbic acid treatment. Ascorbic acid treatment also increased HDL cholesterol in women but not in men (Fotherby et al, 2000).

Ascorbic acid 500 mg per day reduced systolic, diastolic, and mean blood pressure in healthy hypertensive individuals. In a randomized, double-blind trial, 39 hypertensive patients were given ascorbic acid 500 mg or placebo for 1 month. At the end of treatment, systolic blood pressure had been reduced from 155 to 142 mm Hg in the ascorbic acid group (p<0.001) and mean blood pressure from 110 to 100 mm Hg (p<0.001). The changes were significantly greater than those in the placebo group (p=0.03 and p=0.02, respectively). Heart rate was not affected by ascorbic acid treatment (Duffy et al, 1999).

Trauma Support

Early administration of vitamin C and vitamin E to critically ill patients who had experienced trauma or were to undergo surgery reduced the incidence of multiple organ failure and the length of time required in the intensive care unit (ICU). Eligible patients (n=595) were randomized within 24 hours of injury or emergency operation to receive antioxidant supplementation or standard care. d,l-alpha-tocopheryl acetate 1000 IU was given by naso- or orogastric tube every 8 hours, and ascorbic acid 1000 mg was given intravenously in 100 mL D5W (5% dextrose in water) every 8 hours for the shorter of either 28 days or the time in the ICU. The relative risk of pulmonary morbidity (acute respiratory distress syndrome or pneumonia) in patients receiving antioxidants was 0.81 (95% confidence interval (CI) 0.6-1.1). The relative risk of multiple organ failure was 0.43 (95% CI, 0.19-0.96). Patients in the antioxidant group required 1.2 fewer days in the ICU (95% CI, 0.81-1.5) and 0.4 fewer days in the hospital (95% CI: -0.2- 1.0). There were no difference between groups in occurrence of renal failure, and there were no other adverse effects attributable to the antioxidants (Nathens et al, 2002).

INDICATIONS AND USAGE
FDA-approved:

- Prophylaxis of Vitamin C deficiency
- Iron absorption.

Unproven Uses: Vitamin C has been used in the prevention of heart disease, pneumonia, sunburn, and hyperlipidemia, and for cancer prevention, muscle soreness, asthma, common cold, erythema (after CO2 laser skin resurfacing), fluorosis, wound healing after severe trauma, and as an antioxidant.

PRECAUTIONS AND ADVERSE REACTIONS
Avoid rapid intravenous injections. Adverse effects of parenteral vitamin C include faintness or dizziness, hemolysis, renal failure, and injection site pain. Adverse effects of oral vitamin C include diarrhea, esophagitis (rare), and intestinal obstruction (rare).

Use cautiously in patients with preexisting kidney stone disease, erythrocyte G6PD deficiency, hemochromatosis, thalassemia, or sideroblastic anemia.

Avoid supplemental vitamin C before conducting laboratory examinations for acetaminophen, AST (SGOT), bilirubin, carbamazepine, creatinine, glucose, LDH, stool guiac, theophylline, and uric acid.

Drug Interactions
Antacids: Increased risk of aluminum toxicity with concomitant use. *Clinical Management:* Concurrent administration is not recommended, especially in patients with renal insufficiency. If concurrent use cannot be avoided, monitor patients for possible acute aluminum toxicity (e.g., encephalopathy, seizures, or coma) and adjust the doses accordingly.

Aspirin: Increased ascorbic requirements with concomitant use. *Clinical Management:* Increased dietary or supplemental vitamin C intake (100 to 200 mg daily) should be considered for patients on chronic high-dose aspirin.

Cyanocobalmin: Reduced the absorption and bioavailability of cyanocobalmin with concomitant use. *Clinical Management:* Vitamin C should be administered 2 or more hours after a meal.

DOSAGE
Mode of Administration: oral, intramuscular, intravenous

How Supplied: capsule, injectable, lozenge, solution, tablet

Daily Dosage: The following chart lists the Recommended Dietary Allowance (RDA) for vitamin C. Individuals who smoke require an additional 35 mg/day of vitamin C over the established RDA.

Age	Males	Females	Pregnancy	Lactation
0 to 6 months	40 mg/day	40 mg/day		
7 to 12 months	50 mg/day	50 mg/day		
1 to 3 years	15 mg/day	15 mg/day		
4 to 8 years	25 mg/day	25 mg/day		
9 to 13 years	45 mg/day	45 mg/day	80 mg/day	115 mg/day
14 to 18 years	75 mg/day	65 mg/day	80 mg/day	115 mg/day
19 years and older	90 mg/day	75 mg/day	85 mg/day	120 mg/day

ADULTS

Oral

Antioxidant effects: 120 to 450 mg/day (Girodon et al, 1997; Clemens et al, 1997).

Asthma: 500 to 2000 mg/day or prior to exercise (Cohen et al, 1997; Bielory & Gandhi, 1994).

Atherosclerosis prevention: 45 to 1000 mg/day (Jialal & Fuller, 1995; Gale et al, 1995; Kritchevsky et al, 1995).

Delayed-onset muscle soreness: 3000 mg/day (Kaminski & Boal, 1992).

Gastric cancer: 50 mg/day (Anon, 1993).

Histamine detoxification: 2000 mg/day (Johnston et al, 1992).

Hypercholesterolemia: 300 to 3000 mg/day (Simon, 1992).

Respiratory Infection: 1000 to 2000 mg/day (Hemila, 1997a; Hemila, 1997b).

Scurvy: The recommended dose for the treatment of scurvy is 1 to 2 g administered intravenously or orally for the first 2 days, then 500 mg intravenously or orally daily for a week (Oeffinger, 1993). However, the AMA recommends 100 mg 3 times a day for 1 week then 100 mg daily for several weeks until tissue saturation is normal (AMA, 1990).

Sunburn prevention: 2000 mg/day (Eberlein-Konig et al, 1998).

Urine acidification: 3 to 12 g/day titrated to desired effect (Krupp & Chatton, 1980) and given as divided doses every 4 hours (AMA, 1980).

Wound healing: 1000 to 1500 mg/day (Mazzotta, 1994).

Intramuscular

Scurvy: The recommended dose for the treatment of scurvy in adults and children is 100 mg 3 times a day for 1 week, then 100 mg daily for several weeks until tissue saturation is normal. This dosage can be administered intramuscularly, intravenously, or orally (AMA, 1990).

Vitamin deficiency: 100 to 500 milligrams/day (Krupp & Chatton, 1980).

Intravenous

Cancer: A dosing protocol for adjunctive therapy for cancer, based on more than 20 years of experience and isolated case reports (Riordan et al, 2003) is as follows: By intravenous (IV) drip (not push) week 1: 15 g/d IV 2 to 3 times/week ; week 2: 30 g/day IV 2 to 3 times/week; week 3: 65 g/day IV 2 to 3 times/week; week 4: 100 g/day IV 2 to 3 times/week; The dose should then be adjusted to achieve transient plasma concentrations of 400 mg/dL, or 200 mg/dL if lipoic acid (300 mg twice daily) is also being given. This protocol should be continued for at least a year. Patients are advised to supplement orally with at least 5 g daily when no infusion is given to maintain basal tissue levels and to prevent a rare but possible rebound scurvy.

Scurvy: The recommended dose for the treatment of scurvy is 1 to 2 g administered intravenously or orally for the first 2 days then 500 mg orally or intravenously daily for a week (Oeffinger, 1993). However, the American Medical Association recommends 100 mg 3 times a day for 1 week then 100 mg daily for several weeks until tissue saturation is normal (AMA, 1990).

Topical

Topical wound healing, skin erythema, aqueous solution: 10% solution applied once daily (Alster & West, 1998).

PEDIATRICS

Oral

The recommended prophylactic dose for infants on formula feedings is 35 mg/day orally or intramuscularly for the first few weeks of life. If the formula contains 2 to 3 times the amount of protein in human milk, the dose should be 50 mg/day orally or intramuscularly (AMA, 1980).

Infants and children require 30 to 60 mg of crystalline ascorbic acid daily. This may be taken as oral tablets or as part of the normal diet (i.e., 2 to 4 oz. of orange juice) (AMA, 1980).

Flourosis: 500 mg/day (Gupta et al, 1996).

Scurvy: The recommended dose for the treatment of scurvy in adults and children is 100 mg 3 times a day for 1 week, then 100 mg daily for several weeks until tissue saturation is normal. The regimen may be administered intramuscularly, intravenously, or orally (AMA, 1990).

Intramuscular

Scurvy: See Adult Dosage. The recommended prophylactic dose for infants on formula feedings is 35 mg/day orally or intramuscularly for the first few weeks of life. If the formula contains 2 to 3 times the amount of protein in human milk, the dose should be 50 mg/day orally or intramuscularly (AMA, 1980).

Intravenous

Scurvy: See Adult Dosage. In patients 17 years and younger, ascorbic acid should be diluted in at least an equal volume of fluid and infused over a minimum of 10 minutes. Direct intravenous push is not recommended. The final solution should be protected from light (Anon, 1984). The maximum recommended intravenous dose for ascorbic acid in pediatric patients (17 years and younger) is 100 mg/kg/day up to 6 g/day (Anon, 1984).

LITERATURE

Alster TS & West TB. Effect of topical vitamin C on postoperative carbon dioxide laser resurfacing erythema. *Dermatol Surg*; 24(3):331-334. 1998

AMA Council on Drugs. AMA Drug Evaluations, 4th ed. American Medical Association, Chicago, IL, USA, 1980.

AMA. AMA Drug Evaluations Subscription, vol 2. American Medical Association, Chicago, IL, USA, 1990.

AMA Department of Drugs. AMA Drug Evaluations, 6th ed. American Medical Association, Chicago, IL, USA, 1986.

Angel J, Alfred B, Leichfter J et al. Effect of oral administration of large quantities of ascorbic acid on blood levels and urinary excretion of ascorbic acid in healthy men. *J Vitam Nutr Res*; 45(2):237-243. 1975

Anon. "Little doubt" over gastric cancer link with diet low in vitamin C. *Pharm J*; 830. 1993

Anon. Guidelines for Administration of Intravenous Medications to Pediatric Patients, 2nd ed. American Society of Hospital Pharmacists, Bethesda, MD, USA, 1984a.

Clemens MR, Waladkhani AR, Bublitz K et al. Supplementation with antioxidants prior to bone marrow transplantation. *Wien Klin Wochenschr*; 109(19):771-776. 1997

Cohen HA, Neuman I & Nahum H. Blocking effect of vitamin C in exercise-induced asthma. *Arch Pediatr Adolesc Med*; 151(4):367-370. 1997

Dawson EB, Harris WA, Rankin WE et al. Effect of ascorbic acid on male infertility. *Ann NY Acad Sci*; 498:312-323. 1987

Duffy SJ, Gokce N, Holbrook M et al. Treatment of hypertension with ascorbic acid (letter). *Lancet*; 354(9195):2048-2049. 1999

Fotherby MD, Williams JC, Forster LA et al. Effect of vitamin C on ambulatory blood pressure and plasma lipids in older persons. *J Hypertens*; 18(4):411-415. 2000

Gale CR, Martyn CN, Winter PD et al. Vitamin C and risk of death from stroke and coronary heart disease in cohorts of elderly people. *BMJ*; 310(6994):1563-1566. 1995

Girodon F, Blache D, Monget AL et al. Effect of a two-year supplementation with low doses of antioxidant vitamins and/or minerals in elderly subjects on levels of nutrients and antioxidant defense parameters. *J Am Coll Nutr*; 16(4):357-365. 1997

Gupta SK, Gupta RC, Seth AK et al. Reversal of fluorosis in children. *Acta Paediatr Jpn*; 38(5):513-519. 1996

Hemila H. Vitamin C intake and susceptibility. *Pediatr Infect Dis J*; 16(9):836-837. 1997b

Hemila H. Vitamin C supplementation and the common cold - was Linus Pauling right or wrong? *Int J Vitam Nutr Res*; 67(5):329-335. 1997a

Jialal I & Fuller CJ. Effect of vitamin E, vitamin C and beta-carotene on LDL oxidation and atherosclerosis. *Can J Cardiol*; 11(suppl G):97G-103G. 1995

Johnston CS, Retrum KR & Srilakshmi JC. Antihistamine effects and complications of supplemental vitamin C. *J Am Diet Assoc*; 92(8):988-989. 1992

Kaminski M & Boal R. An effect of ascorbic acid on delayed-onset muscle soreness. *Pain*; 50(3):317-321. 1992

Kodama H, Yamaguchi R, Fukuda J et al. Increased oxidative deoxyribonucleic acid damage in the spermatozoa of infertile male patients. *Fertil Steril*; 68(3):519-524. 1997

Kritchevsky SB, Shimikawa T, Tell GS et al. Dietary antioxidants and carotid artery wall thickness: the ARIC Study. *Circulation*; 92(8):2142-2150. 1995

Krupp MA & Chatton MJ. Current Medical Diagnosis and Treatment. Lange Medical Publications, Los Altos, CA, USA, 1980.

Mazzotta MY. Nutrition and wound healing. *J Am Podiatr Med Assoc*; 84(9):456-462. 1994

Mullan BA, Young IS, Fee H et al. Ascorbic acid reduces blood pressure and arterial stiffness in type 2 diabetes. *Hypertension*; 40:804-809. 2002

Nathens AB, Neff MJ, Jurkovich GJ et al. Randomized, prospective trial of antioxidant supplementation in critically ill surgical patients. *Ann Surg*;236(6):814-822. 2002

Nyyssonen K, Parviainen MT, Salonen R et al. Vitamin C deficiency and risk of myocardial infarction: prospective population study of men from eastern Finland. *BMJ*; 314(7081):634-638. 1997

Oeffinger KC. Scurvy: more than historical relevance. *Am Fam Physician*; 48(4):609-613. 1993

Riordan HD, Hunninghake RB, Riordan NH et al. Intravenous ascorbic acid: protocol for its application and use. *Puerto Rico Health Sci J*; 22(3):2003. 2003

Schorah CJ, Tormey WP, Brooks GH et al. The effect of vitamin C supplement on body weight, serum proteins, and general health of an elderly populatin. *Am J Clin Nutr*; 34(5):871-876. 1981

Simon JA. Vitamin C and cardiovascular disease: a review. *J Am Coll Nutr*, 11(2):107-125. 1992

Vilter RW. Nutritional aspects of ascorbic acid: uses and abuses. *West J Med*; 133(6):485-492. 1980

White JD: No ill effects from high-dose vitamin C (letter). *N Engl J Med*; 304(24):1491-1492. 1981

Will JC & Byers T. Does diabetes mellitus increase the requirement for vitamin C? *Nutr Rev*; 54(7):193-202. 11. 1996

Zandi PP, Anthony JC, Khachaturian AS et al. Reduced risk of Alzheimer disease in users of antioxidant vitamin supplements. *Arch Neurol*; 61:82-88. 2004

Vitamin E

DESCRIPTION

Vitamin E is a fat-soluble vitamin chemically known as tocopherol. Vitamin E is extremely versatile in both preventive and therapeutic applications, though it is rarely used alone. In prevention, vitamin E may be the most important nutrient supplement, as apparently effective doses are quite beyond maximum dietary intake. Vitamin E appears to be extremely safe, except when normal coagulation mechanisms are impaired. While the synthetic vitamin has been effective when used in clinical trials, the natural stereoisomer may be superior in bioavailability.

Several forms of vitamin E exist: Alpha-tocopherol (Farrell & Roberts, 1994); d-alpha tocopherol (also termed RRR-alpha tocopherol) is an unesterified natural product derived from soybean oil; d-alpha tocopheryl (acetate or succinate) is an esterified form of the natural product; dl-alpha tocopheryl (acetate or succinate) is an esterified form of synthetic vitamin E (also termed all-rac-alpha tocopherol). Mixed tocopherols is a mixture of unesterified natural isomers including alpha, beta, delta, and gamma tocopherol.

Tocopherol Equivalents (Farrell & Roberts, 1994):

1 mg dl-alpha tocopheryl acetate = 1 IU
1 mg dl-alpha tocopherol = 1.1 IU
1 mg d-alpha tocopheryl acetate = 1.36 IU
1 mg d-alpha tocopherol = 1.49 IU
1 mg d-alpha tocopheryl acid succinate = 1.21 IU
1 mg dl-alpha tocopheryl acid succinate = 0.89 IU

Other Names: Alpha-tocopherol, D-alpha tocopherol, D-alpha tocopheryl acid succinate, Dl-alpha tocopheryl acetate, D-alpha tocopherol,Dl-alpha tocopheryl acid succinate, D-alpha tocopheryl acetate

ACTIONS AND PHARMACOLOGY
EFFECTS

Vitamin E has antioxidant, immunomodulation, and antiplatelet effects.

Antioxidant Effects: Vitamin E appears to act as an antioxidant within membranes by preventing propagated oxidation of unsaturated fatty acids (Spielberg et al, 1979). Vitamin E is hypothesized to reduce atherosclerosis and subsequent coronary heart disease by preventing oxidative changes to low-density lipoproteins (LDL). Oxidized LDL particles are more readily converted by macrophages than native LDL to the cholesterol-loaded foam cells found in the fatty streak of early atherosclerosis. Atherogenesis may also be promoted by oxidized LDL's chemotactic action on monocytes, its cytotoxicity to endothelial cells, its stimulation of the release of growth factors and cytokines, its immunogenicity, and its possible arterial vasoconstrictor actions (Rimm et al, 1993; Stampfer et al, 1993).

Immunomodulating Effects: Vitamin E appears to enhance lymphocyte proliferation, decrease production of immunosuppressive prostaglandin E2, and decrease levels of immunosuppressive serum lipid peroxides (Meydani, 1995b).

Antiplatelet Effects: Vitamin E inhibits platelet adhesion measured in a laminar flow chamber using blood from patients who have taken vitamin E supplements. This effect appears to be related to a reduction in the development of pseudopodia, which normally occurs upon platelet activation. This effect of vitamin E may be related to changes in fatty acylation of structural platelet proteins. Although vitamin E inhibits platelet aggregation in vitro, its effect in vivo has not been consistently shown. Thromboembolic disease may be prevented with vitamin E supplementation (Calzada et al, 1997; Steiner, 1993).

Platelet Adhesion Effects: Vitamin E administration at 200 IU daily for 2 weeks has resulted in reduction of platelet adhesion by 44% to 75%. After an additional 2 weeks at a dose of 400 IU, platelet adhesion reduction was 77% to 82% (Steiner, 1993; Jandak et al, 1989). A related study found no dose-dependent downward trend in platelet adhesion at vitamin E doses between 400 IU and 1600 IU (Jandak et al, 1988). The effects of vitamin E on platelet adhesion appear to be independent of the effects of aspirin on platelet aggregation (Steiner et al, 1995).

CLINICAL TRIALS
Alzheimer's Disease

Vitamin C and vitamin E supplements in combination were associated with reduced prevalence and incidence of Alzheimer's disease (AD) in a cross-sectional, prospective study. A population of 4,740 adults 65 years of age and older were assessed for cognitive status, and their use of vitamin supplements was determined. Vitamin C users were those who took at least 500 mg of ascorbic acid, either as a single supplement or as part of a multivitamin preparation. Vitamin E users were defined as those who took a multivitamin preparation or an individual vitamin E supplement providing more than 400 IU per day. Multiple vitamin users were those whose preparation provided lower amounts of vitamin E and vitamin C. There were 200 prevalent cases of AD in the starting population. At the end of follow-up (up to 5 years), there were 104 incident cases of AD and 3,123 subjects who were free of dementia. The group of 1,429 people lost to follow-up comprised individuals who were older, less educated, and had performed less well on their cognitive screen than those who completed the protocol. Hence, AD incidence during the follow-up period may have been underestimated. After adjustment for age, sex, education, and apolipoprotein E genotype, prevalence analysis showed a significant inverse relation between prevalence of AD and vitamin E and multivitamin use. Vitamin E alone, vitamin C alone, or vitamin C in combination with multivitamins were not associated with AD prevalence. The strongest association was with the combination of vitamin E and vitamin C, with or without multivitamins (multivariate adjusted odds ratio, 0.22; 95% confidence interval (CI), 0.05 to 0.6). The combination of vitamin E and vitamin C also apparently reduced incidence (adjusted hazard ratio, 0.36; 95% CI, 0.09 to 0.99). For incidence, associations were not significant for vitamin E alone, vitamin C alone, multivitamin use alone or in combination (Zandi et al, 2004).

In an epidemiological study of elderly Japanese-American men, long-term use of vitamin E and/or vitamin C was associated with reduced incidence of vascular and mixed dementia and with higher cognitive function among those without dementia; however, there was no effect of vitamin usage on frequency of development of Alzheimer's dementia. Supplemental vitamin use was determined from an examination given between 1980 and 1982 and again in a questionnaire administered in 1988. Cognitive function and dementia were assessed between 1991 and 1993. Combined vitamin E and C supplement use was associated with an 88% reduction in the frequency of subsequent vascular dementia. Use of either vitamin resulted in better cognitive performance among non-demented subjects (OR, 1.25, 95% confidence interval, 0.995 to 1.5) (Masaki et al, 2000).

Antioxidation

Supplementation of vitamin E intake of smokers decreased susceptibility of their erythrocytes to hydrogen peroxide-induced lipid peroxidation. Fifty male smokers were given daily supplements of 70, 140, 560, or 1050 mg of d-alpha-tocopheryl acetate for 20 weeks. Erythrocyte vitamin E levels rose in a dose-dependent manner, and peroxidizability of erythrocytes decreased significantly with each dose (p<0.001). Nonsmokers also showed decreased erythrocyte peroxidizability with increasing vitamin E, except at the 1050-mg dose, at which they displayed significantly increased peroxidizability (p<0.001). Increases in red-cell vitamin E were associated with decreases in plasma ascorbate. The percentage increase in red cell peroxidizability was positively correlated with the percentage decrease in plasma ascorbate (r=0.767, p<0.001) in nonsmokers consuming 1050 mg d-alpha-tocopheryl acetate daily for 20 weeks (Brown et al, 1997).

Supplementation with antioxidant vitamins, including vitamin E, prior to conditioning therapy (chemotherapy and radiation) for bone marrow transplantation resulted in less of a rise in plasma lipid hydroperoxides than did conditioning therapy without presupplementation. Sixteen patients with leukemia were supplemented with alpha-tocopherol 825 mg, beta-carotene 45 mg, and ascorbic acid 450 mg for 3 weeks before beginning conditioning therapy. Ten other patients received conditioning therapy without supplementation with antioxidant vitamins. The rise in plasma lipid hydroperoxide level between the start of conditioning therapy and the completion of transplantation was from 20.1 to 36.2 mmol/liter in the supplemented group and from 23.3 to 83.5 mmol/liter in the unsupplemented group. The increase was significant (p<0.05) only in the unsupplemented group. Conditioning therapy causes delayed toxic effects in several tissues, which are thought to be caused by free-radical damage. The authors

speculated that reducing lipid peroxide formation may reduce the toxicity of conditioning therapy (Clemens et al, 1997).

The addition of vitamin E to aspirin therapy reduced the incidence of ischemic cerebrovascular events among patients with a history of transient ischemic attacks (TIAs). One hundred TIA patients randomly received either aspirin 325 mg per day plus placebo or aspirin plus vitamin E 400 IU daily in a double-blind fashion. After 2 years, the aspirin-only group had experienced 6 ischemic attacks and 2 recurrent TIAs while the combination treatment group experienced 1 ischemic attack and 1 recurrent TIA (p less than 0.05). There was no difference in incidence of hemorrhagic events (Steiner et al, 1995).

Atherosclerosis

The combination of vitamin E and vitamin C slowed the progression of atherosclerosis in hypercholesterolemic subjects. In the Antioxidant Supplementation in Atherosclerosis Prevention (ASAP) study, 520 smoking and nonsmoking men and postmenopausal women aged 45 to 69 years with serum cholesterol above 193 mg/dL were stratified by sex and smoking habits and then randomly assigned to receive twice daily, with a meal, alpha-tocopherol 91 mg (136 IU of vitamin E), slow-release ascorbic acid (vitamin C) 250 mg, the combination of both vitamin doses, or placebo. Administration was double-blinded for 3 years. At the end of 3 years, all supplemented subjects were eligible to continue open supplementation with the combination for 3 more years. The placebo subjects continued without supplementation. Four hundred forty subjects were included in the intent-to-treat analysis at 6 years. Over 6 years, the mean annual increase in the common carotid artery intima-media thickness (CCA-IMT) (difference of first and last measures) was 0.0162 mm/yr in nonsupplemented males and 0.0103 mm/yr in supplemented males, a 37% treatment effect (p=0.028). In women, CCA-IMT increased 0.0111 mm/yr in the nonsupplemented group and 0.0102 in the supplemented group (p=0.625), a 14% treatment effect (not significant). When the first and second 3-year periods were compared, the treatment effect in men was significant only in the second period (p=0.029). The treatment effect was greater in subjects who already had plaques at baseline than in those without. The treatment effect was principally confined to subjects who had baseline plasma vitamin C levels below the median (less than 71 mmol/liter) (Salonen et al, 2003).

Platelet Aggregation

Vitamin E at daily dosages of 400 IU to 1200 IU for 6 weeks produced no significant effects on platelet aggregation induced by collagen, ADP, or epinephrine in a controlled study of 47 healthy volunteers (Steiner, 1983). However, another controlled study of 40 healthy subjects found that vitamin E 300 mg daily for 8 weeks significantly decreased platelet aggregation in response to ADP and arachidonic acid, increased platelet sensitivity to inhibition by PGE1, decreased plasma beta-thromboglobulin concentration, and decreased ATP secretion (Calzada et al, 1997).

Cardiovascular Disease, Prevention of

A meta-analysis of large studies investigating the use of vitamin E for the prevention of cardiovascular disease showed no benefit relative to placebo for mortality. Seven trials involving vitamin E alone or in combination with other antioxidants were analyzed. Daily doses of vitamin E ranged from 50 IU to 800 IU. Duration of studies ranged from 1.4 to 12 years. All studies were randomized, placebo-controlled trials with intention-to-treat analyses and included 1,000 or more subjects each (total number of subjects = 81,788). Vitamin E did not lower all-cause mortality (11.3% vs

11.1%; odds ratio (OR) 1.02, 95% confidence interval (CI) 0.98-1.06) or cardiovascular mortality (6.0% vs 6.0%; OR 1, 95% CI 0.96-1.06) relative to placebo. The incidence of cerebrovascular accidents did not differ between vitamin E-treated and placebo-treated patients (3.6% vs 3.5%; OR 1.02, 95% CI 0.92-1.12). When primary and secondary prevention studies were analyzed separately, no improvement in all-cause mortality was observed with vitamin E treatment for either category (Vivekananthan et al, 2003).

Higher dietary intake of vitamin E and high plasma levels of vitamin E were weakly associated with lowered risk of atherosclerosis in men but not in women. No benefit was seen from supplemental antioxidant vitamin use. In a study of more than 1,000 asymptomatic subjects, with equal numbers in age deciles of 27 to 77 years, the relationships of carotid intima-media wall thickness (IMT) and focal plaque to dietary intake of antioxidant vitamins and plasma vitamin concentrations were examined. In men, there was a progressive decrease in mean IMT with increasing quartiles of dietary vitamin E intake (p=0.02) and a nonsignificant trend for women (p=0.10). There were no significant relationships between dietary vitamin A, beta-carotene, or vitamin C and IMT. Plasma levels of lycopene were inversely correlated with mean carotid artery IMT in women (p=0.047). The prevalence of carotid artery plaque decreased with increasing quartiles of dietary vitamin E in women (p=0.03), but there was no significant association between plaque and dietary intake of any antioxidant vitamin in men. The prevalence of carotid artery plaque decreased with increasing plasma levels of alpha-carotene (p=0.03) and lycopene (p=0.001) in women and with vitamin A (p=0.02) and lycopene (p=0.001) in men. However, when adjusted for other risk factors (eg, age, smoking, hypertension, total energy intake), there were no residual associations between any dietary or plasma antioxidant vitamins or supplemental vitamin use and the risk of focal plaque in men and women (McQuillan et al, 2001).

High-dose vitamin E from natural sources (400 IU daily) for an average of 4.5 years did not reduce the incidence of cardiovascular events in subjects at high risk. In a double-blind, randomized, 2-by-2 factorial design study (the Heart Outcomes Prevention Evaluation (HOPE) Study), 9,541 subjects were given vitamin E (from natural sources) or placebo and ramipril or placebo. Primary cardiovascular events (myocardial infarction, stroke, and death from cardiovascular causes) occurred in 16.2% of patients who received vitamin E and 15.5% of those who received placebo (relative risk 1.05; 95 percent confidence interval, 0.95 to 1.16). There were no significant differences due to vitamin E treatment for any of the specific cardiovascular events. Likewise, there were no differences due to vitamin E with respect to secondary outcomes (death from any cause, unstable angina, congestive heart failure, revascularization or limb amputation, nephropathy or the need for dialysis) (Anon, 2000).

INDICATIONS AND USAGE
Accepted Uses: Supplementation is indicated for prevention and treatment of vitamin E deficiency. However, dietary improvement is preferred for prophylaxis, while vitamin E supplements are preferred for treating a deficiency (USP DI 2004).

Unproven Uses: Vitamin E is used to prevent coronary heart disease, ischemic cerebrovascular events (in conjunction with aspirin), and cancer of the oropharynx, prostate, and upper gastrointestinal tract. Vitamin E is also used to prevent exercise-induced tissue damage, nitrate tolerance, sunburn, some types of senile cataracts, other cancers, as well as to enhance immune function in the elderly, intermittent claudication, osteoarthritis, and some types of male infertility. Along with other therapies,

vitamin E may be an important adjunctive treatment in Alzheimer's disease, diabetes, hemodialysis, premenstrual syndrome, tardive dyskinesia, and some cases of variant angina. Conditions such as dysmenorrhea, epilepsy, fibromyalgia, rheumatoid arthritis, and vasomotor menopausal symptoms may respond to vitamin E, but further investigation is needed into these applications.

CONTRAINDICATIONS
Oral use is contraindicated in coagulation disorders or anticoagulant therapy. Topical use is contraindicated after recent chemical peel or dermabrasion.

PRECAUTIONS AND ADVERSE REACTIONS
Thrombophlebitis has been reported in patients at risk of small-vessel disease who were taking 400 IU or more. In patients with blood clotting disorders or those taking anticoagulant medication, bleeding time should be monitored (Kappus & Diplock, 1992)

Drug Interactions
Anticoagulants: Concomitant use may potentiate the effect of anticoagulants. *Clinical Management:* Concomitant use of oral anticoagulants and vitamin E should be avoided if possible. If these drugs are used together, monitor carefully.

Colestipol: Concomitant use may reduce vitamin E absorption. *Clinical Management:* Since colestipol may interfere with absorption of vitamin E, try to separate administration of doses as much as possible.

Orlistat: Concomitant use may reduce vitamin E absorption. *Clinical Management:* Patients should be instructed to space the administration of orlistat and vitamin E by at least two hours.

OVERDOSAGE
Vitamin E plasma concentrations greater than 3.5 mg/dL may result in toxicity (Lemons & Maisels, 1985). Prolonged vitamin E plasma levels of approximately 4.5 mg/dL were associated with an increased incidence of bacterial sepsis and necrotizing enterocolitis (Meyers et al, 1986).

DOSAGE
Mode of Administration: Oral, topical, intramuscular

How Supplied: Tablet, capsule, ointment, suspension

Daily Dosage: 1 mg of alpha-tocopherol is approximately equal to 1.5 International Units (IU). Recommended Dietary Allowance (RDA): *adults and adolescents 14 years and older* — 15 mg (22 IU) daily. *During pregnancy* — 15 mg/day; *during lactation* — 19 mg/day. *Infants and children: 0 to 6 months* — 4 mg/day; *7 to 12 months* — 5 mg/day; *1 to 3 years* — 6 mg/day; *4 to 8 years* — 7 mg/day; *9 to 13 years* — 11 mg/day.

ADULTS

Deficiency: 32 to 50 mg daily. The usual oral dose for vitamin E deficiency is 4 to 5 times the RDA. Doses as high as 300 mg may be necessary (Gilman et al, 1985; Alpers et al, 1983).

Alzheimer's disease: 2000 IU daily (Sano et al, 1997).

Anemia in hemodialysis patients: 500 mg/day (Cristol et al, 1997).

Angina pectoris: 50 to 300 mg/day (Rapola et al, 1996; Miwa et al, 1996).

Antioxidant effects: 100 to 800 mg/day (Brown et al, 1997; Clemens et al, 1997; Girodon, et al, 1997; Prieme et al, 1997).

Antiplatelet effects: 200 to 400 IU/day (Calzada et al, 1997; Steiner, 1993).

Cerebrovascular disease: 400 IU/day with aspirin 325 mg/day (Steiner et al, 1995).

Colorectal cancer prevention: 50 mg/day (Anon, 1994).

Coronary heart disease prevention: 100 to 800 IU/day (Kushi et al, 1996; Azen et al, 1996; Stephens et al, 1996; Takamatsu et al, 1995; Rimm et al, 1993; Stampfer et al, 1993).

Cystic fibrosis: 50 mg/day for correction of anemia (Anon, 1988; Nasr et al, 1993).

Diabetes: 100 to 900 IU/day for improving glucose tolerance and reducing protein glycation in insulin-dependent (and some non-insulin dependent) diabetics (Jain et al, 1996; Duntas et al, 1996; Paolisso et al, 1993; Paolisso et al, 1993a).

Dysmenorrhea: 150 mg/day (Butler & McKnight, 1955).

Exercise-induced tissue damage, prevention: 500 to 1200 IU/day (McBride et al, 1998; Rokitzki et al, 1994; Meydani et al, 1993).

Exercise performance at high altitude: 400 mg/day (Simon-Schnass & Pabst, 1988).

Fibromyalgia: 300 IU/day (Steinberg, 1949).

Immune system support in geriatric patients: 200 mg daily (Meydani et al, 1997).

Infertility, male: 200 to 300 mg/day (Kodama et al, 1997; Suleiman et al, 1996; Geva et al, 1996).

Intermittent claudication: 600 to 1600 mg/day (Piesse, 1984; Williams et al, 1971; Williams et al, 1962; Livingstone & Jones, 1958).

Menopause: 75 to 100 mg/day (Finkler, 1949; Rubenstein, 1948).

Nitrate tolerance: 600 mg/day (Watanabe et al, 1997).

Oral leukoplakia and oropharyngeal cancer (prevention): 800 IU/day (Benner et al, 1993; Gridley et al, 1992). Osteoarthritis: 400 to 1200 IU/day (Scherak et al, 1990; Blankenhorn, 1986; Machtey & Ouaknine, 1978).

Premenstrual symptoms: 150 to 600 IU/day (London et al, 1987; London et al, 1983a; London et al, 1983b).

Prostate cancer, prevention: 50 mg/day (Heinonen et al, 1998; Anon, 1994).

Rheumatoid arthritis: 800 to 1200 IU/day (Edmonds et al, 1997; Kolarz et al, 1990).

Stomach and esophageal cancer, prevention: 30 mg/day with 15 mg beta-carotene and 50 micrograms selenium (Taylor et al, 1994; Blot et al, 1993).

Sunburn, prevention: 1000 IU/day with 2000 mg vitamin C (Eberlein-Konig et al, 1998).

Tardive dyskinesia: 1200 to 1600 IU/day (Lohr & Caligiuri, 1996; Egan et al, 1992; Elkashef et al, 1990; Lohr et al, 1987).

PEDIATRICS

Premature or low-birth-weight neonates: vitamin E 25 to 50 units/day results in normal plasma tocopherol levels in 1 week (Taketomo et al, 2003). (1 unit = 1 mg alpha tocopheryl acetate).

Children with malabsorption syndrome: water-miscible vitamin E 1 unit/kg/day (to raise plasma tocopherol to within the normal range within 2 months and to maintain normal plasma concentrations) (Taketomo et al, 2003).

LITERATURE

Anon: Vitamin E supplementation and cardiovascular events in high-risk patients. *N Engl J Med*; 342(3):154-160. 2000

Anon. Vitamin E therapy in cystic fibrosis. Nutr Rev 1988; 46(8):289-290. 89. Jain SK, McVie R, Jaramillo JJ et al. Effect of modest vitamin E supplementation on blood glycated

hemoglobin and triglyceride levels and red cell indices in type 1 diabetic patients. *J Am Coll Nutr*; 15(5):458-461. 1996

Benner SE, Winn RJ, Lippman SM et al. Regression of oral leukoplakia with alpha-tocopherol: a Community Clinical Oncology Program Chemoprevention study. *J Natl Cancer Inst*; 85(1):44-47. 1993

Blankenhorn G. Clinical effectiveness of Spondyvit (Vitamin E) in activated arthroses: a multicenter placebo-controlled double-blind study (German). *Z Orthop*; 124(3):340-343. 1986

Blot WJ, Li JY, Taylor PR, et al. Nutrition intervention trials in Linxian, China: supplementation with specific vitamin/mineral combinations, cancer incidence, and disease-specific mortality in the general population. *J Natl Cancer Inst*; 85(18):1483-1492. 1993

Brown KM, Morrice PC & Duthie GG. Erythrocyte vitamin E and plasma ascorbate concentrations in relation to erythrocyte peroxidation in smokers and nonsmokers: dose response to vitamin E supplementation. *Am J Clin Nutr*; 65(2):496-502. 1997

Butler EB & McKnight E. Vitamin E in the treatment of primary dysmenorrhea. *Lancet*; 1(Apr Jun 2):844-847. 1955

Calzada C, Bruckdorfer KR, Rice-Evans CA. The influence of antioxidant nutrients on platelet function in healthy volunteers. *Atherosclerosis*; 128(1):97-105. 1997

Clemens MR, Waladkhani AR, Bublitz K et al. Supplementation with antioxidants prior to bone marrow transplantation. *Wien Klin Wochenschr*; 101(19):771-776. 1997

Cristol JP, Bosc JY, Badiou S et al. Erythropoietin and oxidative stress in haemodialysis: beneficial effects of vitamin E supplementation. *Nephrol Dial Transplant*; 12(11):2312-2317. 1997

Duntas L, Kemmer TP, Vorberg B et al. Administration of d-alpha-tocopherol in patients with insulin-dependent diabetes mellitus. *Curr Ther Res Clin Exp*; 57(9):682-690. 1996

Eberlein-Konig B, Placzek M & Przybilla B. Protective effect against sunburn of combined systemic ascorbic acid (vitamin C) and d-alpha-tocopherol (vitamin E). *J Am Acad Dermatol*; 38(1):45-48. 1998

Edmonds SE, Winyard PG, Guo R et al. Putative analgesic activity of repeated oral doses of vitamin E in the treatment of rheumatoid arthritis: results of a prospective placebo controlled double blind trial. *Ann Rheum Dis*; 56(11):649-655. 1997

Egan MF, Hyde TM, Albers GW et al. Treatment of tardive dyskinesia with vitamin E. *Am J Psychiatry*; 149(6):773-777. 1992

Elkashef AM, Ruskin PE, Bacher N et al. Vitamin E in the treatment of tardive dyskinesia. *Am J Psychiatry*; 147(4):505-506. 1990

Farrell PM & Roberts RJ. Vitamin E, in Shils ME, Olsen JA & Shike M (eds): Modern Nutrition in Health and Disease, 8th ed. Lea & Febiger, Philadelphia, PA, USA, 1994:326-341.

Finkler RS. The effect of vitamin E in the menopause. *J Clin Endocrinol Metab*; 9(1):89-94. 1949

Geva E, Bartoov B Zabludovsky N et al. The effect of antioxidant treatment on human spermatazoa and fertilization rate in an in vitro fertilization program. *Fertil Steril*; 66(3):430-434. 1996

Gilman AG, Goodman LS, Rall TW et al (eds). Goodman and Gilman's The Pharmacological Basis of Therapeutics, 7th ed. Macmillan Publishing Co, New York, NY, USA, 1985.

Girodon F, Blache D, Monget AL et al. Effect of a two-year supplementation with low doses of antioxidant vitamins and/or minerals in elderly subjects on levels of nutrients and antioxidant defense parameters. *J Am Coll Nutr*; 16(4):357-365. 1997

Gridley G, McLaughlin JK, Block G et al. Vitamin supplementation use and reduced risk of oral and pharyngeal cancer. *Am J Epidemiol*; 135(10):1083-1092. 1992

Heinonen OP, Albanes D, Virtamo J et al. Prostate cancer and supplementation with alpha-tocopherol and beta-carotene: incidence and mortality in a controlled trial. *J Natl Cancer Inst*; 90(6):440-446. 1998

Kappus H & Diplock AT: Tolerance and safety of vitamin E: a toxicological position report. Free Radic Biol Med 1992; 13(1):55-74.

Kodama H, Yamaguchi R & Fukuda J et al. Increased oxidative deoxyribonucleic acid damage in the spermatozoa of infertile male patients. *Fertil Steril*; 68(3):519-524. 1997

Kolarz G, Scherak O, El-Shohoumi M et al. High dose vitamin E in rheumatoid arthritis (German). *Aktuel Rheumatol*; 15(6):233-237. 1990

Kushi LH, Folsom AR, Prineas RJ et al. Dietary antioxidant vitamins and death from coronary heart disease in postmenopausal women. *N Engl J Med*; 334(18):1156-1162. 1996

Lemons JA & Maisels MJ. Vitamin E-how much is too much? *Pediatrics*; 76(4):625-627. 1985

Livingstone PD & Jones C. Treatment of intermittent claudication with vitamin E. *Lancet*; 2(1 Sept):602-604. 1958

Lohr JB & Caligiuri MP. A double-blind placebo controlled study of vitamin E treatment of tardive dyskinesia. *J Clin Psychiatry*; 57(4):167-173. 1996

Lohr JB, Cadet JL, Lohr MA et al. Alpha-tocopherol in tardive dyskinesia (letter). *Lancet*; 1(8538):213-214. 1987

London RS, Murphy L, Kitlowski KE et al. Efficacy of alpha-tocopherol in the treatment of the premenstrual syndrome. *J Reprod Med*; 32(6):400-404. 1987

London RS, Sundaram GS, Murphy L et al. Evaluation and treatment of breast symptoms in patients with the premenstrual syndrome. *J Reprod Med*; 28(8):503-508. 1983a

London RS, Sundaram GS, Murphy L et al. The effect of alpha-tocopherol on premenstrual symptomatology: a double-blind study. *J Am Coll Nutr*; 2(2):115-122. 1983b

London RS, Sundaram GS, Murphy L et al. The effect of vitamin E on mammary dysplasia: a double-blind study. *Obstet Gynecol*; 65(1):104-106. 1985

Machtey I & Ouaknine L. Tocopherol in osteoarthritis: a controlled pilot study. J Am Geriatr Soc; 26(7):328-330. 1978

McBride JM, Kraemer WJ, Triplett-McBride T et al. Effect of resistance exercise on free radical production. *Med Sci Sports Exerc*; 30(1):67-72. 1998

McQuillan BM, Hung J, Beilby JP et al. Antioxidant vitamins and the risk of carotid atherosclerosis: The Perth Carotid Ultrasound Disease Assessment Study (CUDAS). *J Am Coll Cardiol*; 38(7):1788-1794. 2001

Meydani M, Evans WJ, Handelman et al. Protective effect of vitamin E on exercise-induced oxidative damage in young and older adults. *Am J Physiol*; 264(5 pt 2):R992-R998. 1993

Meydani SN, Meydani M, Blumberg JB et al. Vitamin E supplementation and in vivo immune response in healthy elderly subjects: a randomized controlled trial. *JAMA*; 277(17):1380-1386. 1997

Meydani SN. Vitamin E enhancement of T-cell mediated function in healthy elderly: mechanisms of action. *Nutr Rev*; 53(4 pt 2):S52-S58. 1995b

Miwa K, Miyagi Y, Igawa A et al. Vitamin E deficiency in variant angina. *Circulation*; 94(1):14-18. 1996

Ogunmekan AO. Plasma vitamin E (alpha-tocopherol) levels in normal children and in epileptic children with and without anticonvulsant drug therapy. *Trop Geogr Med*; 37:175-177. 1985

Paolisso G, D'Amore A, Galzerano D et al. Daily vitamin E supplements improve metabolic control but not insulin secretion in elderly type II diabetic patients. *Diabetes Care*; 16(11):1433-1437. 1993a

Paolisso G, D'Amore A, Giugliano D et al. Pharmacologic doses of vitamin E improve insulin action in healthy subjects and non-insulin-dependent diabetic patients. *Am J Clin Nutr*; 57(5):650-656. 1993

Piesse JW. Vitamin E and peripheral vascular disease. *Int Clin Nutr Rev*; 4(4):178-182. 1984

Prieme H, Loft S, Nyssonen K et al. No effect of supplementation with vitamin E, ascorbic acid, or coenzyme Q10 on oxidative DNA damage estimated by 8-oxo-7,8-dihydro-2'-deoxyguanosine excretion in smokers. *Am J Clin Nutr*; 65(2):503-507. 1997

Rapola JM, Virtamo J, Haukka JK et al. Effect of vitamin E and beta carotene on the incidence of angina pectoris: a randomized, double-blind, controlled trial. *JAMA*; 275(9):693-698. 1996

Rimm EB, Stamper MJ, Ascherio A et al: Vitamin E consumption and the risk of coronary heart disease in men. *N Engl J Med*; 328(20):1450-1456. 1993

Rokitzki L, Logemann E, Huber G et al. Alpha-tocopherol supplementation in racing cyclists during extreme endurance *training*. *Int J Sport Nutr*; 4(3):253-264. 1994

Rubenstein BB. Vitamin E diminishes the vasomotor symptoms of menopause (abstract). *Fed Proc*; 7:106. 1948

Salonen RM, Nyyssonen K, Kaikkonen J et al. Six-year effect of combined vitamin C and E supplementation on atherosclerotic progression. *Circulation*; 107:947-953. 2003

Sano M, Ernesto C, Thomas RG et al. A controlled trial of selegiline, alpha-tocopherol, or both as treatment for Alzheimer's disease: the Alzhmeier's Disease Cooperative Study. *N Engl J Med*; 336(17):1216-1222. 1997

Scherak O & Kolarz G. Vitamin E and rheumatoid arthritis (letter). *Arthritis Rheum*; 34(9):1205-1206. 1991

Simon-Schnass I & Pabst H. Influence of vitamin E on physical performance. *Int J Vitam Nutr Res*; 58(1):49-54. 1988

Spielberg SP, Boxer LA, Corash LM et al. Improved erythrocyte survival with high-dose vitamin E in chronic hemolyzing G6PD and glutathione synthetase deficiencies. *Ann Intern Med*; 90(1):53-54. 1979

Stampfer MJ, Hennekens CH, Manson JE et al. Vitamin E consumption and the risk of coronary disease in women. *N Engl J Med*; 328(20):1444-1449. 1993

Steinberg CL. Vitamin E and collagen in the rheumatic diseases. *Ann NY Acad Sci*; 52(3):380-389. 1949

Steiner M, Glantz M & Lekos A. Vitamin E plus aspirin compared with aspirin alone in patients with transient ischemic attacks. *Am J Clin Nutr*; 62(6 suppl):1381S-1384S. 1995

Steiner M. Vitamin E: more than an antioxidant. *Clin Cardiol*; 16(4 suppl 1):I16-I18. 1993

Stephens NG, Parsons A, Schofield PM et al. Randomized controlled trial of vitamin E in patients with coronary disease: Cambridge Heart Antioxidant Study (CHAOS). *Lancet*; 347(9004):781-786. 1996

Suleiman SA, Ali ME, Zaki ZM et al. Lipid peroxidation and human sperm motility: protective role of vitamin E. *J Androl*; 17(5):530-537. 1996

Takamatsu S, Takamatsu M, Satoh K et al. Effects on health of dietary supplementation with 100 mg d-alpha tocopheryl acetate daily for 6 years. *J Intern Med Res*; 23(5):342-357. 1995

Taketomo CK, Hodding JH & Kraus DM (eds). Pediatric Dosage Handbook, 9th edition, 2002-2003. Lexi-Comp, Inc.

Taylor PR, Li B, Dawsey SM et al. Prevention of esophageal cancer: the nutrition intervention trials in Linxian, China, Linxian Nutrition Intervention Trials Study Group. *Cancer Res*; 54(7 suppl):2029S-2031S. 1994

Vivekananthan DP, Penn MS, Sapp SK et al. Use of antioxidant vitamins for the prevention of cardiovascular disease: meta-analysis of randomised trials. *Lancet*; 361:2017-2023. 2003

Watanabe H, Kakihana M, Ohtsuka S et al. Randomized, double, blind, placebo-controlled study of supplemental vitamin E on attenuation of the development of nitrate tolerance. *Circulation*; 96(8):2545-2550 1997

Williams HT, Clein LJ & Macbeth RA. Alpha tocopherol in the treatment of intermittent claudication. *Can Med Assoc J*; 87(10):538-540. 1962

Williams HT, Fenna D & Macbeth RA. Alpha tocopherol in the treatment of intermittent claudication. *Surg Gynecol Obstet*; 132(4):662-666. 1971

Zandi PP, Anthony JC, Khachaturian AS et al. Reduced risk of Alzheimer disease in users of antioxidant vitamin supplements. *Arch Neurol*; 61:82-88. 2004

Zinc

DESCRIPTION

Zinc is an essential trace element. Zinc salts are used for supplementation to correct zinc-deficiency conditions such as acrodermatitis enteropathica, as an astringent to relieve minor eye irritations, and for therapy with penicillamine (e.g., such as that used for Wilson's disease). Other disease entities associated with zinc-depletion are anorexia nervosa, arthritis, diarrhea, eczema, recurrent infections, and recalcitrant skin problems. Other illnesses where efficacy, safety, and standardized dose of zinc have yet to be established include sickle cell disease, thalassemia, senile dementia, the common cold, diabetes mellitus, virile potency disturbances, acne vulgaris, neoplasia, and infertili-

ty. However, the mechanisms of action of zinc have to be further clarified and more studies are needed to determine its specific place in therapy.

Other Names: Zinc can be administered as zinc sulfate, zinc acetate, zinc chloride, zinc-D-gluconate, zinc carbonate, zinc oxide, zinc aspartate, bis(L-histidinato)zinc or zinc orotate. A 220-mg dose of zinc sulfate is equivalent to 50 mg of elemental Zinc (Alpers et al, 1995).

ACTIONS AND PHARMACOLOGY
EFFECTS

Zinc is thought to have antimicrobial, anti-sickling, cell-protective, copper-absorbing, enzyme-regulating, and growth-stimulating effects.

Antimicrobial Effects: Zinc may reduce the growth rate of plaque bacteria and thus decrease oral plaque growth (Cohen et al, 1986; Harrap et al, 1984).

Anti-sickling Effects: Zinc increases the filterability of partially deoxygenated cells in vitro. It decreases calcium-induced hemo-globin binding to red cell membranes and antagonizes the echino-cyte-promoting effect of calcium. Thus, it can be used as an anti-sickling agent (Gupta & Choubey, 1987).

Cell-Protective Effects: Zinc exerts a protective effect in maintaining the integrity of both cellular and organelle membranes. Zinc deficiency can cause increased membrane peroxidation and subsequent membrane damage and abnormalities of cellular transport with decreased enzyme activity (Gupta & Choubey, 1987).

Copper-Absorbing Effects: Zinc inhibits copper absorption and induces a negative copper balance, which is the primary goal in the treatment of Wilson's disease (Hoogenraad & Van Hattum, 1988). It is thought that zinc causes copper malabsorption by preventing serosal transfer of copper secondary to induction of the intestinal copper-binding protein metallothionein and the copper is thus excreted in the feces (Friedman, 1993; Brewer et al, 1987).

Enzyme-Regulating Effects: Zinc is an integral part of several enzymes necessary for protein and carbohydrate metabolism. It is required for synthesis and mobilization of retinol-binding protein.

Growth-Stimulating Effects: Zinc supplementation may increase hepatic synthesis of somatomedin-C; it may accelerate growth response to growth hormone, or it can be involved directly in promoting growth. Studies are needed to establish the relationship of growth hormone, somatomedin, and zinc in beta thalasemia major (Arcasoy et al, 1987).

CLINICAL TRIALS
Common Cold

Zinc lozenges have been reported to be effective in some studies and ineffective in others. Efficacy may depend on whether the zinc is provided in a molecular form. A meta-analysis of 6 clinical trials was conducted to evaluate the effectiveness of zinc salts lozenges in the common cold. All studies had consistent moderate quality scores. The summary odds ratio for the incidence of any cold symptom was reported to be 0.50, but this did not reach statistical significance. It remains questionable if zinc therapy of the common cold is beneficial (Jackson et al, 1997).

Positive results were reported in a double-blind, placebo-controlled study of 100 patients. Zinc gluconate therapy was initiated within 24 hours of symptom onset. One zinc gluconate lozenge containing 13.3 mg of zinc was administered every 2 hours while awake for the duration of cold symptoms in 50 patients. The zinc-treated group had a significantly shorter time to symptom resolution than the placebo group (4.4 versus 7.6 days, p<0.001). Coughing, headache, hoarseness, nasal congestion and drainage, and sore throat were the symptoms that responded to zinc treatment. Nausea (10 vs 2 patients) and bad-taste reactions (39 vs 15 patients) were significantly more common in the zinc-treated group than the placebo group; one zinc-treated patient withdrew because of intolerance to the lozenge (Mossad et al, 1996).

Herpes Simplex Virus

A solution of 0.25% zinc sulfate can cause clearing of Herpes simplex lesions, but solutions of 0.025% to 0.05% were ineffective as treatment for acute attacks or as prophylaxis for recurrent infections. Zinc sulfate gel 103 mg/g applied topically every 2 hours was more effective than placebo in clearing herpes simplex labialis infections in a controlled double-blind trial with 80 patients. Symptoms were milder and lesions healed more rapidly with zinc sulfate gel than with placebo gel. (Kneist et al, 1995)

In another study, 200 patients with Herpes simplex showed clearing of lesions within 3 to 6 days of treatment with 0.25% zinc sulfate in camphor water USP applied 8 to 10 times per day beginning within 24 hours after the appearance of the lesions (Finnerty, 1986).

Immune Function

Zinc supplementation may improve cell-mediated immunity and leukocyte chemotaxis independently of zinc depletion. The cell-mediated immune response determined by CD4, DR, T-cells and cytotoxic T-lymphocytes was improved after zinc supplementation in a randomized, double-blind, placebo-controlled study of 118 patients older than 65 years. Patients received 25 mg of zinc sulfate per day; 800 mcg of retinol palmitate; 25 mg of zinc per day plus 800 mcg of retinol palmitate; or placebo. Significant increases in the zinc group were observed for CD4+DR+T-cells (P=0.016) and cytotoxic t-lymphocytes (P=0.005). For vitamin A, reductions in the counts of CD3+T-cells (P=0.012) and CD4+T-cells (P=0.0129) were reported (Fortes et al, 1998).

The rate of infection was significantly reduced by zinc and selenium supplementation in a 2-year randomized, placebo-controlled study of 81 institutionalized elderly patients. Daily doses of 20 mg of zinc plus 100 mcg of selenium or the same doses of trace elements plus daily doses of 120 mg of vitamin C, 6 mg of beta-carotene, and 15 mg of alpha-tocopherol were equally effective in correcting deficiencies after 6 months and in preventing infectious events (Girodon et al, 1997).

Macular Degeneration

Zinc supplementation has yet to be proved useful in age-related macular degeneration (ARMD). Prospective, randomized, controlled trials have been conducted investigating the role of zinc in ARMD using doses 5.3 times RDA of zinc for men and 6.7 times the RDA of zinc for women. Beneficial results from one small trial could not be confirmed in the much larger AREDS trial (see below), which failed to find a significant reduction in visual acuity loss after zinc therapy.

The Age-Related Eye Disease Study report 8 (AREDS) was an 11-center, double-blind, prospective trial designed to evaluate the effect of high-dose vitamins C and E, beta-carotene, and zinc supplementation on ARMD progression and visual acuity. Three thousand six hundred forty (3,640) participants aged 55 to 80 years were enrolled. All subjects had extensive small drusen, intermediate drusen, large drusen, noncentral geographic atrophy,

or pigment abnormalities in one or both eyes, or advanced ARMD or vision loss due to ARMD in one eye. At least one eye had best corrected visual acuity of 20/32 or better. Participants were randomized to 1 of 4 treatment groups: antioxidants (500 mg vitamin C, 400 IU vitamin E, and 15 mg beta-carotene daily); zinc oxide and cupric oxide (80 mg elemental zinc and 2 mg elemental copper daily); antioxidants plus zinc; or placebo. The total daily dosage of each supplement was taken orally by each participant in 2 divided doses with food to avoid potential gastrointestinal irritation by zinc. The main outcome measures included photographic assessment of progression to or treatment for advanced ARMD and at least moderate visual acuity loss from baseline (15 or more letters from the Snellen eye chart). Comparison with placebo demonstrated a statistically significant odds ratio (OR) reduction for the development of advanced AMD with antioxidants plus zinc (0.72, 99% confidence interval (CI) 0.52-0.98, p<0.007). The ORs for zinc alone (0.75, 99% CI 0.55-1.03, p<0.02) and antioxidants alone (0.80, 99% CI 0.59-1.09, p less than 0.07) were not found to be statistically significant (Anon, 2001b).

INDICATIONS AND USAGE
Approved by the FDA for:

■ Zinc deficiency

Unproven Uses: Zinc supplements are used for numerous conditions, including the following: acne vulgaris, acrodermatitis enteropathica, Alzheimer's disease, common cold, dental hygiene, diabetes mellitus, diarrhea, eczema, eye irritation, growth, Hansen's disease, herpes simplex infection, hypertension, hypogeusia (decreased sense of taste), immunodeficiency, impotence, infertility, leg ulcers, lipid peroxidation, macular degeneration, necrolytic migratory erythema, parasites, peptic ulcer disease, psoriasis, scalp dermatoses, schistosomiasis, sepsis, sickle cell anemia, stomatitis, thalassemia major, trichomoniasis, Wilson's disease, and wound healing.

PRECAUTIONS AND ADVERSE REACTIONS
Zinc ophthalmic solution should be used cautiously in patients with glaucoma.

Side effects include gastrointestinal discomfort, nausea, vomiting, headaches, drowsiness, and metallic taste. Do not use zinc ophthalmic solutions that have changed color.

Breastfeeding: Zinc should not be used in doses greater than the RDA during lactation.

Drug Interactions

Copper or Iron: Concurrent administration with zinc inhibits the absorption of copper and iron. *Clinical Management:* Optimal dosage separation time has not been determined. Space administration of zinc and copper or iron as far apart as possible.

Penicillamine: Concurrent administration with zinc reduces zinc absorption. *Clinical Management:* Optimal dosage separation time has not been determined. Space administration of zinc and penicillamine as far apart as possible.

Quinolones: Zinc decreases absorption of quinolone antibiotics. *Clinical Management:* Zinc salts or vitamins containing zinc should be given 2 hours after or 6 hours before antibiotics.

Tetracycline: Concurrent administration results in decreased tetracycline effectiveness. *Clinical Management:* Administer tetracycline at least 2 hours before or 3 hours after zinc.

Drug-Food Interactions

Caffeine: Concurrent administration with zinc reduces zinc absorption.

Foods containing high amounts of phosphorous, calcium (dairy), or phytates (e.g., bran, brown bread) may reduce absorption.

OVERDOSAGE

Intravenous overdose has been associated with thrombocytopenia, hypotension, cardiac arrhythmias, oliguria, hyperamylasemia, diarrhea, jaundice, and pulmonary edema, sideroblastic anemia, microcytic anemia secondary to zinc-induced copper deficiency anemia, copper deficiency, hemorrhagic gastric erosions, and lymphocytoma cutis.

DOSAGE

Mode of Administration: oral, topical, intramuscular

How Supplied: tablet, cream, gel

Daily Dosage: Recommended Dietary Allowance (RDA): *Men and adolescent boys 14 and older* — 11 mg/day; *adolescent girls 14 to 18 years* — 9 mg/day; *women 19 years and older* — 8 mg/day; *pregnancy (19 years and older)* — 11 mg/day; *lactation (19 years and older)* — 12 mg/day. *Infants and children: 7 months to 3 years* — 3 mg/day; *4 to 8 years* — 5 mg/day; *9 to 13 years* — 8 mg/day.

ADULTS

Dietary supplement: daily oral doses range from 9 to 25 mg

Acne and dermatitis: a topical preparation (cream or gel) of 10 mg zinc sulfate per gram or 27 to 30 mg zinc oxide per gram used several times daily.

Acne : 90 to 135 mg orally daily

Zinc deficiency/acrodermatitis: maximum doses up to 40 mg orally daily

Wilson's Disease, tablet: 300 mg to 1200 mg orally daily in divided doses

PEDIATRICS

Acne: 135 mg orally daily.

Zinc deficiency: daily doses ranging from 1.5 to 12 mg, depending on age.

Supplementation (intramuscular injection): 100 mcg per kg body weight per day for children up to 5 years old.

Wilson's disease (intramuscular injection): 25 mg 3 times daily for children 10 years and older.

LITERATURE

Alpers DH, Stenson WF & Bier DM. Manual of Nutritional Therapeutics, 3rd ed. Little, Brown & Co, Boston, MA, 1995

Anon. A randomized, placebo-controlled, clinical trial of high-dose supplementation with vitamins C and E, beta-carotene, and zinc for age-related macular degeneration and vision loss: AREDS report no. 8. *Arch Ophthalmol*; 119(10):1417-1436. 2001

Arcasoy A, Cavdar A, Cin S et al. Effects of zinc supplementation on linear growth in beta-thalasemia (a new approach). *Am J Hematol*; 24(2):127-136. 1987

Brewer GJ, Yuzbasiyan-Gurkan V, Johnson V et al. Treatment of Wilson's disease with zinc, XII: dose regimen requirements. *Am J Med Sci*; 305(4):199-202. 1993

Cohen DW, Hangorsky U, Emling RC et al. Clinical evaluations of a zinc sulfate/ascorbic acid mouthrinse. *Clin Prev Dent*; 8(6):5-12. 1986

Finnerty EF. Topical zinc in the treatment of herpes simplex. Cutis 1986; 37(2):130-131.

Fortes C, Forastiere F, Agabiti N et al. The effect of zinc and vitamin A supplementation on immune response in an older population. *J Am Geriatr Soc*; 46(1):19-26. 1998

Friedman LS. Zinc in the treatment of Wilson's disease: how it works. *Gastroenterology*; 10495):1566-1575. 1993

Fung EB, Ritchie LD, Woodhouse LR et al. Zinc absorption in women during pregnancy and lactation: a longitudinal study. *Am J Clin Nutr*; 66(1):80-88. 1997

Girodon F, Lombard M, Galan P et al. Effect of micronutrient supplementation on infection in institutionalized elderly subjects: a controlled trial. *Ann Nutr Metab*; 41(2):98-107. 1997

Gupta VL & Choubey BS. RBC survival, zinc deficiency, and efficacy of zinc therapy in sickle cell disease. *Birth Defects*; 23(5A):477-483. 1987

Haeger K, Lanner E & Magnusson PO. Oral zinc sulfate in the treatement of venous leg ulcers, in Pories WJ, Strain WH, Hwu JM et al (eds): Clinical applications of zinc metabolism. CC Thomas, Springfield, IL:158-167. 1974

Harrap GJ, Best JS & Saxton CA. Human oral retention of zinc from mouthwashes containing zinc salts and its relevance to dental plaque control. *Arch Oral Biol*; 29(2):87-91. 1984

Henderson LM, Brewer GJ, Dressman JB et al. Effect of intragastric pH on the absorption of oral zinc acetate and zinc oxide in young healthy volunteers. *J Parenter Enteral Nutr*; 19(5):393-397. 1995

Jackson JL, Peterson C & Lesho E. A meta-analysis of zinc salts lozenges and the common cold. *Arch Intern Med*; 157(20):2373-2376. 1997

Kneist W, Hempel B & Borelli S. Klinische Doppelblindpruefung mit Zinksulfat topisch bei Herpes labialis recidivans (German). *Arzneimittelforschung*; 45(5):624-626. 1995

Krieger I. Picolinic acid in the treatment of disorders requiring zinc supplementation. *Nutr Rev*; 38(4):148-149. 1980

Mossad SB, Macknin ML, Medendorp SV et al. Zinc gluconate lozenges for treating the common cold: a randomized, double-blind, placebo-controlled study. *Ann Intern Med*; 125(2):81-88. 1996

Naveh Y, Schapira D, Ravel Y et al. Zinc metabolism in rheumatoid arthritis: plasma and urinary zinc and relationship to disease activity. *J Rheumatol*; 24(4):643-646. 1997

Product Information: Galzin®, zinc acetate. Gate Pharmaceuticals, Sellersville, PA, USA, 1997

Product Information. Visine AC®, zinc sulfate and tetrahydrozoline hydrochloride. Pfizer Consumer Health Care, Parsippany, NJ, USA, 1994

Wood RJ & Zheng JJ. High dietary calcium intakes reduce zinc absorption and balance in humans. *Am J Clin Nutr*; 65(6):1803-1809. 1997

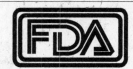

U.S. FOOD AND DRUG ADMINISTRATION

Medical Product Reporting Programs

MedWatch (24-hour service)..**800-332-1088**
Reporting of problems with drugs, devices, biologics (except vaccines), medical foods, and dietary supplements.

Vaccine Adverse Event Reporting System (24-hour service) **800-822-7967**
Reporting of vaccine-related problems.

Mandatory Medical Device Reporting **240-276-3000**
Reporting required from user facilities regarding device-related deaths and serious injuries.

Veterinary Adverse Drug Reaction Program **888-332-8387**
Reporting of adverse drug events in animals.

Division of Drug Marketing, Advertising, and Communication (DDMAC) **301-827-2828**
Inquiries from health professionals regarding product promotion.

USP Medication Errors **800-233-7767**
Reporting of medication errors or near-errors to help avoid future problems through improvement in product names and packaging.

Information for Health Professionals

Center for Drug Evaluation and (CDER) Research Drug Information Hotline........................**301-827-4573**
Information on human drugs including hormones.

Center for Biologics Office of Communications...**301-827-2000**
Information on biological products including vaccines and blood.

Emergency Operations..**301-443-1240**
Emergencies involving FDA-regulated products, tampering reports, and emergency Investigational New Drug requests.

Office of Orphan Products Development **301-827-3666**
Information on products for rare diseases.

General Information

General Consumer Inquiries **888-463-6332**
Consumer information on regulated products/issues.

Freedom of Information..**301-827-6500**
Requests for publicly available FDA documents.

Office of Public Affairs..**301-827-6250**
Interviews/press inquiries on FDA activities.

Center for Food Safety and Applied Nutrition..**888-723-3366**
Information on food safety, seafood, dietary supplements, women's nutrition, and cosmetics.

Consumer Information Service, Center for Devices and Radiological Health **301-443-4190**
Information on medical devices, mammography facilities, and radiation-emitting products.